Model of Human Occupation:
Theory and Application

Fourth Edition

Model of Human Occupation: Theory and Application

Fourth Edition

Gary Kielhofner, DrPH, OTR, FAOTA

Professor and Wade/Meyer Chair

Department of Occupational Therapy

College of Applied Health Sciences

University of Illinois at Chicago

Chicago, Illinois

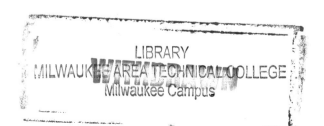

Acquisitions Editor: Emily J. Lupash
Managing Editor: Matthew J. Hauber
Marketing Manager: Allison M. Noplock
Production Editor: Paula C. Williams
Designer: Risa J. Clow
Compositor: Maryland Composition, Inc.

Fourth Edition

Copyright © 2008, 2002, Lippincott Williams & Wilkins, a Wolters Kluwer business.

351 West Camden Street   530 Walnut Street
Baltimore, MD 21201   Philadelphia, PA 19106

Printed in China.

9 8 7 6 5 4 3 2

Library of Congress Cataloging-in-Publication Data

CIP Data is available: ISBN 13: 978-0-7817-6996-9
                       ISBN 10: 0-7817-6996-5

DISCLAIMER

Care has been taken to confirm the accuracy of the information present and to describe generally accepted practices. However, the authors, editors, and publisher are not responsible for errors or omissions or for any consequences from application of the information in this book and make no warranty, expressed or implied, with respect to the currency, completeness, or accuracy of the contents of the publication. Application of this information in a particular situation remains the professional responsibility of the practi-tioner; the clinical treatments described and recommended may not be considered absolute and universal recommendations.

The authors, editors, and publisher have exerted every effort to ensure that drug selection and dosage set forth in this text are in accordance with the current recommendations and practice at the time of publi-cation. However, in view of ongoing research, changes in government regulations, and the constant flow of information relating to drug therapy and drug reactions, the reader is urged to check the package insert for each drug for any change in indications and dosage and for added warnings and precautions. This is particularly important when the recommended agent is a new or infrequently employed drug.

Some drugs and medical devices presented in this publication have Food and Drug Administration (FDA) clearance for limited use in restricted research settings. It is the responsibility of the health care provider to ascertain the FDA status of each drug or device planned for use in their clinical practice.

To purchase additional copies of this book, call our customer service department at **(800) 638-3030** or fax orders to **(301) 223-2320**. International customers should call **(301) 223-2300**.

Visit Lippincott Williams & Wilkins on the Internet: http://www.lww.com. Lippincott Williams & Wilkins cus-tomer service representatives are available from 8:30 am to 6:00 pm, EST.

To the community of therapists around the world who have contributed to the development of the Model of Human Occupation.

ACKNOWLEDGMENTS

This fourth edition of *Model of Human Occupation* goes to press over three decades after work on the model first began. The idea that took shape in my graduate work in the early 1970s has become more than I could have imagined then. This is due to literally hundreds of persons who have contributed to the development of various aspects of the model. It is simply impossible to recount all of them. Nonetheless, I am grateful for each of them.

Putting together a book like this one takes a great deal of time and effort from many people. Each time I have undertaken to write an edition of *Model of Human Occupation*, I have had the uncommon good fortune of working with an outstanding team of people. The reader will recognize that authors from many corners of the world have directly contributed to the contents of this book. It has been a pleasure to work with each of them and to see the ways in which therapists have expanded and applied the model's concepts.

The members of my team at the University of Illinois at Chicago, Emily Ashpole, Jessica Kramer, Kathleen Kramer, Sun Wook Lee, Annie Ploszaj, and Dr. Patricia Bowyer have not only helped with the inevitable logistics of writing a text, but have also been a source of input and feedback that has shaped the contents. They all have my deepest gratitude. I am also indebted to all the therapists who provided case materials and anecdotes for this book.

In so many ways, disabled people have lent their stories and voices to this volume. Since *Model of Human Occupation* grows out of a professional and personal desire to positively impact the lives of those who experience disability, I hope the book is worthy of what they have lent us of themselves. I also hope each rendering of a part of someone's life herein is both faithful and a tribute to them.

CONTRIBUTORS

Susan Andersen, MS, OTR/L
Occupational Therapist
Marklund Hyde Center
Geneva, IL

Ana Laura Auzmendia, TO
Instructor
Department of Occupational Therapy
Universidad Nacional de Mar del Plata
Mar del Plata, Argentina

Tal Baz, MS, OTR/L
Private Practice
Somerville, MA

René Bélanger, OTR, MBA
Clinical Professor
Rehabilitation Department
Hôtel-Dieu de Lévis Hospital and Laval University
Lévis, Quebec, Canada

Melinda Blondis, MS, OTR/L
Occupational Therapist
Proviso Area for Exceptional Children
Brookfield, Illinois

Lena Borell, PhD, OT (reg.)
Professor of Occupational Therapy
Karolinska Institutet
Stockholm, Sweden

Patricia Bowyer, EdD, OTR/L, BCN
Assistant Professor, Program Director
School of Occupational Therapy, Houston Center
Texas Woman's University
Houston, TX

Brent Braveman, PhD, OTR/L, FAOTA
Clinical Associate Professor
Director of Professional Education
Department of Occupational Therapy
University of Illinois at Chicago
Chicago, Illinois

Jutta Brettschneider, OTR
Hebrew Home of Greater Washington
Rockville, Maryland

Susan M. Cahill, MAEA, OTR/L
Clinical Assistant Professor
Department of Occupational Therapy
University of Illinois at Chicago
Chicago, Illinois

Christine Clay, AA
Teacher Assistant
Chicago Lighthouse for the Blind
Chicago, Illinois

Carmen Gloria de las Heras, MS, OTR
Private Practice
Santiago, Chile

Brad E. Egan, OTD, OTR/L
Occupational Therapy Supervisor
Alexian Brothers Bonaventure House
Chicago, Illinois

Elin Ekladh, MSc, OT (reg.)
PhD Student
Section of Occupational Therapy
Linköping University
Linköping, Sweden

Kirsty Forsyth, PhD, BSc, MSc
Senior Lecturer
Occupational Therapy Department
Queen Margaret University College
Edinburgh, Scotland

Lena Haglund, PhD, MScOT, OT (reg.)
Associate Professor
Section of Occupational Therapy
Linköping University
Linköping, Sweden

Helena Hemmingsson, PhD, OT (reg.)
Associated Professor
Division of Occupational Therapy
Department of Neurobiology, Caring Sciences and
    Society
Karolinska Institutet
Stokholm, Sweden

Alexis D. Henry, ScD, OTR/L, FAOTA
Research Assistant Professor
Center for Health Policy and Research
University of Massachusetts Medical School
Shrewsbury, Massachusetts

Renee Hinson-Smith, MSOT, OTR/L
Director
Generations Adult and Child Daycare
Fort Lauderdale, Florida

Roberta Holzmueller, PhD
Associate Professor
Institute for Juvenile Research
University of Illinois at Chicago
Chicago, Illinois

Jennifer Hutson, MS, OTR/L, ATP
Clinical Occupational Therapist
Evanston Northwestern Hospital
Evanston, Illinois

Hans Jonsson, PhD, OT (reg.)
Associate Professor
Director of Master Courses
Division of Occupational Therapy
Department of Neurobiology, Care Sciences and
    Society
Karolinska Institutet
Stockholm, Sweden

Staffan Josephsson, PhD, OT (reg.)
Associate Professor
Division of Occupational Therapy
Karolinska Institutet
Stockholm, Sweden

Riitta Keponen, MSc, OTR
Helsinki Polytechnic Stadia
Helsinki, Finland

Jessica M. Kramer, MS, OTR/L
PhD Student, Disabilities Studies
Head Research Assistant MOHO Clearinghouse
Department of Occupational Therapy
University of Illinois at Chicago
Chicago, Illinois

Kathleen Kramer, BBA
MS/C Student in Occupational Therapy
Department of Occupational Therapy
University of Illinois at Chicago
Chicago, Illinois

Dalleen Last, Dip COT, SROT
Clinical Specialist in Occupational Therapy
Oxford City Learning Disability Team
Oxfordshire Learning Disability National Health
    Service Trust
Oxfordshire, England

Sun Wook Lee
PhD student, Disability Studies
MOHO Clearinghouse
Department of Occupational Therapy
University of Illinois at Chicago
Chicago, Illinois

Mara Levin, MS, OTR/L
PhD Student, Disabilities Studies
Visiting Project Coordinator
Department of Occupational Therapy
University of Illinois at Chicago
Chicago, Illinois

Jane Melton, MSc, Dip COT
Consultant Occupational Therapist in
    Mental Health
Gloucestershire Partnership NHS Trust
Gloucester, United Kingdom

Christiane Mentrup, MScOT
Head of Institute for Occupational Therapy
School of Health Studies
Zurich University of Applied Sciences
Winterthur, Switzerland

Claudia Miranda, Lic T.O.
Magíster Social Psicology Instructor
Department of Occupational Therapy
Researcher
Nacional Univercity de Mar del Plata
Mar del Plata, Argentina

Alice Moody, BSc(Hons)OT
Occupational Therapist
Mental Health Services for Older People
Gloucestershire Partnership Trust
Cheltenham, England.

Kelly Munger, MS
PhD Student, Disabilities Studies
University of Illinois at Chicago
Chicago, Illinois

Hiromi Nakamura-Thomas, MOT, OTR
Lecturer
Saitama Prefectural University
Department of Occupational Therapy
Koshigaya-city, Saitama prefecture, Japan

Louise Nygård, PhD, OT (reg.)
Associate Professor, Senior Researcher
Division of Occupational Therapy
Karolinska Institutet
Stockholm, Sweden

Linda Olson, MS, OTR/L
Assistant Professor, Program Specialist
Department of Occupational Therapy
Rush University
Chicago, Illinois

Ay-Woan Pan, PhD, OTR/C (Taiwan)
Associate Professor
School of Occupational Therapy
College of Medicine
National Taiwan University
Taipei, Taiwan

Sue Parkinson, BA, Dip COT
Occupational Therapist
Derbyshire Mental Health Services
Derbyshire, England

Annie Ploszaj, BA
OTD Student in Occupational Therapy
Department of Occupational Therapy
University of Illinois at Chicago
Chicago, Illinois

Susan Prior, BSc
Practitioner Lecturer
NHS Lothian & Queen Margaret University College
Edinburgh, UK

Christine Raber, PhD, OTR/L
Assistant Professor
Department of Occupational Therapy
Shawnee State University
Portsmouth, Ohio

Júnia Rjeille Cordeiro, BAOT, MSc
Occupational Therapist
Pulmonary Rehabilitation Center at the Federal
   University of São Paulo,
Brazil

Laurie Rockwell-Dylla, MS, OTR/L
Lemont Center & Palos Home Health
Lemont, Illinois

Deborah M. Roitman, MSc, OTR
Independent Geriatric Practice
Shoham, Israel

Daniela Schulte, OT
Occupational Therapist
St. Vinzenz Krankenhaus
Haseluenne, Germany

Jayne Shepherd, MS, OTR/L, FAOTA
Associate Professor
Assistant Chair, Post Professional Education
Virginia Commonwealth University
Richmond, Virginia

Camille Skubik-Peplaski, MS, OTR/L, BCP
Occupational Therapy Practice Coordinator
Cardinal Hill Healthcare System
Lexington, KY

Meghan O. Suman, MS, OTR/L
Pediatric Occupational Therapy
University of Illinois Medical Center
Chicago, Illinois

Kerstin Tham, PhD
Associate Professor,
Head of the Division of Occupational Therapy
Karolinska Institutet
Stockholm, Sweden

Luc Vercruysse, OT
Head of Occupational Therapy Department
University Psychiatric Centre
UPC Katholieke Universiteit Leuven
Campus Kortenberg
Belgium

Takashi Yamada, PhD
Department of Occupational Therapy
Tokyo Metropolitan University of Health Sciences
Tokyo, Japan

Noga Ziv, MScOT
Department of Occupational Therapy, School of
  Health Professions
Tel-Aviv University
Yehud, Israel

Case and Photo Contributors

Erin Boodey, MS, OTR/L
Pediatric Occupational Therapy
University of Illinois Medical Center at Chicago

Susan M. Cahill, MAEA, OTR/L
Department of Occupational Therapy
University of Illinois at Chicago

Bridget Caruso, OTR/L
Occupational Therapy
University of Illinois Medical Center at Chicago

Lisa Castle, MBA, OTR/L
Director of Occupational Therapy
University of Illinois Medical Center at Chicago

Jane Clifford O'Brien, PhD, OTR/L
Department of Occupational Therapy
University of New England

Cathleen Conway Jensen, OTR/L
Adult Physical Disabilities, Occupational Therapy
University of Illinois Medical Center at Chicago

William Croninger, MS, OTR/L
Department of Occupational Therapy
University of New England

Emma Dobson, BSc (Hons)
Senior Occupational Therapist
SWITCH Partnership, Lanarkshire

Sanet du Toit, Master in OT, MSc
Department of Occupational Therapy
University of the Free State

Elena Espiritu, MA, OTR/L
Occupational Therapy
University of Illinois Medical Center at Chicago

Joaquim Faias, OTR/L
Head of the Scientific Area of Occupational Therapy
    at the Escola Superior de Tecnologia da Saúde do
    Porto
Instituto Politécnico do Porto - Portugal

Ana Cristina Farinha, OT (lic.)
Unidade de Ambulatório de Recuperação Global
Hospital Miguel Bombarda - Lisboa, Portugal

Gail Fisher, MPA, OTR/L
Department of Occupational Therapy
University of Illinois at Chicago

Maria Kapanadze, MA
Occupational Therapy Student
Tbilisi State I. Chavchavadze University

Riitta Keponen, MSc, OTR
Helsinki Polytechnic Stadia

Leon Kieschner, OTR/L
New York City Department of Education

Eunyoung Kim, MS, OT
Children's Center for Developmental Support
Ewha Womans University

Tunde Koncz, OTR/L
Occupational Therapy
University of Illinois Medical Center at Chicago

Jessica M. Kramer, MS, OTR/L
Department of Occupational Therapy
University of Illinois at Chicago

Dalleen Last, Dip COT, SROT
Oxford City Learning Disability Team
Oxfordshire Learning Disability National Health
    Service Trust

Mike Littleton, MPH, OTR/L, CHT
Occupational Therapy
University of Illinois Medical Center at Chicago

Stephanie McCammon, MS, OTR/L
Comprehensive Assessment and Treatment Unit for
    Adolescents
University of Illinois Medical Center at Chicago

Christiane Mentrup, MScOT
Institute of Occupational Therapy
Zurich University of Applied Sciences

Kristjana Olafsdottir, BS, OTR
Kopavogur County schools
Kopavogur, Iceland

Ay-Woan Pan, PhD, OTR/L
School of Occupational Therapy
College of Medicine
National Taiwan University

Geneviève Pépin, PhD, OT (reg.)
Rehabilitation Department
Faculty of Medicine, Laval University

Christine Raber, PhD, OTR/L
Department of Occupational Therapy
Shawnee State University

Susan L. Roberts, M.Div., OTR/L
Changes Occupational Therapy

Catalina Edith Sánchez Galicia
Student of the Master Program of Occupational
    Therapy
Instituto de Terapia Ocupacional

Supriya Sen, MS, OTR/L
Department of Occupational Therapy
University of Illinois at Chicago
University of Illinois Medical Center at Chicago

Michele Shapiro, MS
Beit Issie Shapiro

Dianne F. Simons, PhD, OTR
Department of Occupational Therapy
Virginia Commonwealth University

Meghan O. Suman, MS, OTR/L
Pediatric Occupational Therapy
University of Illinois Medical Center at Chicago

Erla B. Sveinbjornsdottir, BS, OTR
Medferdarteymi barna;
Heilsugaeslustod Grafarvogs
Kopavogur, Iceland

Laura Vidaña Moya
Neuro-rehabilitation Department
Parc Taulí Hospital

Naomi Weintraub, PhD, OTR
School of Occupational Therapy
Hadassah and the Hebrew University of
    Jerusalem, Israel

Laura White, Dip COT
South Birmingham Primary Care Trust

Takashi Yamada, PhD
Department of Occupational Therapy
Tokyo Metropolitan University of Health Sciences

Farzaneh Yazdani, PhD
Faculty of Rehabilitation
University of Jordan

Occupational therapists in the Northumberland,
    Tyne, and Wear Mental Health NHS Trust, United
    Kingdom

Members of UK Core

Contents

Chapter 1   Introduction to the Model of Human Occupation   1
Kielhofner

I   Explaining Human Occupation   9

Chapter 2   The Basic Concepts of Human Occupation   11
Kielhofner

Chapter 3   The Dynamics of Human Occupation   24
Kielhofner

Chapter 4   Volition   32
Kielhofner

Chapter 5   Habituation: Patterns of Daily Occupation   51
Kielhofner

Chapter 6   Performance Capacity and Lived Body   68
Kielhofner, Tham, Baz, Hutson

Chapter 7   The Environment and Human Occupation   85
Kielhofner

Chapter 8   Dimensions of Doing   101
Kielhofner

Chapter 9   Crafting Occupational Life   110
Kielhofner, Borell, Holzmueller, Jonsson, Josephsson, Keponin, Melton, Munger, Nygård

Chapter 10   Doing and Becoming: Occupational Change and Development   126
Kielhofner

II   Applying MOHO: The Therapy Process and Therapeutic Reasoning   141

Chapter 11   Therapeutic Reasoning: Planning, Implementing, and Evaluating the Outcomes of Therapy   143
Kielhofner, Forysth

Chapter 12   Assessment: Choosing and Using Structured and Unstructured Means of Gathering Information   155
Kielhofner, Forsyth

Chapter 13   Occupational Engagement: How Clients Achieve Change   171
Kielhofner, Forsyth

Chapter 14   Therapeutic Strategies for Enabling Change   185
Kielhofner, Forsyth

SECTION II THERAPEUTIC REASONING TABLE   204
Forsyth, Kielhofner

 Assessments: Structured Methods for Gathering Client Information   215

Chapter 15   Observational Assessments   217
Kielhofner, Cahill, Forsyth, de las Heras, Melton, Raber, Prior

Chapter 16   Self-Reports: Eliciting Client's Perspectives   237
Kielhofner, Forsyth, Suman, J. Kramer, Nakamura-Thomas, Yamada, Rjeille-Cordeiro, Keponen, Pan, Henry

Chapter 17   Talking With Clients: Assessments That Collect Information   262
Kielhofner, Forsyth, Clay, Ekbladh, Haglund, Hemmingsson, Keponen, Olson

Chapter 18   Assessments Combining Methods of Information Gathering   288
Forsyth, Kielhofner, Bowyer, K. Kramer, Ploszaj, Blondis, Hinson-Smith, Parkinson

 Case Illustrations   311

Chapter 19   Recrafting Occupational Narratives   313
Auzmendia, de las Heras, Kielhofner, Miranda

Chapter 20   Applying MOHO to Clients Who Are Cognitively Impaired   337
Kielhofner, Andersen, Last, Roitman, Brettschneider, Vercruysse, Ziv

Chapter 21   Facilitating Participation Through Community-Based Interventions   355
Kielhofner, Levin, Egan, Moody, Skubik-Peplaski, Rockwell-Dylla

Chapter 22   Enabling Clients to Reconstruct Their Occupational Lives in Long-Term Settings   379
Kielhofner, Mentrup, Miranda, Schulte, Shepherd

 Resources for Applying and Developing MOHO   405

Chapter 23   Communication and Documentation   407
Forsyth, Kielhofner

Chapter 24   Program Development   442
Braveman, Kielhofner, Bélanger

Chapter 25   Evidence for Practice from the Model of Human Occupation   466
J. Kramer, Bowyer, Kielhofner

Chapter 26   Research: Investigating MOHO   506
Kielhofner

Chapter 27   The Model of Human Occupation, the ICF, and the Occupational Therapy Practice
Framework: Connections to Support Best Practice Around the World   519
J. Kramer, Bowyer, Kielhofner

Appendix   532

Appendix A   Bibliography   532
Appendix B   Introduction to the MOHO Clearinghouse and Web Site   550
Lee, Ploszaj

Index   557

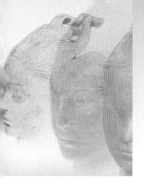

1

Introduction to the Model of Human Occupation

● Gary Kielhofner

The model of human occupation (MOHO) was first published in 1980 as a series of four articles in the *American Journal of Occupational Therapy* (Kielhofner, 1980a, b; Kielhofner & Burke, 1980; Kielhofner Burke, & Heard, 1980). It was the product of three occupational therapy practitioners attempting to articulate concepts that guided their practice. In the three decades since MOHO was first being formulated, countless contributions of practitioners and researchers have augmented its development. This book aims to capture their efforts and provide an overview of the current status of the model's theory, research, and application.

There is evidence that MOHO has become the most widely used occupation-focused model in occupational therapy practice internationally (Haglund, Ekbladh, Thorell, & Hallberg, 2000; National Board for Certification in Occupational Therapy, 2004; Law & McColl, 1989). In a recent nationwide random study of occupational therapists in the United States (Lee et al., in press) 80% of therapists indicated they used MOHO in their practice. These therapists indicated that they chose MOHO because it fit with their view of occupational therapy and reflected their clients' needs. Moreover, the vast majority of these therapists indicated that in their experience MOHO:

● Supports occupation-focused practice
● Helps prioritize clients' needs
● Provides a holistic view of clients
● Offers a client-centered approach

● Affords a strong base for generating treatment goals
● Supplies a rationale for intervention.

These views of practitioners coincide with many of the aims that have guided the development of MOHO over the past 3 decades.

The vision for MOHO has been to support practice throughout the world that is occupation-focused, client-centered, holistic, evidence-based, and complementary to practice based on other occupational therapy models and interdisciplinary theories. Each of these elements is discussed in this chapter.

Multinational and Multicultural

MOHO has received much attention, including criticism, elaboration, application, and empirical testing by occupational therapists throughout the world. Attempts to apply and test MOHO in different cultures and under different national conditions have provided priceless feedback about how its theoretical arguments

> *The vision for MOHO has been to support practice throughout the world that is occupation-focused, client-centered, holistic, evidence-based, and complementary to practice based on other occupational therapy models and interdisciplinary theories.*

and technology for application can best be developed to transcend cultural differences and national boundaries. MOHO incorporates a respect for each client's individuality and cultural background, and many MOHO assessments capture a client's unique cultural perspective. Successful applications of MOHO throughout the world point to its broad relevance. For instance, MOHO-based assessments and publications are available now in more than 20 languages. Most important, however, is that members of the occupational therapy profession throughout the world are now making important contributions to the development of MOHO, so that its concepts and application increasingly reflect multiple perspectives.

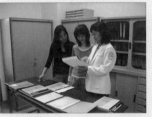

Dr. Ay-Woan Pan (on the right) discusses MOHO center assessments with research assistants at National Taiwan University. A poster outside the MOHO research center explains the purpose of MOHO to visitors.

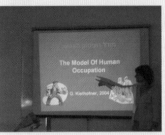

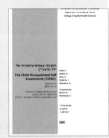

At Hebrew University, Israel, researchers introduce students to MOHO and translate MOHO tools to support the use of MOHO in practice, including the Child Occupational Self Assessment (COSA). Translated MOHO assessments are then used as measures in a variety of research projects.

*S*cholars around the world conduct MOHO based research and disseminate resources to support the use of MOHO in practice[1]

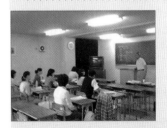

Dr. Tak Yamada in Japan teaches clinicians and students MOHO concepts. Dr. Yamada collaborates with national and international researchers and conducts research to demonstrate the cross-cultural application of MOHO concepts and assessments.

At Quebec's Centre de Référence du Modèle de L'Occupation Humaine (CRMOH), OT researchers, including Dr. Geneviève Pépin, collaborate with psychiatrists and

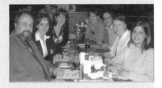

nurses in a longitudinal study comparing the Remotivation Process with traditional service delivery for clients with depression. This study also seeks to determine the effects of the Remotivation Process on volition and functioning. Here, the researchers are celebrating the launch of this groundbreaking project over dinner (from left to right, Francis Guerette, OT, Brigitte Lefebvre, OT and chief of rehabilitation services, Genevieve Pepin, OT and researcher, Chantale Theriault, nurse, Paul Jacques, psychiatrist, Claire Blouin, OT and Karine Mercier, OT.).

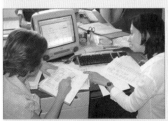

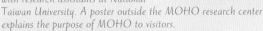
Centro de Estudos de Ocupação Humana

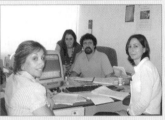

At the Centro de Estudos de Ocupação Humana in Portugal, the research team is developing a Portuguese translation of the OPHI-II. Here, they are preparing the translated assessment for a review by a panel of experts (From the left in the first picture: Helena Sousa and Maria Joo Ramos Pinto). The team has also worked to translate several other MOHO assessments, including the SSI, the MOHOST, and the ACIS, to support Portuguese therapists to use MOHO in practice (from the left in the second picture: Helena Sousa, Paula Portugal, Joaquim Faias, and Maria Joo Ramos Pinto.).

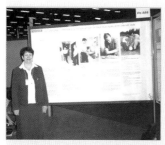

Riitta Keponen, a researcher and clinician from Finland, presents at the WFOT congress in Stocholm (2002) with a poster presenting the results of an analysis of OPHI-II narratives of men living with chronic pain. Her research demonstrates how MOHO assessments can be used in occupational therapy practice and research to understand client's life circumstances.

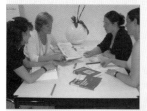

Christiane Mentrup, second from left, introduces MOHO to some colleagues at the Zuercher Hochschule Winterthur, the first university based OT program in the German part of Switzerland.

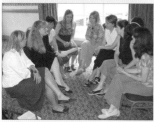
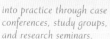

Researchers and practitioners come together at the United Kingdom Center of Outcomes Research and Education (UKCORE) to integrate MOHO theory into practice through case conferences, study groups, and research seminars.

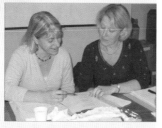

[1] *Special thanks to those who provided pictures, including: Dr. Tak Yamanda, Department of Occupational Therapy, Metropolitan University of Health Sciences, Tokyo, Japan; Dr. Geneviève Pépin, Faculty of Medicine, Laval University, Quebec, Canada; Dr. Ay-Woan Pan, Associate Professor, Department of Occupational Therapy, National Taiwan University, & Department of Psychiatry, National Taiwan University Hospital, & Department of Occupational Therapy, Fu-Zen University, Taipei, Taiwan; Dr. Naomi Weintraub, Deputy Chair, School of Occupational Therapy of Hadassah and the Hebrew University, Jerusalem, Israel; Joaquim Faias, Adjunct Professor and Coordinator of the Occupational Therapy Department, School of Health Technology of Porto, Instituto Politecnico do Porto, Portugal; Riitta Keponen, Helsinki Polytechnic Stadia, Helsinki, Finland; Christiane Mentrup, Zuercher Hochschule Winterthur, Switzerland; Dr. Kirsty Forsyth, Senior Lecturer, Occupational Therapy, Queen Margaret University College.*

Practice Oriented

When therapists use concepts from MOHO, they must link them to the specific client or client group to whom they are providing services. MOHO provides a wide range of resources (assessments, case examples, intervention protocols, and programs) to aid therapists to make this link. Moreover, an important emphasis underlying the development of MOHO has been to ensure that it is grounded in the real-world situations of everyday practice (Kielhofner, 2005a; Forsyth, Summerfield-Mann, & Kielhofner, 2005). Thus, this model has strongly emphasized involving practitioners and consumers in research and development efforts to ensure that they are grounded in practice and relevant to those who receive services.

Occupation-Focused

MOHO was the first contemporary model to articulate a focus on occupation in practice. It was designed as a conceptual model that provided guidelines of occupation-focused practice. Its theory addresses three practical concerns related to this focus:

- How occupation is motivated, organized into everyday life patterns, and performed in the context of the environment
- What happens in the face of impairments, illness, and other factors that create occupational problems
- How occupational therapy enables people to engage in occupations that provide meaning and satisfaction and that support their physical and emotional well-being.

Client-Centered

Even before the emergence of client-centered concepts in occupational therapy, MOHO stressed the importance of incorporating the client's perspective and desires in shaping therapy. Thus, MOHO is recognized as consistent with concepts of client-centered practice (Law, 1998). MOHO is inherently a client-centered model in two important ways. First, it focuses the therapist on the client's uniqueness and provides concepts that allow the therapist to more deeply appreciate the client's perspective and situation. MOHO-based practice requires a client-therapist relationship in which the therapist must understand, respect, and support the client's values, sense of capacity and efficacy, roles, habits, performance experience, and personal environment. Second, since MOHO conceptualizes the client's own doing, thinking, and feeling as the central dynamic of therapy, the client's choice, action, and experience must be central to the therapy process.

Additionally, MOHO has been influenced by many of the ideas emerging from disabilities studies (Albrecht, Seelman, & Bury 2001; Kielhofner, 2005b; Longmore, 1995; Oliver, 1994; Scotch, 1988; Shapiro, 1994), which argue that theory must be informed more fully by the perspectives of those with disabilities. MOHO has always been consistent with the idea of informing theory and practice with clients' viewpoints. However, in the past decade, a special effort has been made to have the model resonate with the voices of disabled persons and emphasize the experience of disability. Also in concert with the disability studies theme that disability occurs because of a misfit between person and environment, MOHO pays close attention to the environment as both an enabler of and a barrier to occupation.

Holistic

MOHO seeks to explain how occupation is motivated, patterned, and performed. By offering explanations of such diverse phenomena, MOHO provides a broad and integrative view of human occupation. For example, two of the phenomena addressed in MOHO, motivation and performance, are not typically considered together in the same theoretical framework. That is, occupational therapy theories that concentrate on physical performance have generally attended to the bodily components (brain and musculoskeletal system) involved in physical doing, while motives have been seen as part of a separate mental domain.

There is growing recognition of the importance of considering body and mind together in explaining phenomena (Trombly, 1995). After all, motivation for a task can influence the extent of physical effort directed to that task (Riccio, Nelson, & Bush, 1990), while physical impairments can weigh down the desire to do things (Toombs, 1992). MOHO concepts seek to avoid dividing humans into separate physical

and mental components. Rather, body and mind are viewed as integrated aspects of the total human being.

Evidence-Based

MOHO is supported by a substantial body of research generated over the past 3 decades, and new research is developing at a rapid pace. To date, more than 100 studies of MOHO have been published in English. Collectively these studies have accomplished the following:

- Supported the validity of the concepts offered in the model
- Confirmed the reliability and validity of MOHO assessments
- Documented the process and outcomes of interventions based on MOHO.

Therapists who wish to use an evidence-based model can find substantial empirical support for MOHO, as discussed in Chapter 25. To facilitate access, an evidence-based search engine can be found at www.moho.uic.edu.

Designed to Complement Other Models and Theories

MOHO was developed when most models in occupational therapy focused on impairment and when the importance of occupation was being rediscovered (Kielhofner, 2004). The intention of the model was to fill a gap that existed in occupational therapy knowledge and to complement the focus on impairment with an understanding of the client's motivation and lifestyle and the environmental context. The model was always intended to be used alongside other occupational therapy models and interdisciplinary concepts. It is recognized that MOHO rarely addresses all of the problems faced by a client, which requires therapists to actively use other models and concepts. Most therapists who use MOHO use it in combination with other models, such as the biomechanical, sensory integration, and motor control models. The latter models provide a focus on performance components not provided in MOHO. Thus, use of these models in combination allows a comprehensive approach to meeting clients' needs.

A **Definition of Human Occupation**

. . . .

MOHO was specifically developed to focus theory, research, and practice on occupation. The concept, human occupation, refers to the doing of work, play, or activities of daily living within a temporal, physical, and sociocultural context that characterizes much of human life. Each of the components of this definition is discussed below.

Humans are characterized by an intense need to do things (Fidler & Fidler, 1983; Nelson, 1988). Human occupation comprises three broad areas of doing: activities of daily living, play, and productivity. **Activities of daily living** are the typical life tasks required for self-care and self-maintenance, such as grooming, bathing, eating, cleaning the house, and doing laundry. **Play** refers to activities freely undertaken for their own sake; it includes exploring, pretending, celebrating, engaging in games or sports, and pursuing hobbies (Reilly, 1974). **Productivity** refers to activities (both paid and unpaid) that provide services or commodities to others such as ideas, knowledge, help, information-sharing, entertainment, utilitarian or artistic objects, and protection (Shannon, 1970). Activities such as studying, practicing, and apprenticing improve abilities for productive performance. Thus, productivity includes activities engaged in as a student, employee, volunteer, parent, serious hobbyist, and amateur.

Human doing exists in the framework of time. Humans are moved to occupy time with the things they do (Meyer, 1922). This doing marks time's passing and fills the present. It resonates with the cycles of time that shape the recurring patterns of doing (Young, 1988). Occupation also anticipates the future and shapes the course of lives over time (Kerby, 1991). From the early struggle to move against gravity to the mastery of a complex world of places and objects, humans also occupy a physical world (Ayres, 1979; Reilly, 1962). They traverse, manipulate, and transform their physical surroundings.

Humans are sociocultural creatures who share common worlds of action and meaning. Occupation involves doing things among and with others (Rogers, 1983). Occupation expresses and maintains the social fabric that surrounds us. People make places for themselves in the social world by what they do. In turn, these social positions influence what we, as people, are ex-

pected to do. Culture is the medium through which humans make sense of their doing. Culture generates a whole range of things to do and gives them shape and significance. Members of a culture realize the significance of what they are doing by virtue of how their culture views and makes sense of it (Yerxa et al., 1989).

In sum, occupation encompasses a wide range of doing that occurs in the context of time, space, society, and culture. Temporal, physical, social, and cultural contexts pose conditions that invite, shape, and inform human occupation. The things humans do, why and how they do them, and what they think and feel about them all derive from the intersecting conditions and influences of time, space, society, and culture.

Approaching This Book

As noted earlier, this book aims to provide an overview of contemporary MOHO theory, application, and research. It is divided into four sections. Section 1 covers MOHO theory. Section 2 covers such topics as therapeutic reasoning, assessments, and planning and documenting therapy. Section 3 illustrates the application of MOHO in therapy by providing a series of in-depth cases. Section 4 contains resources for program development, research, and further exploration of MOHO.

In addition to the several contributing authors, there are many implicit and explicit voices here. They include those of colleagues from around the world who have helped to conceptualize MOHO, those of persons who have told their stories of living with disabilities, and those of therapists who have created practical means of applying MOHO. We hope that these voices have come together in an interesting, instructive, and instrumentally useful way.

Key Terms

Activities of daily living: The typical life tasks required for self-care and self-maintenance, such as grooming, bathing, eating, cleaning the house, and doing laundry.

Human occupation: The doing of work, play, or activities of daily living within a temporal, physical, and sociocultural context that characterizes much of human life.

Play: Activities undertaken for their own sake.

Work: Activities (both paid and unpaid) that provide services or commodities to others such as ideas, knowledge, help, information sharing, entertainment, utilitarian or artistic objects, and protection.

References

Albrecht, G. L., Seelman, K. D., & Bury, M. (2001). *Handbook of disability studies*. Thousand Oaks, CA: Sage.

Ayres, A. J. (1979). *Sensory integration and the child*. Los Angeles: Western Psychological Services.

Fidler, G., & Fidler, J. (1983). Doing and becoming: The occupational therapy experience. In G. Kielhofner (Ed.), *Health through occupation: Theory and practice in occupational therapy*. Philadelphia: FA Davis.

Forsyth, K., Summerfield-Mann, L., & Kielhofner, G. (2005). A Scholarship of practice: Making occupation-focused, theory-driven, evidence-based practice a reality. *British Journal of Occupational Therapy, 68*, 261–268.

Haglund, L., Ekbladh, E., Thorell, L. H., and Hallberg, I. R.(2000). Practice models in Swedish psychiatric occupational therapy. *Scandinavian Journal of Occupational Therapy, 7*,107–113.

Kerby, A. P. (1991). *Narrative and the self*. Bloomington: Indiana University.

Kielhofner, G. (1980a). A model of human occupation, part two. Ontogenesis from the perspective of temporal adaptation. *American Journal of Occupational Therapy, 34*, 657–663.

Kielhofner, G. (1980b). A model of human occupation, part three. Benign and vicious cycles. *American Journal of Occupational Therapy, 34*, 731–737.

Kielhofner, G. (2004). *Conceptual foundations of occupational therapy* (3rd ed.). Philadelphia: FA Davis.

Kielhofner, G. (2005a). A scholarship of practice: Creating discourse between theory, research and practice. *Occupational Therapy in Health Care , 19*, 7–17.

Kielhofner, G. (2005b). Rethinking disability and what to do about it: Disability studies and its implications for occupational therapy. *American Journal of Occupational Therapy, 59*, 487–496.

Kielhofner, G., & Burke, J. (1980). A model of human occupation, part one. Conceptual framework and content. *American Journal of Occupational Therapy, 34*, 572–581.

Kielhofner, G., Burke, J., & Heard, I. C. (1980). A model of human occupation, part four. Assessment and intervention. *American Journal of Occupational Therapy, 34*, 777–788.

Law, M. (1998). *Client centered occupational therapy*. Thorofare, NJ: Slack.

Law, M. & McColl, M. A. (1989). Knowledge and use of theory among occupational therapists: A Canadian survey. *Canadian Journal of Occupational Therapy, 56*(4), 198–204.

Lee, S., Taylor, R., Kielhofner, G., & Fisher, G. (in press). Theory use in practice: A national survey of therapists who use the Model of Human Occupation. American Journal of Occupational Therapy.

Longmore, P.K. (1995). The second phase: From disability rights to disability culture. *The Disability Rag & Resource, Sept/Oct,* 4–11.

Meyer, A. (1922). The philosophy of occupational therapy. *Archives of Occupational Therapy, 1*: 1.

Nelson, D. (1988). Occupation: Form and performance. *American Journal of Occupational Therapy, 38*, 777–788.

National Board for Certification in Occupational Therapy. (2004). A practice analysis study of entry-level occupational therapist registered and certified occupational therapy assistant practice. *OTJR, Occupation, Participation and Health*. Spring, Volume 24, Supplement 1, S3–31.

Oliver, M. (1994). The social model in context. In *Understanding Disability: From theory to practice*. London: Macmillan.

Reilly, M. (1962). Occupational therapy can be one of the great ideas of 20th century medicine. *American Journal of Occupational Therapy, 16*, 1–9.

Reilly, M. (1974). *Play as exploratory learning*. Beverly Hills, CA: Sage.

Riccio, C. M., Nelson, D. L., & Bush, M. A. (1990). Adding purpose to the repetitive exercise of elderly women. *American Journal of Occupational Therapy, 44*, 714–719.

Rogers, J. (1983). The study of human occupation. In G. Kielhofner (Ed.), *Health through occupation: Theory and practice in occupational therapy*. Philadelphia: FA Davis.

Scotch, R. (1988). Disability as a basis for a social movement: Advocacy and the politics of definition. *Journal of Social Issues, 44*(1), 159–172.

Shannon, P. (1970). The work-play model: A basis for occupational therapy programming. *American Journal of Occupational Therapy, 24*, 215–218.

Shapiro, J. (1994). *No pity: People with disabilities forging a new civil rights movement*. New York: Times Books.

Toombs, K. (1992). *The meaning of illness: A phenomenological account of the different perspectives of physician and patient.* Boston: Kluwer Academic.

Trombly, C. (1995). Occupation: Purposefulness and meaningfulness as therapeutic mechanisms. *American Journal of Occupational Therapy, 49,* 960–972.

Yerxa, E. J., Clark, F., Frank, G., Jackson, J., Parham, D., Pierce, D., Stein, C., & Zemke, R. (1989). An introduction to occupation science: A foundation for occupational therapy in the 21st century. *Occupational Therapy in Health Care, 6*(4), 1–17.

Young, M. (1988). *The metronomic society: Natural rhythms and human timetables.* Cambridge, MA: Harvard University.

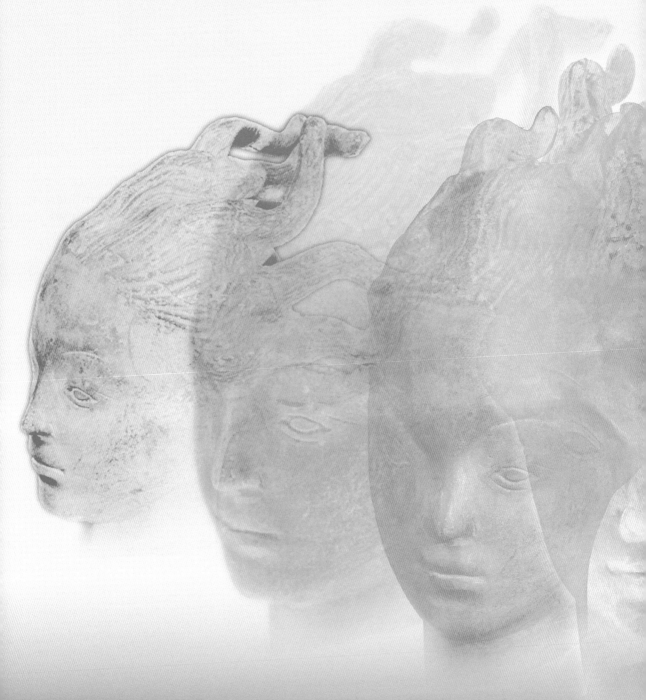

Explaining Human Occupation

Introduction to Section I

Chapters 2 to 10 present MOHO theory. Chapter 2 introduces concepts aimed at explaining how occupation is motivated, patterned, and performed. Chapter 3 provides a framework for integrating the concepts of the previous chapter into coherent understanding of human occupation. Chapters 4 to 6 expand on how occupation is motivated, patterned, and performed. Chapter 7 discusses the environmental context of occupational behavior, explaining what aspects of the environment influence occupation and how they exert this influence. Chapter 8 identifies levels at which we can examine occupation and discusses how occupation shapes a person's identity and competence over time. Chapter 9 builds on Chapter 8 by focusing on how persons construct their occupational lives as stories unfolding over time. Chapter 10 examines how occupation changes and gives an overview of typical occupational changes through the life course.

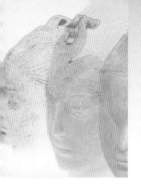

2

The Basic Concepts of Human Occupation

● Gary Kielhofner

Drew[2-1]

is a first grader who lives in a large American city. The youngest of three, he attends the same school as his siblings. This year Drew has the same teacher that his older sister and brother previously had. Drew's teacher regularly reminds him of how smart his sister and brother are and that she expects him to achieve at the same level. However, Drew has some challenges keeping his attention focused in the classroom and when doing homework. At the beginning of the school year, he did poorly

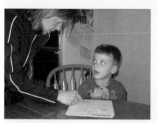

Drew's mother provides encouragement and support as he completes his homework.

on his last homework assignment which added to Drew's feelings of ineffectiveness as a student. He doesn't want to let his parents down because he knows how much they value doing well in school, but he increasingly dreads going to school. However, Drew recently started dealing with all the pressures of being a student by ignoring some of his homework assignments. Concerned about Drew's increasing difficulty in school, his mother has been making Drew study during the evening time with his siblings, a time when he usually plays with neighborhood friends.

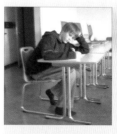

Oli[2-2]

Oli struggles to complete his classwork.

is an Icelandic teenage boy. He is having school difficulties. His low muscle tone contributes to his poor posture and difficulty with completing fine motor tasks such as written school work. These difficulties are complicated by the fact that the desk in his classroom is too small for him. Overall Oli is feeling badly about himself since he receives a lot of negative feedback about his school performance both in the classroom and elsewhere. As a consequence he doesn't see much value in trying to do his schoolwork. On the other hand, Oli is very motivated by his two passions: playing the drums and karate. He is looking forward to playing the drums in a school concert; he especially likes being able to be competent around his classmates.

Carlos[2-3]

is 26 years old and lives in Mexico. As a child he was diagnosed as developmentally delayed. He is independent in his personal care, but is unable to cross the streets or manage money by himself. He enjoys music, but otherwise has few interests or pastimes. He wants to work like other young men and

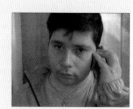

Carlos practices calling a friend on his cell phone.

attends a sheltered workshop two times a week where he packages products. In the workshop he has trouble with new tasks that involve following directions and does not get along well with his supervisor. Carlos feels frustrated that he is not able to control more aspects of his life and do things that others his age are able to do.

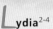ydia[2-4]

is an 83-year-old Sesotho resident of the dementia care unit in Bloemfontein, South Africa. She loves young people as she raised 6 children of her own. She treats any younger person as if they were her offspring, offering food or assistance. Most

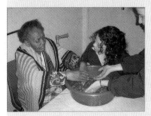

people humor her or gently decline her offers, to which Lydia always responds, "How will I ever get you to grow up?" Lydia's caring nature and strong religious beliefs makes her a favorite among the unit staff. She

Lydia interacts with occupational therapy students during a therapy session.

willingly engages in any of the occupational therapy groups offered in the unit. She is friendly and kind to all and often sits by herself and softly sings hymns. Although she is seldom reality orientated, she loves to pray for others. She attempts to communicate in Sotho, Xhosa, Afrikaans and / or English, depending on the language preference of the person with whom she is interacting.

[2-1] Susan Cahill, Clinical Instructor at University of Illinois at Chicago, provided the case of Drew for this chapter.

[2-2] Erla B. Sveinbjornsdottir and Kristjana Olafsdottir, occupational therapists in Kopavogur, Iceland provided the case of Oli for this chapter.

[2-3] Catalina Edith Sanchez Galicia, student of the Master of Occupational Therapy program at Instituto de Terapia Ocupacional in Mexico City, Mexico provided the case of Carlos for this chapter.

[2-4] Sanet du Toit from University of the Free State in Blomenfontein, South Africa, provided the case of Lydia for this chapter.

Each of these individuals differ in how they are motivated toward and choose to do things, in their patterns of everyday life, and in their individual capacities. In order to have a common way to understand all their circumstances, concepts that explain how they select, organize, and undertake their occupations are needed. In MOHO, humans are conceptualized as being made up of three interrelated components:

- Volition
- Habituation
- Performance capacity.

Volition refers to the motivation for occupation. Habituation refers to the process by which occupation is organized into patterns or routines. Performance capacity refers to the physical and mental abilities that underlie skilled occupational performance. Although the following sections discuss these components separately, it is important to keep in mind that they are three different aspects of the total person.

Within MOHO, consideration of any aspect of the person (volition, habituation, or performance) always includes how the environment is influencing the person's motivation, pattern, and performance. The environment is a constant influence on occupation, and persons' occupational circumstances cannot be appreciated without an understanding of their environments.

Volition

Humans possess a complex nervous system that gives them an intense and pervasive need to act (Berlyne, 1960; Florey, 1969; McClelland, 1961; Reilly, 1962; Shibutani, 1968; Smith, 1969; White, 1959). Moreover, humans have a body capable of action. Finally, humans have an awareness of their potential for doing things (DeCharms, 1968). Together, these factors result in a need for action that is the underlying motive for occupation. Other motives are sometimes involved in an occupation (Nelson, 1988). For example, financial rewards may partly motivate work. Daily living tasks are partly in the service of basic drives such as hunger, and recreational activities such as dating have a sexual dimension. Nonetheless, the desire for action manifests itself throughout occupation and is its dominant motive.

Volitional Thoughts and Feelings

In addition to the need or desire to act, each person has distinct feelings and thoughts about doing things that are essential to volition. These thoughts and feelings are responses to these questions: Am I good at this? Is this worth doing? Do I like this? Thus, volitional thoughts and feelings are about the following:

- Personal capacity and effectiveness
- Importance or worth attached to what one does
- Enjoyment or satisfaction one experiences in doing things.

Thus, while humans are all energized by a universal drive toward action, they want to do the things that they value, feel competent to do, and find satisfying.

Personal Causation, Values, and Interests

In MOHO, these volitional thoughts and feelings are referred to as personal causation, values, and interests (*Fig. 2.1*). **Personal causation** refers to one's sense of capacity and effectiveness. **Values** refer to what one finds important and meaningful to do. **Interests** refer to what one finds enjoyable or satisfying to do. In everyday life, personal causation, values, and interests are interwoven. For example, Drew's volition can be seen in the values he has internalized about the importance of school performance and his sense of feeling

FIGURE 2.1 The content of volitional thoughts and feelings.

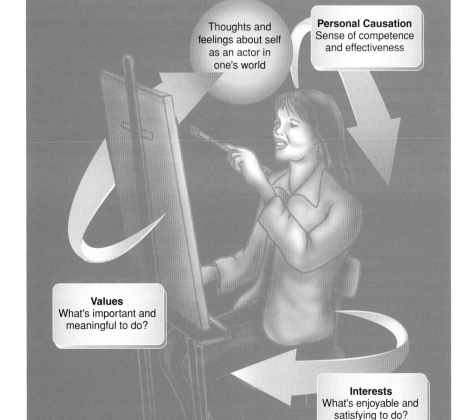

Thoughts and feelings about self as an actor in one's world

Personal Causation
Sense of competence and effectiveness

Values
What's important and meaningful to do?

Interests
What's enjoyable and satisfying to do?

ineffective in doing well in school. Carlos's volition is reflected in his interest in music, the value he has of wanting to be like other young adults, and his feelings that he does not control his life as he would like to. Oli's volition is a picture of contrasts that includes his feeling bad about and alienated from academic aspects of school along with his passion for paying the drums and doing karate. Lydia's volition is still apparent through the veil of her dementia. Her love of children and her religious values still radiate. As each of these examples illustrate, volition is reflected in the wide range of thoughts and feelings people have about the things they have done, are doing, or might do.

Volitional Processes

Volition is an ongoing process. That is, volitional thoughts and feelings occur over time as people experience, interpret, anticipate, and choose occupations.

EXPERIENCE

Whenever we do something, a whole range of experiences is possible. We may, for example, feel pleasure, anxiety, comfort, challenge, or boredom. Moreover, we may have thoughts of self-doubt or self-confidence. We may proceed deliberately, with solid convictions about why we are doing what we are doing, or hesitantly, worrying that our actions are futile or meaningless. **Experience** refers, then, to the immediate thoughts and feelings that emerge in the midst of and in response to performance. These include, for instance, the joy Oli feels when playing the drums or the anxiety Drew has when facing homework.

INTERPRETATION

Of course, we not only experience what we do but also reflect on and interpret that experience. A person may do this in a variety of ways, and the following are some examples. Carlos feels bad about an encounter with his supervisor and recalls the incident to consider whether he should have behaved differently. After receiving less

than optimal feedback on some aspect of school performance, Oli thinks to himself that he just can't seem to do well at school. Drew asks his mother whether she thinks he has improved doing his homework. Whenever people reflect on or discuss with others how they performed, what it was like to do something, and whether it is worth doing, they are engaged in the volitional process of interpretation. **Interpretation** is thus defined as recalling and reflecting on performance in terms of its significance for oneself and one's world.

ANTICIPATION

The world presents us with immediate and future possibilities for action. Whether we pay attention to them and how we react to the opportunities and expectations for action is also part of the volitional process. The following are examples. Oli walks into a classroom and dreads an upcoming exam. Drew peers out the window to see whether friends are gathered yet in the park. Lydia looks around the dayroom for a "young person" she can help out.

Anticipation always considers what we might be doing in the immediate or distant future. The world presents us possibilities and expectations for action, but which ones we notice and how we think and feel about them are influenced by what we like and feel competent and obligated to do. Consequently, **anticipation** is defined as the process of noticing and reacting to potentials or expectations for action.

ACTIVITY AND OCCUPATIONAL CHOICES

Our daily lives are influenced by what we choose to do next, later on, and tomorrow. These **activity choices** are defined as short-term, deliberate decisions to enter and exit occupational activities. Examples of activity choices include deciding to go for a morning walk, have lunch with a friend later in the day, and clean one's apartment this coming Saturday morning. While activity choices require only brief deliberation, they determine a significant amount of what we actually do.

Individuals also make larger choices concerning occupations that will become an extended or permanent part of their lives. These occupational choices (Heard, 1977; Matsutsuyu, 1971) are commitments to enter into a course of action or to sustain regular performance over time. They include taking on a new role, establishing a new activity as part of one's permanent

> *Volition is reflected in the wide range of thoughts and feelings people have about the things they have done, are doing, or might do.*

routine, and undertaking a project. Examples of occupational choices are starting a job, joining a club, taking up a new hobby, and deciding to tend a summer garden. Ordinarily, occupational choices require some deliberation and may involve information gathering, reflection, imagining possibilities, and considering alternatives. Occupational choices also involve commitment, since they require doing over time. **Occupational choices** are thus defined as deliberate commitments to enter an occupational role, acquire a new habit, or undertake a personal project.

Together, activity choices and occupational choices influence, to a large extent, what kinds of occupational performance make up our daily lives. These choices are the function of volition. They reflect our personal causation, our interests, and our values.

Summary and Definition of Volition

The cycle of experience, interpretation, anticipation, and choice is an integrated process. As shown in *Figure 2.2*, each process flows into the next. One chooses action, the doing of which stimulates experience. One re-

FIGURE 2.2 Volitional processes.

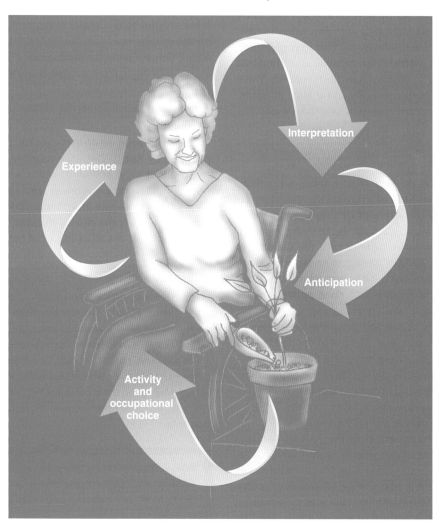

calls and reflects on experience to interpret what was done. Finally, the meanings generated from such reflections lead to the next choices.

Thus we can say that **volition** is a pattern of thoughts and feelings about oneself as an actor in one's world which occurs as one anticipates, chooses, experiences, and interprets what one does. Volitional thoughts and feelings include personal causation, values, and interests.

Through the cycle of anticipating, choosing, experiencing, and interpreting, volition tends to perpetuate itself. For example, once we experience ourselves as competent in an occupation, we will tend to anticipate that occupation with positive feelings and choose to do it again. Volition is also an unfolding process in which changes take place. As we develop and age and as we encounter new environments with new opportunities and demands for action, we may find new pleasures, lose old interests, discover new capabilities, or find that we are no longer so adept at a particular activity. There are elements of both continuity and change in values, interests, and personal causation over the lifespan.

Habituation

Much of what we do belongs to a taken-for-granted round of daily life. Most of us repeat the same familiar weekday morning routine of getting up, grooming, and heading to work or school. On the way, we walk, ride, or drive the same route or take the same train, subway, or bus without having to consciously think about what we are doing. Once arrived, we set about doing tasks we previously have done multiple times, undertaking them in much the same way as before. We encounter others, saying and doing the same types of things with them that we have done in the past. We do these things unreflectively, and doing them feels familiar, locating us in our ordinary, taken-for-granted life. Moreover, by engaging in certain routine behaviors we reaffirm ourselves as having a certain identity. These aspects of routine daily life unfold automatically.

The term **habituation** refers to this semiautonomous pattern of behavior in concert with our familiar temporal, physical, and social habitats as shown in *Figure 2.3*. Habituation allows us to recognize and respond to temporal cues and time frames. (e.g., the recurring pattern of weeks), to our familiar physical worlds (e.g., the physical layout of our home, workplace, school, and neighborhood), and to the social customs and the patterns that make up our own culture.

The world around us, our habitat, has a certain stability; we, in return, also have a habituated tendency to act in consistent, patterned ways. That we do so is a function of habits and roles.

Habits

Habits preserve ways of doing things that we have internalized through repeated performance. We generate habits by consistently doing the same thing in the same context. What once required attention and concentration eventually becomes automatic. Thus, **habits** are defined as acquired tendencies to respond and perform in certain consistent ways in familiar environments or situations. Consequently, for habits to exist:

- We must repeat action sufficiently to establish the pattern
- Consistent environmental circumstances must be present.

Much of what we do in the course of a day or week is guided by habits. Our daily routine, our manner of going about most anything we do, and the peculiar ways we always do a given task are all reflected in our habits. Drew's struggle to do homework regularly, Oli's regular practicing the drums, the way Carlos does his packaging tasks, are all examples of habits.

Internalized Roles

Our patterns of action also reflect roles that we have internalized. That is, we identify with and behave in ways that we have learned to associate with a particular social status or identity. For example, when people act as a spouse, parent, worker, or student, they exhibit patterns of behavior that reflect that socially identified status. Moreover, their behavior will tend to be along the lines of what others expect them to do as part of that role.

The world around us, our habitat, has a certain stability; we, in return, also have a habituated tendency to act in consistent, patterned ways.

FIGURE 2.3 Habituation shapes interaction with our habitats.

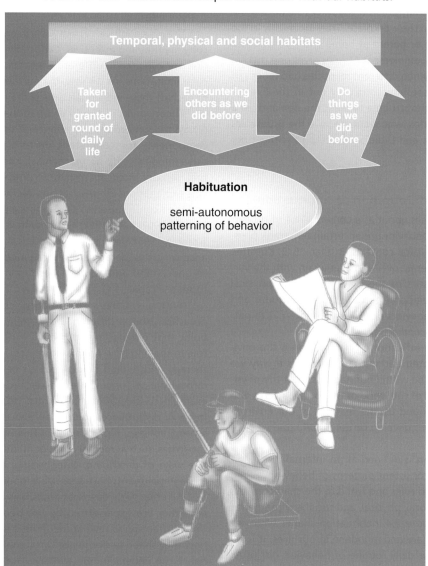

Through a process of socialization, people acquire roles that derive from social status. Socialization involves interacting over time with explicit and implicit definitions and expectations for the role. As a result, one internalizes a sense of self, attitudes, and behaviors that correspond to the social definition and expectations of the role. Other roles are self-defined and shaped by the interrelated and ongoing nature of a set of tasks for which one feels responsibility. Such roles arise out of personal circumstances or necessity. They are established as one engages in a pattern of related actions and assumes an identity connected to them.

Given these considerations, the **internalized role** can be defined as incorporation of a socially and/or personally defined status and a related cluster of attitudes and behaviors. People ordinarily have several roles that occupy routine times and spaces. For example, people generally are in the worker role during the workweek and in the workplace. They are mostly in the role of a spouse or parent at home and outside work hours. Having a complement of roles gives one rhythm and change between different identities and modes of doing. We can see how roles play out in the lives of Drew and Oli, who struggle to meet the demands of a student role; Carlos, who wants to have the usual roles of young adults; and Lydia, who seeks to reenact her role as a parent.

Summary and Definition of Habituation

Habituation comes about as a consequence of repeating patterns of behavior under certain temporal, physical, and sociocultural contexts (Bruner, 1973; Koestler, 1969). As we interact over and over again with the various characteristics of these contexts (e.g., physical arrangement, temporal patterns, social attitudes and expectations, behaviors of others), we internalize patterns of attitude and action.

A pervasive influence on habituation is the environment. As noted earlier, habituation is a way we have learned to be within our habitats. Be it the physical arrangement of the world or the social patterns and norms that surround us, the features of our environments shape us to develop certain habituated ways of doing things.

Habituation is defined as an internalized readiness to exhibit consistent patterns of behavior guided by our habits and roles and fitted to the characteristics of routine temporal, physical, and social environments. As shown in *Figure 2.4*, habituation shapes what we take to be ordinary and mundane in our lives. It is responsible for our daily routine of behavior; our usual way of going about doing things; the various routes we take in going about our homes, neighborhoods, and larger community; and our patterns of involvement with others.

Performance Capacity

The capacity to do things depends on these factors:

- Musculoskeletal, neurologic, cardiopulmonary, and other bodily systems that are used when acting on the world

- Mental or cognitive abilities, such as memory and planning.

Drew's cognitive capacity is affected by his difficulty maintaining attention. Carlos's and Lydia's cognition are impaired in different ways. Oli has neuromuscular limitations. As we saw, the performance capacity of each of these individuals affects their occupation.

Theory and practice in occupational therapy have always recognized the importance of these underlying components for competent performance. Notably, other models (e.g., biomechanical, cognitive-perceptual, sensory integration, motor control) provide specific explanations of physical and mental components and their contribution to performance (Bundy, Lane, & Murray, 2002; Katz, 1992; Mathiowetz & Haugen, 1994; Trombly, 1995). Because other models address performance capacity, therapists use these models as a means to understand and address specific problems of performance capacity.

Within MOHO, performance capacity is approached from a different but complementary viewpoint that emphasizes subjective experience and its role in shaping how people do things. In occupational therapy and related fields, people's performance and difficulty in performing are approached objectively. For example, consideration may be given to understanding losses or disturbances of ordinary movement capacity; sensory abilities, such as sight or hearing; or cognitive capacities, such as memory or judgment. Various objective ways of describing, categorizing, and measuring these impairments have been developed.

All objectively describable abilities and limitations of ability are experienced by the people who have them. Attention to the nature of these experiences and how they shape performance can complement and enhance the understanding we have from the objective approach to performance capacity.

Therefore, within MOHO, the concept of **performance capacity** is defined as the ability to do things provided by the status of underlying objective physical and

> *All objectively describable abilities and limitations of ability are experienced by the people who have them.*

FIGURE 2.4 Habituation: habits and roles influencing behavior in familiar environments and situations.

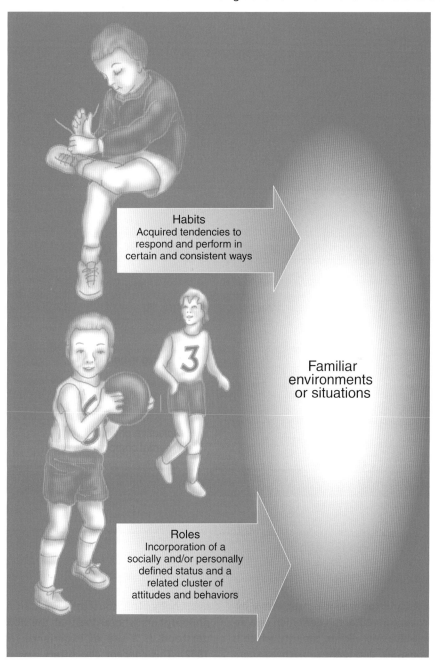

FIGURE 2.5 Objective and subjective components of performance capacity.

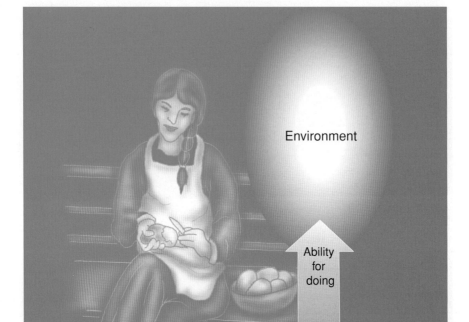

mental components and corresponding subjective experience. As shown in *Figure 2.5*, this definition calls attention to the objective approach to capacity, which is the focus of other models, and to the subjective experiential focus on capacity that we emphasize.

In discussing the experiential aspect of performance capacity, we employ a concept referred to as the *lived body*. This concept derives from the work of philosophers who argue that the body must be understood as a site of experience (Merleau-Ponty, 1962). This concept also offers new ways of understanding both how we are able to perform and how disease or impairment is experienced and affects performance.

> *Occupation is always located in, influenced, and given meaning by its physical and sociocultural context.*

The Environment

All occupation occurs in a complex, multilayered environment. Occupation is always located in, influenced, and given meaning by its physical and sociocultural context.

Thus the environment includes the spaces humans occupy, the objects they use, the people with whom they interact, and the possibilities and meanings for doing that exist in the human collective of which they are a part. Each environment offers potential opportunities and resources, demands and constraints. How the characteristics of a given environment interact with each person's values, interests, personal causation, roles, habits, and performance capacities will determine what influence the environment has for that person. The opportunity, support, demand, and constraint that the physical and social aspects of the environment have on a particular individual is referred to as **environmental impact**. This impact can enable or disable the individual. The environment is often the critical dimension that either supports or interferes with an individual's occupation. Drew's school environment presents expectations he finds difficult to meet. Oli has mixed opportunities and challenges in his school environment (i.e., the school band versus classroom work). Lydia has necessary supports that allow her to function at her level and be safe despite her dementia.

Conclusion

At the beginning of this chapter, it was indicated that volition, habituation, and performance capacity are integrated parts of each person. As shown in *Figure 2.6*, they operate seamlessly, forming a coherent whole. Volition, habituation, and performance ca-

pacity each contribute different but complementary functions to what we do and how we experience our doing. We cannot fully understand the occupations of people like Drew, Oli, Carlos, and Lydia without reference to all three contributing factors and without reference to the environment. Taking this broader view recognizes the complexity inherent in human occupation.

Key Terms

Activity choices: Short-term, deliberate decisions to enter and exit occupational activities.

Anticipation: Noticing and reacting to potentials or expectations for action.

Experience: The immediate thoughts and feelings that emerge in the midst of and in response to performance.

Habits: Acquired tendencies to respond and perform in certain consistent ways in familiar environments or situations.

Habituation: Internalized readiness to exhibit consistent patterns of behavior guided by habits and roles and fitted to the characteristics of routine temporal, physical, and social environments.

Environmental impact: the opportunity, support, demand, and constraint of the physical and social aspects of the environment on a particular individual.

Interests: What one finds enjoyable or satisfying.

Internalized role: Incorporation of a socially and/or personally defined status and a related cluster of attitudes and behaviors.

Interpretation: Recalling and reflecting on performance in terms of its significance for oneself and one's world.

Occupational choices: Deliberate commitments to enter an occupational role, acquire a new habit, or undertake a personal project.

Performance capacity: Ability to do things provided by the status of underlying objective physical and mental components and corresponding subjective experience.

Personal causation: Sense of capacity and effectiveness.

Values: What one finds important and meaningful.

Volition: Pattern of thoughts and feelings about oneself as an actor in one's world which occur as one anticipates, chooses, experiences, and interprets what one does.

FIGURE 2.6 Integration of volition, habituation, and performance capacity into the whole person.

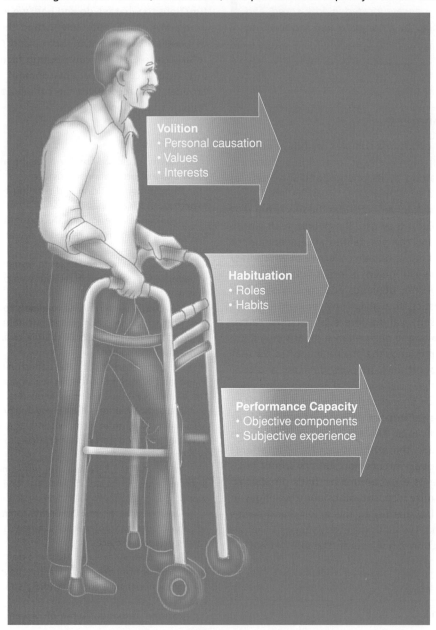

References

Berlyne, D. E. (1960). *Conflict, arousal, and curiosity*. New York: McGraw-Hill.

Bruner, J. (1973). Organization of early skilled action. *Child Development, 44*, 1–11.

Bundy, A.C., Lane, S.J., & Murray, E.A. (2002). *Sensory integration: Theory and practice* (2nd ed.). Philadelphia: FA Davis.

DeCharms, R. E. (1968). *Personal causation: The internal affective determinants of behaviors*. New York: Academic.

Florey, L. L. (1969). Intrinsic motivation: The dynamics of occupational therapy theory. *American Journal of Occupational Therapy, 23*, 319–322.

Heard, C. (1977). Occupational role acquisition: A perspective on the chronically disabled. *American Journal of Occupational Therapy, 41*, 243–247.

Katz, N. (1992). *Cognitive rehabilitation: Models for intervention in occupational therapy*. Boston: Andover Medical.

Koestler, A. (1969). Beyond atomism and holism: The concept of the holon. In A. Koestler & J. R. Smythies (Eds.), *Beyond reductionism*. Boston: Beacon.

Mathiowetz, V., & Haugen, J. B. (1994). Motor behavior research: Implications for therapeutic approaches to central nervous system dysfunction. *American Journal of Occupational Therapy, 48*, 733–745.

Matsutsuyu, J. (1971). Occupational behavior: A perspective on work and play. *American Journal of Occupational Therapy, 25*, 291–294.

McClelland, D. (1961). *The achieving society*. New York: Free Press.

Merleau-Ponty, M. (1962). *Phenomenology of perception* (C. Smith, trans.). London: Routledge & Kegan Paul. (Original work published 1945.)

Nelson, D. (1988). Occupation: Form and performance. *American Journal of Occupational Therapy, 34*, 777–788.

Reilly, M. (1962). Occupational therapy can be one of the great ideas of 20th century medicine. *American Journal of Occupational Therapy, 16*, 1–9.

Shibutani, T. (1968). A cybernetic approach to motivation. In W. Buckley (Ed.), *Modern systems research for the behavioral scientist*. Chicago: Aldine.

Smith, M. B. (1969). *Social psychology and human values*. Chicago: Aldine.

Trombly, C. (1995). Occupation: Purposefulness and meaningfulness as therapeutic mechanisms. *American Journal of Occupational Therapy, 49,* 960–972.

White, R. W. (1959). Excerpts from motivation reconsidered: The concept of competence. *Psychological Review, 66*, 126–134.

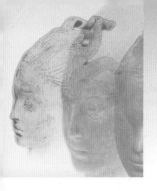

3

The Dynamics of Human Occupation

● Gary Kielhofner

hapter 2 proposed that occupation is motivated by volitional thoughts and feelings (i.e., personal causation, values, and interests), shaped by the habits and roles that make up habituation, and made possible by performance capacities. This chapter will explain how volition, habituation, and performance capacity are integrated together and how they relate to one's environment. Concepts from systems theory[1] will be introduced and used to state a number of principles that explicate the dynamics of occupation. Following this, implications for occupational therapy will be discussed.

How Occupation Occurs

A highly organized process unfolds as people go about their everyday occupations. Consider, for example, Rigo doing his morning routine of getting washed up, groomed, and dressed. After getting out of bed, he puts on some coffee, takes a shower and shaves, and then dons his work clothes. During much of this time Rigo is thinking about a fishing trip that he is taking on the weekend with his best friend, Carlos. During his drive to the construction site where he is foreman of a plumbing crew, he plans how the crew will finish up the job. As he pulls into the construction site, he calls

Carlos to remind him to stop by the bait and tackle shop after work to buy fishing supplies.

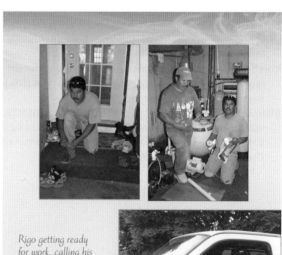

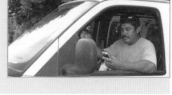

Rigo getting ready for work, calling his friend Carlos to make weekend plans, and working with his crew.

This short scenario illustrates several aspects of volition, habituation, and performance capacity. For instance, Rigo's habits guide his morning routine and free him to engage in volitional anticipation of the upcoming fishing trip. Similarly, while his habit of driving to work unfolds, his awareness of the responsibilities of his foreman role stimulates him to plan the activities of the work crew. During this time, Rigo's physical and mental capacities are being called upon as he engages and ties his shoes, watches the traffic as he drives, and plans an

---

[1]Systems theory refers to a large and changing body of literature that has evolved over the past half-century. The model of human occupation was originally based on concepts of open systems and general systems theory (e.g., von Bertalanffy, 1968a, b; Koestler, 1969). As these original systems ideas were expanded and revised in more recent dynamical systems theory (e.g., Kelso, & Tuller, 1984; Thelen & Ulrich, 1991), the use of systems concepts in MOHO has evolved. The intention of this chapter is to draw from the tradition of systems thinking the concepts that are useful for thinking about how volition, habituation, performance capacity, and the environment interact and influence occupation and about how change takes place.

errand after work. As this small slice of Rigo's occupational life illustrates, occupation always involves an ongoing interplay of volition, habituation, performance capacity, and the environmental context. This interplay reflects two important systems concepts, heterarchy and emergence.

Heterarchy is the principle that aspects of a person and that person's environment are linked into a dynamic whole (Capra, 1997; Clarke, 1997; Thelen & Ulrich, 1991; Turvey, 1990). In a heterarchy, each component contributes something to a total dynamic. For instance, as shown in *Figure 3.1*, Rigo's habits for going about his morning routine provide a tendency to manifest a sequence of behaviors. Rigo's performance capacity makes possible certain abilities that are called upon when habitual self-care unfolds. Rigo's interests (i.e., his love of fishing) and his values (i.e., doing a good job) are also at play. Each of these elements contributes something to the total dynamic of the morning routine.

Importantly, the environment is central to these dynamics (Clarke, 1997). For example, Rigo's activities of daily living involve and are shaped by the objects and spaces that make up his home. Moreover, while Rigo's memory may provide him with rough instructions for driving to the construction site, he must rely on the physical environment to give him cues about when to speed up, slow down or stop, how to steer on the road, and when to turn at an intersection.

What Rigo does, thinks, and feels emerges out of the collective conditions created by the interaction of these personal and environmental elements. **Emergence** is the principle that complex actions, thoughts, and feelings spontaneously arise out of the interactions of several components (Clarke 1997; Haken, 1987; Kelso & Tuller, 1984). As shown in *Figure 3.1*, Rigo's thoughts, emotions, and actions in the morning routine emerge from the dynamic interaction of his volition, habituation, performance capacity, and environ-

FIGURE 3.1 Heterarchical contributions of volition, habituation, performance capacity, and environment to an occupation.

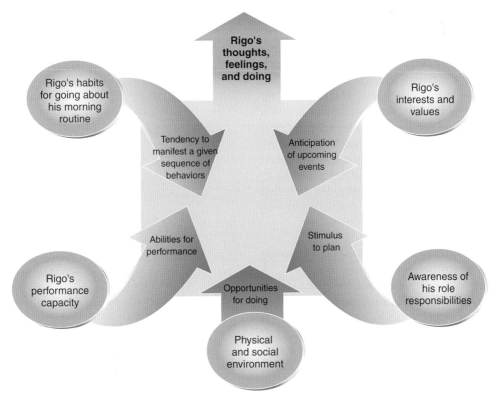

ment. The concepts of heterarchy and emergence allow the following principle to be stated:

> *Occupational actions, thoughts and emotions always arise out of the dynamic interaction of volition, habituation, performance capacity, and environmental context.*

This means that no single causal factor can ever account fully for emergent behavior, thought, or feeling. A corollary to this principle is that volition, habituation, performance capacity, and the environment do not always make synergistic contributions. For example:

- Anxiety from a lack of belief in capacity can interfere with performance even when a person has the necessary underlying capacities
- Old habits can resist new volitional choices
- The pull of values can keep one going despite pain and fatigue.

In these and other circumstances, values, interests, personal causation, roles, habits, performance capacity, and the environment may produce a complex dynamic in which some factors support and others constrain a particular behavior, emotion, or thought. It is always the summation of their total contributions to the dynamic whole that results in the outcome.

Another systems concept indicates that a critical change in one of the factors can shift the total dynamic and result in a different emergent behavior. This change in one of the factors that creates a new dynamic and shifts thought, emotion, and/or action is known as a **control parameter** (Thelen & Ulrich, 1991; Turvey, 1990). A control parameter sufficiently changes the total dynamic to result in the emergence of something different. For instance, if Rigo had a flare-up of his arthritic condition, if a storm damaged or destroyed his house, if his friend called to say a family emergency

meant he could not go on the fishing trip, or if Rigo lost his job, his actions, thoughts, and feelings during the morning routine would be quite different. Thus, a second principle can be stated:

> *Change in any aspect of volition, habituation, performance capacity, and/or the environment can result in a change in the thoughts, feelings, and doing that make up one's occupation.*

---

*U*nderstanding Occupation

The concepts of heterarchy and emergence can be used to generate a comprehensive understanding of all aspects of occupation. For example, to understand what kind of occupational task a person will choose, it is necessary to consider that it is a function of the interaction of the following factors:

- The kind of things a person feels effective in doing
- What the person likes to do
- What the person finds valuable or meaningful to do
- The opportunities or expectations in the environment for doing things.

For example, whether a person with chronic mental illness will be motivated and choose to enter the worker role will be influenced by factors such as these:

- The extent to which the person feels capable of doing work based on past experiences
- Whether and what kinds of work tasks the person has enjoyed doing in the past
- How important work, and other factors either positively or negatively associated with work, are to this person
- The kinds of jobs available to the person and whether they match the felt capacity, interests, and values of the person
- The other factors in the environment that are affected by working (e.g., the availability of disability income or medical insurance)
- The extent to which others in the environment expect and want the person to work.

> *Values, interests, personal causation, roles, habits, performance capacity, and the environment may produce a complex dynamic in which some factors support and others constrain a particular behavior, emotion, or thought. It is always the summation of their total contributions to the dynamic whole that results in the outcome.*

In the same way, the quality of a person's performance in doing the task will be influenced by these interactions:

- The person's underlying capacity for the performance
- The complexity and demands of the task itself
- The kinds of objects present in the environment for engaging in the task.

For example, whether and how a child with severe motor problems can use a computer depends on:

- How the child's impairments affect fine motor movements
- Whether adapted keyboards or other adapted interfaces are available and appropriate
- Whether the child has developed the habit of using these adaptive objects.

Every instance of human occupation reflects a unique configuration of such elements that together determine what a person chooses to do, how that person performs, and the outcome of the performance.

Human Organization and Change

Human beings are highly organized systems that are maintained by underlying physiological, mental, affective, and behavioral processes (Brent, 1978; Sameroff, 1983). Thus, a third important principle is:

> *Volition, habituation, and performance capacity are maintained and changed through what one does and what one thinks and feels about doing.*

How people change and develop over time depends on their ongoing occupation. As noted in Chapter 2, humans are endowed with a need to act. Consequently, from the time we enter this world, we set about doing things. Within the first weeks of life, we have begun a course of occupation that has already established some performance capacity, given us a rudimentary sense of ourselves and of the world around us, and created a basic daily routine. From then on, we per-

sist in a process of doing that continually shapes and re-shapes ourselves (Capra, 1997; Wolf 1987).

People thus shape themselves through their occupations. Consider, for instance, what happened to Jane's volition, habituation, and performance capacity when she took up jogging.[2]

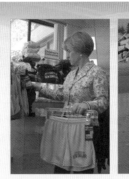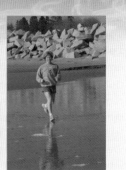

Jane shopping for running clothes as part of her role as a runner, and running along the beachfront.

Repeated jogging reshaped her existing physical, psychological, and social structures. Her aerobic capacity increased, the muscles she used to run gained strength, and the image of herself as capable of jogging was enhanced. Also, her public identity as a jogger was affirmed when she swapped stories and tips about jogging with others, shopped for jogging clothes, joined a friend for a regular run after work, and participated in organized races.

When Jane took up and repeated jogging and related behaviors, her actions and the associated thoughts and feelings rearranged her personal causation, role, and performance capacity into that of a jogger. She became what she did. Moreover, as long as she sustained these occupations, the corresponding organization was maintained. However, if Jane were to abandon the behavior for long enough, her aerobic capacity would diminish, her muscles would weaken, and her confidence for running and her jogger role identity would wane. As this illustrates, one can also unbecome when one ceases to do.

---

[2]Jane Clifford O'Brien and William Croninger, associate professors in the occupational therapy department at the University of New England, provided the case and photos of Jane for this chapter.

To consider how this process continues to unfold throughout life, we address two questions: How do we maintain our organized patterns? How do we change? The remainder of this chapter discusses some basic answers to these questions.

Maintaining Occupational Patterns

Across time, people do exhibit certain constancy in who they are and what they do. Maintaining these organized patterns of emotion, thought, choice, and behavior always involves the following elements:

- Our existing volition, habituation, and performance capacity (which we previously generated through our doing) provide certain resources, limitations, and tendencies for emoting, thinking, and behaving
- We encounter consistent environmental conditions, seek them out, or create them
- Given the interaction of internal resources, limitations, and tendencies with consistent environmental conditions, we repeat what we have done before, sustaining an organized pattern of behaving and of the thoughts and feelings that accompany behavior.

Thus the fourth principle about how occupation maintains patterns can be stated:

> *A particular pattern of volition, habituation, and performance capacity will be maintained so long as the underlying thoughts, feelings, and actions are consistently repeated in a supporting environment.*

Importantly, this organized pattern represents a way of operating with its own internal coherence that resists change. Once we have a way of feeling, thinking, and behaving, we tend to behave so as to preserve it. For example, a study of women with chronic pain revealed four distinct patterns of doing, thinking, and feeling (Keponen & Kielhofner, 2006). For instance, one group of women saw themselves as moving on. They emphasized recognizing the limitations imposed by their chronic pain, making decisions about what occupations were important to them, asking others to understand and assist them to live their lives as positively as possible, and having plans for the future. Another group saw themselves as fighting. They tried to hide their pain from others and gave priority to do-

ing the things they felt obligated to do, often sacrificing their own interests and life satisfaction. These women found it impossible to imagine the future. Women in both groups saw their way of living with chronic pain as the only option. They persisted in behavior that reinforced their thoughts and feelings. As the example illustrates, each individual "actively constructs his or her view of self" (Gergen & Gergen, 1983, p. 255). Once a person's volition, habituation, or performance capacity has been organized in a particular way, it tends to stay that way. Nonetheless, change does occur. The next section considers how.

Change

Earlier in this chapter, it was noted that alteration of any single internal or external component in a heterarchy can contribute something new to the total dynamic out of which new thoughts, feelings, and actions may emerge. Therefore, a shift in volition, habituation, performance capacity, or the environment can alter the overall dynamics, leading to the emergence of something new.

Thus, a key element in change is some alteration in internal or external circumstances that results in the emergence of novel thoughts, feelings, and behaviors.

The next requirement for change is that the novel thoughts, feelings, and behaviors must continue over time. Only by repetition do we begin to reshape ourselves. Repetition of new behaviors, thoughts, and feelings requires supportive environmental conditions. However, if the new pattern is repeated enough, volition, habituation, and performance capacity will coalesce toward a new organization. Therefore, we can specify a fifth principle:

> *Change requires that novel thoughts, feelings, and actions be sufficiently repeated in a consistent environment to coalesce into a new organized pattern.*

> *A shift in volition, habituation, performance capacity, or the environment can alter the overall dynamics, leading to the emergence of something new.*

Ordinarily, there is a natural history of new behaviors, thoughts, and emotions over time, in which volition, habituation, and performance capacity together are altered incrementally together over time. Throughout this natural history of change, these elements resonate with each other, each taking turns in contributing something new to the mix of components that spur on the ongoing changes process.

Implications for Therapy

The systems concepts discussed in this chapter have important implications for the process of occupational therapy. First, they indicate that assessment (the goal of which is to understand a person's needs, problems, and concerns (AOTA, 2002) requires consideration of how volition, habituation, performance capacity, and environmental factors contribute to the client's circumstance. Without assessing all of these factors one cannot fully understand a client's situation. The purpose of evaluation is to understand and consider how all the factors that make up the total dynamic are affecting the client's doing, thinking, and feeling. This means that the assessment process should be holistic and dynamic. To be holistic, it should to the extent possible consider the status of performance capacity, habits, roles, personal causation, values, interests, and environmental circumstance. To be dynamic, it should consider how these factors are interacting to create the total situation of the client. No single factor is necessarily the most important to consider first in assessment. Rather, it important to have adequate information to determine how each is influencing the client's occupational life.[3]

Most often several factors are involved simultaneously. For example, if Rigo, discussed earlier, sustained a spinal cord injury in a car accident, a new set of dynamics would emerge, as shown in *Figure 3-2*. While the most obvious change in Rigo would be a major loss of sensory and motor capacity following the spinal cord injury, a cascade of other factors would also be involved.

Rigo's values and interests may no longer be consistent with what he is capable of doing. He may lose his physically demanding job. His old friend might feel uncomfortable and avoid Rigo. The once familiar environments of his home, truck, and work sites would all be physically inaccessible to him. The habitual ways he had learned to do things would no long work in the face of his motor and sensory impairments. Without consideration of all these factors, one cannot fully understand the nature of a person's occupational problems.

Second, since many factors contribute to the emergence of occupational behaviors, thoughts, and feelings, it is important to consider multiple possibilities for addressing a client's problems and challenges. For example, when a person has some limitation of capacity (e.g., mobility, strength, attention, or memory), therapy can use strategies that increase or restore capacity. However, there are other possibilities. They include, for instance:

- Compensating for loss of one's capacity by modifying the ways necessary activities are done
- Altering the environment to provide supports for doing
- Making new choices for action so that the things that can no longer be done are replaced by an alternative activity.

Successful occupational therapy often involves a combination of strategies. Treatment planning requires an ongoing process of deciding, in collaboration with the client, what combination can best create a positive dynamic out of which positive actions, thoughts, and feelings can emerge.

Third, therapy should, to the extent possible, consider and address all of the factors contributing to the client's occupational dynamic. This means that such factors as diminished performance capacity, problematic habits, lost roles, a sense of inefficacy, problems operationalizing values and interests, and environmental barriers are all factors that may be addressed in therapy. Addressing some factors and not others can result in less than optimal outcomes of therapy. Nonetheless, it is important that the process of deciding what factors to address be client-centered, meaning that those factors most important to the client should be addressed first or given the most emphasis. Therapists should, when appropriate, assist clients to understand how all relevant factors may affect their occupational lives.

---

[3]Contemporary occupational therapy calls for a top-down approach to assessment (Coster, 1998) that begins with consideration of the person's occupation and then proceeds to consideration of underlying performance capacity. What is being suggested here is not a top-down but a dynamic approach to assessment ensuring that all factors (volition, habituation, performance capacity, and environment) are examined and considered simultaneously.

FIGURE 3.2 Altered heterarchical contributions of volition, habituation, performance capacity, and environment following a traumatic onset of a disability.

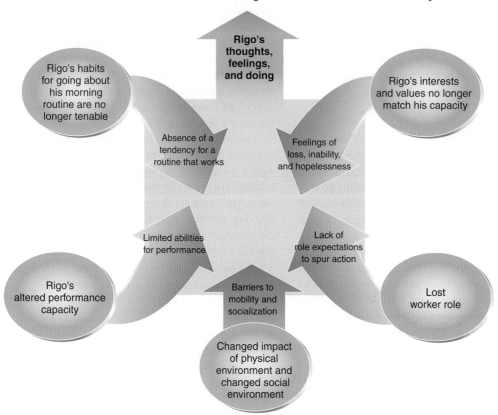

Fourth, because the aim of therapy is always to achieve a new and positive pattern of occupational life, it requires sustained occupational engagement in a supportive environment. Therapy must support the client to engage in new forms of doing, thinking, and feeling that can reorganize volition, habituation, performance capacity, and the environment into a new and positive dynamic. This process is ordinarily begun during therapy and continues on even beyond the period of intervention.

Conclusion

This chapter used systems concepts to explain how volition, habituation, and performance capacity are integrated together and how they relate to the environ-ment. Five key postulates (*Table 3.1*) were proposed to explain the dynamics of occupation. Finally, the chapter offered a discussion of the implications of systems concepts for therapy. The concepts and postulates discussed in this chapter will be reflected and integrated throughout this text.

Key Terms

Emergence: the principle that complex actions, thoughts and feelings spontaneously arise out of the interactions of several components.

Heterarchy: the principle that aspects of a person and that person's environment are linked into a dynamic whole.

Table 3.1   Key Postulates Derived from Systems Concepts

1. Occupational actions, thoughts, and emotions arise out of the interaction of volition, habituation, performance capacity, and environmental context.
2. Change in any aspect of volition, habituation, performance capacity, and/or the environment can result in a change in thought, feeling, and doing.
3. Volition, habituation, and performance capacity are maintained and changed through what one does and what one thinks and feels about doing.
4. A particular pattern of volition, habituation, and performance capacity will be maintained so long as the underlying thoughts, feelings, and actions are consistently repeated in a supporting environment.
5. Change requires that novel thoughts, feelings, and actions emerge and be sufficiently repeated in a supportive environment to coalesce into a new organized pattern.

Control parameter: change in a factor that creates a new dynamic and shifts thought, emotion, and/or action.

References

American Occupational Therapy Association (AOTA) (2002). Occupational therapy practice framework: Domain and process. *American Journal of Occupational Therapy, 56,* 609–639.

Brent, S. B. (1978). Motivation, steady-state, and structural development. *Motivation and Emotion, 2,* 299–332.

Capra, F. (1997). *The web of life.* London: HarperCollins.

Clarke, A. (1997). *Being there: Putting brain, body and world together again.* Cambridge, MA: MIT.

Coster, W. (1998). Occupation-centered assessment of children. *American Journal of Occupational Therapy, 52,* 337–434.

Gergen, K. J., & Gergen, M. M. (1983). Narratives of the self. In T. R. Sarbin & K. E. Scheibe (Eds.), *Studies in social identity.* New York: Praeger.

Haken, H. (1987). Synergetics: An approach to self-organization. In F. E. Yates (Ed.), *Self-organizing systems: The emergence of order.* New York: Plenum.

Kelso, J. A. S., & Tuller, B. (1984). A dynamical basis for action systems. In M. S. Gazzaniga (Ed.), *Handbook of cognitive neuroscience.* New York: Plenum.

Keponen, R. & Kielhofner, G. (2006). Occupation and meaning in the lives of women with chronic pain. *Scandinavian Journal of Occupational Therapy, 13*(4), 211–220.

Koestler, A. (1969). Beyond atomism and holism: The concept of the holon. In A. Koestler & J. R. Smythies (Eds.), *Beyond reductionism.* Boston: Beacon.

Sameroff, A. J. (1983). Developmental systems: Contexts and evolution. In P. H. Mussen (Ed.), *Handbook of child psychology.* New York: Wiley.

Thelen, E., & Ulrich, B. D. (1991). Hidden skills: A dynamic systems analysis of treadmill stepping during the first year. *Monographs of the Society for Research in Child Development, 56* (1, Serial No. 223).

Turvey, M. T. (1990). Coordination. *American Psychologist, 45,* 938–953.

von Bertalanffy, L. (1968a). General system theory: A critical review. In W. Buckley (Ed.), *Modern systems research for the behavioral scientist.* Chicago: Aldine.

von Bertalanffy, L. (1968b). *General systems theory.* New York: George Braziller.

Wolf, P. H. (1987). *The development of behavioral states and expression of emotion in early infancy.* Chicago: University of Chicago.

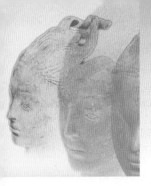

Volition

- Gary Kielhofner

Jiyeon

Jiyeon,[1] aged 8, has a diagnosis of cerebral palsy. Like many children her age in Korea, she is very interested in playing a game, gong-gi nolyi, that involves 5 small marbles. Jiyeon also very much wants to use chopsticks, since Koreans customarily use a spoon for eating rice and chopsticks for the side dishes. Because of her strong desire to play marbles and use chopsticks like other children in her culture, she is frustrated with her inabilities in these areas.

Jiyeon's occupational therapist is helping her achieve these goals. Jiyeon's fine motor skills do not allow her to play the marble game according to its usual rules (i.e., tossing one marble in the air and then grabbing a marble off the floor before catching the tossed marble). Therefore, the occupational therapist has arranged a modified version of the game that allows Jiyeon to engage in an activity of interest while developing better fine motor skills. She has responded well to this adaptation of the game. The occupational therapist also devised an activity to allow Jiyeon to work toward being able to use chopsticks. They began using wooden thongs that resemble chopsticks to pick up and move objects and later to eat side dishes. By harnessing things that Jiyeon valued and found enjoyable, the therapist was able not only to help Jiyeon increase skills but also to develop greater belief in her ability to do things.

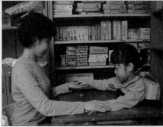

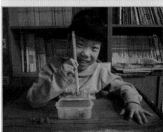

Jiyeon playing an adapted version of the Korean marble game, gong-gi nolyi with her occupational therapist and and using tong to develop fine motor skills for handling chopsticks.

Elizabeth

Elizabeth[2] is 14 and has just begun attending high school in a Midwestern American city. She feels a great deal of pressure from her peers to wear the latest fashions in clothes. Because of her insecurity about her own competence and being accepted by peers, she feels strongly compelled to fall in line with her peers' values about clothes. Because her family has fewer resources than many of her peers' families in the school she attends, Elizabeth often feels she cannot keep up materi-

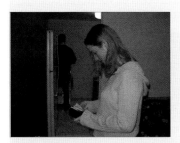

Elizabeth takes some of her brother's funds without permission in order to buy new clothes.

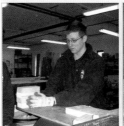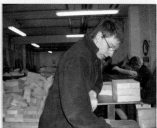

Richard at work.

ally with her classmates. In the past her brother lent her money to buy trendy clothes, but lately he has refused. Elizabeth was hoping to buy a new pair of jeans to wear to school. Feeling that she had no other way to get the resources, Elizabeth decided to just take the money and try to replace it somehow in the future. After taking her brother's money without permission, Elizabeth feels even more out of control and remorseful that she did something she knew was not honest.

Richard

Richard,[3] 17 years old, lives in a small English village. He very much wants to be successful like his older brother, who is an officer in the military. He recently left school after not doing very well and wants to work. He has secured a position at a job center that employs persons with disabilities, but he is struggling. Richard has a right-sided weakness and trouble with attention due to a neurological condition. Thus, he tires quickly and sometimes is unable to follow sequences. Because Richard wants to be seen as competent, he often pushes himself when fatigued instead of resting, which causes him to make mistakes. For the same reason, Richard will not ask for assistance when he is unsure how to complete work tasks and consequently sometimes does them incorrectly. These behaviors, although intended to make himself appear more competent, paradoxically result in Richard receiving negative feedback. This only increases Richard's sense of inefficacy on the job.

Driekie

Driekie[4] is a 72-year-old resident of a specialized care unit in South Africa. She is the seventh member of her family to be diagnosed with Alzheimer's disease. Driekie is a trained nurse who spent a substantial amount of her working years in a local hospital when she lived in Zambia with her family. Her caring nature is still evident, as she is preoccupied with any of the residents on the ward who are bedridden. Under supervision of staff she spends a lot of time fidgeting with these residents' bedclothes, as she tugs

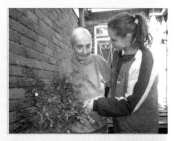

Drieike interacting with occupational therapy students and exploring the multisensory garden.

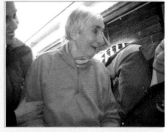

and pulls at them, apparently in an effort to "straighten her patients' beds." Despite lacking verbal communication, she welcomes all newcomers on the ward by approaching them and speaking incoherently. She also likes to take fellow residents by the hand and lead them up and down the ward hall. Finally, one of Driekie's favorite occupations is to explore the ward's multisensory garden.

[1]Eunyoung Kim, Occupational Therapist at Children's Center for Developmental Support, Ewha Womans University in Seoul, Republic of Korea, provided the case of Jiyeon for this chapter.

[2]Susan Cahill, clinical instructor at the University of Illinois at Chicago, provided the case of Elizabeth for this chapter.

[3]Dalleen Last, clinical specialist in occupational therapy at Oxfordshire Learning Disability National Health Service Trust in Oxford, England, provided the case of Richard for this chapter.

[4]Sanet du Toit of the University of the Free State in Bloemfontein, South Africa, provided the case of Driekie for this chapter.

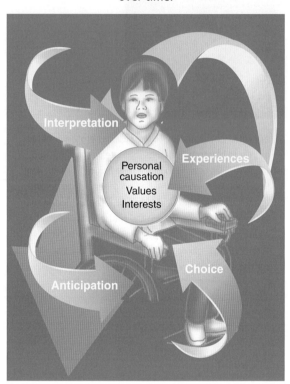

FIGURE 4.1 The process of volitional change over time.

Each of these scenarios illustrates volition. They demonstrate how volition involves thoughts and feelings about what one holds important (values), perceives as personal capacity and effectiveness (personal causation), and finds enjoyable (interests). They also illustrate aspects of the volitional cycle (*Fig. 4.1*) of anticipating, choosing, experiencing, and interpreting what one does. As this cycle is repeated, it maintains or reshapes one's values, personal causation, and interests. With each new experience and reflection, people come to think and feel about themselves and their lives in similar or in slightly different ways. Then they anticipate possibilities for and make decisions to do things accordingly, and the cycle repeats itself. For example, Jiyeon's values and interests lead her to choose to be involved in the tasks described. The experience of feeling successful in doing these things may lead her to reflect about how she can have more control over her life and shape her orientation to the world and the choices she makes.

Culture and Volition

Although values and personal causation are universal human concerns, how persons think and feel about

personal effectiveness and assign significance to what they do will greatly depend on culture. Culture shapes what kinds of abilities are important, what kinds of meanings are tied to actions, what pastimes are enjoyed, and what one should strive after in life (Bruner, 1990; Gergen & Gergen, 1983, 1988; Markus, 1983). How culture shapes volitional thoughts and feelings can be appreciated by considering Elizabeth's dilemma. Her culture emphasizes certain ways of dressing, and she feels deeply obligated to conform. At the same time she has incorporated values from her family about honesty and justice. These two sets of values clash when she finds herself trying to fit in with the values of her peers. Moreover, her cycle of anticipating, choosing, experiencing, and interpreting what she does threatens to spiral Elizabeth toward a greater and greater sense of failure and being out of control.

Personal Circumstances and History

Each person has unique volitional thoughts and feelings. Volition begins with biological propensities, such as one's level of arousal, preferred sensory modes, and temperaments, and sometimes impairments. These personal inclinations influence what capacities one develops, what one enjoys, and what one considers important. Additionally, as life unfolds, each person accumulates a personal history of doing, experience, and reflection that shape volition. These experiences

- Afford one the opportunity to learn what one can and cannot do well
- Provide occasions to discover what one enjoys doing
- Shape what one considers important to do.

At any point in time a person's volition will reflect a unique personal history and circumstances that have shaped and continue to shape it. For example, Richard's experiences of following a highly successful older brother, his living with a neurological impairment, and his reflecting difficulties in school and recently at work all combine in his unique volition. His volition includes, among other things, the following:

- A strong value of performing well like his brother
- Feelings of incapacity and failure.

These aspects of his volition lead Richard to choose to ignore his own difficulties in an effort to make himself appear competent. These choices, however, only generate further difficulties that keep him locked in a cycle of poor choices and negative experiences. When Richard's occupational therapist recognized this dynamic, she was able to help Richard learn to ask for help and support when he needed it in order to have more positive experiences at work. In time this led Richard to accumulate positive feedback that built up his sense of efficacy at work.

> *At any point in time a person's volition will reflect a unique personal history and circumstances that have shaped and continue to shape it.*

Confluence of Personal Causation, Values, and Interests

Thoughts and feelings about competence, enjoyment, and value are always interwoven. People want to be competent at doing the things they value. They tend to find enjoyable the things they do well and to dislike those that overtax them. They feel bad when they cannot do the things they care about deeply. Consequently, a person's volition can be understood fully only after examination of the dynamic relationship among personal causation, values, and interests. While the following sections discuss each separately, one should be mindful that personal causation, values, and interests are each aspects of a larger volitional whole.

Personal Causation

One of the first discoveries of life is that one can be a cause (i.e., do things that produce results) (Bruner, 1973; Burke, 1977; DeCharms, 1968). Throughout early development, individuals become increasingly aware that they can make things happen. For example, infants come to realize that their movements can make objects move and create noises. This awareness that one can cause things to happen is the beginning of personal causation (DeCharms, 1968). Over time as one engages in a wider and wider range of action, one discovers:

- What one is capable of doing
- What kinds of effects one's doing can produce.

Two Dimensions of Personal Causation

As the previous statement indicated, personal causation involves two components: a sense of one's personal capacity and knowledge of one's self-efficacy in the world. The **sense of personal capacity** is an assessment of one's physical, intellectual, and social abilities (Harter, 1983, 1985; Harter & Connel, 1984). The second dimension, **self-efficacy**, refers to one's sense of effectiveness in using personal capacities to achieve desired outcomes in life (Lefcourt, 1981; Rotter, 1960). Self-efficacy is specific to different spheres of life (Connel, 1985; Fiske & Taylor, 1985; Lefcourt, 1981; Skinner, Chapman, & Baltes, 1988); that is, we feel more able to control outcomes in certain circumstances than in others.

Persons who feel capable and effective seek out opportunities, use feedback to correct performance, and persevere to achieve goals. In contrast, individuals who feel incapable and lack a sense of efficacy shy away from opportunity, avoid feedback, and have trouble persisting (Burke, 1977; DeCharms, 1968; Goodman, 1960). Consequently, personal causation influences how one is motivated toward doing things.

As shown in *Figure 4.2*, personal causation can be conceptualized as growing out of the original awareness of being a cause and developing over time—through a continuing cycle of anticipation, choice, experience, and interpretation—into the sense of personal capacity and self-efficacy. The following sections consider these two components of personal causation.

FIGURE 4.2 The development of personal causation over time as one encounters the world.

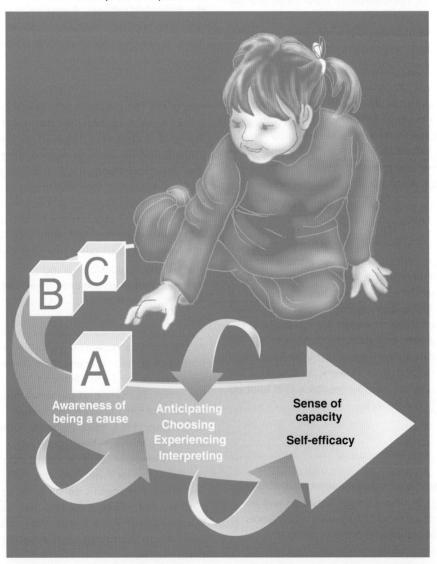

> *The sense of capacity is an active awareness of one's capabilities for carrying out the life one wants to live.*

Sense of Capacity

People observe themselves through the common sense lens of their culture, building up a store of knowledge about what kind of capacities they have for doing the things that matter.

The sense of capacity is an active awareness of one's capabilities for carrying out the life one wants to live. Moreover, as one proceeds through life, new experiences can alter one's sense of capacity.

Challenges to a Sense of Capacity

While all people must realize the limits of their capacities, having an impairment uniquely challenges the view of self as capable (Molnar, 1989; Wright, 1960). As shown at the beginning of the chapter, both Jiyeon and Richard are facing challenges to their sense of capacity related to their unique impairments. These challenges are felt particularly when the impairments limit their ability to do things that they want to do.

Pain, fatigue, and limitations of sensation, cognition, or movement can constrain people to achieve less than they desire (Werner-Beland, 1980). Sienkiewicz-Mercer & Kaplan (1989) write about their experience of cerebral palsy as being trapped in a body that "followed few directions of its mind and ignored the simple commands of speech and movement that nearly everyone takes for granted" (p. 64).

Similarly, Deegan (1991) writes about her experience of schizophrenia and its impact on everyday tasks: "I remember being asked to come into the kitchen to help knead some bread dough. I got up, went into the kitchen, and looked at the dough for what seemed an eternity. Then I walked back to my chair and wept. The task seemed overwhelming to me" (p. 49).

Another woman describes how chronic pain interferes with doing housework:

> Hanging the washing on the line. The arms ache. I might get about four things on the line, then it starts to ache. Washing up I can start. I can't do the saucepans, because of the scrubbing. Cooking—

oh, I can do a bit of cooking, but I can't lift heavy saucepans. I have dropped them. I have burnt myself. (Ewan, Lowy, & Reid, 1991, p. 178)

Murphy (1987), a professor, describes how his progressive paralysis made lecturing increasingly problematic as his voice "lost timbre and resonance, no longer projecting as well as it did" (p. 80). As these examples illustrate, incapacity is experienced as difficulty doing the things that matter in one's life.

The knowledge that one is less capable than others or than one once was can be a source of considerable emotional pain. For this reason some persons go out of their way to avoid situations that provide occasions for failure (Cromwell, 1963; Moss, 1958). For example, emotionally disturbed adolescents indicate feelings of incompetence and often prefer solitary tasks whose results are not judged by others (American Psychiatric Association, 2000; Smyntek, 1983). Adults with developmental disabilities are often plagued with doubts about their abilities and go to great lengths to disguise their limitations (Edgerton, 1967; Kielhofner, 1983). For example, Doris, a middle-aged woman who spent much of her childhood and young adulthood in a state hospital after being diagnosed as mentally retarded, was haunted by concerns about her capacity. She carried and often showed her (decade old) discharge papers as proof that she was competent (Kielhofner, 1980). When shame or fear of failure governs a person's sense of capacity, there is disincentive to take risks, to learn new skills, or to make the best use of what one has. A negative sense of capacity can be even more limiting than the impairments on which it is based.

People are disposed to undertake that for which they feel capable and to avoid that which threatens them with failure. The close link between the sense of capacity and the desire to act accordingly is underscored by Murphy's (1987) observation that "With all bodily stimuli to movement muted and almost forgotten, one gradually loses the volition for physical activity" (p. 193). The sense of capacity readies one to anticipate, choose, experience, and interpret behavior. Those who see themselves to be capable are disposed

> *incapacity is experienced as difficulty doing the things that matter in one's life.*

to act and generate further evidence of their capacity. Those who view themselves as incapable feel compelled in the opposite direction.

SELF-EFFICACY

Self-efficacy includes one's perception of the following:

- Self-control
- How much one is able to bring about what one wants.

Through experience, people generate images of how effective they are in using their capacities and of how compliant or resistant life is to their efforts. Persons' beliefs about whether they can use their capacities to influence the course of events or circumstances in the external world are also powerful motivators. People will only put their efforts where they believe they will be effective.

Self-Control

Self-efficacy begins with self-control. To use one's capacities effectively, one must be able to shape or contain emotions and thoughts and exercise control over one's decisions and actions. A strong sense of efficacy is impossible if one believes that one is at the mercy of overwhelming emotions or uncontrollable thoughts. Conversely, a strong sense of self-control can greatly enhance how persons adapt, as illustrated in the following passage from a young woman with quadriplegia:

> The ability to say my mind is in charge here. Not this environment. Not what's happening to me—it's not in charge. What determines what I will do and how I will handle things is right here [pointing to her head], and I do have control over it. That's the important thing, that events can't shake you, physical environments can't shake you as long as you are able to say, "my mind is in control here . . . " (Patsy & Kielhofner, 1989)

Impact of Efforts

Self-efficacy also concerns whether one's efforts are sufficient to accomplish desired ends. The ability to achieve wanted outcomes in life can be challenged in a number of ways by impairments. That disease and trauma arrive uninvited and with negative consequences readily engenders feelings of being controlled by outside factors (Burish & Bradley, 1983; Triesch-

mann, 1989). Children who grow up with impairments learn that they cannot do what others do and are prone to develop feelings of ineffectiveness (Molnar, 1989). Such children may become unnecessarily dependent on others because they do not see their own actions as the most effective route for achieving their desires (Wasserman, 1986). Feeling helpless is concomitant with many forms of mental illness (American Psychiatric Association, 2000; Meissner, 1982). Persons with mental illness often lack a sense of control over life outcomes (Lovejoy, 1982; Wylie, 1979; Youkilis & Bootzin, 1979). Depression in particular is associated with the belief that one lacks control (Becker & Lesiak, 1977; Lefcourt, 1976; Leggett & Archer, 1979).

The loss of abilities significantly affects self-efficacy. Hull (1990) gives a poignant description of how loss of sight took away personal control:

> I just sit here. The creatures emitting the noise have to engage in some activity. They have to scrape, bang, hit, club, strike surface upon surface, impact, make their vocal cords vibrate. They must take the initiative in announcing their presence to me. For my part, I have no power to explore them. I cannot penetrate them or discover them without their active cooperation. (p. 83)

Such constant reminders of one's inability to control the external world can result in feelings of powerlessness. Countering them requires extraordinary effort (Miller & Oertel, 1983; Murphy, 1987).

Dependence on medical personnel, family, or friends can exacerbate feelings of inefficacy. The patient role itself can contribute to a decreased sense of efficacy (Goffman, 1961). As persons are hospitalized and lose responsibility for their daily occupations, they may come to doubt whether they can manage their own lives. As Delaney-Naumoff (1980) notes, "The patient feels he has lost power, direction, and goals—behaviors that characterize the mature adult in his interactions with others. Rather than feeling that he is in the center of activity, he feels pushed to the periphery. He becomes an outsider dependent upon the ministrations of others" (p. 87).

Disabled persons frequently note that the challenge of maintaining appropriate feelings of efficacy is complex and difficult. For example, Sienkiewicz-Mercer, who has cerebral palsy, describes her own struggle with self-efficacy. After the disappointments of not being able to stand and feed herself, being able to talk was the one area in which she kept up hope, since it was "something that was infinitely more important to me than anything else" (Sienkiewicz-Mercer & Kaplan, 1989, p.12). Although she had to go on to deal with not being able to speak, she found her voice in her autobiography, *I Raise My Eyes To Say Yes*.

Self-efficacy can be complicated by important and consequential factors that might take away personal control in the future. For example, Thelma, who has bipolar disorder, discusses the uncertainty surrounding her disease and social welfare:

> And if I ever got a job [then] I got to pay full fee for my [subsidized] apartment . . . I don't want to be making the wrong move and then I'll be stuck with nothing, you know . . . You see, you may get [a job] and then you may get sick again, or have a relapse. You're out in the cold again trying to get back on disability. (Helfrich, Kielhofner, & Mattingly, 1994, p. 316)

As Thelma illustrates, it is difficult to have a sense of self-efficacy when illness or the vagaries of a welfare system may foil one's efforts to achieve a better life.

Disabled persons must often achieve a fine balance between necessary hope for the future and unrealistic expectations. The search for efficacy involves knowing disappointment, realizing what one cannot control, and finding and emphasizing what one is able to influence. Finding such a balanced view is not easy (Burish & Bradley, 1983).

APPRAISING THE SELF

How people judge their own capacity and efficacy is a matter of great importance and consequence. Thoughts and feelings about personal capacity and control incur strong emotions. So just how accurately can people assess themselves?

A number of factors influence self-appraisals. Cognitive limitations may impair comprehension of one's capacity. The psychological pain of acknowledging limitations and failures invites denial, avoidance, and projection (Valient, 1994). On the other hand, secondary gains related to being incapacitated (e.g., freedom from unsatisfying work conditions) may bias persons toward overestimating their limitations.

Persons who exaggerate their limitations may unnecessarily limit their actions. Those who overestimate their capacities may make choices that can lead to injury, exacerbation of symptoms, and failure in performance. The view of personal capacity and efficacy can also affect therapy. For example, Krefting (1989) discusses a young man with a head injury that produced cognitive and communication deficits. He insisted that his only problem was walking and as a consequence "saw no need to compensate for his deficits" (p. 74).

Achieving an accurate view of one's capabilities and efficacy is not always easy. Persons with newly acquired impairments have not yet discovered what their capacities will be. Similarly, persons with progressive conditions or those who have exacerbations and remissions cannot anticipate what abilities they will have in the future. In the face of a disability, personal causation is a highly individualized process of discovering how impairment may curtail or complicate the things one must and wants to do. This discovery may be ongoing as one's impairment and life changes.

Values

Over the course of development, people acquire beliefs and commitments about what is good, right, and important to do (Grossack & Gardner, 1970; Kalish & Collier, 1981; Klavins, 1972; Lee, 1971; Smith, 1969). These values are derived from culture, which specifies what things matter, communicating how one ought to act and what goals or aspirations are desirable (Bellah, Madsen, Sullivan, Swidler, & Tipton, 1985).

These cultural messages commit people to a way of life and impart common sense meaning to the lives they lead. Thus, values are convictions that carry with them a strong disposition to act accordingly. As shown in *Figure 4.3*, the process of anticipating, choosing, experiencing, and interpreting in our cultural context generates personal convictions and the sense of obligation that goes with them.

Importantly, values influence the sense of self-worth that one derives from doing certain things. Since values involve commitments to performing in culturally

> *These cultural messages commit people to a way of life and impart common sense meaning to the lives they lead.*

FIGURE 4.3 The emergence of values from interactions with the cultural milieu.

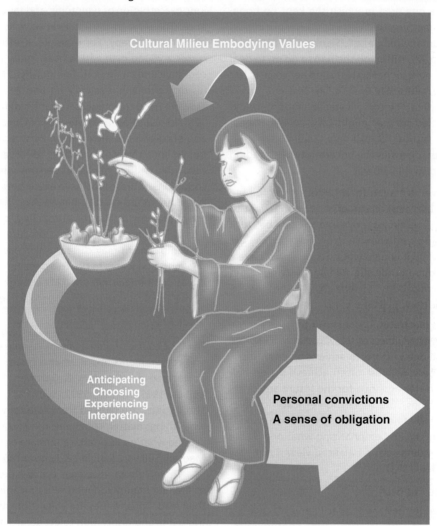

meaningful and sanctioned ways, one experiences a sense of belonging and appropriateness when following values (Lee, 1971). Moreover, one does not act contrary to one's values without a feeling of shame, guilt, failure, or inadequacy, as illustrated by the example of Elizabeth at the beginning of this chapter.

Personal Convictions

All values are part of a coherent world view about which people feel deeply (Bruner 1990; Gergen & Gergen, 1988; Mitchell, 1983). These **personal convictions** are strongly held views of life that define what matters. For example, personal convictions may be organized around a fundamental religious viewpoint of right and wrong that defines what is a good life. A very different set of convictions underlie a street-smart adolescent who learns a code of gang solidarity, territoriality, and survival by aggression. While these two sets of convictions are vastly different, each represents a deeply held way of viewing the world.

Sense of Obligation

Values bind people to action (Bruner, 1990; Fein, 1990). Because values evoke powerful feelings of importance, security, worthiness, belonging, and purpose, they create a sense of obligation to perform in ways consistent with those values. This sense of obligation may include such things as how time should be spent, what one should do, how one should do something, what constitutes adequate effort or outcomes, and what goals one should pursue (Cottle, 1971; Hall, 1959; Kluckholn, 1951). In sum, the **sense of obligation** is a strong emotional disposition to follow perceived right ways to act.

Values and Impairment

The interface of impairment and value is complex and multifaceted. Values shape how persons experience impairments. Values that conflict with what one is able to do can lead one to self-devaluation. Finally, an impairment may challenge one's values.

Persons with disabilities often find that their very condition is in conflict with mainstream cultural values. As Murphy (1987) notes, "The disabled, individually and as a group, contravene all the values of youth, virility, activity, and physical beauty" (pp. 116–117).

Similarly, DeLoach, Wilkins, and Walker (1983) note that the American work ethic has "tended to discredit anyone who does not or cannot work" (p. 14). Indeed, persons with acquired disabilities often find themselves devalued by the very standards they have held all their lives.

A discontinuity between one's capacity and what one values can lower self-esteem (Zane & Lowenthal, 1960). A woman with functional limitations imposed by repetitive strain injury notes: "I got to the stage where you felt that you weren't worth anything, you were good for nothing. You couldn't do anything. What's the good of me? I can't do anything" (Ewan, Lowy, & Reid, 1991, p. 184). Loss of capacity can mean either rejecting old values or devaluing self as unable to live up to old values (Rabinowitz & Mitsos, 1964; Vash, 1981).

Values can commit one to impossible ideals (Fein, 1990). Persons with disabilities sometimes struggle futilely to achieve values inconsistent with their capacities. For example, Mike, throughout his adolescence and young adulthood, accepted his parents' vision that he would follow in the footsteps of his father, a suc-

cessful surgeon. In college, he found the coursework overwhelming, failed his classes, became withdrawn and inactive, and finally required hospitalization for depression. Following this, he worked in a blue-collar position, which he enjoyed. Plagued with the idea that he was not living up to his parents' ideal, he returned to college only to repeat the pattern of failure, depression, and hospitalization. Twice more he repeated the same cycle, needing hospitalization each time. Only after these repeated failures was he able to admit that the values he had pursued were not consistent with his abilities or his interests.

Like Mike, individuals may strive after certain values in the belief that their lives will not be fulfilled or that they will not have worth unless they somehow realize those values. In such instances, values can drive individuals toward choices that make life disappointing or difficult to bear.

Disability can radically challenge the whole view of life in which one's values are embedded. Consider, for example, persons who have made sense of their hard work as a means to a valued promotion and career development. In the face of a progressively disabling disease, their ideal of the progressive work career would no longer be viable.

As the previous example illustrates, the future as one imagined it may be partially or totally invalidated by disability. Without an image of what life will be like, it is more difficult to manage the taxing problems imposed by disability (Litman, 1972; Rogers & Figone, 1978, 1979). Without a sense of some valued future goal or state toward which one is striving, persons may question the worth of life and/or find themselves alienated and without a sense of purpose (Frankl, 1978; Korner, 1970; Menninger, 1962; Mitchell, 1975; Schiamberg, 1973).

Disability Values

While preexisting values can have an important influence on what a disability means to an individual, the existence of a disability can also be the critical occasion for development of new values. This is not easy, since most cultures devalue disability and persons with disabilities (Longmore, 1995b; Oliver, 1996; Scotch, 1988; Shapiro, 1994). Indeed, one of the consistent messages that persons with disabilities receive is that the part of the self that is disabled is essentially "bad" and must be

> *Because dominant societal values tend to denigrate persons with disabilities, a growing community of disabled persons emphasizes a different valuation of disability.*

balanced or overcome with the parts that are still "good," or not disabled (Gill, 1997).

Because dominant societal values tend to denigrate persons with disabilities, a growing community of disabled persons emphasizes a different valuation of disability. They identify their disability as a positive value rather than an aberration from what is good or right. A disability culture is beginning to emerge that extols ideals such as disability pride and encourages exhibiting rather than hiding one's disability (Gill, 1994, 1997).

Having a disability may serve as the impetus for a person to develop a new consciousness. For example, Snyder (2002) illustrate how many artists' visions were shaped by their experience of disability and how their art carried explicit messages aimed at questioning or contradicting societal values.

Exposure to others who share common experiences and positive disability values is important for disabled persons (Gill, 1994, 1997). Such exposure can be hampered by the fact that people with disabilities are a diverse group, and a single disability culture does not yet exist (Hahn, 1985). Until a disability culture and the values it extols become more widespread, disabled persons will continue to carry the burden of mainstream cultural values that demean them.

VALUES, DISABILITY, AND CHOICE

By rendering many of the things one used to do as impossible, impairment may force persons to examine what is most important to them. For example, Roberts (1989) recalls of his own experience:

> One of my therapists insisted that I learn to feed myself. Meals took hours, and I was always exhausted. After, I realized then that I could either use my time to feed myself or have an attendant feed me, allowing me to spend the time saved to go to school. I went to school. (p. 234)

Another example is Melanie, who had arthritis. She routinely entertained her husband's business associates in their home, highly valuing her ability as a gourmet cook and expert hostess. However, after the onset of arthritis she found that her routine of shopping for products, preparing a complex meal, dressing appropriately, and then decorating the home for guests was no longer feasible. Her pain was so great by the time guests arrived that she could not enjoy the evening. Although she valued all components of the routine, she had to choose which aspects would be dropped or modified. She chose to have meals catered so that she would have the energy and relative freedom from pain to be a good hostess.

Disability can become a source of rethinking personal values and one's fundamental view of life. Wright (1960) argues that to adjust to disability persons may need to enlarge the scope of their values to incorporate behaviors for which they are still capable. In addition, persons may need to learn new values that judge their performance given their capacities and reject old values that compare one's performance to that of others without disabilities. Since impairments typically invalidate some aspect of one's values, adjusting to disability almost invariably means a quest for new ways of viewing and valuing life.

One important example is the way the disability community has critiqued the Western value of independence. They note that independence is typically thought of only in terms of functional capacity of persons to take care of themselves, with insufficient attention to enabling self-determination though the exercise of free choice (Brisenden, 1986; Longmore, 1995a; Oliver, 1993; Scheer & Luborsky, 1991). Moreover, as pointed out by Longmore (1995b), interdependence is a much more acceptable value for many disabled persons. Thus, personal choice and interdependence are proposed as values preferable to independence.

Interests

Interests are what one finds enjoyable or satisfying to do. Thus, interests reveal themselves both as the enjoyment of doing something and as a preference for doing certain things over others (Matsutsuyu, 1969). As shown in *Figure 4.4*, interests reflect highly individual tastes generated from the cycle of anticipating, choosing, experiencing, and interpreting one's actions. Dreikie provides a moving example of

FIGURE 4.4 Interests.

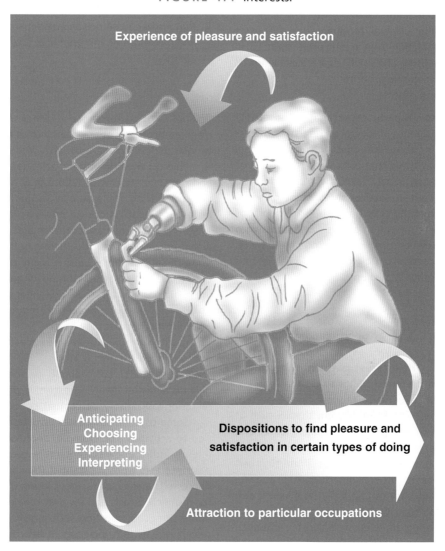

how interests can continue to energize volition even in the midst of severe cognitive decline. She reenacts as best she can the activities that gave her enjoyment and satisfaction as a nurse (straightening out patients' beds, greeting new patients, and leading them about the ward).

Enjoyment

The enjoyment of doing things ranges from the simple satisfaction derived from small daily rituals to the in- tense pleasure people feel in pursuing their driving passions. The feeling of enjoyment may come from a wide range of factors. These include:

> *The enjoyment of doing things ranges from the simple satisfaction derived from small daily rituals to the intense pleasure people feel in pursuing their driving passions.*

- Bodily pleasure associated with physical exertion
- Handling certain materials or objects
- Fulfillment of intellectual intrigue
- Aesthetic satisfaction from artistic production
- Fulfillment of using one's skill to face a challenge
- Creation of a pleasing product
- Fellowship with others.

Attraction to any particular occupation most likely represents a confluence of several such factors. The occupations that evoke the strongest feelings of attraction are generally those that evoke several sources of enjoyment. Csikszentmihalyi (1990) describes a form of ultimate enjoyment in physical, intellectual, or social occupations, which he calls flow. The experience of flow is a complete saturation of one's awareness with the positive experience of performing the activity. According to his research, flow occurs when a person's capacities are optimally challenged.

Pattern

Since we do not engage in all occupations with equal pleasure or satisfaction, we each develop a unique pattern of interests. The **interest pattern** is the unique configuration of preferred things to do that one has accumulated from experience. In some cases, a pattern of interests will reflect an underlying theme, such as athletic interest or cultural interests like theater and art. On the other hand, persons may have very diverse and seemingly unrelated preferences. Preferring certain occupations to others allows one to choose. Feeling a preference for certain activities makes it easier to select what to do. Consequently, one's pattern of interests is usually paralleled by a routine in which one's interests are at least partially indulged.

Impairment and Interests

Although it is commonly overlooked, one of the most pervasive effects of impairment on occupation is its influence on the experience of satisfaction and pleasure in life. The daily pleasures, comforts, and enjoyments that enliven existence and help maintain energy and mood can be threatened or altered by disability.

Children with disabilities may have been given fewer opportunities to develop normal investment and satisfaction in occupational performance. Further, dif-

> *The daily pleasures, comforts, and enjoyments that enliven existence and help maintain energy and mood can be threatened or altered by disability.*

ficulties with performance and fear of being recognized as incompetent may lead a child to avoid opportunities to develop a sense of attraction to occupations.

Physical impairments and attendant fatigue, pain, and preoccupation with failure may reduce or eliminate the feeling of pleasure in occupations. Physical or procedural adaptations necessary to allow performance may negatively affect the ambiance and spirit of activities, making it difficult to experience the same sense of satisfaction as before. Many persons with acquired disabilities say that it is no longer worth engaging in old pastimes. They are no longer enjoyable or do not warrant the additional effort required.

Further, persons may be prevented by limitations of capacity from participating in activities they previously enjoyed (Rogers & Figone, 1978; Trieschmann, 1989; Vash, 1981). For example, persons may have to give up activities involving excessive physical stress or requiring lost sensory, perceptual, or cognitive abilities.

Some psychiatric illnesses involve a loss of attraction to activities. For example, depressed persons frequently indicate few current interests even when their past interests were substantial (Neville, 1987). Many depressed persons speak about losing their enthusiasm for former interests and say that they no longer enjoy doing things. Supporting such individual reports, research reveals that increases in depressed mood and decreases in enjoyment in activities go hand in hand (Neville, 1987; Turner, Ward, & Turner, 1979). Research also suggests that persons with psychiatric problems engage in few interests (Grob & Singer, 1974; Spivak, Siegel, Sklaver, Deuschle, & Garrett, 1982). Jack, who is psychiatrically disabled, indicates the kind of limbo some people inhabit when they are able neither to establish nor to be guided by interests:

> I don't have any drive. There's nothing I really feel like working for. I guess I wouldn't mind being a songwriter. But I never wrote anything worthwhile. No, I'd like to be an architect. I'd like to

design bizarre houses. I'll never do it, because I'd lose interest. I'd like to do something with my life, but what I don't know. (Estroff, 1981, p. 142)

In discussing how persons with spinal cord injury may experience changes in interests, Trieschmann (1989) notes, "Reduced access to satisfying activity can certainly lower mood, which tends to lower a person's interest in activity, which further lowers mood. Thus, a vicious circle evolves" (p. 242).

Her argument is supported by the finding that when persons increase their activities, their mood improves as well (Turner, Ward, & Turner, 1979). Thus, it appears that the reduction in interest and attraction associated with many forms of disability may reflect a complex process in which decreased feelings of attraction, decreases in activity, and demoralization interrelate in a downward spiral.

Thus, one of the challenges presented by disability is often to find new interests or new avenues for channeling one's interests. One of my earliest client encounters was a young man who had great promise as a swimmer and diver. He had won regional and national championships and was an Olympic hopeful. He broke his neck in a diving accident and was rendered a high-level quadriplegic. Fortunately, he discovered that he was also a talented writer and speaker and was able to channel his interest in sports toward sports journalism. Others do not so easily redirect their interests. Another client I knew at the same time had been an accomplished dancer in a nationally famous dance troupe. Following her spinal cord injury, she became despondent over her loss of ability and slipped into chronic substance abuse.

When Interests Fail

Persons may develop preferences that lead to problematic activity choices. For example, there is evidence to suggest that some adolescents with psychosocial difficulties may be attracted to socially unacceptable interests (Lambert, Rothschild, Atland, & Green, 1978; Werthman, 1976). As another example, adults with developmental disabilities tend to have mainly solitary and sedentary interests (Cheseldine & Jeffree, 1981; Coyne, 1980; Matthews, 1980; Mitic & Stevenson, 1981). As a consequence of their interests, these persons made choices to do things that isolated them-

selves, led to chronic physical inactivity, or got them into trouble.

Other research has found that persons with alcoholism are less likely to pursue their stated interests (Scaffa, 1982). Some persons appear to substitute the pleasure induced by substance abuse for the enjoyment of doing things. Others feel they cannot enjoy themselves without the assistance of drugs or alcohol.

A prospective study of more than 3000 aircraft workers found that those who hardly ever enjoyed their job tasks were 2.5 times more likely to report a back injury than subjects who almost always enjoyed their job tasks (Bigos et al., 1991). Whereas there is some reason to suspect that many workers today may feel disaffected from their work (Kielhofner, 1993), this may be true particularly when one has a disability. For example, Alice, who has a psychiatric disability, notes:

I hate my job. I just hate it. It takes the mind of a seven-year-old to work there. It's boring. My supervisor is like a slave driver. I tried so many Civil Service jobs you wouldn't believe it. Sometimes two to three job interviews a week. But no one would hire me. No one. They never did tell me why. I bet I'll be stuck at Goodwill forever . . . (Estroff, 1981, p. 136)

Since work is a fact of life for so many adults, the degree of interest persons find in their work is no small issue.

Interest as Inspiration

Interests can infuse life with meaning and energy, as illustrated in a story told by Christi Brown in his autobiography, *My Left Foot*. Brown, severely disabled with cerebral palsy, explains that as a 10-year-old boy he became depressed and despondent. With a set of watercolors bartered from his brother, he learned to paint with his foot. He explains, "I didn't know it then, but I had found a way to be happy. Slowly I begin to lose my early depression. I had a feeling of pure joy while I painted, a feeling I had never experienced before which seemed almost to lift me above myself" (Brown, 1990, pp. 57).

Brown's characterization of painting as a way to be happy underscores an important point about interests. The process of finding pleasure and satisfaction in doing things is a central component of adapting in occupational life. The contentment we find in doing things gives us positive emotional experiences. Even more important, we must find some enthusiasm for doing particular things that urges us to action and gives us something to which we can look forward. Interest gives life much of its appeal.

Volitional Processes

The previous sections examined personal causation, values, and interests independently. As noted at the outset of this chapter, these three elements are woven together in one's thoughts and feelings about one's actions and the world. Moreover, it is noted at the beginning of this chapter that volition is a dynamic process involving a cycle of anticipation, making choices, experience while doing, and subsequent evaluation or interpretation. This last section examines the dynamic process of volition. In doing so, it considers how personal causation, values, and interests are part of a coherent pattern of thoughts and feelings unfolding in everyday life.

Anticipation

People's interests, values, and personal causation influence how they anticipate action—that is, what they notice and search out in the world and what they feel and think about prospects for doing things. People tend to be unaware of things in which they have no volitional investment. Conversely, they notice what corresponds to their competence, interests, and commitments. What is out there in the world for anyone is very much a function of volition. For example, Dreikie notices things on the dementia ward that reflect opportunities for her to enact the nursing behaviors that give her satisfaction.

Making Choices

People's choices for action shape their everyday doing and influence the course of their lives. These choices involve complex contributions from all components of volition. Thus choices are shaped by one's interests, personal causation, and values. Activity choices shape the immediate future. They involve decisions to begin or terminate activities and how to go about them. Thus they commence, shape, and terminate what one does. Occupational choices (i.e., decisions to begin or end

roles, alter a habit pattern, or undertake a personal project) occur much less frequently than activity choices, but they have a much farther-reaching impact on our lives. In fact, what most characterizes an occupational choice is that it changes something fundamental about one's life. Consequently, most occupational choices are made over a period of deliberation as one considers what they mean for one's life. The onset of an acquired disability is often an occasion for occupational choice. When a disability interferes with role performance, requires extra time to do things, or makes old habits or projects no longer viable, people must make a series of different occupational choices to find a new pattern of behavior. The success of such choices will have a great deal to do with how well a person adapts to the circumstance of having a disability. Richard's desire to enter a worker role and Jiyeon's efforts to learn the tasks that her peers do are both examples of the importance of this process of making choices.

Experience

Volition also influences how we experience what we do. When we engage in occupations, our volition determines what we find more or less enjoyable or valuable. It also determines the extent of confidence or anxiety we feel. Volition leads each of us to experience action in our own unique way.

Our experience in performing is closely linked to our quality of life. After all, how we experience the things we do—be it enjoyment, boredom, fulfillment, angst, triumph, or disappointment—determines much of what we get out of life. Finding harmony between our volition and what we actually get to do in the course of daily life contributes to life satisfaction. For instance, the fact that Driekie's environment allows her to continue to do occupations that satisfy her allows her to achieve a measure of life satisfaction despite her severe impairment.

Finally, experience is also a critical dimension of therapy. The therapeutic transformation that comes from doing things depends on what we experience in the midst of performance. Research has shown that volition is an important determinant of how therapy is experienced and a critical factor in whether clients benefit from therapy (Barrett, Beer, & Kielhofner, 1999; Helfrich & Kielhofner, 1994; Kielhofner & Barrett, 1998).

Interpretation

Volition influences how we interpret our actions. Our personal causation, values, and interests have an important influence on the significance we assign to what we have done. For example, Richard's commitment to achieving a productive life like his brother will influence how he makes sense of everyday experiences on the job. Elizabeth's feelings of insecurity and inefficacy around her peers influences the way she views her interpersonal performance. As these examples show, volition provides the framework by which people make sense of their actions.

Conclusion

Volition has a pervasive influence on occupational life. It shapes how people see the world and the opportunities and challenges it presents. It guides the activity and occupational choices that together determine much of what we do. It determines the experience of doing. It shapes how people make sense of what they have done, including effectiveness in achieving desired ends and success in realizing important values. To a large extent, how people experience life and how they regard themselves and their world has to do with volition.

Key Terms

Enjoyment: The feeling of pleasure or satisfaction that comes from doing things.

Interest pattern: The unique configuration of preferred things to do that one has accumulated from experience.

Interests: What one finds enjoyable or satisfying to do.

Personal causation: One's sense of competence and effectiveness.

Personal convictions: Views of life that define what matters.

Self-efficacy: Thoughts and feelings concerning perceived effectiveness in using personal abilities to achieve desired outcomes in life.

Sense of obligation: Strong emotional dispositions to follow what are perceived as right ways to act.

Sense of personal capacity: Assessment of one's physical, intellectual, and social abilities.

Values: What one finds important and meaningful to do.

Volition: Pattern of thoughts and feelings about oneself as an actor in one's world which occur as one anticipates, chooses, experiences, and interprets what one does.

References

American Psychiatric Association. (2000). *Diagnostic and statistical manual of mental disorders* (4th ed., text revision). Washington, DC: Author.

Barrett, L., Beer, D., & Kielhofner, G. (1999). The importance of volitional narrative in treatment: An ethnographic case study in a work program. *Work, 12,* 79–92.

Becker, E. W., & Lesiak, W. J. (1977). Feelings of hostility and personal control as related to depression. *Journal of Clinical Psychology, 33,* 654–657.

Bellah, R., Madsen, R., Sullivan, W., Swidler, A., & Tipton, S. (1985). *Habits of the heart.* Berkeley: University of California.

Bigos, S. J., Battie, M. C., Spengler, M. D., Fisher, L. D., Fordyce, W. E., Hansson, T. H., Nachemson, A. L., & Wortley, M. D. (1991). A prospective study of work perceptions and psychosocial factors affecting the report of back injury. *Spine, 16,* 1–6.

Brisenden, S. (1986). Independent living and the medical model of disability. *Disability, Handicap, and Society, 1,* 173–178.

Brown, C. (1990). *My left foot.* London: Minerva.

Bruner, J. (1973). Organization of early skilled action. *Child Development, 44,* 1–11.

Bruner, J. (1990). *Acts of meaning.* Cambridge, MA: Harvard University.

Burish, T. G., & Bradley, L. A. (1983). *Coping with chronic disease: Research and applications.* New York: Academic.

Burke, J. P. (1977). A clinical perspective on motivation: Pawn versus origin. *American Journal of Occupational Therapy, 31,* 254–258.

Cheseldine, S., & Jeffree, D. (1981). Mentally handicapped adolescents: Their use of leisure time. *Journal of Mental Health Deficiency Research, 25,* 49–59.

Connel, J. P. (1985). A new multidimensional measure of children's perceptions of control. *Child Development, 56,* 1018–1041.

Cottle, T. J. (1971). *Time's children: Impressions of youth.* Boston: Little, Brown.

Coyne, P. (1980). Developing social skills in the developmentally disabled adolescent and young adult: A recreation and social/sexual approach. *Journal of Leisure, 7,* 70–76.

Cromwell, R. L. (1963). A social learning approach to mental retardation. In N. R. Ellis (Ed.), *Handbook of mental deficiency*. New York: McGraw-Hill.

Csikszentmihalyi, M. (1990). *Flow: The psychology of optimal experience*. New York: Harper & Row.

DeCharms, R.E. (1968). *Personal causation: The internal affective determinants of behaviors*. New York: Academic.

Deegan, P. (1991). Recovery: The lived experience of rehabilitation. In R. P. Marinelli & A. E. Dell Orto (Eds.), *The psychological and social impact of disability* (3rd ed.). New York: Springer-Verlag.

Delaney-Naumoff, M. (1980). Loss of heart. In J. A. Werner-Beland (Ed.), *Grief responses to long-term illness and disability*. Reston, VA: Reston.

DeLoach, C. P., Wilkins, R. D., & Walker, G. W. (1983). *Independent living: Philosophy, process, and services*. Baltimore: University Park.

Edgerton, R. B. (1967). *The cloak of competence: Stigma in the lives of the mentally retarded*. Berkeley: University of California.

Estroff, S. E. (1981). *Making it crazy*. Berkeley: University of California.

Ewan, C., Lowy, E., & Reid, J. (1991). "Falling out of culture": The effects of repetition strain injury on sufferers' roles and identity. *Sociology of Health and Illness, 13*, 168–192.

Fein, M. L. (1990). *Role change: A resocialization perspective*. New York: Praeger.

Fiske, S., & Taylor, S. E. (1985). *Social cognition*. New York: Random House.

Frankl, V. E. (1978). *The unheard cry for meaning*. New York: Touchstone.

Gergen, K. J., & Gergen, M. M. (1983). Narratives of the self. In T. R. Sarbin & K. E. Scheibe (Eds.), *Studies in social identity*. New York: Praeger.

Gergen, K. J., & Gergen, M. M. (1988). Narrative and the self as relationship. In L. Berkowitz (Ed.), *Advances in experimental social psychology* (pp. 17–56). San Diego: Academic.

Gill, C. (1994). A bicultural framework for understanding disability. *The Family Psychologist, Fall,* 13–16.

Gill, C. (1997). Four types of integration in disability identity development. *Journal of Vocational Rehabilitation, 9*, 39–46.

Goffman, E. (1961). *Asylums*. New York: Doubleday.

Goodman, P. (1960). *Growing up absurd*. New York: Vintage.

Grob, M., & Singer, J. (1974). *Adolescent patients in transition: Impact and outcome of psychiatric hospitalization*. New York: Behavioral.

Grossack, M., & Gardner, H. (1970). *Man and men: Social psychology as social science*. Scranton, PA: International Textbook.

Hahn, H. (1985). Disability policy and the problem of discrimination. *American Behavioral Scientist, 28,* 293–318.

Hall, E. T. (1959). *The silent language*. Greenwich, CT: Fawcett.

Harter, S. (1983). The development of the self-system. In M. Hetherington (Ed.), *Handbook of child psychology: Social and personality development* (Vol. 4). New York: Wiley.

Harter, S. (1985). Competence as a dimension of self-evaluation: Toward a comprehensive model of self-worth. In R. L. Leahy (Ed.), *The development of the self*. Orlando, FL: Academic.

Harter, S., & Connel, J. P. (1984). A model of relationships among children's academic achievement and self-perceptions of competence, control, and motivation. In J. Nicholls (Ed.), *The development of achievement motivation*. Greenwich, CT: JAI.

Helfrich, C., & Kielhofner, G. (1994). Volitional narratives and the meaning of therapy. *American Journal of Occupational Therapy, 48*, 318–326.

Helfrich, C., Kielhofner, G., & Mattingly, C. (1994). Volition as narrative: Understanding motivation in chronic illness. *American Journal of Occupational Therapy, 48*, 311–317.

Hull, J. M. (1990). *Touching the rock: An experience of blindness*. New York: Vintage.

Kalish, R. A., & Collier, K. W. (1981). *Exploring human values*. Monterey, CA: Brooks/Cole.

Kielhofner, G. (1980). *Evaluating deinstitutionalization: An ethnographic study of social policy*. Unpublished doctoral dissertation, University of California at Los Angeles.

Kielhofner, G. (1983). "Teaching" retarded adults: Paradoxical effects of a pedagogical enterprise. *Urban Life, 12*, 307–326.

Kielhofner, G. (1993). Functional assessment: Toward a dialectical view of person-environment relations. *American Journal of Occupational Therapy, 47*, 248–251.

Kielhofner, G., & Barrett, L. (1998). Meaning and misunderstanding in occupational forms: A study of therapeutic goal-setting. *American Journal of Occupational Therapy, 52*, 345–353.

Klavins, R. (1972). Work-play behavior: Cultural influences. *American Journal of Occupational Therapy, 26*, 176–179.

Kluckholn, C. (1951). Values and value orientations in the theory of action: An exploration in definition and classification. In T. Parsons & E. Shils (Eds.), *Toward a general theory of action*. Cambridge, MA: Harvard University.

Korner, I. (1970). Hope as a method of coping. *Journal of Consulting and Clinical Psychology, 34*, 134–139.

Krefting, L. (1989). Reintegration into the community after head injury: The results of an ethnographic study. *Occupational Therapy Journal of Research, 9*, 67–83.

Lambert, B. G., Rothschild, B. F., Atland, R., & Green, L. B. (1978). *Adolescence: Transition from childhood to maturity* (2nd ed.). Monterey, CA: Brooks/Cole.

Lee, D. (1971). Culture and the experience of value. In A. H. Maslow (Ed.), *Neural knowledge in human values*. Chicago: Henry Regnery.

Lefcourt, H. (1981). *Research with the locus of control construct, Vol. 1: Assessment and methods*. New York: Academic.

Lefcourt, H. M. (1976). *Locus of control: Current trends in theory and research*. Hillsdale, NJ: Erlbaum.

Leggett, J., & Archer, R. P. (1979). Locus of control and depression among psychiatric patients. *Psychology Report, 45*, 835–838.

Litman, T. J. (1972). Physical rehabilitation: A social-psychological approach. In E. G. Jaco (Ed.), *Patients, physicians and illness: A sourcebook in behavioral science and health* (2nd ed.). New York: Free Press.

Longmore, P.K. (1995a). Medical decision making and people with disabilities: A clash of cultures. *Journal of Law, Medicine & Ethics, 23*, 82–87.

Longmore, P. K. (1995b). The second phase: From disability rights to disability culture. *The Disability Rag & Resource, Sept/Oct*, 4–11.

Lovejoy, M. (1982). Expectations and the recovery process. *Schizophrenia Bulletin, 8*, 605–609.

Markus, H. (1983). Self knowledge: An expanded view. *Journal of Personality, 51*, 543–562.

Matsutsuyu, J. (1969). The interest checklist. *American Journal of Occupational Therapy, 23*, 323–328.

Matthews, P. R. (1980). Why the mentally retarded do not participate in certain types of recreational activities. *Therapeutic Recreation Journal, 14*, 44–50.

Meissner, W. W. (1982). Notes on the potential differentiation of borderline conditions. *Psychoanalytic Review, 70*, 179–209.

Menninger, K. (1962). Hope. In S. Doniger (Ed.), *The nature of man in theological and psychological perspective*. New York: Harper Brothers.

Miller, J. F., & Oertel, C. B. (1983). Powerlessness in the elderly: Preventing hopelessness. In J. F. Miller (Ed.), *Coping with chronic illness: Overcoming powerlessness*. Philadelphia: FA Davis.

Mitchell, A. (1983). *The nine American lifestyles*. New York: Macmillan.

Mitchell, J. J. (1975). *The adolescent predicament*. Toronto: Holt, Winston.

Mitic, T. D., & Stevenson, C. L. (1981). Mentally retarded people as a resource to the recreationist in planning for integrated community recreation. *Journal of Leisure Research, 8*, 30–34.

Molnar, G. E. (1989). The influence of psychosocial factors on personality development and emotional health in children with cerebral palsy and spina bifida. In B. W. Heller, L. M. Flohr, & L. S. Zegans (Eds.), *Psychosocial interventions with physically disabled persons*. New Brunswick, NJ: Rutgers University.

Moss, J. W. (1958). *Failure-avoiding and stress-striving behavior in mentally retarded and normal children*. Ann Arbor, MI: University Microfilms.

Murphy, R. (1987). *The body silent*. New York: WW Norton.

Neville, A. M. (1987). *The relationship of locus of control, future time perspective and interest to productivity among individuals with varying degrees of depression*. Unpublished doctoral dissertation, New York University.

Oliver, M. (1993). Disability and dependency: A creation of industrial societies. In J. Swain, V. Finkelstein. French, S., Oliver, M. (Eds). Disabling Barriers—Enabling Environment. London: Sage, 49–60.

Oliver, M. (1996). The social model in context. *Understanding disability from theory to practice*. New York: St. Martin's, pp. 30–42.

Patsy, D., & Kielhofner, G. (1989). *An exploratory study of psychosocial adaptation to spinal cord injury*. Unpublished manuscript.

Rabinowitz, H. S., & Mitsos, S. B. (1964). Rehabilitation as planned social change: A conceptual framework. *Journal of Health and Social Behavior, 5*, 2–13.

Roberts, E. V. (1989). A history of the independent living movement: A founder's perspective. In B. W. Heller, L. M. Flohr, & L. S. Zegans (Eds.), *Psychosocial interventions with physically disabled persons*. New Brunswick, NJ: Rutgers University.

Rogers, J. C., & Figone, J. J. (1978). The avocational pursuits of rehabilitants with traumatic quadriplegia. *American Journal of Occupational Therapy, 32*, 571–576.

Rogers, J. C., & Figone, J. J. (1979). Psychosocial parameters in treating the person with quadriplegia. *American Journal of Occupational Therapy, 33*, 432–439.

Rotter, J. B. (1960). Generalized expectancies for internal versus external control of reinforcement. *Psychological Monographs: General Applications, 80*, 1–28.

Scaffa, M. (1982). *Temporal adaptation and alcoholism.* Unpublished master's thesis, Virginia Commonwealth University, Richmond.

Scheer, J., & Luborsky, M. L. (1991). Post-polio sequelae: The cultural context of polio biographies. *Orthopedics, 14,* 1173-1181.

Schiamberg, L. B. (1973). *Adolescent alienation.* Columbus, OH: Merrill.

Scotch, R. (1988). Disability as a basis for a social movement: Advocacy and the politics of definition. *Journal of Social Issues, 44* (1), 159–172.

Shapiro, J. (1994). No pity: People with disabilities forging a new civil rights movement. New York: Times Books.

Sienkiewicz-Mercer, R., & Kaplan, S. B. (1989). *I raise my eyes to say yes.* New York: Avon.

Skinner, E. A., Chapman, M., & Baltes, P. B. (1988). Control, means-end, and agency beliefs: A new conceptualization and its measurement during childhood. *Journal of Personality and Social Psychology, 54,* 117–133.

Smith, M. B. (1969). *Social psychology and human values.* Chicago: Aldine.

Smyntek, L. E. (1983). *A comparison of occupationally functional and dysfunctional adolescents.* Unpublished master's project, Virginia Commonwealth University, Richmond.

Snyder, S. (2002). Infinities of forms: Disability figures in artistic traditions. In S. Snyder, B. Brueggemann, & R. Thompson (Eds.), Enabling the humanities: A sourcebook in disability studies. New York: Modern Languages Association, 173–196.

Spivak, G., Siegel, J., Sklaver, D., Deuschle, L., & Garrett, L. (1982). The long-term patient in the community: Lifestyle patterns and treatment implications. *Hospital Community Psychiatry, 33,* 291–295.

Trieschmann, R. B. (1989). Psychosocial adjustment to spinal cord injury. In B. W. Heller, L. M. Flohr, & L. S.

Zegans (Eds.), *Psychosocial interventions with physically disabled persons.* New Brunswick, NJ: Rutgers University.

Turner, R. W., Ward, M. F., & Turner, D. J. (1979). Behavioral treatment for depression: An evaluation of therapeutic components. *Journal of Clinical Psychology, 35,* 166–175.

Valient, G. E. (1994). Ego mechanisms of defense and personality psychopathology. *Journal of Abnormal Psychology, 103,* 44–50.

Vash, C. L. (1981). *The psychology of disability.* New York: Springer-Verlag.

Wasserman, G. A. (1986). Affective expression in normal and physically handicapped infants. Situational and developmental effects. *Journal of the American Academy of Child and Adolescent Psychiatry, 25,* 393–399.

Werner-Beland, J. A. (Ed.). (1980). *Grief responses to long-term illness and disability.* Reston, VA: Reston.

Werthman, C. (1976). The function of sociological definitions in the development of the gang boy's career. In R. Giallombardo (Ed.), *Juvenile delinquency: A book of readings* (3rd ed.). New York: Wiley.

Wright, B. A. (1960). *Physical disability: A psychological approach.* New York: Harper & Row.

Wylie, R. (1979). *The self-concept: Theory and research* (2nd ed.). Lincoln: University of Nebraska.

Youkilis, H., & Bootzin, R. (1979). The relationship between adjustment and perceived locus of control in female psychiatric in-patients. *Journal of Genetic Psychology, 135,* 297–299.

Zane, M. D., & Lowenthal, M. (1960). Motivation in rehabilitation of the physically handicapped. *Archive of Physical Medicine and Rehabilitation, 41,* 400–407.

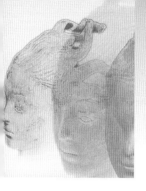

5

Habituation: Patterns of Daily Occupation

- Gary Kielhofner

*W*alt

Walt,[1] a primary school student in a Midwestern American city, struggles with organization of his schoolwork. Despite a folder with numerous pockets provided by his therapist, Walt has developed a habit of placing all of his papers in the same pocket, so he has problems finding the items he needs and getting them out in a timely manner. He has become quite frustrated with the folder solution for keeping his homework assignments and other papers organized.

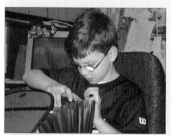

Walt is having difficulty finding a way to use a folder to organize his homework.

*C*hun-Haw

Chun-Haw[2] is a 22-year-old medical student in Taiwan. He is an avid tennis player who participates regularly in this leisure occupation, experiences a great deal of pleasure and satisfaction from it, and has incorporated

tennis playing as a significant part of his identity. When talking about his tennis playing, Chun-Haw also notes that he sees it as beneficial to his physical and psychological health, since it improves his cardiopulmonary function and reduces the stress associated with his strenuous studies. Additionally, playing tennis is a major way that Chun-Haw interacts with peers and builds friendships. Chun-Haw has also gone through an intensive training course and constantly focuses on increasing his tennis skills. By doing this, he has become more self-confident, to the point that he now plans to participate in tennis competitions in the future.

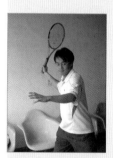

Chun-Haw works on his swing in therapy.

*H*annah

Hannah[3] is a teenager living in an American suburb. She is a starting player on her soccer and softball teams and captain of her basketball team. Her obligations to the numerous sports teams of which she is a member have begun to take time away from her studies. Despite having done poorly on a previous math exam, Hannah feels torn between studying for tomorrow's test and practicing for this weekend's game.

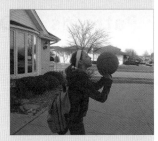

Hannah gets in some basketball practice while waiting for the school bus.

$\mathcal{M}$r. Chen

Mr. Chen[4] is a successful professional who has been able to provide a comfortable life for his family in Taiwan. In the past, Mr. Chen found it challenging to balance the multiple demands associated with being a husband, father, and son with working in a high-pressure job. After a period of significant loss and frustration, Mr. Chen reassessed his life and priorities. Now he is working to maintain more balance and satisfaction from his involvement in his family roles and from his leisure time. He has decided to have more modest life goals, be satisfied with what he does accomplish, and have more time for family, rest, and leisure. One aspect of his changed lifestyle is that Mr. Chen has taken up golf, which he plays regularly with his wife. As a consequence of changes he made in his life, Mr. Chen has a new sense of achievement and pleasure and family connection.

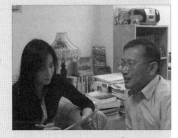

Mr. Chen discusses changes in his lifestyle with his occupational therapist.

[1] Susan Cahill, clinical instructor at the University of Illinois at Chicago, provided the case of Walt for this chapter.

[2] Ay-Woan Pan, Associate Professor at National Taiwan University and Fu-Zen University in Taipai, Taiwan, provided the case of Chun-Haw for this chapter.

[3] Susan Cahill, clinical instructor at the University of Illinois at Chicago, provided the case of Hannah for this chapter.

[4] Ay-Woan Pan, Associate Professor at National Taiwan University and Fu-Zen University in Taipai, Taiwan, provided the case of Chun-Haw for this chapter.

Each of these individuals illustrates the way in which going about everyday life can affect one's success and satisfaction. Walt is struggling with finding a routine way to manage his homework. Chun-Haw is seeking to enrich his life with a new role as a serious tennis player. Hannah is struggling to maintain a balance between her academic and sport involvement. Mr. Chen has decided to alter his daily and weekly routine to have more balance between work and family and leisure pursuits.

Chapter 2 proposes that the organization of routine life is a function of habituation. **Habituation** is an internalized readiness to exhibit consistent patterns of behavior guided by habits and roles and fitted to the characteristics of routine temporal, physical, and social environments. As shown in *Figure 5.1*, habituation allows persons to cooperate with their environments to do the routine actions that make up everyday life.

Interdependency of Habituation and Habitat

The regularity in habituated behavior depends on the reliability of habitats. A degree of sameness in the physical environment provides a stable arena for performance. The recurring temporal patterns—such as day and night, workweek and weekend—provide a stable structure within which routines unfold. Similarly, the social order has sufficient stability to furnish known situations to which a person has ways of responding. Because of the regularity of environments, persons are mostly grounded in the familiar, not having to calculate moves consciously. As Young (1988) notes, habituated performances are "generated and locked into place by recurrences" (p. 79).

Habituation involves the internalization of action-oriented representations that in the words of Clarke

FIGURE 5.1 Habituation.

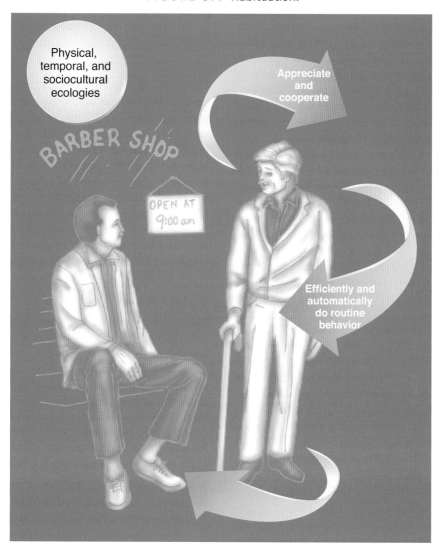

(1997) "simultaneously describe aspects of the world and prescribe possible actions" (p. 49). When we repeat behavior in a constant context, we learn to attend to aspects of the environment that will help sculpt the action that is part of any habit or role.

Habits

Habits can be defined as acquired tendencies to automatically respond and perform in certain consistent ways in familiar environments or situations. Habits regulate behavior by providing a regulated manner of dealing with environmental contingencies (Dewey, 1922; Camic, 1986). Habits guide behavior in the way that grammar organizes language or rules regulate a game (Koestler, 1969; Young, 1988). Bourdieu (1977) underscores that learning a habit is acquiring a set of rules for how to appreciate and act in the world. Appreciating the environment means that we automatically locate ourselves in the midst of familiar environmental features, apprehending their action impli-cations for a habitual behavior we are doing. For exam-ple, in the routine of getting dressed, people automat-ically recognize which piece of clothing goes where and which pieces of clothing need to be donned before others. We attend to and comprehend our environ-ments in terms of their implications for our routine do-ing. Therefore, a large component of any habitual ac-tion will be strategies for incorporating the things, people, and events around us into what we do.

This is exactly the aspect of habit with which Walt is struggling. He has been provided a folder that would allow him to separate different homework assign-ments and keep related materials together. However, to effectively and routinely make use of objects in the environment, most people develop personal habits that capitalize on the features of the environment. Until Walt is able to practice and acquire a new set of rules for placing materials in his folder in an orderly and systematic fashion, it will not provide a solution to his homework woes.

So long as we experience the world as familiar, habits operate smoothly and without need of attention. It is the unfamiliar (i.e., that for which we do not have in-ternalized rules) that extricates us from our habitual way of doing things. Consequently, habits operate as inter-nalized, appreciative capacities for recognizing familiar events and contexts and for guiding action. Habits pro-vide a way to appreciate and construct action appropri-ate to what is going on in the world around us.

Effectiveness and Efficiency of Habits

Habits preserve a learned way to do something from earlier performance in a given environment. Habits will incorporate ways of doing things that have a certain value within the environment in which they are per-formed. This does not mean that all habits are effective in every way. Walt's habit of dumping his papers into one section of the folder may serve some purpose, such as avoiding the challenging process of sorting them out, but it does not help him be well organized in his approach to homework. Adaptive habits allow persons to complete routine activities in a consistent and effec-tive manner (Camic, 1986).

Habits hold together the patterns of ordinary ac-tion that give life its familiar character. Young (1988) argues that habits serve as a kind of self-perpetuating flywheel conserving patterns of action. Once launched,

> *Habits hold together the patterns of ordinary ac-tion that give life its familiar character.*

habits provide momentum that allows action to unfold on its own. This frees up conscious attention for other purposes (James, 1950). Habits can also allow two or more behaviors to occur simultaneously. While one is performing habituated behaviors (e.g., getting dressed in the morning, driving home after work) it is possible to engage in other thoughts and behaviors (e.g., making a phone call, planning a meeting, or listening to the ra-dio). Therefore, habits decrease the effort required for occupational performance not only by reducing the amount of conscious attention required but also freeing up persons for other simultaneous activity.

Social Relevance of Habits

Habits also serve a purpose for society. Young (1988) notes that habits shared by a group of people constitute social customs. Thus, by acquiring habits humans be-come carriers and messengers of the customs that make up the way of life of a particular group. Moreover, in a social group one person's habitual behavior may be part of the environmental context necessary for an-other's habits. For example, Rowles (1991) provided the following description of a group of elderly men engag-ing in the habit of gathering at the post office:

> Every morning, shortly before 10:00 A.M., Walter takes a leisurely 400-yard stroll down the hill from his house to the trailer that serves as the post office to "pick up the mail." He traces exactly the same path each day. Several male age peers from different lo-cations within Colton embark on the same trip at about the same time.... Picking up the mail provides a rationale for an informal gathering of the elderly men of the community at the bench outside the Colton Store, which is located adjacent to the post office. The men generally linger throughout the morning. They watch the passing traffic, converse with patrons of the store, and discuss events of the day. Then, around lunchtime, the group disperses and Walter winds his way home again. (p. 268)

Walter's habit of getting the mail and meeting with other older residents illustrates how habits guide us to take advantage of and be in harmony with others' behavior (Cardwell, 1971).

Typical behaviors are to a large extent those recognized, expected, and depended on by others in the environment. For example, the habits of punctuality and industriousness reflect typical expectations of Western society. One is to be at work, meetings, and appointments at scheduled times and to focus on the task at hand during periods so designated. A person who is not punctual or attentive to work tasks will not be in synchrony with such an environment. Conse-quently, habits also allow a person to be integrated into the smooth functioning of society. This point is illustrated by Mr.

Chen's alteration of his routine, which allowed him to come into a more harmonious relationship with his family. Whereas his previous habits of working kept him away from leisure activities with family members, his new routine allowed more contact with family.

Three Influences of Habits in Daily Occupations

The influence of habits on everyday behavior is pervasive (Camic, 1986). What one does, when one does it, and how one goes about it reflects ones habits. As shown in *Figure 5.2*, we can recognize three influences of habits:

FIGURE 5.2 Influences of habits on occupation.

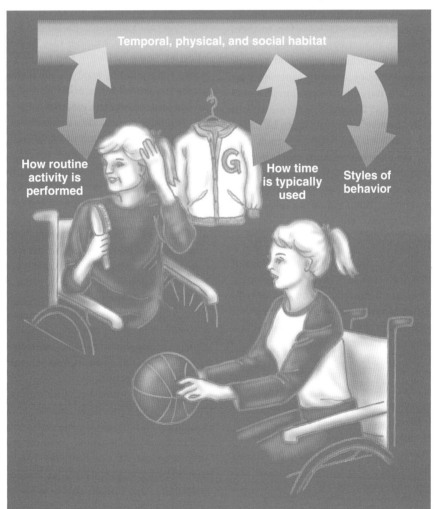

- Habits impact how routine activity is performed
- Habits regulate how time is typically used
- Habits generate styles of behavior that characterize a range of occupational performances.

HABITS OF OCCUPATIONAL PERFORMANCE

Each person has his or her own way of performing routine activities, such as grooming and dressing, making the bed, preparing morning coffee, taking out the dog, paying bills, and going to work or school. Habits may fit with ideas about proper etiquette or form. They may reflect the way a parent or mentor taught. They may simply emanate from what is simplest and most efficient. Whatever the reasons, people tend to be firmly entrenched in their particular ways of doing familiar activities.

Seamon (1980) noted that habits ordinarily involve a sequence of physical movements. He refers to them as body ballets, noting that they are "a set of integrated behaviors which sustain a particular task or aim" (p. 157). Habitual ways of performing ordinary activities organize actions together to accomplish a goal under routine conditions. Dewey (1922) referred to such daily habits as "passive tools waiting to be called into action" (p. 24). Indeed, our habits are tools of a sort that we call upon to get done what we do in ordinary life. Although the habitual ways of doing almost everything we do go largely unnoticed, getting through the day without them would be unbearably cumbersome.

HABITS OF ROUTINE

The influence of habits is also found in routine use of time. Seamon (1980) refers to such habits as time–space routines, since they are ordinarily linked not only to what time it is but also to where a person is or how that person is moving through space. He offers the following description of such a routine:

> *Although the habitual ways of doing almost everything we do go largely unnoticed, getting through the day without them would be unbearably cumbersome.*

> He would be up at seven-thirty, make his bed, perform his morning toilet, and be out of his house by eight. He would then walk to the corner cafe up the street, pick up the newspaper (which *had* to be the *New York Times*), order his usual fare (one scrambled egg, toast, and coffee), and stay there until around nine when he would walk to his nearby office. (p. 158)

Each of us will recognize similar routine use of time that characterizes our everyday patterns.

Chapin (1968) points out that routines include not only daily habits but habits within a variety of temporal cycles: " … cooking, eating and washing dishes during the twenty-four hour period of a day; the work, school, shopping, recreation or socializing routine during a seven day week; visiting out-of-town relatives and family vacation or other holiday outing routines during a year's time … " (p. 13)

Consequently, routines may be linked to a variety of cycles. Some cycles are tied to the kind of work one does. For example, teachers have changing routines across the school term, and farmers' routines depend on the seasons and the weather.

Routines do provide a degree of structure and predictability to life. In a longitudinal study of retirement, one of the greatest challenges for older persons was to find a new routine after working (Jonsson, Josephsson, & Kielhofner, 2001). While no two days are exactly the same, most persons have and can identify a routine that is typical for a given day of the week. In industrialized societies persons generally have patterns that characterize schooldays and workdays as well as alternative patterns that characterize days off from work or school. The degree of consistency in a routine depends on one's environment. Some environments demand a fixed routine, such as the grade school or factory schedule, which requires persons to show up, do certain tasks, take lunch and breaks, and terminate the day at specific times. Other environments require a more flexible pattern of action.

Habits of routine help locate us effectively within the stream of time. They enable us to be where we should be and get done what we should be doing over the course of daily, weekly, and other life cycles. To a very large extent, our everyday lives are defined and shaped by these cyclical routines. They create the overall pattern by which we go about our various occupations.

HABITS OF STYLE

Dewey (1922) noted that one's habits were reflected in a typical "style of … being-in-the-world" (p. 20). Such characteristics as being big picture versus detail oriented, quick versus plodding, or prompt versus procrastinating are examples of styles of performance regulated by habits. Habits of style are also found in our interpersonal behavior. Whether we tend to be quiet or talkative, direct or evasive, trusting or cautious, and formal or informal are examples of social habits of style.

Habits of style are manifest across a whole range of activities. That is, we tend to bring our personal styles to the performance of all that we do. Camic (1986) defines such habits thus: "The durable and generalized disposition that suffuses a person's action throughout an entire domain of life or, in the extreme instance, throughout all of life—in which case the term comes to mean the whole manner, turn, cast, or mold of the personality" (p. 1045).

Indeed, habits of style give a unique and stable character to performance.

Habit Formation and Change

Children come into the world without internal regulators of patterned behavior, save perhaps certain biorhythms. Soon, however, they are integrated into the rhythms, routines, and customs that make up the physical, social, and temporal world. Children first acquire routines through parental guidance and support. These are routines of day and night with the attending patterns of sleeping, waking, eating, bathing, and so on. Over the course of development, as routines, customs, and ways of doing things are experienced again and again, the child develops complex habit patterns.

A number of these patterns, such as sleeping and eating patterns, remain somewhat stable throughout life. Others change with the attainment of developmental stages, such as entering the student or worker roles. Interestingly, each new environmental context has its own regular rhythms that encourage individuals to internalize a pattern of action like that of others in the social system. Eventually, a number of rhythms may interweave, such as the rhythms and patterns of home life and those of school or work life.

All habits serve to preserve patterns of action, so they are naturally resistant to change. Whenever we make alterations in our schedules or environments, we encounter the tenacity of old habits. We show up at old appointed times, or we visit the wrong cabinet or office for some time after we have rearranged our belongings or relocated our work.

Habits resist change because they are based on our most fundamental certainties about how the world is constructed (Berger & Luckman, 1966). Habits presuppose a particular order in the physical, temporal, and social world. When habits and their background assumptions are disrupted or altered, a feeling of disorientation or unreality follows. For example, when our sleep patterns are disrupted or altered, we can find ourselves waking up without the usual sense of being firmly anchored in the temporal world (i.e., thinking it is dawn when it is really dusk). A similar feeling of disorientation can occur when we are in the midst of a familiar task and lose our place (e.g., suddenly realizing we do not recognize where we are on the road when driving to a familiar destination). In such cases, we are shocked into sudden consciousness with no clear footing in what is ordinarily a familiar and taken-for-granted world.

Habits and Disability

Habits organize our use of underlying performance capacity so that we can perform within our environment. The fit of our habits to our performance capacity and to our environment will determine how effective we are in our everyday routines. Habits play an especially important role when persons face the challenges of a disability. As the following discussions show, habits may either contribute to a disability or effectively compensate for underlying impairments.

DYSFUNCTIONAL HABITS

We intuitively know that the wrong habits can negatively affect us. All of us have possessed habits we would rather have been without. Sometimes, however, dysfunctional habits become more than a nuisance. They become a serious liability threatening one's welfare (Kielhofner, Barris, & Watts, 1982).

Acquired impairments can lead to an erosion of habits that further exacerbate the consequences of these functional limitations. For example, persons facing depression may be unable to pursue their routines because of limited motivation and energy (American

Psychiatric Association, 2000). Over time, this can lead to an erosion of habits that contributes to inactivity (Melges, 1982). When this happens and the person loses previously effective and satisfying routines, mood and energy can be further degraded. In such cases, the disruption of habits becomes part of a downward spiral. Impairments negatively affect habits, and their disruption further exacerbates the symptoms and/or consequences of the underlying condition.

Another habit problem associated with disability is that persons may learn dysfunctional habits from their environments. For example, the inactivity imposed by hospitalization can contribute to the loss of habits. Unfortunately, opportunities for persons to practice old or new habits are often not provided during rehabilitation (Shillam, Beeman, & Loshin, 1983). Many persons with severe emotional and cognitive impairments are placed in institutional environments. In such settings the routines can result in residents learning habits of passivity and inactivity that do not serve them well in the institution or later, when they return to the larger community (Borell, Gustausson, Sandman, & Kielhofner, 1994; Kielhofner, 1979, 1981, 1983).

Impact of Impairments on Habits

When capacities are diminished, previously established habits can be severely disrupted. One may be forced to develop new habits for many or most aspects of everyday life. Alterations in a person's functional status can totally disrupt the effectiveness of an existing habit. Zola (1982) illustrates this in his description of trying to complete his morning routine from the new viewpoint of a wheelchair:

> Washing up was a mess. Though the sink was low enough, I nevertheless managed to soak myself thoroughly. In retrospect, I should not have worn anything. Ordinarily when washing my face, chest, and arms, I would lean over the sink, and any excess water from my splashing would drip into it. My body angle in a wheel-chair was different. I could not extend over the sink very far without tipping. Thus, much of the water dripped down my neck onto me. Splashing with water was out, and the use of a damp washcloth, what I once called a "sponge bath," was in. (p. 64)

When impairments are pronounced, so are the complications of everyday routines. When persons have to make extensive use of adaptive equipment or require assistance from other persons, entirely new routines must be acquired. Sometimes new habits related to the management of the disability are required. For example, people may need to learn new habits for bowel and bladder care, for joint protection and energy conservation, or for following complicated medication regimens. Remissions and exacerbations or progressive decreases in physical functioning can make acquiring these necessary new habits difficult.

Disabled persons whose abilities are variable may need to develop extremely flexible habits. For example, persons with unpredictable impairments must be ready to capitalize on those times when things are better, such as the following gentleman with Parkinson's disease: "I cram in to the periods when I'm flexible all the things I would have liked to have done the rest of the day … One day I may be nine-tenths of the day free, although that's very rare, and another much less. There's nothing I can do about it" (Pinder, 1988, p. 79).

On the other hand, steadily progressive impairments may mean that habits are to an extent replaced with conscious strategies. For example, Murphy (1987) explains how his progressive paralysis meant that everyday routines had to be calculated. As he notes, the routine of transferring from wheelchair to toilet required him to figure out how to get up, "choosing … supports with care, calculating the number of steps it would take to reach [the toilet]" (p. 76). When habits cannot automatically regulate what one does, additional effort and concentration are required, taking away the ease and efficiency that ordinarily accompany everyday routines.

Disruption of Space and Time

The onset of a severe impairment can radically alter the spatial and temporal dimensions of routine performance. For example, the spinal cord–injured person must

> *When habits cannot automatically regulate what one does, additional effort and concentration are required, taking away the ease and efficiency that ordinarily accompany everyday routines.*

learn to organize behavior around the constraints of where one can go in a wheelchair and how long it will take (Paap, 1972). With the onset of a disability, the entire relationship of persons with their environments may change in dramatic ways, resulting in the need for new habits. In this regard Hull (1990) notes: "On the whole, my experience has been that, if I have a bad habit, it … is naturally corrected …. In other words, blindness itself imposes an iron law upon the user of the white cane. Lampposts, curbs, and stairways are the best teachers" (p. 15).

In similar fashion, wheelchairs and other devices to assist walking require their users to choose not simply the closest route to a destination but rather the route with friendly ramps, curbs, and surfaces. The habits that accommodate a new disability must not only deal with altered performance capacity but must also grapple with a physical world whose implications for action are radically changed. Also, people can become more vulnerable to external contingencies, such as bad weather and crowded public places.

Time also becomes a different matter. When their impairments necessitate additional time to conduct routine tasks, persons must develop daily routines that involve doing fewer things. Such temporal challenges can be further constrained by the necessity of adding new self-care habits to the daily routine.

Reconstructing Habits

As the foregoing discussions illustrate, the task of organizing daily life in the face of disability means reconstructing one's habits. Accommodations and trade-offs must take place. Some activities may have to be eliminated. New ways of doing things must be discovered and learned. Finally, one may have to delegate some tasks to family members or an attendant to have time for other more valued activities.

As Williams (1984) notes, "If the disabled individual is to move toward 'mere' impairment, eventually alternative ways of accomplishing the tasks of everyday life will be committed to memory and habit, ingrained in relationships with a new world which is once again 'had'" (p. 110).

The path to these new habits involves leaving behind a once familiar world that has been invalidated by disability. As Merleau-Ponty (1945/1962)

notes, "It is precisely when my customary world arouses in me habitual intentions that I can no longer, if I have lost a limb, be effectively drawn into it: the utilizable objects, precisely in so far as they present themselves as utilizable, appeal to a hand I no longer have" (p. 82).

Only by reencountering the world with one's altered condition can a new relationship to the world emerge and once again become familiar and taken for granted. DeLoach and Greer describe this transformation (1981) in the following way:

> A person begins to learn new ways of doing what she did before—and ways of accomplishing, as well, some brand-new things. These new, different ways are, at first, awkward, stress-producing, and frustrating … little by little, a person gets accustomed to a new modus operandi. What at first was awkward, painful, or embarrassing becomes just a regular part of living, incorporated into one's routine. After such habituation, the person begins to concentrate more on participation in life now rather than on what used to be or what might have been. (p. 251)

As they indicate, the transformation of habits is a necessary pathway through which persons find their way back to the participation in everyday activities of daily living, work, and leisure.

Internalized Roles

Routine action is influenced by the fact that each of us belongs to and acts in social systems. Much of what we do is done as a spouse, parent, worker, student, and so on. Having internalized such roles, we act in ways that reflect our role status (Fein, 1990). Internalizing the role means taking on an identity, an outlook, and actions that belong to the role. Consequently, an **internalized role** is the incorporation of a socially and/or personally defined status and a related cluster of attitudes and actions. Chun-Haw's tennis playing is an example of this process of internalizing a role. He sees himself as and has acquired equipment and clothes that signify he is a tennis player. He has sought out training to improve his game. He interacts with others who share this role and is working toward involvement in formal competitions that will allow him to publicly enact the role in new contexts.

Internalizing a role involves gaining a sense of one's relationships to others and of expected behaviors. As Sarbin and Scheibe (1983) note, effective action depends on the "correct placements of self in the world of occurrences" (p. 8). Consequently, internalized roles give us the necessary social bearings to act effectively.

Role Identification

We see ourselves as students, workers, parents, and so on because we recognize ourselves as occupying certain statuses or positions and also because we experience ourselves acting as someone who holds these roles. According to Sarbin and Scheibe (1983), "a person's identity at any time is a function of his or her validated social positions" (p. 7). We identify with our roles in part because we see ourselves reflected in the attitudes and actions of others toward us. Consequently, role identity is generated when others recognize and respond to us as occupying a particular status. Who we are is intertwined with the roles we inhabit (Cardwell, 1971; Ruddock, 1976; Schein, 1971; Turner, 1962).

Identifying with any role means internalizing both what attributes society assigns to the role and one's personal interpretation of that role (Fein, 1990). For example, one person may develop a student role identity that stresses being an intellectual. For such a person being a student may resonate with the volitional sense of having intellectual capacity, interests, and values. Another student, whose interest and values lie elsewhere, may view the student role as only instrumental to gaining a credential. Both inhabit the student role, but the ways in which they internalize it, identify with it, and enact its expectations differ significantly.

Whatever way we come to think of and experience ourselves in a role becomes part of our self-understanding. To an extent, we see ourselves and judge our actions in terms of our own perception of the roles we inhabit. As Miller (1983) argues, personal identity reflects our awareness of all our various roles. Integrating one's various roles into a personal identity involves assigning centrality or importance to some roles over others. This process is dynamic and changes over time as different roles assume different places in our lives or demand extra effort or attention (Hall, Stevens, & Meleis, 1992; Hammel, 1999). Mr. Chen is an example of someone who has redefined his worker, leisure, and family roles.

However, not all roles have a clearly defined social status. Some roles are informal. Some arise out of personal circumstances (Hammel, 1999; Rosow, 1976). One informal role without a clear social status is caregiver for a disabled spouse or parent (Schumacher, 1995). Such roles that do not correspond to a formal social status have ambiguous meanings and expectations attached to them. Consequently, internalization of such roles requires more improvisation. Persons are often left to impart their definition on the role and to find social partners who will recognize and validate the role. This is one of the reasons that support groups are so popular. They often provide persons access to others who, like themselves, occupy a role that is not well defined. In such groups persons find validation for their role and sort out what are reasonable expectations for the role.

People know how to act in a given role because of an internalized script that guides how they perceive themselves and their role partners (Fein, 1990; Miller,1983; Mancuso & Sarbin, 1983). The script allows one to tacitly appreciate how one should proceed. For example, how we perform a greeting is guided by the role relationship with the other person. Depending on whether a pair is parent and child, worker and boss, student and teacher, or two close friends, the greeting may take on quite different forms.

Influences of Roles on Occupation

As shown in *Figure 5.3*, roles organize action in three main ways. First, they influence the manner and content of our actions. Moving from one role to another is often demarcated by such changes as how we dress, our manner of speech, and our way of relating to others. Second, each role carries with it a range of actions that makes up that role. Consequently, roles shape what kinds of things we do. For example, a student is

> *Internalizing a role involves gaining a sense of one's relationships to others and of expected behaviors.*

FIGURE 5.3 Influences of roles on occupation.

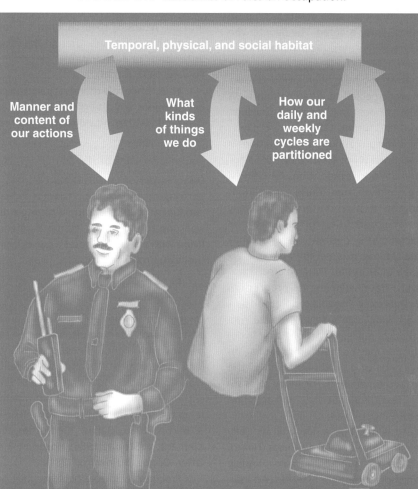

expected to attend class, take notes, ask questions, read articles or books, complete assignments, study, and take tests. The actions expected for a role are clearly defined by some social groups. In other situations, persons must negotiate or define for themselves what actions make up the role.

Third, roles partition our daily and weekly cycles into times when we inhabit certain roles. The course of each day ordinarily involves a succession or overlap of roles. Any parent who has attempted to talk on the phone with a coworker while holding a fussy baby and watching food on the stove will immediately appreciate how roles can overlap. Across our days, weeks, and lives, roles are social spaces that we enter, enact, and exit.

> *Across our days, weeks, and lives, roles are social spaces that we enter, enact, and exit.*

Socialization and Role Change

Beginning in childhood, we perceive others to fill positions that everyone takes for granted. The people who occupy such positions as mothers, teachers, and baby sitters tend to behave in predictable ways. As time goes on, we discover that we too have been assigned roles. We learn that we are expected to act in certain ways because of the roles we occupy (Grossack & Gardner, 1970; Katz & Kahn, 1966; Turner, 1962).

The process of communicating role expectations is referred to as socialization (Brim & Wheeler, 1966). For example, as children develop, expectations for being a family member are communicated. These expectations involve where and how to play, conformity to family routines, and the responsibilities for self-care and chores. These expectations for performance as a family member are generally more informal than the role expectations that come later in life. Thus, role socialization generally involves a developmental progression from informal to formal roles. This role progression parallels the child's growing ability to internalize role scripts and to use them as guides for action. Later in development, socialization may be much more formal, including education, practicing or apprenticing in the role, credentialing, and supervision. For many roles society goes to great lengths to socialize and regulate those who fill the role.

Persons being socialized into a new role typically negotiate their role in a give-and-take process (Heard, 1977; Schein, 1971). Each person fulfills a role uniquely but is also bound by how others are affected. An individual who enacts a role in ways that negatively affect others invites their invectives to conform to the role's expectations.

Socialization is an ongoing process because roles change throughout life. Society expects and structures role transitions at various life stages, such as entering and leaving the student role, beginning work, and retiring. Persons also choose to enter and leave roles. Finally, role change is sometimes thrust on people by circumstances.

Role change is complex, involving alterations of one's identity, one's relationships to others, the tasks one is expected to perform, and how one's lifestyle is organized. An example of the complexity of role change is the experience of family members when aging parents require children to take care of them. This circumstance entails "a clear reversal of roles as the older generation loses power, and the authority to make the most personal kinds of decisions gravitates into the hands of their children .... Roles need to be thoroughly redefined, often in the face of stiff resistance and understandable resentment" (Hage & Powers, 1992, p. 118).

Thus, while role change is part and parcel of human development, it is often the occasion of significant reorganization within individuals and their social systems.

Roles and Disability

Disabled persons may be barred from, have difficulty performing, or lack opportunities to learn or enter occupational roles. In addition, having a disability can assign one to unwanted, marginal roles. Consequently, living with a disability poses a number of challenges for occupying roles.

ROLE PERFORMANCE DIFFICULTIES ASSOCIATED WITH DISABILITY

Disability often presents itself as a problem with role performance. For example, a common factor that leads persons with mental illness or substance abuse problems to enter mental health care is a failure in school or work roles (Black, 1976; Mechanic, 1980). Adolescents with mental illness have more problems in academic, leisure, and work roles than their peers (Barris, Dickie, & Baron, 1988; Barris, Kielhofner, Burch, Gelinas, Klement, & Schultz,1986; Holzman & Grinker, 1974; Offer, Ostrov, & Howard, 1981).

Problems with role behavior may occur when one has not internalized appropriate role scripts and therefore one does not meet the expectations of the social group. By virtue of having a disability, people may have fewer experiences in which to acquire role scripts (Smith, 1972; Versluys, 1983). For example, persons with cognitive impairments are often denied access to opportunities to learn adult roles (Guskin, 1963; Kielhofner, 1983; Wolfensberger, 1975). In such cases, limitations of capacity are magnified by the lack of learning experiences.

Limitations of physical capacity may disrupt or terminate role performance. In other cases, a person may be able to retain a role only by making major modifications in how the role is enacted. For example, a person who acquires a disability may continue as a worker but must engage in a new type of work. In many instances, this can mean moving to a lesser-paying job.

A disability may create problems of role performance such as being unable to discharge the role in ways consistent with one's own or others' expectations for the role. For example, persons whose impairments are not visible to others may be viewed by friends, family, or coworkers as malingering (Schiffer, Rudick, & Herndon, 1983). In other cases the conflict may be between one's own view of the role and how one is able to perform. For example, one gentleman who has multiple sclerosis notes of his family roles: "I feel left out of discipline over the children because I am static in an armchair and cannot even phone the school. I had lost the ability to be a real father and husband" (Robinson, 1988, p. 60). Hull (1990) similarly describes how being blind has robbed him of the ability to supervise and to participate in play with his children, eroding and constricting what kind of father he can be. Such shifts in the identity and function of ongoing roles can be sources of conflict and self-devaluation.

Role strain may occur when a person cannot meet the multiple obligations or aspirations represented in several roles (Beutell & Greenhaus, 1983; Coser, 1974; Gerson, 1976; Gray; 1972). Impairments may require persons to exert more time and energy on maintaining such major life roles as work or homemaking, requiring them to relinquish other roles (Hallet, Zasler, Maurer, & Cash, 1994; Hammel, 1999). Overall, persons with disabilities tend to occupy fewer roles than their nondisabled counterparts (Dickerson, & Oakely, 1995; Ebb, Coster, & Duncombe, 1989).

SOCIAL BARRIERS TO ROLES

Although impairments may contribute to difficulties in role performance, among the most significant obstacles for persons with disabilities are social barriers (Hahn, 1985, 1988). For many people, the presence of a visible disability creates immediate difficulties of access to ordinary roles. Beginning in childhood, persons with disabilities may be discouraged or prevented from exploring, learning, and occupying roles. Such persons may be chronically frustrated because they are unable to attain a series of roles (Kielhofner, 1979, 1981). Social barriers to roles range from subtle attitudinal barriers that make access difficult, to policies whose consequence is to make roles inaccessible to persons with disabilities.

Sometimes barriers to roles are evident, as when people refuse to admit those with disabilities into various social groups. One of the most dramatic examples is employment. Despite legislation in most industrialized countries that assures some equal access to the marketplace, persons with disabilities still have a harder time finding employment (Erikson, 1973; Trieschmann, 1989). In the United States fewer than one-third of severely disabled persons of working age work (Hale, Hayghe, & McNeil, 1998; Louis Harris and Associates, 1998; Trupin, Sebesta, Yelin, & LaPlante, 1997). Barriers to work include discrimination in the workplace and public policy that often penalizes persons financially or in terms of health benefits if they seek employment (Brandt & Pope, 1997; National Council on Disability, 1996).

CONSEQUENCES OF ROLE LOSS AND ROLELESSNESS

Research suggests that involvement in too few roles is even more likely to be detrimental to psychosocial well-being than having too many role demands (Marks, 1977; Seiber, 1974; Spreitzer, Snyder, & Larson, 1979). Without sufficient roles one lacks identity, purpose, and structure in everyday life. Unemployment has been linked to suicide, depression, stress-related physical health problems, child abuse, and increased substance abuse (Borrero, 1980; Briar, 1980).

A loss of identity and self-esteem may occur as persons take on roles they believe to be relatively unimportant or as they lose roles (Thomas, 1966; Werner-Beland, 1980). For example, Krefting (1989) notes:

> Most head-injured people remember parts of their old selves and recognize that the old self is gone. But they have nothing upon which to build a new self-identity. This is largely a result of lack of opportunity to fill legitimate roles in society. If an individual's personhood is not acknowledged by others, it is difficult for him or her to develop a sense of self-identity. (p. 76)

This view is echoed throughout accounts given by persons with disabilities. There is a substantial cost to personal identity when persons no longer are recognized as the fathers, mothers, spouses, students, workers, caretakers, or friends that they used to be.

SICK AND DISABLED ROLES

Disability may not only remove or bar people from occupational roles but also relegate them to sick and deviant roles (Bogdan & Taylor, 1989; Parsons, 1953;

> *There is a substantial cost to personal identity when persons no longer are recognized as the fathers, mothers, spouses, students, workers, caretakers, or friends that they used to be.*

Werner-Beland, 1980). When a person is ill and incapacitated, normal role expectations are typically suspended and the person is relegated to the sick role and expected to do what is necessary to get well (Parsons, 1953; McKeen, 1992). The sick role and its expectations for passivity and compliance can be problematic for persons with a long-term illness or disability.

A case in point is Bill, diagnosed with sarcoma that required him to leave his job as a mechanic to undergo a regimen of surgery and chemotherapy over 3 years. Bill became accustomed to the sick role, in which others made decisions about the care that dominated his life. His identity as a cancer patient overshadowed other aspects of his identity. His interactions with others and his daily routine centered on his patient role. At the end of 3 years, Bill was left with an able body but found it overwhelming to consider reentry into work and other adult roles.

The reactions of others can cast a person in a disabled role (Asch, 1998; Toombs, 1987; Werner-Beland, 1980). For example, others may unnecessarily lower their expectations, become overprotective or overly helpful, or consider the person to be disabled beyond his or her actual limitations. Zola (1982) discusses how using a wheelchair transformed his social interactions:

> As soon as I sat in the wheelchair I was no longer seen as a person who could fend for himself. Although Metz has known me well for nine months, and had never before done anything physical for me without asking, now he took over without permission. Suddenly, in his eyes, I was no longer able to carry things, reach for objects, or even push myself around. Though I was perfectly capable of doing all these things, I was being wheeled around, and things were being brought to me—all without my asking. Most frightening was my own compliance, my alienation from myself and from the process. (p. 52)

As he suggests, the identity of being disabled can itself trigger new expectations and behaviors. This dramatic transformation validated the sensibleness of Zola's earlier attempts to avoid being cast into the role of a disabled person: "I had separated myself early from the physically handicapped by refusing to attend a special residential school. Later, I had simply never socialized with anyone who had a chronic disease or physical handicap. I too had been seeking to gain a different identity through my associations" (Zola, 1982, p. 75).

Distancing oneself from the disabled role is understandable in light of social reactions to disability. However, by doing so, people with disabilities are less likely to develop a positive identity as a disabled person or to engage in social and political action that might ameliorate social prejudice toward disability (Gill, 1997).

Conclusion

This chapter explained how occupation is patterned by habituation. The habits and internalized roles that make up habituation plants people in the familiar territory of everyday life, ready to interact with our physical, temporal, and social ecology. When habituation is challenged by impairments and/or environmental circumstances, people can lose a great deal of what has given life familiarity, consistency, and relative ease. One of the major tasks of living with disability is to reconstruct habits and roles.

Key Terms

Habits: Acquired tendencies to respond automatically and perform in certain consistent ways in familiar environments or situations.

Habituation: Internalized readiness to exhibit consistent patterns of behavior guided by habits and roles and fitted to the characteristics of routine temporal, physical, and social environments.

Internalized role: The incorporation of a socially and/or personally defined status and a related cluster of attitudes and actions.

References

American Psychiatric Association. (2000). *Diagnostic and statistical manual of mental disorders* (4th ed., text revision). Washington, DC: Author.

Asch, A. (1998). Distracted by disability. The "difference" of disability in the medical setting. *Cambridge Quarterly of Healthcare Ethics, 7,* 77–87.

Barris, R., Dickie, V., & Baron, K. (1988). A comparison of psychiatric patients and normal subjects based on the model of human occupation. *Occupational Therapy Journal of Research, 8,* 3–37.

Barris, R., Kielhofner, G., Burch, R. M., Gelinas, I., Klement, M., & Schultz, B. (1986). Occupational function and dysfunction in three groups of adolescents. *Occupational Therapy Journal of Research, 6,* 301–317.

Berger, P. L., & Luckman, T. (1966). *The social construction of reality.* New York: Doubleday/Anchor.

Beutell, N. J., & Greenhaus, J. H. (1983). Integration of home and nonhome roles: Women's conflict and coping behavior. *Journal of Applied Psychology, 68,* 43–48.

Black, M. (1976). The occupational career. *American Journal of Occupational Therapy, 30,* 225–228.

Bogdan, R., & Taylor, S. J. (1989). The social construction of humanness: Relationships with severely disabled people. *Social Problems, 36,* 135–148.

Borell, L., Gustavsson, A., Sandman, P.-O., & Kielhofner, G. (1994). Occupational Programming in a day hospital for patients with dementia. *The Occupational Therapy Journal of Research, 14*(4), 219–238.

Borrero, I. M. (1980). Psychological and emotional impact of unemployment. *Journal of Sociology and Social Welfare, 7,* 916–934.

Bourdieu, P. (1977). *Outline of a theory of practice* (R. Nice, Trans.). London: Cambridge University.

Brandt, E. N., & Pope, A. M. (Eds.). (1997). *Enabling America: Assessing the role of rehabilitation science and engineering.* Washington, DC: National Academy.

Briar, K. H. (1980). Helping the unemployed client. *Journal of Sociology and Social Welfare, 7,* 895–906.

Brim, O. J., & Wheeler, S. (1966). *Socialization after childhood: Two essays.* New York: Wiley.

Camic, C. (1986). The matter of habit. *American Journal of Sociology, 91,* 1039–1087.

Cardwell, J. D. (1971). *Social psychology: A symbolic interaction perspective.* Philadelphia: FA Davis.

Chapin, F. S. (1968). Activity systems and urban structure: A working schema. *Journal of the American Institute of Planners, 34,* 11–18.

Clarke, A. (1997). *Being there: Putting brain, body and world together again.* Cambridge, MA: MIT.

Coser, L. (1974). *Greedy institutions.* New York: Free Press.

DeLoach, C. P., & Greer, B. G. (1981). *Adjustment to severe physical disability: A metamorphosis.* New York: McGraw-Hill.

Dewey, J. (1922). *Human nature and conduct.* New York: Henry Holt.

Dickerson, A. E., & Oakely, F. (1995). Comparing the roles of community-living persons and patient populations. *American Journal of Occupational Therapy, 49,* 221–228.

Ebb, E. W., Coster, W., & Duncombe, L. (1989). Comparison of normal and psychosocially dysfunctional male adolescents. *Occupational Therapy in Mental Health, 9,* 53–74.

Erikson, K. T. (1973). Notes on the sociology of deviance. In H. S. Becker (Ed.), *The other side: Perspectives on deviance.* New York: Free Press.

Fein, M. L. (1990). *Role change: A resocialization perspective.* New York: Praeger.

Gerson, E. M. (1976). On "quality of life." *American Sociological Review, 41,* 793–806.

Gill, C. J. (1997). Four types of integration in disability identity development. *Journal of Vocational Rehabilitation, 9,* 39–46.

Gray, M. (1972). Effects of hospitalization on work-play behavior. *American Journal of Occupational Therapy, 26,* 180–185.

Grossack, M., & Gardner, H. (1970). *Man and men: Social psychology as social science.* Scranton, PA: International Textbook.

Guskin, S. L. (1963). Social psychologies of mental deficiency. In N. R. Ellis (Ed.), *Handbook of mental deficiency.* New York: McGraw-Hill.

Hage, G., & Powers, C. H. (1992). *Post-industrial lives: Roles & relationships in the 21st Century.* Newbury Park, NJ: Sage.

Hahn, H. (1985). Disability policy and the problem of discrimination. *American Behavioral Scientist, 28,* 293–318.

Hahn, H. (1988). Toward a politics of disability: Definitions, disciplines and policies. *Social Science Journal, 22,* 87–105.

Hale, T. W., Hayghe, H. W., & McNeil, J. M. (1998). Persons with disabilities: Labor market activities, 1994. *Monthly Labor Review, 121* (9), 3–12.

Hall, J. M., Stevens, P. E., & Meleis, A. I. (1992). Developing the construct of role integration: A narrative analysis of women clerical workers' daily lives. *Research in Nursing & Health, 15,* 447–457.

Hallet, J., Zasler, N., Maurer, P. & Cash, S. (1994). Role change after traumatic brain injury in adults. *American Journal of Occupational Therapy, 48,* 241–246.

Hammel, J. (1999). The life rope: A transactional approach to exploring worker and life role development. *Work, 12,* 47–60.

Heard, C. (1977). Occupational role acquisition: A perspective on the chronically disabled. *American Journal of Occupational Therapy, 41,* 243–247.

Holzman, P., & Grinker, R. (1974). Schizophrenia in adolescence. *Journal of Youth and Adolescence, 3,* 267–279.

Hull, J. M. (1990). *Touching the rock: An experience of blindness.* New York: Vintage.

James, W. (1950). *The principles of psychology.* New York: Dover.

Jonsson, H., Josephsson, S., & Kielhofner, G. (2001). Narratives and experience in an occupational transition: A longitudinal study of the retirement process. *American Journal of Occupational Therapy, 55,* 424–432.

Katz, D., & Kahn, R. L. (1966). *The social psychology of organizations.* New York: Wiley.

Kielhofner, G. (1979). The temporal dimension in the lives of retarded adults. *American Journal of Occupational Therapy, 33,* 161–168.

Kielhofner, G. (1981). An ethnographic study of deinstitutionalized adults: Their community settings and daily life experiences. *Occupational Therapy Journal of Research, 1,* 125–141.

Kielhofner, G. (1983). "Teaching" retarded adults: Paradoxical effects of a pedagogical enterprise. *Urban Life, 12,* 307–326.

Kielhofner, G., Barris, R., & Watts, J. (1982). Habits and habit dysfunction: A clinical perspective for psychosocial occupational therapy. *Occupational Therapy Mental Health, 2,* 1–22.

Koestler, A. (1969). Beyond atomism and holism: The concept of the holon. In A. Koestler & J. R. Smythies (Eds.), *Beyond reductionism.* Boston: Beacon.

Krefting, L. (1989). Reintegration into the community after head injury: The results of an ethnographic study. *Occupational Therapy Journal of Research, 9,* 67–83.

Louis Harris and Associates. (1998). *Highlights of the N.O.D/Harris 1998 Survey of Americans with Disabilities.* Washington, DC: National Organization on Disability.

Mancuso, J. C., & Sarbin, T. R. (1983). The self-narrative in the enactment of roles. In T. R. Sarbin & K. E. Scheibe (Eds.), *Studies in social identity.* New York: Praeger.

Marks, S. R. (1977). Multiple roles and role strain: Some notes on human energy, time, and commitment. *American Sociological Review, 42,* 921–936.

Mechanic, D. (1980). *Mental health and social policy* (2nd ed.). Englewood Cliffs, NJ: Prentice-Hall.

Melges, F. T. (1982). *Time and inner future: A temporal approach to psychiatric disorders.* New York: Wiley.

Merleau-Ponty, M. (1962). *Phenomenology of perception.* (C. Smith, Trans.). London: Routledge & Kegan Paul. (Original work published 1945.)

McKeen, D. G. (1992). Such a good little patient. *Disability Rag, July/August,* 43.

Miller, D. R. (1983). Self, symptom and social control. In T. R. Sarbin & K. E. Scheibe (Eds.), *Studies in social identity.* New York: Praeger.

Murphy, R. F. (1987). *The body silent.* New York: WW Norton.

National Council on Disability. (1996). *Achieving independence: The challenge for the 21st century.* Washington, DC: Author.

Offer, D., Ostrov, E., & Howard, K. (1981). *The adolescent: A psychological self-report.* New York: Basic Books.

Paap, W. R. (1972). The social reconstruction of reality: The rehabilitation of paraplegics and quadriplegics. *Dissertation Abstracts International, 33,* 45-A. (University Microfilms No. 72-19, 234).

Parsons, T. (1953). Illness and the role of the physician: A sociological perspective. In C. Kluckhohn, H. Murray, & O. Schneider (Eds.), *Personality in nature, society, and culture* (2nd ed.). New York: Alfred A. Knopf.

Pinder, R. (1988). Striking balances: Living with Parkinson's disease. In R. Anderson & M. Bury (Eds.), *Living with chronic illness: The experience of patients and their families.* London: Unwin Hyman.

Robinson, I. (1988). Reconstructing lives: Negotiating the meaning of multiple sclerosis. In R. Anderson & M. Bury (Eds.), *Living with chronic illness: The experience of patients and their families.* London: Unwin Hyman.

Rosow, I. (1976). Status and role change through the life span. In R.H. Binstock and E. Shanas (Eds.), *Handbook of Aging and the Social Sciences.* New York: Van Nostrand Reinhold.

Rowles, G. D. (1991). Beyond performance: Being in place as a component of occupational therapy. *American Journal of Occupational Therapy, 45,* 265–272.

Ruddock, R. (1976). *Roles and relationships.* London: Routledge & Kegan Paul.

Sarbin, T. R., & Scheibe, K. E. (1983). A model of social identity. In T. R. Sarbin & K. E. Scheibe (Eds.), *Studies in social identity.* New York: Praeger.

Schein, E. H. (1971). The individual, the organization, and the career: A conceptual scheme. *Journal of Applied Behavioral Science, 7,* 401–426.

Schiffer, R. B., Rudick, R. A., & Herndon, R. M. (1983). Psychologic aspects of multiple sclerosis. *New York State Journal of Medicine, 3,* 312–316.

Schumacher, K. L. (1995). Family caregiver role acquisition: Role-making through situated interaction. *Scholarly Inquiry for Nursing Practice: An International Journal, 9,* 211–226.

Seamon, D. (1980). Body-subject, time-space routines, and place-ballets. In A. Buttimer & D. Seamon (Eds.), *The hu-*

man experience of space and place. London: Croom Helm.

Seiber, S. D. (1974). Toward a theory of role accumulation. *American Sociological Review, 39*, 567–578.

Shillam, L. L., Beeman, C., & Loshin, P. (1983). Effect of occupational therapy intervention on bathing independence of disabled persons. *American Journal of Occupational Therapy, 37*, 744–748.

Smith, C. A. (1972). Body image changes after myocardial infarction. *Nursing Clinics of North America, 7*, 663–668.

Spreitzer, E., Snyder, E. E., & Larson, D. L. (1979). Multiple roles and psychological well-being. *Social Focus, 12*, 141–148.

Thomas, E. J. (1966). Problems of disability from the perspective of role theory. *Journal of Health and Human Behavior, 7*, 2–14.

Toombs, S. K. (1987). The meaning of illness: A phenomenological approach to the patient-physician relationship. *Journal of Medicine & Philosophy, 12,* (3), 219–240.

Trieschmann, R. B. (1989). Psychosocial adjustment to spinal cord injury. In B. W. Heller, L. M. Flohr, & L. S. Zegans (Eds.), *Psychosocial interventions with physically disabled persons*. New Brunswick, NJ: Rutgers University.

Trupin, L. D., Sebesta, S., Yelin, E., & LaPlante, M. P. (1997). Trends in labor force participation among persons with disabilities, 1993–94. *Disability Statistics Report, 10,* 1–39.

Turner, R. (1962). Role-taking, process versus conformity. In M. Rose (Ed.), *Human behavior and social processes*. Boston: Houghton Mifflin.

Versluys, H. P. (1983). Psychosocial adjustment to physical disability. In C. A. Trombly (Ed.), *Occupational therapy for physical dysfunction* (2nd ed.). Baltimore: Williams & Wilkins.

Werner-Beland, J. A. (Ed.) (1980). *Grief responses to long-term illness and disability*. Reston, VA: Reston.

Williams, R. S. (1984). Ability, disability and rehabilitation: A phenomenological description. *Journal of Medicine and Philosophy, 9*, 93–112.

Wolfensberger, W. (1975). *The origin and nature of our institutional models*. Syracuse, NY: Human Policy.

Young, M. (1988). *The metronomic society: Natural rhythms and human timetables*. Cambridge, MA: Harvard University.

Zola, I. K. (1982). *Missing pieces: A chronicle of living with a disability*. Philadelphia: Temple University.

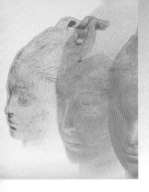

6

Performance Capacity and the Lived Body

- Gary Kielhofner
- Kerstin Tham
- Tal Baz
- Jennifer Hutson

Performance Capacity

The multitude of things people do require them to sense and interpret the world, move their bodies in space, manipulate objects, plan actions, and communicate and interact with others. Even the most ordinary occupation reflects the complex and exquisite organization of the human capacity to perform. As noted in Chapter 2, **performance capacity** is the ability to do things provided by the status of underlying objective physical and mental components and corresponding subjective experience (*Fig. 6.1*). This definition highlights that capacity involves both objective and subjective aspects.

Objective Components of Performance Capacity

Performance depends on musculoskeletal, neurologic, cardiopulmonary, and other body systems. The capacity to perform also depends on cognitive abilities, such as memory. When people do things, they exercise these capacities.

Other conceptual practice models in occupational therapy provide detailed explanations of specific performance capacities. These models address such phenomena as the biomechanics of movement, motor control processes, organization of sensory information, and perceptual and cognitive processes (Bundy, Lane, and Murray, 2002; Katz, 2005; Trombly and Radomski, 2002). Collectively, these models address performance

capacity by objective study of physical (e.g., muscle, bone, nerve, brain) and psychological (e.g., memory, perception, cognition) phenomena. These models explain performance as a function of the status of objective performance capacities. Objective description uses language to name, classify, and measure systems that appraise capacity by systematically observing performance. For example, we can speak about joint range of motion measured in degrees of movement or cognition measured by test scores.

This objective approach is typically coupled with an effort to explain problems of function in terms of disturbances to underlying structures and functions. For instance, limitations of movement might be attributed to loss of muscle strength and damage to joints. Similarly, limitations in problem solving might be attributed to disturbances of attention resulting from brain damage. Such depictions of impairments are important and helpful because the objective understanding of their nature can provide useful cues to how they may be remediated or their negative consequences minimized.

Subjective Approach to Performance Capacity

Objectively describable abilities and limitations of ability are also experienced by those who have them. However, the objective approach generally views these experiences as only consequences of the real problem, which must be appraised from an outsider's detached

FIGURE 6.1 Objective and subjective components of performance capacity.

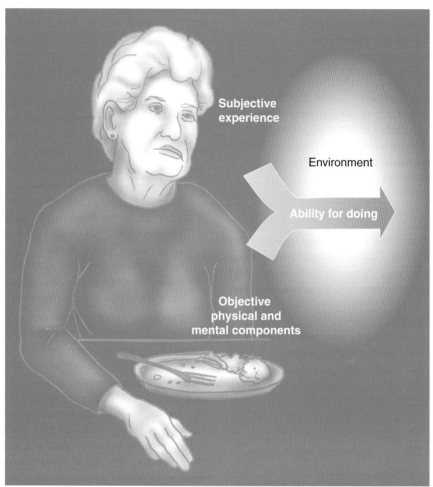

viewpoint. Even when therapists using this approach ask people about their subjective experience, they do so with an eye toward building an objective picture of performance capacity.

Nonetheless, subjective experience also shapes how people perform (Kielhofner, 1995). Paying careful attention to subjective experience in its own right can reveal a great deal about performance capacity and limitations of performance. It can also reveal important information about how to undertake therapy.

Focusing on the subjective aspect of performance capacity is complementary to the traditional objective approach. As shown in *Figure 6.2*, the objective ap-

proach provides a view of performance capacity from the outside, while the approach offered in this chapter provides a view of performance capacity from the inside. Both the observer's objective perspective and the performer's subjective experience have something to tell us about performance capacity. Neither perspective fully accounts for the other. The objective and the subjective are bound together in any instant of performance, and both contribute to the performance.

For example, in moving one's arm to reach out for something, there is both how it is to perform the movement and how the arm moves in space. Both tell something about what is involved in reaching. The objective

> *The objective and the subjective are bound to-*
> *gether in any instant of performance, and both*
> *contribute to the performance.*

approach provides a picture of how muscle contractions generate forces across joints producing degrees of extension and rotation that carry the arm through the trajectory of movement for reaching. The subjective experience tells another story. This chapter is mainly about the nature of that story.

The Lived Body

The concept of the lived body ultimately emanates from the work of the philosopher Merleau-Ponty (1945/1962), whose view of human performance paid careful attention to the nature of experience. He used

FIGURE 6.2 Complementary objective and subjective views of performance.

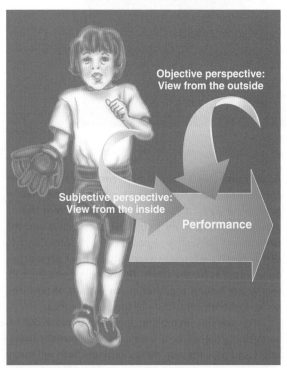

experience as a central concept in explaining how performance was possible. Unlike the objective approach, which describes performance from a detached, objective perspective, he emphasized a phenomenological approach that considered subjective experience as fundamental to understanding human perception, cognition, and action.

Using this phenomenological approach, Leder (1990) employed the term *lived body* to emphasize how we experience, that is, live through our body. He describes the lived body as follows:

> Human experience is incarnated. I receive the surrounding world through my eyes, my ears, my hands.... My legs carry me toward a desired goal seen across the distance. My hands reach out to take up tools.... My actions are motivated by emotions, needs, desires, that well up from a corporeal self. Relations with others are based upon our mutuality of gaze and touch, our speech, our resonances of feeling and perspective. (p. 1)

Following Leder's (1990) utilization, we employ the concept of the **lived body** to refer to the experience of being and knowing the world through a particular body. The concept of the lived body applies both to human embodiment in general and to unique specific forms of embodiment associated with disability.

The lived body concept underscores two fundamental ideas. First, mind and body are seen not as separate phenomena but as part of a single unitary entity—namely, the lived body. Second, subjective experience of performance is not simply an artifact of performing. Rather, it is fundamental to how we perform. That is, in doing things and learning how to do things, we call on not only the objective components that make up performance capacity but also the experience of exercising our capacities. The following sections discuss these two aspects of the lived body.

Mind-Body Unity

The tendency to view body and mind as separate has been a dominant force in Western science and culture. It began with the philosopher Descartes, who observed that the body was an object like other objects in the physical world and therefore subject to the same causal laws (Leder, 1984). According to his classic and influential argument, the workings of the human body should be understood through the same objective methods with which other objects in the physical world can be investigated and understood. The other side of Descartes's philosophical argument was that the mind was immaterial and thus operated according to different, abstract principles. Hence, Cartesian dualism proclaimed that the body and mind represented completely separate realms and that understanding them required radically different approaches.

To cease regarding the body and mind as two separate entities and instead to see them as dual aspects of a single entity is not easy. Dualism is deeply ingrained in our way of thinking. Nonetheless, we can begin to understand mind-body unity by paying attention both to how the body is experienced and how the mind is embodied.

BODILY EXPERIENCE

We can experience our own bodies as objects in the way of Descartes. For example, we can look at our hands just as we gaze at other things in the world. In such looking, our experience is directed to our hands (Leder, 1990). However, this is neither the only nor the dominant way in which we experience our hands. Rather, we routinely experience from our hands that which is outside ourselves.

When we reach into a purse for coins, grasp a door handle, pull on our socks, pat our dog, wave to our friends, or caress our loved ones, we are attending and acting to the world and from our hands. In those instances our hands are subjects, not objects. Our hands are, in these instances, our point of view for reaching, grasping, pulling, patting, waving, and caressing.

Thus, the fundamental difference between experiencing our body as object and as subject goes like this: When I experience some part of my body as an object in the world, I am attending to that body part and am distinguishing between my body and myself. When I am attending to the world from my body, there is no distinction between self and body. As Sartre (1970) noted, one does not just have one's body, one is one's body.

Leder (1990) describes this phenomena in the following way. He notes that when we are doing things, our bodies disappear to us. Our experience is directed to that part of the world with which we are interact-

> *In the course of our daily occupational lives, our bodies are an invisible viewpoint from which we experience and act upon the world.*

ing, and our bodies recede from our awareness. Moreover, our bodies are that from which our attention and action is focused to what is outside us. Thus, in the course of our daily occupational lives, our bodies are an invisible viewpoint from which we experience and act upon the world.

We experience our bodies "as an attitude directed towards a certain existing or possible task" (Merleau-Ponty, 1945/1962, p. 100).

Because of this experience, it can seem that the body is not really part of conscious experience. For example, we experience reading a book as a mental activity, unaware that we are holding it with our hands and seeing it with our eyes. It is the body that is doing the reading.

In everyday life, the body is the taken-for-granted place from which we exist and from which we attend to and act on the world. We may become aware of our bodies as objects when we perceive fatigue or pain and therefore attend to the tired or aching limb. For the most part, however, doing things requires that we attend from our bodies to what we are doing.

Because our bodies are in use much of the time, our experience of our bodies is grounded in doing things. Consequently, we each experience the body as the self that is always taking in the world around us and doing things in that world. Moreover, we experience our body not as "a collection of adjacent organs, but as a synergic system, all the functions of which are exercised and linked together in the general action of being in the world ... " (Merleau-Ponty, 1945/1962, p. 234). For example, when we are walking outside and

> *... we experience our body not as "a collection of adjacent organs, but as a synergic system, all the functions of which are exercised and linked together in the general action of being in the world ... "*

viewing the scenery, we have no separate awareness of the movements of legs and arms in walking or the orientation of our head and eyes in attending to the things around us. When we raise our hand above our eyes to shade the sun, it is simply part of looking, not a separate act by a separate part of the body. We experience all of the parts of the body as a unified whole engaged in the action of walking and looking. Moreover, most of our experience of our bodies is awareness of doing things as a body. We can imagine a walk outside, but it is only a facsimile (and a poor one at that) of feeling the sun on our brow and the ground at our feet, of apprehending the world in the midst of moving around within it. We are most aware when we are bodies in the midst of action.

When we consider the body in this way, we cannot readily separate it from what we call mind. Further, we can see that awareness is not something belonging to a separate mind and imposed on the body. Rather, the body is an intimate part of how we are aware.

Embodied Mind

Whatever else we might attribute to mind, it consists of knowing about things and knowing how to do things. Descartes posited knowledge as what distinguished the mind from the body. However, knowing is seated in the body. We do not mean simply that knowledge is stored or processed biochemically in the brain. Rather, we mean that the whole of the body is the way we apprehend and thus know how to do things. The body is the existential medium of knowing.

Knowing Things

What we know about the world around us begins with our body looking at, touching, and probing the world (Merleau-Ponty, 1945/1962).

Abstract properties we attribute to various objects in the world echo how our body experiences those objects. For example:

> How do I know that the ball is spherical, solid, and leathery? My moving, throwing and pressing hands reveal these properties ... [that] do not exist solely in the ball and not at all in my hands. It is only when my hands touch the ball that these properties are revealed to me. (Engelbrecht, 1968, p.12)

Sartre (1970) elaborates this notion in the following example of how bodily action gives us an experience of the world: "We never have any sensation of our effort.... We perceive the resistance of things. What I perceive when I want to lift this glass to my mouth is not my effort but the heaviness of the glass" (p. 231).

When we do things, we generate bodily experiences of the world that we come to interpret as properties of that world. Nevertheless, the world we know is always on the other end of something we are doing with our bodies.

Perception is not simply the registration and evaluation of sense data, but rather an active taking hold of the world. When we perceive objects and their characteristics, the foundation of our knowing them always has to do with how our bodies encounter and engage them. Once again, we are speaking here not of the objective ways sensory data are taken in by sensory organs and networked through the central nervous system. Instead, we are referring to the body as a way of generating experience in response to its own questions posed as forms of acting toward and in the world. What the mind asks of the world and the answers that make up the mind's accumulated knowledge are asked, in large measure, through bodily action.

Even abstract knowledge grows out of bodily experiences. For example, only by using the body to do things—touching, grasping, lifting, shoving, observing, and listening to the world—do we gain access to experiences that give meaning to concepts of distance, direction, temporality, clarity, resistance, resilience, and obscurity (Leder, 1990; Merleau-Ponty, 1945/1962;

> *Abstract properties we attribute to various objects in the world echo how our body experiences those objects.*

> *Perception is not simply the registration and evaluation of sense data, but rather an active taking hold of the world.*

Sudnow, 1979). Thought itself builds on what the body does and experiences. As Sudnow (1979) argues:

> When I sit before the piano keyboard, I am directly aligned to its center…. I sit down and there I am, as exactly middled as before the dinner plate, the steering wheel, the bathroom faucets—before whatever action moves out from the center. Dividing in half all the body's ways, is part of the calculus, topography, trigonometry, and algebra that my body does…. Mathematics is perhaps the purest form of human thought, not because its pictures struggle toward a perfect concept of nature, but because its pictures have their origin in the ways of the body … (p. 79)

The structure and content of mental operations are always based on the body's way of comprehending the world. As Leder (1990) notes, abstract cognition "may sublimate but never fully escapes its inherence in a perceiving, active body" (p. 7).

Knowing How To Do Things

When typing or playing the piano, one's fingers instinctively know where to go for the right letter or note (Sudnow, 1979). For example, the most efficient strategy for locating the H key on a computer keyboard is to begin to type a word beginning with that letter. Without consciously thinking about its location, the right index finger will begin to move to the center right of the keyboard, to the H key. What is also notable in this and other instances of bodily knowing is that the body instinctively knows which part of itself should perform any action.

Our bodies readily perform all manner of things that we cannot readily describe how to do. Imagine doing any ordinary action such as a dance step, a swim stroke, whistling a tune, or tying a shoe. Describing the action only gives us a vague trace of what it is. We must typically watch our bodies do things to notice exactly what we are doing. Compare thinking about how to tie a shoe to actually tying the shoe to see how much the knowing is in the body.

Subjective Experience and Performance

As noted previously, every action we perform is objectively describable. It can be divided into so much flex-

ion, extension, or rotation at joints. It can be described in terms of the trajectory, speed, and the efficiency with which movement is accomplished.

Such bodily action is known differently from within. When we reach for a cup of coffee, open a door, walk to the bus, or drive a car, we do not objectively know or do the movements involved. Instead, we are inside the movements and experience them from that vantage point. Consequently, when we use our bodies to do things, we aim for the subjective experience of doing them. Indeed, we cannot fully attend to the objective features of our performance without disrupting it. For example, if we concentrate too much on how to move our hands in tying our shoes, we will interrupt our performance.

When learning to do something, we may at first aim for the objective movements. For example, when learning to hold silverware or chopsticks, we first attend to how they are placed in the hand and how the fingers should be positioned. But learning to do something means that we must grasp the experience—learn how it feels.

Most of us also recall that when learning to ride a bicycle, roller skate, ski, or any other skilled form of doing, we began with a sense of what was objectively involved and ended up learning what the right movement felt like. Once we have grasped the feeling of how it is to do something, repeating the performance is altogether different. After that feeling is achieved, we no longer pay attention to the objective aspects of doing the action. Rather, we focus on the experience and use it as our guide to performing. As Sudnow (1978) describes it, "When one first gets the knack of a complex skill … the hang of it has been glimpsed … the experience is tasted. All prior ways of being seem thoroughly lacking, and the new way is encountered with a `this is it' feeling, almost as a revelation" (p. 83).

Being inside any performance allows us to assess it in a uniquely subjective way (Clark, 1993). When we are about to reach somewhere or step somewhere, we appraise the kind of getting there that the distance en-

> *Learning to do something means that we must grasp the experience—learn how it feels.*

> We aim toward the experience of a performance, not the objective features of performance.

tails. In moving our bodies, we do not estimate distances as so much objective distance to be traversed but rather as so much traveling to do.

We aim toward the experience of a performance, not the objective features of performance. Consequently, learning to perform involves finding the right experience, and performance involves aiming for that experience.

The Lived Body in Perspective

Although a great deal of objective knowledge about performance capacity has been generated, the subjective experience of performance has been largely neglected. The previous section highlighted subjective experience of the lived body. The discussion covered two important themes. First, physical and mental aspects of performance do not represent separate realms. Both moving one's body to accomplish a task and planning the steps in the task are functions of a lived body that is at once both physical and mental. Second, the nature of subjective experience and its role in performance were examined. It was argued that experience is not simply an artifact or consequence of doing but rather that experience is central to how we manage to perform. To learn any performance, we must find the experience of it—how it feels. To do any performance we are guided not by the objective features of what is involved but by how it feels to do it. Understanding both performance and limitations of performance requires attention to these features of the lived body.

Disability and the Lived Body

Although there is little systematic study of the embodied experience of disability, a number of writers who have disabilities have offered important insights to their experiences. Toombs (1992), who has multiple sclerosis, reminds us that a particular experience goes with a disability. It is often radically different from experience in a nondisabled state. She notes that with a

physical impairment, "My attention is focused on my hand as hand. I must observe how it is that my fingers grasp the handle of the cup and I am conscious of my hand's unaccustomed ineffectiveness as an instrument of my action. In illness the body intrudes itself into experience" (p. 71).

Zasetsky describes the challenges of trying to write following his traumatic brain injury:

> I didn't have enough of a vocabulary or mind left to write well…. I'd spend ages hunting for the right words. I had to remember and turn up words that were are at least fairly similar or close enough to what I wanted to say. But after I'd put together these second choices, I still wasn't able to start writing until I figured out how to compose a sentence. (in Luria, 1972, pp. 78–79)

Others write about how the world is transformed. For example, Sechehaye (1968) describes her experience of schizophrenia as transforming the world into a place where there:

> reigned an implacable light, blinding, leaving no place for shadow; an immense place without boundary, limitless, flat; a mineral, lunar country, cold as the wastes of the North Pole. In this stretching emptiness, all is unchangeable, immobile, congealed, crystallized. Objects are strange trappings, placed here and there, geometric cubes without meaning. (p. 44)

Similarly, Williams (1994) describes how her experiences as a child with autism placed her in a extraordinary world: "I discovered the air was full of spots. If you looked into nothingness, there were spots. People would walk by, obstructing my magical view of nothingness. I'd move past them" (p. 3).

Others have written about the alteration of experiences that comes with medical treatments. For example, Jamison (1995) describes living with the consequences of taking lithium necessary to control her bipolar illness. In addition to feeling "less lively, less energetic, less high spirited" (p. 92) she also found that some of her ability to read was impaired: "I had to read the same lines repeatedly and take copious notes before I could comprehend the meaning. Even so, what I read often disappeared from my mind like snow on a hot pavement" (p. 95).

Such testimonies from persons with various impairments offer important windows into the experience of limitations or alterations of capacity. Systematic descriptions of the experience of impairments and the course of change over time also have the potential to offer us new ways of understanding and intervening. In what follows, we examine this potential more closely.

Understanding Transformations in the Lived Body

Collectively, we have undertaken three studies to examine the experience of the lived body among persons with disabilities. Each focuses on these factors:

- Nature of the experience
- Contribution of experience to disability
- Evolution of experience over time
- Role of experience in changes in performance capacity

The following sections briefly describe the findings from the three studies. Following this is a discussion of their implications for better understanding the nature of experience in disability and how experience can be used in the therapeutic process.

Recapturing Half of Self and the World

Brain damage often significantly alters experience. One of the more dramatic alterations is unilateral neglect following cerebrovascular accident. Objectively, persons with unilateral neglect are unable to orient their attention toward the left hemispace and are often unaware of the left half of their body (Bisiach & Vallar, 1988).

A study of four Swedish women with unilateral neglect (Tham, Borell, & Gustavsson, 2000) described the unfolding of lived body experiences as they lost and then slowly began to recapture half of themselves and their world. Many are oblivious to their neglect (McGlynn & Schacter, 1989; Tham, Borell, & Gustavsson, 2000). The following are highlights of their discoveries.

Initially, the left half of the women's world did not exist for them. They lived and acted only in the remaining right half of the world, with no sense that the left half of the world had disappeared. Rather, they experienced their half-world as complete.

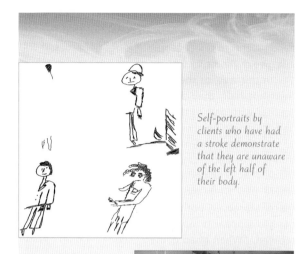
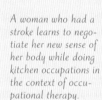

Self-portraits by clients who have had a stroke demonstrate that they are unaware of the left half of their body.

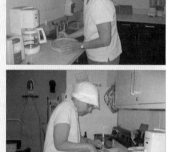

A woman who had a stroke learns to negotiate her new sense of her body while doing kitchen occupations in the context of occupational therapy.

Only with time, as the women began to perform previously familiar tasks, did they begin to sense something vaguely unfamiliar. Their bodies, and their perceptions of space and time, felt oddly different.

As they encountered the left half of the body, it didn't feel as though it belonged to them. Each woman's arm and leg simply didn't seem like part of the self. They felt instead like objects apart from the self. One woman reported that she had to trace her left arm with her right hand to the shoulder to realize that it was really attached to her. Another woman, referring to her hand placed on the table in front of her, said her fingers seemed to her like five sausages just lying there. All four women spoke about the left side of the body in the third person, characterizing it as estranged and cold. One woman lamented that her left hand "wants to reject people. It is not generous. It will just give chilliness."

In this way, as the women first became aware of their left half, they did not experience it as an encounter with part of the self. Rather they saw the left half as something alien, not belonging to them.

As these women began to move about and do things, they also found that they were disoriented to space. They repeatedly found that they did not know where they were and could not orient themselves in space. Moreover, both people and objects could suddenly disappear or appear. For example, one woman recalled, "When I had dinner, I suddenly didn't know where my husband went. He just disappeared."

They also found that they could no longer rely on previously automatic ways of doing things. While they were still unaware of their neglect at this point, they could discern its consequences. They found these consequences of neglect confusing and could not fathom why they had problems in performing certain tasks. They could not link their problems of performance to the neglect, since it did not yet exist for them.

Over time, they began to recognize familiar problems in performance, though they still did not comprehend that they were missing half the world. Bumping into things with their wheelchair was a common problem. While they couldn't perceive what was happening on their left side, they could perceive certain features of the collision, such as the crashing sound and the sudden stopping of the wheelchair.

As such neglect-related experiences accumulated, they began to reflect upon them, searching for explanations for these difficulties. At first, their explanations were still not grounded in neglect. For instance, they attributed their inability to find objects to unfamiliarity with the rehabilitation environment, expecting to find it much easier to locate objects at home. At this point, they could not consciously use any strategies to compensate for their neglect, since they were unaware of their unawareness of the left half of the surrounding world.

As they regained movement in their left side, the sense of that side as belonging to the self began to return. Because improvements in mobility occurred first in the legs, the four women first felt that their left leg

mostly belonged to them, although alienation of the left arm persisted.

Despite its continued estrangement, they began to feel a responsibility to the arm. One women described the experience like this:

> I have to accept it, because it is sitting here on my body. All the time when I am doing something I have to think of it, and to bring it with me. It is like I am carrying a baby all the time, a baby you can't leave on a table and then go your way. You have to bring it with you. You can't forget your hand because everything can go wrong if you do that. Instead, you bring your baby and it is the same with your hand, you can't ignore the hand, because you have it, and in the future you will need it.

While the women began to own responsibility for the left arm, they still did not own it as a part of themselves. This was highlighted by the fact that they could lose the left side of the body, as one woman noted:

> Always when I am going to bed I think that I need a pillow for my arm and if the arm is not lying there, I get scared to death. I think something is wrong because I must always have my arm with me. If I don't have that, it will become swollen. If I can't find my arm, I use the alarm to call someone and ask, 'can you find my bad arm?' And, of course, they always can.

At this point, before they could actually use it, the left hand began to reemerge as a point of view for doing things. As one woman said:

> Suddenly I forget that I can't use my left hand, especially when I am eating. For example if I find some crumbs at the table, beside my plate, I want to clean them up and to put them together. So I try to put the crumbs in my left hand, even if I know that I can't use it.

Such regaining of intentionality in the neglected side was also reflected in their beginning efforts to incorporate the left body parts in their daily life.

Next, they began to comprehend that they were missing the left half of the environment. The understanding was objective, however, and they still did not have any direct experience of this limitation. Importantly, this realization came about as others (therapists, nurses, family members, aides) told them about their neglect, explained how problems were related to neglect, or demonstrated that there were objects to the left by coaching them to search there. Thus, for these women, neglect was first understood as an objective fact, related to them by others.

Armed with this objective knowledge of their neglect and its consequences, they wanted to improve their ability to find objects and to orient to the left half of the environment. The four women gradually became more and more able to use conscious strategies to perform better by compensating for their unilateral neglect.

There appeared to emerge for each woman a kind of existential pull from the left, when objects there were part of an occupation in which they were engaged or when circumstances on their left needed their attention. For example, one woman, while working in the kitchen, suddenly saw the toaster on her left side when she noticed that its electrical cord was hanging over the sink. She noted, "I could see the electrical cord to the left because I know it is unsafe to have it over the sink. The electricity can short, and that is dangerous."

They could also more readily locate objects that they knew should be present. One woman described searching for lotion and toothpaste in her dressing case: "I look and I look. At first I can't see the things but I know that they should be there. Then I move my eyes and I turn my head so I really can see everything because I know that the things should be there."

Increasingly, the women developed a way of reasoning that considered how things should be so that they could compare it with what they perceived. This proved effective in overcoming some problems posed by the neglect. One woman noted:

> Sometimes when I am eating I think, but God, didn't I get the fish? They told us that we should be served fish today. But of course, it is placed on the left side of the plate, I think. So I begin to search to the left, and then I can see it.

Sometimes they were able to anticipate problems caused by the neglect and use a strategy to avoid them. For example, one woman surveyed and memorized any new environment before she began to move around with the wheelchair. She could use her mental map to avoid crashing into objects that she would not see once she was moving along.

By 5 months after their strokes, the four women had accumulated substantial experience using such conscious compensatory strategies. Their understanding and awareness of their neglect became deeper, and their compensatory strategies became habitual.

Thus, while they still did not naturally have access to the left half of the world, they were aware that it existed outside of their immediate experience. They began to spontaneously remember to access this world. They used a number of strategies for gaining access to what was present or going on in the left half of the world. They would, for instance, use sounds that came from the left. They would search to the left by reaching and feeling for things. Finally they could actively visually search to the left. As one woman put it: "Look to the left, look to the left, I tell myself, and then when I look to the left, I can find the thing that I am looking for."

In the end, the left half of the world existed for them, but not as before their cerebrovascular accidents. It was not an immediate presence like the rest of the world. It was a hidden place that had consequences for action, where things resided unseen. Through special efforts, objects in the left half of the world could be found and its arrangement, although unseen, could be imagined. Thus, they regained the lost half of the world in pragmatic terms, although it was forever lost to them in immediate experience.

Learning to Cycle: A Therapeutic Passage to Embodiment

Tom was a 10-year-old boy diagnosed with a regulatory disorder (i.e., difficulty in regulating his behavior and his sensory, attentional, motor, and affective processes) and somatosensory dyspraxia (i.e., difficulty formulating a plan of action necessary to sequencing and carrying out skilled motor acts). Through observation and interviews, Baz (1998) documented Tom's experience of disability and change over eight weekly therapy sessions that are characterized in what follows.

While Tom was a bright boy with age-appropriate fine motor skills, he had extreme difficulties moving his body about in space and dealing with moving objects. His favorite occupations were reading and playing on the computer. He called these "brain things." When engaged in these activities, Tom could be static (sitting) and the focus of his attention within a specific, stable frame of acting.

According to his mother, "[Tom] has a lot of fears … he's afraid of a lot of things…. He's scared to death about learning to ride a bike because he [fears he] will fall and hurt himself … and he's had nightmares about it."

Similarly, his occupational therapist notes, "He's got these fears. They're really big in his head. They feel really scary to him and he doesn't seem to be able to meet those fears."

As his mother and therapist attest, Tom's awareness of his body and of the world was dominated by fear. This fear was not only a feeling Tom had about his body; rather, it was a way of being in his body. He experienced himself as a fragile, disjointed collection of bodily parts that did not behave as a whole. Further, he could have the frightening sensation of his physical self literally coming apart.

Tom's disjointed experience of self extended to his distinction between thought and action. When he described doing ordinary things involving thinking and acting, as in the following playground vignette, he separated mind and body, objectifying his body movements: "If you want to go down the slide but the slide's dirty … you gotta think what to do with the slide. Usually what I think is, 'clean the slide,' so I use my arm muscles to move the … dirt or slimy worm, or ants around with the small towel thing."

In another incident, Tom was scratching himself when someone remarked that it might be due to dry skin. He responded, "Well, I think that's why my brain is telling me to itch that." His language for describing himself and his actions is one of discontinuity—among parts of the self and between the self and the world.

Not surprisingly Tom felt alienated from his body. He was not at home in it. His body was not really his thing through which to live. To an unusual extent, he attended to his body rather than from it. For example, his therapist noted:

> He has a tendency to keep his visual field down and low … looking at his hands and feet … as opposed to looking where he is going…. When attending to his body as an object, Tom loses awareness of objects in the world and loses his way in the flow of action.

Ill at ease with his body, Tom encountered things in the world with an underlying attitude of fearfulness. For Tom, fear was woven into his mode of perception. Rather than apprehending, he was apprehensive. Accordingly, things in the world often appeared to him as faceless. Tom did not recognize possibilities for action in them. For instance, when Tom saw an object that he had never seen before, he found it hard to imagine what it would feel like to touch, hold, or manipulate it. He found it difficult to translate his vision to his touch. He could not envision the potential that an object held for action.

Sounds, textures, and sights faded into one amorphous, meaningless background, or they threateningly leaped out of the world. For Tom, the world could be a large abyss. Moving into it was often like stepping into thin air. Moreover, Tom's world could be downright assaulting, with he, its easy victim.

Therefore, Tom often tried to avoid the world. He often did this two ways. First he assumed a disembodied, reflective mode of perception. Not surprisingly, Tom's primary mode of relating to the world was visual. Vision is the sense considered to be closest in nature to intellect (Leder, 1990). By intellectualizing a visual image of the world, Tom was sometimes able to keep it at bay. Second, he would create a mini-world immediately in front of himself where he could engage in well-controlled fine motor actions. To do this Tom became so totally absorbed in his visual analysis and fine motor action that he was unable to respond to other events in the world. Tom's mother recalls:

> I thought he was deaf because he would concentrate so thoroughly on his play with construction toys. I mean, he would build amazing things, but a train could go through the living room and he would not react to it, and certainly not to human voices. Yeah, and it was hard to get him to establish eye contact. Whenever I was feeding him, I would work very hard to sing and be very animated and everything was always bigger and grander to engage him more.

Things were still much the same. For example, Tom describes how it was for him when his brother entered the room during his visual fixation on a toy train: "When Ray came in for a little while, I kind of ignored him, like my eyes were like glued to what I was doing.... I was like, [I] couldn't hear him. And I couldn't understand his thoughts because I couldn't see him."

Tom approached the world analytically, focusing on facts. Unfortunately, facts by themselves do not hold a potential for action. It is not surprising that while Tom readily acquired encyclopedic knowledge about the world, learning a new motor skill for moving about in the world was an arduous process for him.

He approached each new motor task logically and visually. However, he could not do it in his body. Rather, he tended to overconcentrate. He would dart his attention back and forth between the world and his body, trying to direct his action from a disembodied vantage point. When the exigencies of doing a dynamic motor act called for Tom to be in his body as an actor, he faltered, as described by his therapist:

Ask him to walk across a balance beam or to run and kick a ball or anything that has to do with propelling himself and being the agent of action where he's the doer … [he falls apart]. I think it's the idea of him carrying himself and being competent alone and by himself as a physical unit that he hasn't quite gotten.

As the therapist notes, the feeling of being fully within and in control of his body was beyond Tom's experiential grasp at the time.

Despite all this, Tom wanted to learn to ride his bicycle like others his age. When his therapist joined him at home for a first attempt, Tom clutched the bike, feeling it melt out of control in his hands. Throwing it to the ground, he stomped off. Afterward, just thinking about riding the bicycle triggered overwhelming fear. About subsequent attempts on the bike, his therapist notes: "He gets on that thing and just goes limp, he's not doing anything to be active on the bike … he literally falls into me rather than uses his own body to catch himself ."

Underlying Tom's surrender was a lack of knowing how to search for experience. For example, when his therapist demonstrated riding a bicycle, Tom noted that it gave him "no clue about how it would feel to me." When making his feeble attempts at riding, he was in his usual mode of apprehensiveness and intellectualizing that distanced him from being open to bodily experience. As his therapist notes:

It's hard for him to coordinate all the aspects of this [bike riding], the visual part, the postural part, the hand movements and the foot movements all together…. He's really concentrating…. Tom often overconcentrates until he loses the integrity and the flow of the action. He overanalyzes it and then he doesn't have any flow.

Hence for Tom, the bicycle and the prospect of riding it alternately floats obscurely in shadows or looms menacingly.

Claiming His Body

An important step in Tom's transformation took place in the following therapeutic session. According to his therapist, Tom came in the room "melting to the ground." He was unresponsive and avoided eye contact. The therapist had to call his name repeatedly before Tom responded. Tom was feeling ill at ease and retreating from the world into his disembodied visual-intellectual mode. Initially, his therapist's entreaties were a discomfort and a nuisance. Sensing his experience, the therapist invited him to engage in a sequence of gross motor activities that began with jumping on a trampoline and continued with a series of interactions between Tom and her. According to both Tom and the therapist, this activity was a turning point. Here is what happened.

Jumping up and down on the trampoline immediately engaged Tom's entire body in a rapid movement in which he could neither visually fixate nor retreat into his disembodied mode. He was thus shepherded into abandoning his typical objectification of his body. For the duration of jumping, Tom had to act from his body to the routine of jumping. Moreover, the jumping prompted Tom to feel his body as a unified whole. He began to be at home with himself.

At the same time, Tom's slightest movements were immediately echoed by the trampoline. Moreover, the trampoline moved him in response to his movements. Within this dynamic, the world was taking hold of his body and moving him, but doing so in direct response to his actions. This echo of movement also served to abet and attune Tom to his moving. Moreover, because the trampoline resonated with Tom's movements, the boundary between inside and outside faded. They became part of a unitary experience. Additionally, the dynamic of the trampoline presented Tom with a specific rhythm so that he was invited to go along with the natural frequency of the trampoline. Jumping on the trampoline opened for Tom a very immediate way of attuning himself to the world and reciprocating with it. For Tom, the trampoline had the exact characteristics to invite him toward something that had always remained just outside his experiential grasp. It allowed him to begin to glimpse a new way of being in his body and in his world. Tom began to live his body in a new way.

Next, the therapist introduced tossing a basketball that Tom was to catch and toss into a basket while still jumping on the trampoline. As if by magic, Tom saw the oncoming ball not as a threat but as an invitation to act. In his state of attending to the world from his body he was able to apprehend the ball's trajectory and catch it. Later he had the same experience with juggling beanbags. Notably, the therapist was able to sense Tom's readiness to catch and toss and found the rhythm that enabled him to do so.

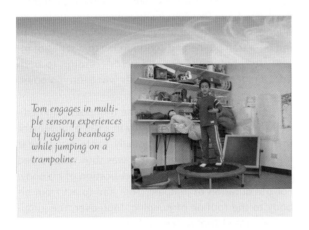

Tom engages in multiple sensory experiences by juggling beanbags while jumping on a trampoline.

In the midst of these experiences Tom's action evolved as follows. Initially Tom's movements were very rigid and constricted. His knees were unbent and locked. His hands hung stiffly alongside his body. His mouth was nearly motionless when he talked, and his intonation was flat. He held his breath in anxiety. He looked away from the therapist.

Gradually, while jumping on the trampoline, his movements became more fluid. His breathing became more rhythmic. His face began to show expression. His intonations grew richer. His language was more and more interactive. He made eye contact with the therapist. Tom's fearful stance turned into one of involvement. He did not wince or fall apart when the ball was thrown to him and even tolerated being occasionally bombarded with beanbags. His eye-hand coordination and timing in catching and throwing steadily improved. He began to take risks in how he moved. He became more humorous and playful.

After the session Tom noted his own surprise at being able to try something new:

> [The therapist got me] from something that I did know about [basketball] to something that I didn't know about [juggling].... I was surprised because before I was afraid to juggle and I was like no, I couldn't do it, but she got me to juggle and now I know that practice makes perfect.

In a later session, when Tom again attempted riding the bicycle, his therapist noted the following changes:

> I was having to do less work. He was doing more. And although he was leaning, it was not as much ... last week I felt like a training wheel. He was just leaning on me like he would lean on a training wheel and I was correcting him out of that, but today ... I could feel him balancing and then leaning more at the end of the motion.

Within a couple of weeks, Tom mastered riding his bicycle. More important, a deeper transformation took place. Tom was beginning to inhabit his body and his world in a new way.

The "Hand and Me," Then "We"

Curtis, a 42-year-old African American, worked for a catering company and routinely clocked more than 40 hours a week. Curtis threw himself into his work, believing that "you should be able to go as far and do as much in anything that you think you want to do." His work was mostly hands on. Of himself, he says, "Um, I'm pretty good with figuring things out ... if you just sit back and think about it for a minute ... it only takes common sense. So, add a little common sense with a little intelligence, What you got? A person that can figure out problems" (Curtis, 7/13/98, first audiotaped interview).

When problems developed at work, Curtis would jump in and solve the problem. He particularly enjoyed accomplishing tasks and solving problems that required using his hands.

One weekend, while replacing the floorboards on his work truck, Curtis lacerated his left hand with a power saw. The cut was so severe that the third, fourth, and fifth digits were almost completely severed. Alone at the time of injury, he explains:

> [I] grabbed a towel, wrapped my hand up, then got some duct tape and taped it up around the towel. Then I went in the house, got my wallet with my insurance card, got my I.D., got my keys, locked the door … moved the stuff out from under the garage door opener because the door wouldn't come down … let the garage door down, got in the truck and drove myself to [the hospital].

In 17 hours of surgery his fingers were successfully reattached. Based on interviews over 2 months, Hutson (1998) chronicled changes in Curtis's embodiment that occurred as a result of his hand amputation and reattachment.

In the days after surgery, Curtis could not move his hand. He felt suddenly plucked out of his usual mode of being, as his hand was no longer available as an immediate and reliable resource for doing things. Just as important as the inability to move his fingers was that he could no longer do many things that used to be automatic:

> "I couldn't do things, and I'm not that type. These [hands] are … these here's my life, right. Without these [hands] I was … so mad and crazy."

In addition to its no longer being available as a potential for action, Curtis noted that the reattached hand:

> Don't feel like a hand. It's hard to describe how it feel. You know how when you crush your fingertip and it gets black at the nail, you know how it throbs. It feels like that. Or, it don't feel like nothin' at all. Nothin'. Or sometimes it's all tingly.

Not only did he find the sensation of the hand different, but Curtis also felt that his hand was no longer part of himself:

> I don't know. I don't consider, for some … for some strange reason I, it, two thing. I think of it as two things now. It's me and the hand. It's not just

me. It's me and the hand. Uh, why I don't know. Well I don't even know how I came up with that but I guess ever since I been, ever since the accident it's been me and the hand.

Later, as Curtis began to be able to move his hand, his relationship to it changed, but it was still not the same as before. He shifted from using the phrase *me and the hand* to *we*. Curtis explains his new use of *we*:

> I guess because I'm gonna have to do it, but the hand gonna have to perform it, I would assume. And if the hand don't perform it then it's just me. But, when the hand start movin', I said we did it. I didn't say I did it. We did it, because the hand still had to move. So ever since then it's been we…. It's always gonna be we.

His language clearly illustrates that while Curtis' hand was reattached and partly functional, it was not part of the self, as it had been before. His distinction between the self that would do and the hand that would perform underscores the separation of the hand that moves from the self that intends the motion. Nonetheless, unlike the nonfunctional hand that was simply not part of himself, he had formed an unusual partnership with the new performing hand.

What kept his hand from being part of the self despite his growing ability to move it in a functional way was that he still attended to the hand instead of from it. This also created practical problems in how he completed tasks. Because Curtis could not use the hand as an automatic point of view for doing things, he had to monitor the hand's action and any objects it held:

> So, I have to squeeze [something I hold] tight enough where I can feel it in my hand because if I don't, it'll just [slip out], and it takes a lot of concentration…. I pick something up with this hand. I have to keep my eye on what I have in this hand. If I take my mind and go someplace else with it, it'll just slip because I won't feel it. It's kind of hard actually. I try to do a lot with it but it's awful hard because you, you have to concentrate too much on this one thing. And you know, like it should be, it's not automatic like what I'm doing right now [with the right hand]. I can still talk to you and hold this cup at the same time. With this left hand I can't do that.

Because Curtis was not able to act from his left hand, many two-handed tasks took too much attention for ease in everyday performance. So while his left hand had objectively regained functional movement, he initially preferred not to use it in routine activities. Instead he learned to do things with his right hand alone:

> I had to learn how to button up my shirt with one hand. But it have to be short sleeve shirt, 'cause I can't button this up right here [referring to the right cuff] I can't do that. I can do this one with this hand [pointing to left cuff] and these right here [front buttons] but I can't do this one [right cuff]. It wasn't difficult, but in a way it was because of the way that, well you know that men are used to buttoning up the sleeve with one hand anyway. So, it, the point of it was I couldn't grab it and get it over. I just had to keep practicing to get it. But now, it's easy.

As Curtis describes it, after an initial period of clumsiness, he mastered and thus achieved ease in putting on his shirt with one hand. This ease was something he could not achieve when the left hand was incorporated into anything he did.

The left hand was uneasy when doing things, and it also needed tending. He had to consciously monitor its involvement in any activity and to make sure it was not exposed to danger. Consequently, it was easier to leave it out of doing things. For a while this is how things were.

After several weeks Curtis approached his occupational therapist about returning to work because he was tired of sitting at home. The therapist, in consultation with the surgeon, determined that Curtis could return to work on light duty. He was instructed to avoid hot and cold and not to lift anything over 15 pounds using the left hand.

Because of his excellent work history, the employer invited Curtis to return to work full-time as the supervisor with responsibility of organizing and managing other workers. Although the new role was actually a promotion, Curtis did not see it positively. For him, doing things with his hands was essential to his satisfaction. Indicating his hands, he notes, "I like to do things with this." Consequently, Curtis experienced much of his new job as still "doin' nothin'." He

explains, "Because I really don't do nothin'. I don't do much. Just driving. I do a lot of deliveries, box lunches, 'cause I do deliver a lot of lunches and a lot of dinners. Mostly driving, but I don't do."

Because he was not much of a paper pusher, Curtis, by his own admission, began to engage in two-handed tasks he "had no business doin'." Despite his recognition of possible danger to his hand and the cumbersome process of having to concentrate on his left hand whenever he used it, he nonetheless began to feel an irresistible urge to use his injured hand at work:

> I have to do things. Okay, uh it's just like telling a new born baby when he gets up and starts to walking and you tell him no, he can't walk. Uh, you holding him down instead of letting him go and explore the world. That is what I'm gonna have to do anyway with this [left] hand, is explore and find. And I'm gonna have to learn how to compensate for things I can't do to come up with a way of doing it anyhow.

Curtis had the growing feeling that if he did not make use of the hand he might as well "just sit around and let the hand die," in which case it would have been better to "just cut the hand on off." Thus, while his injured hand still offered Curtis no experience of operating from it to the world, he nevertheless began to feel a call to involve the hand in doing.

While Curtis still could not experience the hand as part of his intentional self, he decided to breathe a kind of life into the hand by making it part of his doing things.

His final assessment was that "it's always gonna be we." Clearly, he does not expect the hand to become fully part of himself as before. Nonetheless, his references to the hand as a baby worthy of life, needing soothing and the opportunity to explore and grow, suggests that he has found in the metaphor of parent and child a way to exist with this hand. The hand is not fully part of himself but adopted as part of a new "we."

Discussion

These three studies systematically examine the lived body experience. These studies illuminate both the nature of disability experience and the role of experience in how persons manage to overcome or adapt to their impairments.

Disability Experience

Disability always is a particular way of being embodied. This is an altered way of existing that thrusts itself on the person with a disability. Hence, persons with disabilities must live the reality of their embodiment. Moreover, they are challenged to adapt to their experiences. Any change in capacity must often be in terms of those experiences. As Csordas (1994) reminds us, people with disabilities must take up an existential position in the world that reflects their particular embodiment.

Apparently some phenomena are more general to the disability experience and others are particular to a type of impairment. Still others are unique to the individual. For example, all of the subjects in the studies we examined experienced some form of alienation from their bodies or parts of their bodies. Both Murphy (1987) and Sachs (1993) have also described the experience of disability as including alienation from one's own body.

While alienation involves the common feature of not experiencing the body or some part of the body as belonging to the self, the particular experience of alienation varied. For the women with neglect, there was at one stage disbelief that their left side was attached to the rest of them. For Curtis, his hand was clearly attached to his body, but it no longer felt like part of his intentional self. For Tom there was an element of never having fully owned his body or experienced it as a whole.

Despite these differences, all of the subjects had to find ways of coming to terms with this alienation. Tom was able to achieve ownership and integration of his body; the women regained the sense of acting from their left side. Curtis continued to experience his hand as separate from self but decided in the end to bring it into his routine way of doing things. These findings suggest that coming to terms with bodily alienation may be an important task in regaining capacity for a range of persons with disabilities.

Understanding disability in terms of subjective experience is important because it often explains aspects of a person's functional capacity not accounted for in objective approaches. Curtis exemplifies how an objective description of his performance capacity could not fully account for his performance. Whereas part of his performance capacity is reflected in his objectively describable ability to move his hand, how he experienced his hand was equally important to his functional capacity. Curtis's ability to use his hand cannot be described fully from an objective viewpoint alone.

Consequently, we see that how people perform does not only reflect the objective status of performance components. It also emanates from how they experience themselves and their worlds. Altered experience alters performance.

Importance of Experience for Transforming Capacity

Each of these three cases could be described from an objective view of the body and mind. For example, Tom's integration of sensory information can be seen as due to changes in the brain structure; the women's acquisition of ways to deal with neglect can be described in terms of new learning compensatory strategies; and Curtis's hand function can be described as return of strength, range of motion, and sensation. These objective descriptions are certainly valid and important for understanding what happens to such persons as their impairments change over time. However, as the studies clearly illustrate, these descriptions only partly explain how change took place.

In all three studies, it was through the realm of experience that effective strategies of change were discovered. The actual events and human actions that resulted in change were a function of experience. Each of these persons had to use experience as a way of solving their own problems and challenges. For example, only when Tom could locate the experience of being in relationship to the world in another way, only when he could feel the new experience, did he begin to change. Similarly, the women with neglect had to come to know a new reality in which their practical world consisted not just of what they could perceive but also of something outside perception. Learning to exist effectively in such a world meant that they had to come to a way of understanding their new experiences. Both examples indicate how transformation in performance capacity depends on a transformation in experience.

Conclusion

This chapter offered a subjective approach to understanding performance capacity that is complementary to the usual objective approach. The concept of the lived body derived from phenomenology offers a unique way of conceptualizing subjective experience and its role in performance. Through careful attention to this subjective experience we have a way to better understand performance capacity.

Key Terms

Lived body: The experience of being and knowing the world through a particular body.

Performance capacity: Ability to do things provided by the status of underlying objective physical and mental components and corresponding subjective experience.

References

Baz, T. (1998). *The experience of change in therapy*. Masters thesis, Department of Occupational Therapy, University of Illinois at Chicago.

Bisiach, E., & Vallar, G. (1988). Hemi neglect in humans. In F. Boller & J. Grafman (Eds.), *Handbook of neuropsychology*. Amsterdam: Elsevier Science.

Bundy, A.C., Lane, S.J., & Murray, E.A. (2002). *Sensory Integration: Theory and practice* (2nd ed.). Philadelphia: FA Davis.

Clark, F. (1993). Occupation embedded in a real life: Interweaving occupational science and occupational therapy. *American Journal of Occupational Therapy, 47*, 1067–1078.

Csordas, T. (Ed.). (1994). *Embodiment and experience: The existential ground of culture and self*. New York: Cambridge University.

Engelbrecht, F. (1968). *The phenomenology of the human body*. South Africa: Sovenga.

Hutson, J. (1998). *Qualitative study of the experience of an injured worker*. Masters thesis, Department of Occupational Therapy, University of Illinois at Chicago.

Jamison, K. R. (1995). *An unquiet mind: A memoir of moods and madness*. New York: Vintage.

Katz, N. (2005). *Cognition and Occupation Across the Life Span*. Rockville, MD: AOTA.

Kielhofner, G. (1995). A meditation on the use of hands. *Scandinavian Journal of Occupational Therapy, 2*, 153–166.

Leder, D. (1984). Medicine's paradigm of embodiment. *Journal of Medical Philosophy, 9*, 29–43.

Leder, D. (1990). *The absent body*. Chicago: University of Chicago.

Luria, A. R. (1972). *The man with a shattered world: The history of a brain wound*. New York: Basic Books.

McGlynn, S. M., & Schacter, D. L. (1989). Unawareness of deficits in neuropsychological syndromes. *Journal of Clinical Experimental Neuropsychology, 11*, 143–205.

Merleau-Ponty, M. (1962). *Phenomenology of perception*. (C. Smith, Trans.). London: Routledge & Kegan Paul. (Original work published 1945.)

Murphy, R. (1987). *The body silent*. New York: Henry Holt.

Sachs, O. (1993). *A leg to stand on*. New York: Harper Collins.

Sartre, J. P. (1970). The body. In S. F. Spricher (Ed.), *The philosophy of the body: Reflections on Cartesian dualism*. Chicago: Quadrangle Books.

Sechehaye, M. (1968). *Autobiography of a schizophrenic girl: The true story of Renee*. (G. Rubin-Rabson, trans.). New York: Grune & Stratton.

Sudnow, D. (1978). *Ways of the hand: The organization of improvised conduct*. Cambridge: Harvard University.

Sudnow, D. (1979). *Talk's body: A meditation between two keyboards*. New York: Knopf.

Tham, K., Borell, L., & Gustavsson, A. (2000).The discovery of disability: A phenomenological study of unilateral neglect. *American Journal of Occupational Therapy, 54*, 398–406.

Toombs, K. (1992). *The meaning of illness: A phenomenological account of the different perspectives of physician and patient*. Boston: Kluwer Academic.

Trombly, C. A., & Radomski, M. (2002). *Occupation therapy for physical dysfunction* (5th ed.). Philadelphia: Lippincott, Williams, & Wilkins.

Williams, D. (1994). *Nobody nowhere: The extraordinary autobiography of an autistic*. New York: Avon Books.

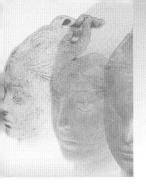

7

The Environment and Human Occupation

● Gary Kielhofner

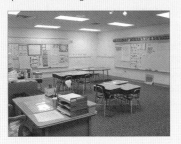

*I*n traditional classrooms students sat in rows facing the teacher and blackboard. Contemporary classrooms often incorporate other formats. For example as shown below, the arrangement of desks in groupings throughout the classroom promotes student interaction and cooperative learning.[1]

A classroom environment that encourages interaction and cooperative learning.

The arrangement of workplaces affects how people perform their work tasks. Like this work environment, many pose difficult physical challenges to workers, and some can put them at risk for injury.[2]

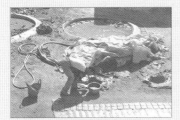

An unsafe work environment.

Children with disabilities often face challenges accessing and using ordinary playgrounds. To address this problem Michele Shapiro, an Israeli occupational therapist, has designed Park Chamverim,[3] an inclusive playground for children of all levels of ability and special needs. In addition to the removal of most physical barriers, the park is organized to teach children who use it to respect each other's needs and to play together. Thus, it seeks to address both physical and social barriers in the environment.

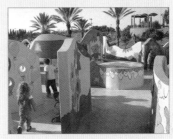

Park Chamverim, an accessible playground.

A group home for persons with intellectual impairments in Chicago[4] provides opportunities for the residents to participate in communal meals, to do tasks necessary to the home, and to complete instrumental activities of daily living such as laundry, as shown in the photographs below. The extent to which a group home

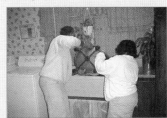

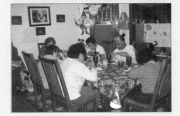

Group home residents do laundry and eat dinner together.

provides opportunities for residents to decorate their space and use the kitchen influences their self-determination and autonomy (Fisher, 2004).

Members and sympathizers of the disability community increasingly engage in marches to raise awareness about disability and to protest against laws and policies that disadvantage persons with disabilities.

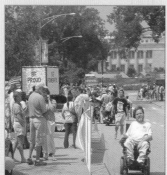

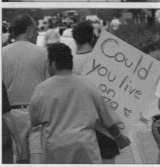

The annual Disability Pride Parade held in Chicago, IL.

[1] Susan Cahill, clinical instructor at University of Illinois at Chicago, provided the photo of the classroom for this chapter.

[2] Supriya Sen, clinical instructor at University of Illinois at Chicago, provided the photo of the work site for this chapter.

[3] Michele Shapiro, from Beit Issie Shapiro, Israel, provided the case about Park Chamverim for this chapter.

[4] Gail Fisher, clinical associate professor at the University of Illinois at Chicago, provided the group home case for this chapter.

As these diverse examples illustrate, the environment can exert an all-important influence on occupation. This chapter provides a conceptualization of the environment and how it affects human occupation as well as how people interact with their environments.

A Definition of the Environment

The **environment** can be defined as the particular physical and social, cultural, economic, and political features of one's contexts that impact upon the motivation, organization, and performance of occupation. As this definition implies, several dimensions of the environment may affect an individual's occupational life. Moreover, most operate in a variety of contexts (e.g., home, neighborhood, school, and workplace). Within these contexts, people encounter different physical spaces, objects, people, expectations, and opportunities for doing things. At the same time, the larger culture, economic conditions, and political factors also exert an influence on occupational life. According to this conceptualization we can envision the environment (*Fig. 7.1*) as including the following dimensions:

- The objects that people use when doing things
- The spaces within which people do things
- The occupational forms or tasks that are available, expected, and/or required by the context
- The social groups (family, friends, coworkers, neighbors) encountered
- The culture that infuses and influences both physical and social aspects of the environment
- The political and economic context that influences such things as freedoms and resources relevant to occupation.

Opportunities and Resources

The environment provides a wide range of opportunities and resources that enable choosing and doing things (Dunn, Brown, & McGuigan, 1994; Gibson, 1979; Law, 1991; Law, Cooper, Strong, Stewart, Rigby, & Letts, 1996; Nelson, 1988; Reed, 1982). Most contexts offer a range of opportunities to choose what to do. For example, a natural resource, such as a lake or forest, may afford opportunities to enjoy the view, to photograph the scene, or to go hiking or swimming. The environment may also provide resources to sustain motivation. For instance, family members and friends may offer emotional support and reassurance to sustain effort toward a goal. In contrast, some retirees who no longer had the expectations of the work environment find it more difficult to maintain their motivation for doing things (Jonsson, Josephsson, & Kielhofner, 2000).

FIGURE 7.1 Dimensions of the environment affecting occupation.

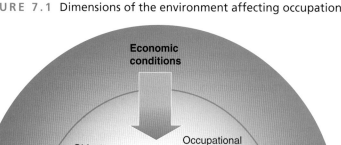

The environment provides resources that may facilitate performance. Tools, instructions, and guidance from others are examples. Familiar aspects of the physical and social environment support routine behaviors. Stable and recurring features of the environment (e.g., the familiar arrangement of spaces and objects and the recurrent events and predictable behavior patterns of others) support habits and roles.

Demands and Constraints

Environments may place limits on or strongly direct action (Dunn et al., 1994; Law, 1991; Law et al., 1996; Lawton, 1980). Such features of the physical environment as fences, walls, steps, walkways, and doorways constrain where one can go or how much effort it takes. Others' expectations, laws and regulations, job requirements, and social norms can affect people's actions, patterns of activity, and even motivation.

Environments thus demand particular behaviors and discourage or disallow others. For example, in an airport the counters and agents, roped areas, security checkpoints, guards, posted rules and announcements, gates, and lines of passengers influence and in part dictate the sequence of things we do. Standing in line, obtaining a boarding pass, checking luggage, passing security, going to the gate, and boarding the plane are all done according to environmental demands and constraints.

Environmental demands and constraints also influence the development of habits and roles. For example, a school's physical arrangement and rules and requirements, combined with teachers, peers, and others' perceptions of the student role, all funnel and shape the attitudes and actions that come to make up each student's role. Demands and constraints of an environment can also negatively constrain motives and action. Many service environments have also been noted to have adverse effects on their occupants. For example, Borell, Gustavsson, Sandman, and Kielhofner (1994) studied how the rules, organized events, and concerns of staff in a day hospital for persons with dementia actually stifled clients' attempts to engage in spontaneous behaviors and encouraged passivity and inactivity.

Environmental Impact

It is important to note the difference between features of an environment and its actual influence on specific persons. As Gitlin and Corcoran (2005) noted, the effect of the environment on daily performance depends on factors such as a person's cognitive and physical abilities, the person's appraisals of role and environmental demands, and the characteristics of ongoing interactions within the environment. **Environmental impact** refers to the opportunity, support, demand, and constraint that the environment has on a particular individual. As shown in *Figure 7.2*, this impact results from the interaction between features of the environment and characteristics of the person. Whether and how environmental opportunities, resources, demands, and constraints are noticed or felt depends on each person's values, interests, personal causation, roles, habits, and performance capacities. For example, environments that challenge a person's capacities tend to evoke involvement, attentiveness, and maximal performance (Csikszentmihalyi, 1990; Kiernat, 1983; Lawton & Nahemow, 1973). On the other hand, when environments demand performance well below capacity, they can evoke boredom and disinterest and even result in "the type of negative affect and behavior seen in sensory deprivation" (Kiernat, 1983, p. 6). When demands are too far beyond capacity, they can make a person feel anxious, overwhelmed, or hopeless. Since persons have different capacities and beliefs in their own abilities, the same environment may engage and excite one person, bore another, and overwhelm a third.

Spaces

Spaces are physical contexts that are bounded and arranged in ways that influence what people do within them. As shown in *Figure 7.3*, these spaces have unique features that shape what we do within them. The physical properties of natural spaces, along with the

weather, offer opportunities, supports, and demands for behavior. Consider, for example, the different possibilities for doing things on a beach during a hot summer day and in a forest during a snowstorm.

Occupations often take place in specific built spaces, such as a school, stadium, shopping mall, or salon. Built spaces reflect and are instrumental to culture. They are readily recognized by members of the culture as having a designated purpose and as intended for certain persons' use (Rubinstein, 1989). Consequently, they offer specific opportunities and constraints for doing. For example, a library invites browsing and reading and discourages speaking aloud, whereas a football stadium encourages spectators to watch and cheer for their team.

Objects

Objects are naturally occurring or fabricated things with which people interact and whose properties influence what they do with them (*Fig. 7.4*). While objects in natural environments occur according to the scheme of nature, those in built environments are placed there by human design. Which objects are present and how they are organized generally depends on the purpose of the space and cultural convention (Rubinstein, 1989).

Objects also strongly influence occupation. For instance, whether children engage in solitary or social play depends on what types of toys and equipment are present (Quilitch & Risley, 1973). Raw materials (boxes, sand, tires) lend themselves to active exploration (Csikszentmihalyi & Rochberg-Halton, 1981), whereas fixed equipment in playgrounds can constrain what play occurs (Haywood, Rothenberg, & Beasley, 1974). Objects also influence behavior simply by virtue of their intrinsic properties (Hocking, 1994). The weight, size, pliability, texture, and other physical attributes of objects may influence whether we toss, carry, bend, or otherwise handle them. Simple and familiar objects may give comfort and invite relaxing behavior, whereas complex objects tend to demand specialized and skilled behavior.

We tend to surround ourselves with objects that reflect our established patterns of interest and activity and that reflect who we are. Adolescents, for example, frequently mention musical instruments and stereo equipment as being their most prized possessions

FIGURE 7.2 Environmental impact depends on the intersection of the social and physical environment with the values, interests, personal causation, habits, roles, and performance capacities of those within the environment.

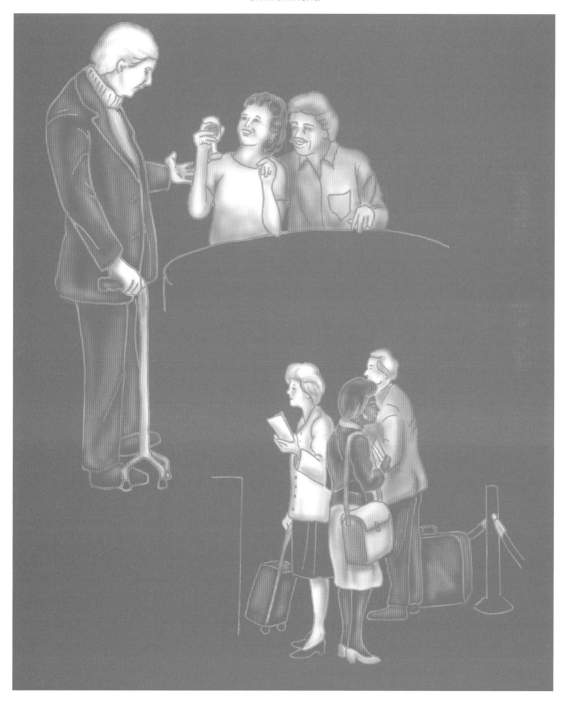

FIGURE 7.3 Natural and built spaces influence what we do.

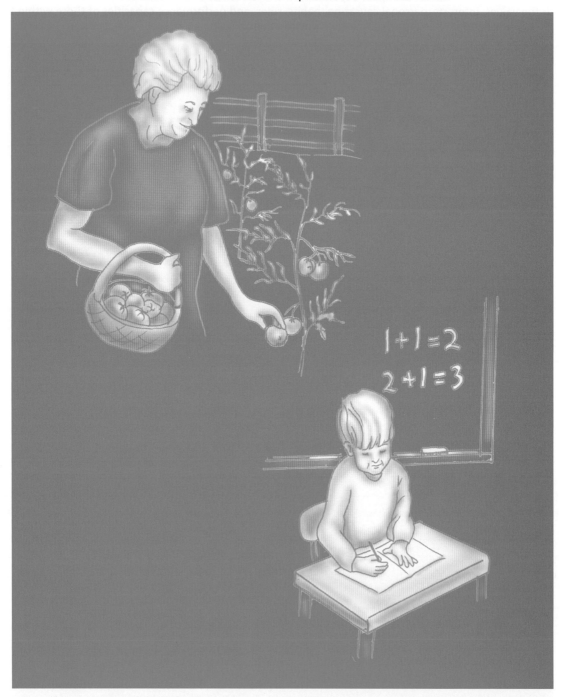

FIGURE 7.4 Objects provide opportunities for doing.

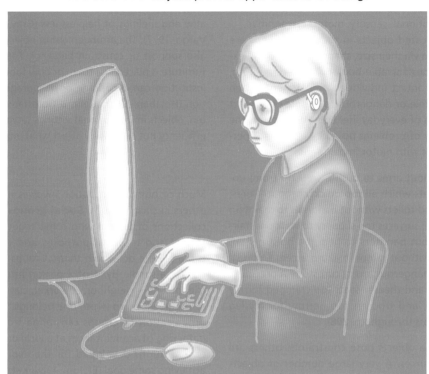

(Csikszentmihalyi & Rochberg-Halton, 1981). Objects often take on the most value when they signify something very personal about one's experiences or accomplishments or one's connections to others (Csikszentmihalyi & Rochberg-Halton, 1981). For example, objects handed down in families may convey the "sense of having roots or of belonging in a particular setting" (Ljungström, 1989). On the other hand, Rubinstein (1989) notes how an elderly woman's collection of figurines "marked and filled her space, gave her sensory pleasure, had a story and gave her stories to tell, and added texture to her rooms" (p. 49).

The symbolic meaning of objects may influence how they support or demand ways of using them. For example, when a car is a symbol of independence and responsibility, the young adult owner may feel increased demands for competence in understanding its maintenance. A practical object with strong sentimental value may be restricted from use to avoid damage or destruction.

IMPACT OF OBJECTS AND SPACES ON PERSONS WITH DISABILITIES

Many people are able to reconfigure their spaces (e.g., home) to accommodate their impairments (Rowles, 1991). Nonetheless, physical spaces often pose multiple problems for persons with disabilities. The most obvious are natural and architectural barriers that interfere with work, play, and daily living tasks. For the person with a physical impairment, an ordinary house can present a multitude of barriers (Rockwell-Dylla, 1992; Murphy, 1987) since much of the built environment is designed without consideration of inhabitants' possible impairments.

Natural spaces similarly can provide a variety of problems for the person with a disability. For example, Hull (1990), who is blind, notes that snow is a particular problem because snow blunts the sounds he relies on and makes use of the cane difficult. As this example illustrates, the kind of problems the physical environment poses will differ depending on whether one's impairment is emotional, sensory, motor, or cognitive.

Most fabricated objects in the environment are naturally geared via their size, shape, weight, complexity, and functions for able-bodied, sighted, hearing, and cognitively intact individuals. Impairments often make it impossible or dangerous to handle or interact with the objects of everyday life. Zola (1982) offers the following litany of problems posed by objects for persons like himself with motor impairments:

> Chairs without arms to push myself up from; unpadded seats which all too quickly produce sores; showers and toilets without handrails to maintain my balance; surfaces too slippery to walk on; staircases without banisters to help me hoist myself; buildings without ramps, making ascent exhausting if not dangerous; every curbstone a precipice; car, plane, and theater seats too cramped for my braced leg; and trousers too narrow for my leg brace to pass through. (p. 208)

While some objects pose constraints, others are important resources. A very large number of objects have been designed and are available to compensate for impairments. Such adaptive aids range from simple tools with built-up handles to compensate for limited grip to complex computer-based systems that control environments and allow communication. Such specialized objects can also carry deep symbolic messages. For instance, Bates, Spencer, Young, and Hopkins-Rintala (1993) chronicle how one spinal cord–injured man, Russell, first saw his wheelchair as a prison and later as a constant reminder that his goal of walking again might not be viable. Over time, he vacillated between wanting to take a blowtorch to the chair and finding it necessary as a means of mobility. The kinds of extraordinary objects that disabled persons use can invoke intense emotional responses. These feelings influence not only what the object means to the individual but also how that individual will learn about and use the object and whether it will be integrated into an acceptable life (Bates et al., 1993).

Everyday objects that provide opportunities for activity choices are also consequential for persons with disabilities (Simmons & Barris, 1984). Specialized settings, such as residential facilities, are frequently devoid of personal belongings, decorations, comfortable furniture, and minor appliances, which can contribute to apathy and feelings of helplessness (Gray, 1972; Magill & Vargo, 1977). The arrangement of objects in a space can also support or constrain behavior. For example, how furniture is placed in a room or how food is served in an institution can encourage or discourage social interaction (Holahan, 1979; Melin & Gotestam, 1981). Too often, objects in institutional settings serve organizational efficiency but negatively affect what inhabitants do.

Social Groups

Much of human occupation involves interacting with others in social groups. **Social groups** are defined as collections of people who come together for various formal and informal purposes and influence what those people do within them. Groups include, for instance, a simple dyad of a person interacting with a friend, family, neighbor, coworker, classmate, or a club or organization to which one belongs. The nature and organization of groups can range from an informal gathering of acquaintances at a local bar to formalized organizations developed for the explicit purpose of achieving some goal (Etzioni, 1964; Katz & Kahn, 1966). Since an enduring climate of values, interests, and activities is characteristic of most groups (Moos, 1974), people tend to acquire the values, interests, and behaviors that characterize the groups to which they belong (Newcomb, 1943; Pervin, 1968). As shown in *Figure 7.5*, they also constitute a social space (Knowles, 1982) in which roles and habits are shaped.

Occupational Forms/Tasks

The environment offers opportunities to do things. These conventionalized ways of doing things are commonly referred to as tasks. In occupational therapy, the term occupational form has also been used to refer to the things people do (Nelson, 1988). The notion of form refers to the specific manner, actions, meanings, and so on that characterize doing something. When we perform, we go through or enact the form. Each culture includes a wide range of occupational forms that constitute the opportunities and demands for doing things that the culture puts on its members.

Each of these forms/tasks has its own internal coherence. That is, the actions and manners that make up

FIGURE 7.5 Groups as social spaces shaping our behavior.

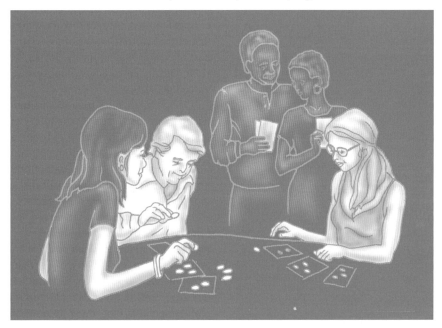

the form are connected to its meaning and purpose. For example, when people are playing a friendly game of cards, their behaviors reflect the purpose or objectives of the game and their attitude will be relaxed and playful. Woodworking, jogging, and shopping are all names for occupational forms. Because occupational forms/tasks are routinely done by members of a group and can be named, they are readily recognized by members of the culture. Consequently, most of the time when we observe others, we are able to say what they are doing. In so doing, we name the task or occupational form they are performing (e.g. cooking, vacuuming, rollerblading, dressing, packing).

Given these considerations, **occupational forms/tasks** can be defined as conventionalized sequences of action that are at once coherent, oriented to a purpose, sustained in collective knowledge, culturally recognizable, and named. They are conventionalized in that there is a typical or correct way of doing them. Cultures specify procedures, outcomes, and standards for doing an occupational form/task that are passed on to those who wish to learn it. Some of these conventions are quite fixed. Taking an examination, for instance, re-

quires someone to be in a particular place at a particular time and to answer a prepared set of questions. Success is contingent on correctly answering a preset percentage of these questions. Some occupational forms/tasks, such as driving, are governed by laws that specify how they are to be done and what is not allowed. In other cases, conventions for doing the form/task are open, such as going for a walk or dressing oneself. However, even occupational forms/tasks that are relatively open-ended conform to recognizable cultural parameters. As shown in *Figure 7.6*, occupational forms/tasks are available in the social environment.

SOCIAL ENVIRONMENT AND DISABILITY

Most social groups have deep ambivalence toward persons with disabilities. Even in societies whose laws, health care, and welfare systems are organized so as to support persons with disabilities, the attitudes of individuals and the practices of groups often betray discomfort with disabled persons (Gill, 1997; Hahn, 1993; Longmore, 1995). Personal accounts of individuals with disabilities are replete with stories of others' negative

FIGURE 7.6 Occupational forms as things we do.

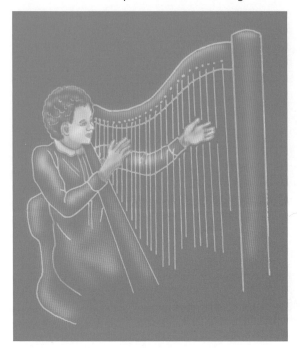

reactions and attitudes and of outright discrimination and rejection.

Onset of a physical disability can transform one's social environment. As Murphy (1987) observes, "The onset of quadriplegia, I discovered, had placed me in a new social dimension" (p. 195).

Emotional or intellectual disabilities can equally set persons apart from the rest of society. Western cultures place a high value on intelligence, so that an implied deficit in this area is tantamount to the most serious kind of personal flaw—something that strikes at the very worth of the individual (Dexter, 1956, 1960; Edgerton, 1967).

Persons who acquire a disability may find themselves temporarily or permanently removed from the groups in which they previously enacted their roles (Sarbin, 1954). Further, the social groups in which the individual does things may be fundamentally changed. For example, coworkers may attribute an injured worker's accident to carelessness and so fear working alongside him or her. Coworkers may resent accommodations made for an emotionally disabled colleague.

Disabled persons may also find their social world shrinking, as old friends and acquaintances are uneasy or unwilling to continue relationships or when the activities that were the basis of association are no longer possible (Hull, 1990; Murphy, Scheer, Murphy, & Mack, 1988; Oliver, Zarb, Silver, Moore, & Salisbury, 1988; Vash, 1981).

The family is both greatly affected by and influential on a member with a disability. For example, parents share in the suffering and grief that may be a part of a child's disability (Kornblum & Anderson, 1982). Household routines, family responsibilities, organization of the physical home, and restraints on family spontaneity, travel, and other factors may all be part and parcel of having a disabled member in the family. Families may be extremely taxed by caring for a disabled family member when political and economic systems constrain availability of services and supports. Activities such as social contact and leisure may suffer (Breslau, 1983). A great deal of stress may be placed on family members who must accommodate the limitations of the person with a disability (Trombly, 1983).

Because persons with disabilities frequently have access to fewer non-kindred relationships, they may depend significantly on the family for emotional, financial, and other forms of support. Consequently, the family can be a vital influence on the disabled person. Families that positively influence their disabled members include them in their routines and rituals and give them meaningful roles in the family (Bogdan & Taylor, 1989).

Disabled persons often end up spending significant portions of their lives in specialized social groups. These groups may include substitutes for home such as halfway houses, residential facilities, or nursing homes. They may be short-term treatment settings, such as hospitals, community mental health centers, and rehabilitation facilities, or long-term social and work settings, such as senior centers and sheltered workshops. Such settings aim to provide services that support or enhance the performance and quality of life of persons with disabilities. However, a variety of factors, from constrained resources to organizational incentives and demands, can result in less than optimal conditions for achieving their ends. Consequently, many of these social groups may contribute to the very problems they seek to alleviate (Edgerton, 1967; Emerson, Rochford,

& Shaw, 1983; Kielhofner, 1983; Scull, 1977; Test & Stein, 1978). For example, Suto and Frank (1994) observed that persons with schizophrenia in a residential setting faced "predominantly passive free time activities, a lack of involvement in traditional social roles, and many hours of free time" (p. 14). The combination of being severed from ordinary social groups and being placed in groups where the normal opportunities for roles and activities are severely restricted can have a profound effect on everyday occupational life.

Most occupational forms/tasks in any culture have been developed without consideration of how persons with impairments may do them. Consequently, the availability of occupational forms can be dramatically altered by disability. Performance limitations can make some occupational forms/tasks impossible. Disabled persons may forgo or relinquish to others what has become impossible to do. The temporal and social nature of occupational forms/tasks may be radically altered. For example, more time may be required for performance. Previously private occupational forms/tasks may require assistance from others. Incorporating necessary adaptive equipment into occupational forms may change their character.

Access to occupational forms/tasks is often unnecessarily restricted for disabled persons. For example, an elderly person who is "asked to make his or her own bed but is capable of much more … feels self-incompetence and helplessness" (Miller & Oertel, 1983, p. 110).

For a variety of reasons disabled persons are given access to occupational forms/tasks that do not challenge them. Zola offers the following reflection on this issue:

> The jobs here were too simple, too fragmented, too mindless, too meaningless. Granted that my fellow residents might have limited physical capacity but why such busy work, why industrial products that were marketable only with a subsidy? Could the workers possibly feel they were doing something worthwhile? Of course, many jobs in the outside world were as repetitive and meaningless but at least those workers may have had a rationalization of the job's being a means to an end. To what end were these tasks oriented? Why was work created from the point of view of the limita-

> tions of the workers rather than their potentialities? (1982, p. 71)

Such questions have been raised repeatedly by both observers and disabled persons. Yet access to occupational forms/tasks that are meaningful and that convey respect all too frequently remains a problem.

Culture

Since the physical and social environments are interpreted and shaped by culture, (Altman & Chemers, 1980) it is important to recognize culture as a pervasive feature of the environment. **Culture** is defined as the beliefs and perceptions, values and norms, customs and behaviors that are shared by a group or society and are passed from one generation to the next through both formal and informal education (Altman & Chemers, 1980; Brake, 1980; Ogbu, 1981; Rapoport, 1980).

Within most cultures there are also a variety of subcultures. For example, American society has urban, rural, ethnic, and other subcultures. Each shows important differences from the dominant culture and in particular influences the organization of various groups.

The impact of culture is not homogeneous. We may experience several different sources of cultural influence, depending on the range of environments in which we do things. I live in a farming community in rural southern Wisconsin, commute to urban Chicago to work, and am responsible for educational and clinical programs whose mission of serving minority populations brings me into contact with Hispanic and African American subcultures. In addition, I travel abroad regularly and count among my friends persons living in Europe, Canada, South America, and Asia. These experiences expose me to a significant range of cultural influences. Although my experience is more diverse than that of many people, it is increasingly probable that persons will experience an array of cultural influences in a world with increasing resources for communication and mobility. The insulated and homogeneous cultural experiences of persons who lived a century ago are less and less likely in today's world (Gergen, 1991).

It is easy to see how the social world, the world of human relationships and activities, is shaped by culture. Nevertheless, there is an equally important influence of culture on the physical environment. Culture deter-

> When we consider any aspect of the physical or social environment, it is important to remember that culture is in the background shaping and defining it.

mines how physical context is organized and what artifacts we are likely to encounter within it. Culture also provides a way of seeing and encountering the physical environment, including the world of nature.

When we consider any aspect of the physical or social environment, it is important to remember that culture is in the background shaping and defining it. Because culture is a pervasive force in the environment, I will repeatedly refer to its role in discussing the physical and social environment. Moreover, it is important to recognize that culture is internalized by people. A person's values, sense of competence, interests, and internalized roles and habits are all reflections of that person's belonging to a particular culture. Culture influences not only what is within the environment but also how a person is predisposed to interact with the environment.

CULTURAL VIEWS OF DISABILITY

Although cultures differ in the way they respond to disability, disabled persons historically generally have been cast as:

> Victims and villains in popular culture, dependent sentimentalized children in charity fund raising, mendicants who should be allowed to beg, "unsightly disgusting objects" who should be banned from public places, potentially dependent or dangerous denizens of society, worthy subjects of poor relief but unworthy citizens of the nation. (Longmore and Goldberger, 2000, p. 5)

As they point out, most cultures have little or no place for disabled persons in the mainstream of society.

Cultural conceptions of disability are generated and perpetuated in oral traditions, art, literature, and film. Mitchell (2002) points out that while narratives freely employ the anomaly of disability as a literary device that embodies and underscores other personal aberrations and social ills, they rarely address disability as either a source of personal knowledge or as a social or political

injustice. Poignant recent examples are the use of physical disfigurement and mobility limitation as a metaphor for malevolence in the books and subsequent films *Hannibal* (Lustig & Scott, 2001) and *The Red Dragon* (Davis & Ratner, 2002). Other films, such as *Million Dollar Baby*, perpetuate the idea that disability is a pitiable state unworthy of sustaining life (Neville-Jan, 2005).

Political and Economic Conditions

Political forces and socioeconomic conditions of a society have an indirect but nonetheless far-reaching influence on the occupation of people in that society.

The extent to which people have resources, access to institutions, freedom to make choices and move about, and opportunities to work are only a few examples of the important consequences of political and economic conditions for occupation. Political conflict and economic injustice have constrained and hindered the occupational lives of persons who are victims of these conditions (Kronenberg, Algado, & Pollard, 2006).

Political and economic conditions have a particularly important impact on the occupational lives of persons with disabilities. Many nations have social philosophies and corresponding policies that treat disabled persons as a negative factor in the economic marketplace (Albrecht & Bury, 2001; Longmore & Goldberger, 2000). The consequence of many of these policies is a form of social oppression that bars disabled persons from access to the labor market and other forms of civil participation (Charlton, 1998). For instance, disabled people fare much worse than non-disabled persons in housing, education, transportation, and employment (Louis Harris & Associates, 1998; McNeil, 1997). Many social policies restrict disabled persons from attaining self-sufficiency (e.g., encouraging nursing home placement over community living) (Charlton, 1998; Hahn,

> The extent to which people have resources, access to institutions, freedom to make choices and move about, and opportunities to work are only a few examples of the important consequences of political and economic conditions for occupation.

1985; Longmore, 1995; Oliver, 1990, 1996; Shapiro, 1993). Finally, economic and social policy influences the extent to which persons with disabilities have access to resources (e.g., rehabilitation services, specialized equipment, environmental modifications) that can enable them to achieve positive occupational lives (Stone, 2005).

Occupational Settings

The physical and social are intertwined in the environments we encounter. Together they constitute occupational settings. An **occupational setting** is a composite of spaces, objects, occupational forms/tasks, and social groups that cohere and constitute a meaningful context for performance. Occupational settings that ordinarily make up the course of daily life are the home, the neighborhood, the workplace, and gathering, recreation, and resource sites (e.g., theaters, churches, temples, beaches, clubs, libraries, galleries, ski lodges, restaurants, health clubs, and stores). A given environment may serve as a different type of occupational setting for different individuals, depending on what they do in it. For example, a restaurant is a workplace for the waiters, cook, and others who labor in it, but a gathering and recreation site for those who frequent it for a meal with family or friends.

For most people, everyday life involves rounds of doing things in a number of occupational settings. As we move from setting to setting, the different spaces, objects, social groups, and occupational forms/tasks we find provide opportunities, resources, demands, and constraints. Much of what we choose to do and how we go about doing it is owing to the features of these settings. Finally, occupational settings are greatly influenced by culture and sociopolitical conditions.

Inseparability of Environment and Occupation

The relationship between humans and their environments is intimate and reciprocal. As has been discussed, the environment affects what people do and how they do it. Humans constantly seek out certain types of environments and seek to change their environments toward their ends. For example, Rubinstein (1989) tells the story of an elderly woman who lives in a studio

apartment and conducts most of her occupational life there. As her day progresses, she meticulously rearranges the apartment to accommodate sleeping, receiving guests, and leisure.

Such modification of the environment to make it suitable for different occupations illustrates how much we depend on context for our experience and action.

The environment also figures centrally in the experience of disability. In fact, a person's degree of access and integration into the physical and social environment can be used as an index of disability (Brandt & Pope, 1997). Disability can be prevented or reduced when the environment is free of barriers and offers adequate support. Consequently, the extent of an individual's disability results in large measure from the surrounding environment (Brandt & Pope, 1997).

In the end, we owe our very humanness and our most essential selves to our environments. As Eisenberg (1977) argues:

> What determines the similarity between my behavior last year and what it is likely to be during the next is not nearly so much a matter of that which is "I" as it is of the social fields of force in which that "I" moves. That is, having acquired a repertoire of behaviors, I maximize their adaptive utility by seeking out the familiar and avoiding the strange in the social world around me. The apparent consistency in the self is the result, not merely of what has gone before, but of the continuation into the future of the same social forces that have given rise to it. (p. 233)

In fact, the environment is so intimately linked with the person that it can be considered "part of the organism" (Sameroff, 1983, p. 242). The central lesson of this chapter is that if we want to understand human occupation, we must also understand the environments in which it takes place. Occupation is, after all, action that occupies a particular social and physical space.

> *Occupation is, after all, action that occupies a particular social and physical space.*

Key Terms

Culture: Beliefs and perceptions, values and norms, customs and behaviors that are shared by a group or society and are passed from one generation to the next through both formal and informal education.

Environment: Particular physical and social features of the specific context in which one does something that impacts upon what one does, and how it is done.

Environmental impact: Actual influence (in the form of opportunity, support, demand, or constraint) that the physical and social aspects of the environment have on a particular individual.

Objects: Naturally occurring or fabricated things with which people interact and whose properties influence what they do with them.

Spaces: physical contexts that are bounded and arranged in ways that influence what people do within them.

Occupational forms/tasks: Conventionalized sequences of action that are coherent, oriented to a purpose, sustained in collective knowledge, culturally recognizable, and named.

Occupational settings: Composite of spaces, objects, occupational forms, and/or social groups that cohere and constitute a meaningful context for performance.

Social groups: Collections of people who come together for various formal and informal purposes and who influence what we do within them.

References

Albrecht, G.L., & Bury, M. (2001). The political economy of the disability marketplace. In G. Albrecht, K. Seelman, & M. Bury (Eds.), *Handbook of Disabilities Studies* (pp. 585–609). Thousand Oaks, CA: Sage.

Altman, I., & Chemers, M. (1980). *Culture and environment*. Monterey, CA: Brooks/Cole.

Bates, P. S., Spencer, J. C., Young, M. E., & Hopkins-Rintala, D. H. (1993). Assistive technology and the newly disabled adult: Adaptation to wheelchair use. *American Journal of Occupational Therapy, 47,* 1014–1021.

Bogdan, R., & Taylor, S. J. (1989). The social construction of humanness: Relationships with severely disabled people. *Social Problems, 36,* 135–148.

Borell, L., Gustavsson, A., Sandman, P., & Kielhofner, G. (1994). Occupational programming in a day hospital for patients with dementia. *Occupational Therapy Journal of Research, 14,* 219–238.

Brake, M. (1980). *The sociology of youth culture and youth cultures*. London: Routledge & Kegan Paul.

Brandt, E. N., & Pope, A. M. (1997). *Enabling America: Assessing the role of rehabilitation science and engineering*. Washington, DC: National Academy.

Breslau, N. (1983). Family care: Effects on siblings and mothers. In G. H. Thompson, I. L. Rubin, & R. M. Belenker (Eds.), *Comprehensive management of cerebral palsy*. New York: Grune & Stratton.

Charlton, J. (1998*). Nothing about us without us.* Berkeley: University of California.

Csikszentmihalyi, M. (1990). *Flow: The psychology of optimal experience*. New York: Harper & Row.

Csikszentmihalyi, M., & Rochberg-Halton, E. (1981). *The meaning of things*. Cambridge, MA: Cambridge University.

Davis, A. (executive producer), & Ratner, B. (director). (2002). *The Red Dragon* [motion picture]. United States: Universal.

Dexter, L. A. (1956). Towards a sociology of mentally defective. *American Journal of Mental Deficiency, 61,* 10–16.

Dexter, L. A. (1960). Research on problems of mental subnormality. *American Journal of Mental Deficiency, 64,* 835–838.

Dunn, W., Brown, C., & McGuigan, A. (1994). The ecology of human performance: A framework for considering the effect of context. *American Journal of Occupational Therapy, 48,* 595–607.

Edgerton, R. B. (1967). *The cloak of competence: Stigma in the lives of the mentally retarded*. Berkeley: University of California.

Eisenberg, L. (1977). Development as a unifying concept in psychiatry. *British Journal of Psychiatry, 131,* 225–237.

Emerson, R. M., Rochford, E. B., & Shaw, L. L. (1983). The micropolitics of trouble in a psychiatric board and care facility. *Urban Life, 12,* 349–366.

Etzioni, A. (1964). *Modern organizations*. Englewood Cliffs, NJ: Prentice-Hall.

Fisher, G. (2004). The Residential Environment Impact Survey. Developmental Disabilities Special Interest Section, *27*(3), 1–4.

Gergen, K. J. (1991). *The saturated self: Dilemmas of identity in contemporary life*. Philadelphia: Basic Books.

Gibson, J. J. (1979). *The ecological approach to visual perception*. Boston: Houghton Mifflin.

Gill, C. J. (1997). Four types of integration in disability identity development. *Journal of Vocational Rehabilitation, 9,* 39–46.

Gitlin, L. N., & Corcoran, M.A. (2005). *Occupational therapy and dementia care: The home environmental skill-building program for individuals and families*. Bethesda, MD: American Occupational Therapy Association.

Gray, M. (1972). Effects of hospitalization on work-play behavior. *American Journal of Occupational Therapy*, *26*, 180–185.

Hahn, H. (1993). The political implications of disability definitions and data. *Journal of Disability Policy Studies, 4 (2)*, 41–52.

Hahn, H. (1985). Disability policy and the problem of discrimination. *American Behavioral Scientist, 28*(3), 293–318.

Haywood, D. G., Rothenberg, M., & Beasley, R. R. (1974). Children's play and urban playground environments. *Environmental Behavior, 6*, 131–168.

Hocking, C. (1994). *Objects in the environment: A critique of the model of human occupation dimensions.* Paper presented at World Federation of Occupational Therapy, Symposium, International Perspectives on the Model of Human Occupation, London.

Holahan, C. J. (1979). Environmental psychology in psychiatric hospital settings. In D. Canter & S. Canter (Eds.), *Designing for therapeutic environments: A review of research.* New York: Wiley.

Hull, J. M. (1990). *Touching the rock: An experience of blindness.* New York: Vintage Books.

Jonsson, H., Josephsson, S., & Kielhofner, G. (2000). Evolving narratives in the course of retirement: A longitudinal study. *American Journal of Occupational Therapy, 54,* 263–270.

Katz, D., & Kahn, R. L. (1966). *The social psychology of organizations.* New York: Wiley.

Kielhofner, G. (1983). "Teaching" retarded adults: Paradoxical effects of a pedagogical enterprise. *Urban Life, 12*, 307–326.

Kiernat, J. M. (1983). Environment: The hidden modality. *Physical & Occupational Therapy in Geriatrics, 2 (1),* 3–12.

Knowles, E. S. (1982). From individuals to group members: A dialectic for the social sciences. In W. Ickes & E. S. Knowles (Eds.), *Personality, roles and social behavior.* New York: Springer-Verlag.

Kornblum, H., & Anderson, B. (1982). Acceptance: Reassessed—a point of view. *Child Psychiatry and Human Development, 12,* 171–178.

Kronenberg, F., Algado, S., & Pollard, N. (2006) *Occupational therapy without borders.* Oxford: Churchill Livingstone.

Law, M. (1991). The environment: A focus for occupational therapy. *Canadian Journal of Occupational Therapy, 58,* 171–179.

Law, M., Cooper, B., Strong, S., Stewart, D., Rigby, P., & Letts, L. (1996). Person-environment occupational model: A transactive approach to occupational performance. *Canadian Journal of Occupational Therapy, 63,* 9–23.

Lawton, M. P. (1980). *Environment and aging.* Monterey, CA: Brooks/Cole.

Lawton, M. P., & Nahemow, L. (1973). Ecology and the aging process. In C. Eisdorfer & M. P. Lawton (Eds.), *Psychology of adult development and aging.* Washington, DC: American Psychological Association.

Ljungström, è. (1989). Craft artifacts: Keys to the past: Narratives from a craft documentation project in Sweden. *Journal of Ethnological Studies, 28*, 75–87.

Longmore, P. K. (1995). The second phase: From disability rights to disability culture. *The Disability Rag and Resource, 16,* 4–11.

Longmore, P.K., & Goldberger, D. (2000). The league of the physically handicapped and the Great Depression: A case study in the new disability history. [Electronic version]. *The Journal of American history, 87* (3), 888–922.

Louis Harris & Associates (1998). *Highlights of the N.O.D./Harris 1998 Survey of Americans with Disabilities.* Washington DC: National Organization on Disability.

Lustig, B. (executive producer), & Scott, R. (director). (2001). *Hannibal* [motion picture]. United States: MGM/Universal.

Magill, J., & Vargo, J. (1977). Helplessness, hope, and the occupational therapist. *Canadian Journal of Occupational Therapy, 44*, 65–69.

McNeil, J.M. (1997). Americans with disabilities: 1994–95. U.S. Bureau of the Census *Current Population Reports.* Washington, DC: U.S. Government Printing Office.

Melin, L., & Gotestam, G. (1981). The effects of rearranging ward routines on communication and eating behaviors of psychogeriatric patients. *Journal of Applied Behavioral Analysis, 14*, 47–51.

Miller, J. F., & Oertel, C. B. (1983). Powerlessness in the elderly: Preventing hopelessness. In J. F. Miller (Ed.), *Coping with chronic illness: Overcoming powerlessness.* Philadelphia: FA Davis.

Mitchell, D. (2002). Narrative prosthesis and the materiality of metaphor. In S.L. Snyder, B.J. Brueggemann, & R. Garland-Thompson (Eds.), *Disability Studies: Enabling the Humanities* (pp. 15–30). New York: Modern Language Association of America.

Moos, R. H. (1974). *Evaluating treatment environments: A social ecological approach.* New York: Wiley.

Murphy, R. F. (1987). *The body silent.* New York: WW Norton.

Murphy, R. F., Scheer, J., Murphy, Y., & Mack, R. (1988). Physical disability and social liminality: A study in the rituals of adversity. *Social Science and Medicine, 26,* 235–242.

Nelson, D. (1988). Occupation: Form and performance. *American Journal of Occupational Therapy, 42*, 633–641.

Neville-Jan, A. (2005). The problem with prevention: The case of spina bifida. *American Journal of Occupational Therapy, 59*, 527–539.

Newcomb, T. M. (1943). *Personality and social change.* New York: Dryden.

Ogbu, J. U. (1981). Origins of human competence: A cultural-ecological perspective. *Child Development, 52*, 413–429.

Oliver, M. (1990). *The politics of disablement.* London: Macmillan.

Oliver, M. (1996). *Understanding disability: From theory to practice.* New York: St. Martin's.

Oliver, M., Zarb, G., Silver, J., Moore, M., & Salisbury, V. (1988). *Walking into darkness: The experience of spinal cord injury.* London: Macmillan.

Pervin, L. A. (1968). Performance and satisfaction as a function of individual-environment fit. *Psychological Bulletin, 69,* 56–68.

Quilitch, H. R., & Risley, T. R. (1973). The effects of play materials on social play. *Journal of Applied Behavioral Analysis, 6,* 573–578.

Rapoport, A. (1980). Cross-cultural aspects of environmental design. In I. Altman, A. Rapoport, & J. F. Wohlwill (Eds.), *Human behavior and environment* (Vol. 4). New York: Plenum.

Reed, E. S. (1982). An outline of a theory of action systems. *Journal of Motor Behavior, 14*, 98–134.

Rockwell-Dylla, L. (1992). *Older adults' meaning of environment: Hospital and home.* Unpublished master's thesis, University of Illinois at Chicago.

Rowles, G. (1991). Beyond performance: Being in place as a component of occupational therapy. *American Journal of Occupational Therapy, 45*, 265–271.

Rubinstein, R. L. (1989). The home environments of older people: A description of the psychosocial processes linking person to place. *Journal of Gerontology, 44*, 45–53.

Sameroff, A. J. (1983). Developmental systems: Contexts and evolution. In P. H. Mussen (Ed.), *Handbook of child psychology.* New York: Wiley.

Sarbin, T. R. (1954). Role theory. In G. Lindzey & E. Aronson (Eds.), *The Hand-book of social psychology* (Vol. 1). Reading, MA: Addison-Wesley.

Scull, A. T. (1977). *Decarceration: Community treatment and the deviant: A radical view.* Englewood Cliffs, NJ: Prentice-Hall.

Shapiro, J. P. (1993). *No pity: People with disabilities forging a new civil rights movement.* New York: Random House.

Simmons, J. E., & Barris, R. (1984). *The relationship between the home environment and the occupational behavior in the post-CVA patient.* Unpublished manuscript.

Stone, G.V.M. (2005). Personal and environmental influences on occupation. In C. H. Christiansen, C. M. Baum, and J. Bass-Haugen (Eds.), *Occupational therapy: Performance, participation, and well-being* (3rd ed.) Thorofare, NJ: Slack.

Suto, M., & Frank, G. (1994). Future time perspective and daily occupations of persons with chronic schizophrenia in a board and care home. *American Journal of Occupational Therapy, 48*, 7–18.

Test, M. A., & Stein, L. I. (1978). Community treatment of the chronic patient: A research overview. *Schizophrenia Bulletin, 4*, 350–364.

Trombly, C. A. (1983). *Occupational therapy for physical dysfunction* (2nd ed.). Baltimore: Williams & Wilkins.

Vash, C. L. (1981). *The psychology of disability.* New York: Springer-Verlag.

Zola, I. K. (1982). *Missing pieces: A chronicle of living with a disability.* Philadelphia: Temple University.

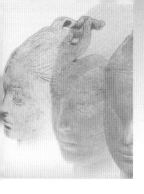

8

Dimensions of Doing

● Gary Kielhofner

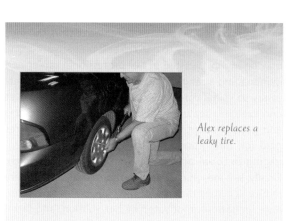

Alex replaces a leaky tire.

Consider Alex, a mechanic, who is replacing a leaking tire.[1] The question, "What is Alex doing?" can be answered in the following ways:

● Alex is making a series of calculated judgments and motor actions.

● Alex is changing a tire.

● Alex is working.

In addition to these responses, we could also answer the question by placing Alex's actions in a larger context and consider how changing a tire fits into the unfolding of his life as an occupational being.

Each of these responses represents a different perspective or vantage point on what a person does when engaged in a specific occupation. This chapter will examine occupation from these different perspectives, offering a cross-sectional and longitudinal perspective.

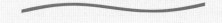

[1] Susan Cahill, clinical instructor at the University of Illinois at Chicago, provided the photo of Alex for this chapter.

A Cross-Section of Occupation: Levels of Doing

When considering what people do in the course of their occupations, one can describe that doing at three levels (Haglund & Henriksson, 1995). These levels correspond to three answers given to the question about what Alex was doing:

● Occupational participation
● Occupational performance
● Occupational skill.

Participation refers to doing in the broadest sense. It attends to engaging in occupation at the level of work, play, and activities of daily living that make up life. Performance denotes the larger chunks of action that make up a coherent undertaking. The concept of skill provides the most detailed or fine-grained look at what a person does, attending to purposeful units of action.

Occupational Participation

The World Health Organization and the Occupational Therapy Practice Framework use the term *participation* to refer to a person's involvement in life situations (American Occupational Therapy Association [AOTA], 2002; World Health Organization [WHO], 2001). Participation connotes persons' taking part in society along with their experiences within their life contexts (WHO, 2001).

Consistent with this usage, the term **occupational participation** refers to engaging in work, play, or activities of daily living that are part of one's sociocultural context and that are desired and/or necessary to one's well-being. Engagement involves not only per-

101

formance but also subjective experience (Yerxa, 1980). Thus, occupational participation connotes doing things with personal and social significance. Examples of occupational participation are volunteering for an organization, working in a full- or part-time job, recreating regularly with friends, doing self-care, maintaining one's living space, and attending school.[2]

Each area of occupational participation involves a cluster of related things that one does. For example, maintaining one's living space may include paying the rent, doing repairs, dusting furniture, decorating, and attending monthly meetings of a resident's association.

Occupational participation is collectively influenced by the following:

- Performance capacities
- Habituation
- Volition
- Environmental conditions.

Thus, occupational participation is both personal and contextual. It is personal in that the types of participation in which a person will engage are influenced by the individual's unique motives, roles, habits, abilities, and limitations. It is contextual in that the environment can either enable or restrict occupational participation.

A 10-year-old's areas of occupational participation may include doing personal hygiene and dressing, routine chores at home, school attendance and homework, participation in sports, family activities, and free play. The child's school attendance and family activities are primarily shaped by societal expectation and social roles assigned to the child. What kind of sports the child plays may depend on capacities, interests, and available opportunities in the environment. Free play activities are a result of choices that reflect the child's personal causation, values, and interests as well as the opportunities provided in the physical and social envi-

ronment. Thus, a complex interaction of personal and environmental factors ultimately shapes the full spectrum of occupational participation in a person's life.

A disability may alter, but need not prevent, occupational participation if adequate environmental supports are in place. For example, consider a young woman with spinal cord injury. Her occupational participation may include doing personal hygiene and grooming with a personal assistant. Use of the personal assistant may reflect both her performance limitations and her volitional choice to dispatch self-care with minimum personal effort and time so she can focus personal resources on work. For the same reason, she may rely on someone else to acquire and prepare food. She may be highly invested in her professional career and in managing a range of health maintenance tasks necessary to spinal cord injury (e.g., ensuring proper diet and exercise, dealing with health providers, accessing and getting adaptive equipment and other resources paid for, hiring and supervising an attendant, or engaging in social activism related to disability rights). Finally, she may pursue discretionary social and solitary leisure activities that are possible within her performance limitations, motivated by her volition, and facilitated by her physical and social environment. As this example indicates, performance limitations may influence, but need not prevent, occupational participation if a person can make volitional choices and has adequate environmental supports.

Occupational Performance

As noted previously, participation in an occupation may involve doing a variety of things. For example, as a mechanic, Alex's work includes not only changing a tire but also a wide range of other tasks/occupational forms, such as tuning an engine and changing oil. Moreover, his leisure occupations include a weekly game of poker, going fishing, bicycling, and attending

---

[2] No single categorization of the areas of occupational participation is proposed here. Readers may wish to examine the WHO classification and the AOTA practice framework classification (AOTA, 2002; WHO, 2001) as examples of ways areas of participation can be identified. Because each person organizes his or her occupational participation into a unique overall life pattern, a useful approach in practice is to pay attention to how the client defines and enacts participation.

> *Performance limitations may influence, but need not prevent, occupational participation if a person can make volitional choices and has adequate environmental supports.*

sports events with friends. His activities of daily living can include such things as taking a shower, dressing, balancing a checkbook, and preparing a meal.

Each time Alex does one of these discrete acts, he is performing (i.e., completing or—literally—going through the form). Thus, **occupational performance** refers to doing an occupational form (Nelson, 1988). Since most performance includes things that are part of everyday routines, habituation has an important influence on performance. Performance is also greatly affected by the environment. Environmental factors are also critical to whether and how impairments affect performance. For example, environmental supports ranging from adapted equipment to memory aids may make it possible for a person to complete an occupational form despite limitations of performance capacity.

Skills

Within any occupational performance, a number of discrete purposeful actions can be discerned. For example, in changing a tire, Alex engages in such purposeful actions as gathering tools for removing the tire, handling the tools, and sequencing the steps necessary to remove and replace the tire. These actions that make up occupational performance are referred to as skills. **Skills** are defined as observable, goal-directed actions that a person uses while performing (Fisher, 1999; Fisher & Kielhofner, 1995; Forsyth, Salamy, Simon, & Kielhofner, 1997). In contrast to performance capacity that refers to underlying ability, skill refers to the concrete actions that are done in the midst of undertaking an occupational form. As shown in *Figure 8.1*, a person's characteristics (including volition, habituation, and performance capacity) interact with the environment, resulting in skill.

Three types of skills are recognized: motor skills, process skills, and communication and interaction skills (*Fig. 8.2*). Detailed taxonomies have been developed as part of creating assessments of motor, process, and communication/interaction skills (see Chapter 15 on observation-based assessments). Fisher and colleagues have developed the taxonomies of motor and process skills, which make up the Assessment of Motor and Process Skills (Berspang & Fisher, 1995; Doble, 1991; Fisher, 1993, 1997). Forsyth and colleagues have devel-

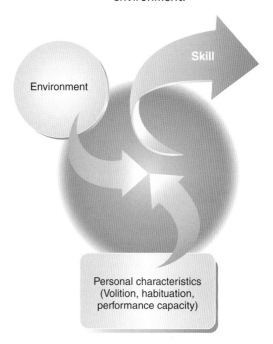

FIGURE 8.1 Skill as a function of the interaction between personal characteristics and the environment.

oped a taxonomy of communication and interaction skills, which make up the Assessment of Communication and Interaction Skills (Forsyth et al., 1997; Forsyth & Kielhofner, 1999).

Motor skills refer to moving self or task objects (Fisher, 1999). They include such actions as stabilizing and bending one's body and manipulating, lifting, and transporting objects. **Process skills** refer to logically sequencing actions over time, selecting and using appropriate tools and materials, and adapting performance when encountering problems (Fisher, 1999). They include such actions as choosing and organizing objects in space as well as initiating and terminating steps in performance. **Communication** and **interaction skills** refer to the ability to convey intentions and needs and to coordinate social action to act together with other people (Forsyth et al., 1997; Forsyth & Kielhofner, 1999). They include such things as gesturing, physically contacting others, speaking, engaging and collaborating with others, and asserting oneself.

FIGURE 8.2 Three types of skills.

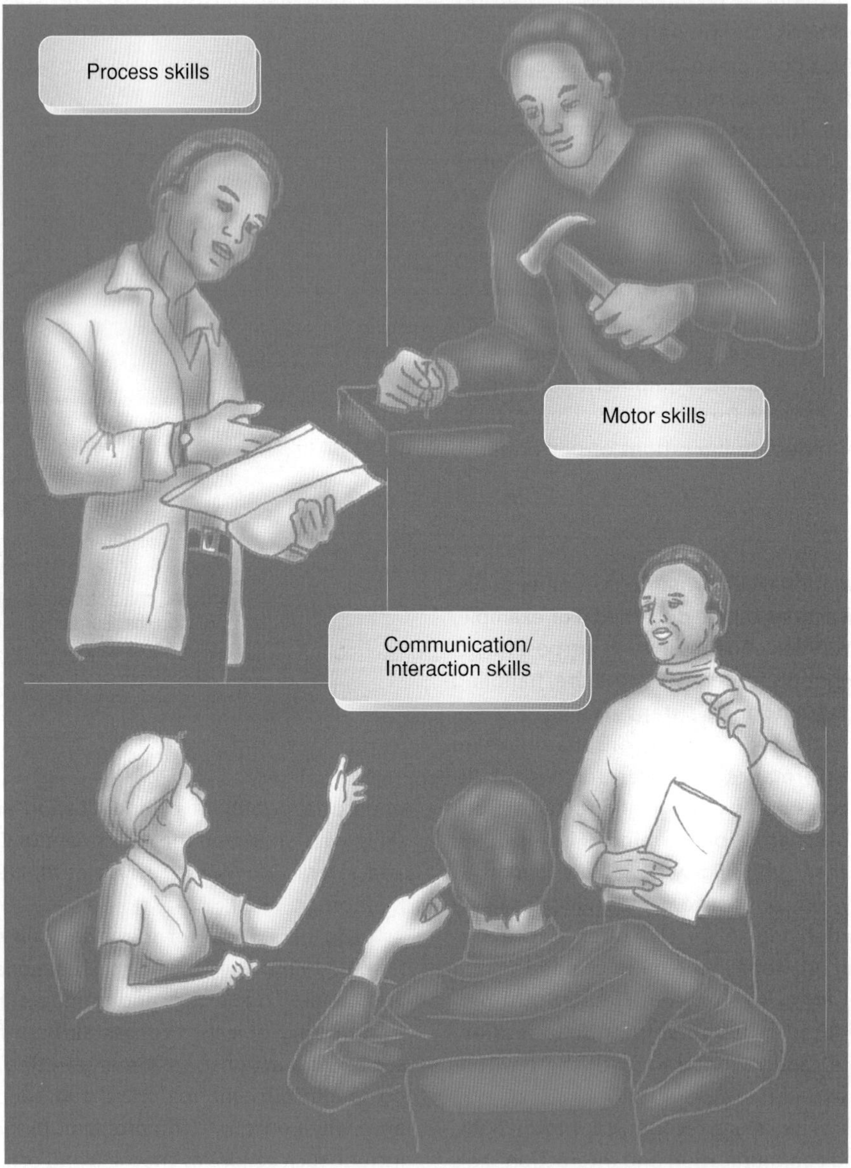

Embedded Levels of Doing

As the previous discussions illustrate, skill is embedded within performance, and the performance is embedded within participation. So whenever persons are partici-

> Skill is embedded within performance, and the performance is embedded within participation.

TABLE 8.1 The Three Levels of Brian's Doing

Level of Examining Doing	Examples		
Occupational participation	Working as a handyman	Taking care of his apartment	Participating in a self-advocacy group
Occupational performance that is a part of the larger area of participation	Mowing the lawn	Cleaning the kitchen	Writing a newsletter
Skills used in the performance	Walking, moving, grasping, sequencing, restoring	Grasping, lifting, sequencing, restoring	Manipulating, sequencing, asking, speaking

pating in occupations, they complete a number of tasks/occupational forms and use a wide range of skills. Let us consider an example, which is illustrated in *Table 8.1* and shown in the photographs.

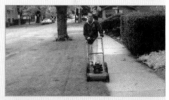

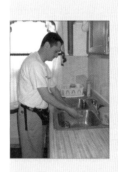

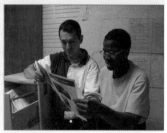

Brian mows the lawn as part of his handyman job, washes the dishes in his apartment, and examines the newsletter he and his girlfriend, Jill, publish for the local advocacy group.

Jessica Kramer, OTR/L, Head Research Assistant in the Model of Human Occupation Clearinghouse at University of Illinois at Chicago, provided the case of Brian for this chapter.

Brian

Brian, who is 39 years old, has an intellectual impairment. Just a year ago, he moved from a group home to his own supervised apartment across the street. He likes his new apartment, where he enjoys playing with his cat, watching television and movies, and listening to music. Brian prepares his own light meals and cleans his apartment. For more than 15 years he has been working as a handyman for a community agency that serves persons with developmental disabilities. His job includes cutting the grass, taking out garbage, changing light bulbs, and painting in several group homes managed by the agency. Additionally, Brian is a member of a self-advocacy organization, along with his girlfriend, whom he has been dating for 3 years. Together, they work on publishing a quarterly newsletter for their local chapter of the self-advocacy group. They also spend time together in their community doing such things as going shopping and going out to eat.

From this example we can see that Brian's occupational participation includes working as a handyman, maintaining his apartment, and being a member of a self-advocacy group along with his girlfriend. Within each of these occupations, Brian completes a number of occupational forms. For example, while working as a handyman, he mows the lawn. While maintaining his apartment, he cleans up the kitchen. While being a part of the self-advocacy group, he works on the newsletter. Within occupational forms/tasks, Brian employs a number of required skills. Thus, several skills make up an occupational performance, just as several occupational performances make up an area of occupational participation.

The extent of success in completing occupational forms depends on proficiency of the skills used to do them. The fullness of a person's participation in work, play, or activities of daily living similarly depends on the degree to which he or she can successfully complete the occupational forms that make up an area of occupational performance. For example, professors' success at lecturing depends primarily on their communication and interaction skills, and their participation in professorial work depends on their success at lecturing and at other occupational forms, such as planning courses, creating and giving examinations, and advising students.

Consequences of Doing: Occupational Identity, Competence, and Adaptation

As the previous discussion demonstrates, most persons' lives consist of several types of occupational participation. This section discusses how over time this participation results in occupational adaptation and its components, occupational identity and competence.

The term *adaptation* has been used in occupational therapy literature to refer to the extent to which persons are able to develop, change in response to challenges, or otherwise achieve a state of well-being through what they do (Fidler & Fidler, 1978; King, 1978; Nelson, 1988; Reilly, 1962). In earlier versions of MOHO, adaptation was defined as meeting personal needs and desires while meeting reasonable environmental expectations through one's occupation (Kielhofner, 1985, 1995).

Schkade and Schultz (1992) first used the term occupational adaptation to refer to "a state of competency in occupational functioning toward which human beings aspire" (p. 831). Their definition suggested that adaptation involved dual aspects of competency and aspiration. Spencer, Davidson, and White (1996) added that occupational adaptation was a cumulative process emanating from one's life history.

Mallinson, Mahaffey, and Kielhofner (1998) reported evidence from a study of life history interviews that a person's adaptation consists of two distinct elements, identity and competence. A subsequent study of life histories generated further evidence of occupational identity and occupational competence as distinct components of occupational adaptation (Kielhofner, Mallinson, Forsyth, & Lai, 2001). Building on this theoretical and empirical work, the following presents a definition of occupational adaptation and its two components, identity and competence.

Occupational Identity

Christiansen (1999) notes that identity refers to a composite definition of the self, including roles and relationships, values, self-concept, and personal desires and goals. He further argues that participation in occupations helps to create identity. Building on his argument, as well as the empirical work referred to earlier, **occupational identity** is defined here as a composite sense of who one is and wishes to become as an occupational being generated from one's history of occupational participation. One's volition, habituation, and experience as a lived body are all integrated into occupational identity.

Consequently, occupational identity includes a composite of the following:

- One's sense of capacity and effectiveness for doing
- What things one finds interesting and satisfying to do
- Who one is, as defined by one's roles and relationships
- What one feels obligated to do and holds as important
- A sense of the familiar routines of life
- Perceptions of one's environment and what it supports and expects.

These elements are garnered over time and become part of one's identity. Their implications for the future are also part of occupational identity.

Thus, occupational identity reflects accumulated life experiences that are organized into an understanding of who one has been and a sense of desired and possible direction for one's future. Occupational identity serves both as a means of self-definition and as a blueprint for upcoming action.

Preliminary evidence suggests that occupational identity is represented in a continuum that begins with self-appraisal and extends toward the more challenging elements of accepting responsibility for and knowing what one wants from life (Kielhofner et al., 2001). Thus, it would appear that building an occupational identity starts with self-knowledge of our capacities and interests from experience and extends to constructing a value-based vision of the future we desire.

Occupational Competence

Occupational competence is the degree to which one sustains a pattern of occupational participation that reflects one's occupational identity. Thus, while identity has to do with the subjective meaning of one's occupational life, competence has to do with putting that identity into action in an ongoing way. Occupational competence includes the following:

- Fulfilling the expectations of one's roles and one's own values and standards for performance
- Maintaining a routine that allows one to discharge responsibilities
- Participating in a range of occupations that provide a sense of ability, control, satisfaction, and fulfillment
- Pursuing one's values and taking action to achieve desired life outcomes.

Competence appears to begin with organizing one's life to meet basic responsibilities and personal standards and extends to meeting role obligations and then achieving a satisfying and interesting life (Kielhofner & Forsyth, 2001).

Occupational Adaptation

Occupational adaptation is defined here as the construction of a positive occupational identity and achieving occupational competence over time in the context of one's environment. This definition acknowledges that occupational adaptation has two distinct and interrelated elements (*Fig. 8.3*). It also specifies that adaptation takes place in a specific context with its opportunities, supports, constraints, and demands.

While occupational identity and competence codevelop over time, one cannot operationalize a view of self and life that one has not developed.

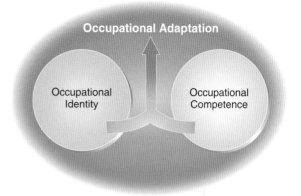

FIGURE 8.3 Occupational adaptation and its two components.

Evidence also suggests that while disability can affect both identity and competence, its effects are more pronounced in competence (Kielhofner et al., 2001; Mallinson et al., 1998).

Development and Threats to Occupational Adaptation

As noted earlier, occupational adaptation is the consequence of one's history of participation in life occupations (*Fig. 8.4*). From the time we learn our first occupational forms and begin to participate in the world around us by doing things, we shape our own volition, habituation, and performance capacity. Throughout this process, we are in constant interaction with the physical and social environment that shapes the development of our volition, habituation, and performance capacity. These personal characteristics, in interaction with the environment, influence our occupational participation.

Over time, we construct our occupational identity and competence through ongoing occupational participation. Occupational identity and competence are realized as we develop and respond to life changes (including illness and impairment). Identity and competence describe, then, the unfolding state in which we find ourselves at any point in our lives.

Our degree of success in occupational adaptation, as reflected in the identities we construct and our extent of competently enacting them, varies over time.

FIGURE 8.4 The process of occupational adaptation.

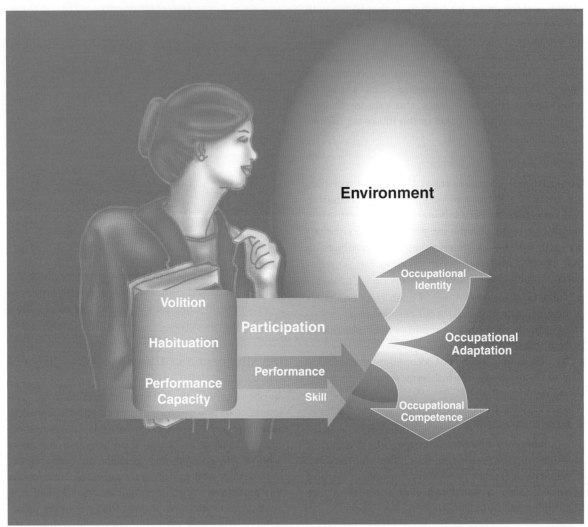

Most people, will, at one time or another, experience a threat to or problems in occupational adaptation requiring the rebuilding of occupational identity and competence. The next chapter examines this process in more depth by considering the occupational adaptation of persons challenged by disability.

> *Most people, will, at one time or another, experience a threat to or problems in occupational adaptation requiring the rebuilding of occupational identity and competence.*

Key Terms

Communication and interaction skills: Conveying intentions and needs and coordinating social action to act together with people.

Motor skills: Moving self or task objects.

Occupational adaptation: Constructing a positive occupational identity and achieving occupational competence over time in the context of one's environment.

Occupational competence: Degree to which one is able to sustain a pattern of occupational participation that reflects one's occupational identity.

Occupational identity: Composite sense of who one is and wishes to become as an occupational being generated from one's history of occupational participation.

Occupational participation: Engagement in work, play, or activities of daily living that are part of one's sociocultural context and that are desired and/or necessary to one's well-being.

Occupational performance: Doing an occupational form/task.

Process skills: Logically sequencing actions over time, selecting and using appropriate tools and materials, and adapting performance when encountering problems.

Skills: Observable, goal-directed actions that a person uses while performing.

References

American Occupational Therapy Association (2002). Occupational Therapy Framework: Domain and process. *American Journal of Occupational Therapy, 56,* 609–639.

Berspang, B., & Fisher, A. G. (1995). Validation of the Assessment of Motor and Process Skills for use in Sweden. *Scandinavian Journal of Occupational therapy, 2,* 3–9.

Christiansen, C. H. (1999). Defining lives: Occupation as identity: An essay on competence, coherence, and the creation of meaning. *American Journal of Occupational Therapy, 53,* 547–558.

Commission on Practice, American Occupational Therapy Association. (2001). *Occupational Therapy Practice Framework.* Unpublished working paper.

Doble, S. (1991). Test-retest and inter-rater reliability of a process skills assessment. *Occupational Therapy Journal of Research, 11,* 8–23.

Fidler, G. S., & Fidler, J. W. (1978). Doing and becoming: Purposeful action and self-actualization. *American Journal of Occupational Therapy, 32,* 305–310.

Fisher, A. G. (1993). The assessment of IADL motor skills: An application of many-faceted Rasch analysis. *American Journal of Occupational Therapy, 47,* 319–338.

Fisher, A. G. (1997). Multifaceted measurement of daily life task performance: Conceptualizing a test of instrumental ADL and validating the addition of personal ADL tasks. *Archives of Physical Medicine and Rehabilitation: State of the Art Reviews, 11,* 289–303.

Fisher A. G. (1999). *Assessment of Motor and Process Skills* (3rd ed.). Ft. Collins, CO: Three Star.

Fisher, A. G., & Kielhofner, G. (1995). Skills in occupational performance. *A model of human occupation: Theory and application* (2nd ed.). Baltimore: Williams & Wilkins.

Forsyth, K., & Kielhofner, G. (1999). Validity of the assessment of communication and interaction skills. *British Journal of Occupational Therapy, 62,* 69–74.

Forsyth, K., Salamy, M., Simon, S., & Kielhofner, G. (1997). *Assessment of communication and interaction skills.* Chicago: University of Illinois, Model of Human Occupation Clearinghouse.

Haglund, L., & Henriksson, C. (1995). Activity—From action to activity. *Scandinavian Journal of Caring Sciences, 9,* 227–234.

Kielhofner, G. (1985). *A model of human occupation: Theory and application.* Baltimore: Williams & Wilkins.

Kielhofner, G. (1995). *A model of human occupation: Theory and application* (2nd ed.). Baltimore: Williams & Wilkins.

Kielhofner, G., & Forsyth, K. (2001). Development of a client self-report for treatment planning and documenting therapy outcomes. *Scandinavian Journal of Occupational Therapy, 8,* 131–139.

Kielhofner, G., Mallinson, T., Forsyth, K., & Lai, J. S. (2001). Psychometric properties of the second version of the Occupational Performance History Interview (OPHI-II). *American Journal of Occupational Therapy, 55,* 260–267.

King, L. J. (1978). Toward a science of adaptive responses. *American Journal of Occupational Therapy, 32,* 429–437.

Mallinson, T., Mahaffey, L., & Kielhofner, G. (1998). The occupational performance history interview: Evidence for three underlying constructs of occupational adaptation. *Canadian Journal of Occupational Therapy, 65,* 219–228.

Nelson, D. (1988). Occupation: Form and performance. *American Journal of Occupational Therapy, 42,* 633.

Reilly, M. (1962). Occupational therapy can be one of the great ideas of 20th century medicine. *American Journal of Occupational Therapy, 16,* 1–9.

Schkade, J. K., & Schultz, S. (1992). Occupational adaptation: Toward a holistic approach for contemporary practice. Part 1. *American Journal of Occupational Therapy, 46,* 829–837.

Spencer, J. C., Davidson, H. A., & White, V. K. (1996). Continuity and change: Past experience as adaptive repertoire in occupational adaptation. *American Journal of Occupational Therapy, 50,* 526–534.

World Health Organization (2001). *International Classification of Functioning, Disability and Health (ICF).* Geneva: World Health Organization.

Yerxa, E. J. (1980). Occupational therapy's role in creating a future climate of caring. *American Journal of Occupational Therapy, 34,* 529–534.

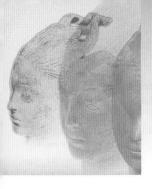

9

Crafting Occupational Life

- Gary Kielhofner
- Lena Borell
- Roberta Holzmueller
- Hans Jonsson
- Staffan Josephsson
- Ritta Keponen
- Jane Melton
- Kelly Munger
- Louise Nygård

Introduction

Chapter 8 notes that occupational identity represents a composite sense of oneself and one's future generated from ongoing occupational participation. It further noted that occupational competence involves sustaining a pattern of participation that reflects one's identity. The purpose of this chapter is to consider further how persons generate and maintain occupational identity and competence—in short, how they craft their occupational lives.

Both occupational identity and competence encompass how volition, habituation, and performance capacity collectively orient each person to his or her own unique life. Consider that this includes the following:

- What one holds as important
- One's unique sense of pleasure and satisfaction in doing things
- Knowledge of one's own capacities, limitations, and relative effectiveness
- Awareness of who one is in reference to the social world
- Familiarity with the rhythms and routines of life
- Lived experience as an embodied being
- Apprehension of the world.

These elements are always in the background, shaping how people craft their ongoing occupational lives in the stream of time. Moreover, they are integrated into each person's unique occupational narrative.

Narrative Organization of Occupational Life

People conduct and draw meaning from life by locating themselves in unfolding narratives that integrate their past, present, and future selves (Geertz, 1986; Gergen & Gergen, 1988; Helfrich, Kielhofner, & Mattingly, 1994; Mattingly, 1991; Schafer, 1981; Spence, 1982; Taylor, 1989). Two important features of narratives—plot and metaphor—synthesize and impart meaning on many elements and episodes of life. The following sections examine these two features of narrative.

Plot

Gergen and Gergen (1988) refer to plot as the forestructure of narrative; it determines how people think

> *People conduct and draw meaning from life by locating themselves in unfolding narratives that integrate their past, present, and future selves.*

and talk when they use stories. The plot of a story is the intersection between the progression of time and the direction (for better or worse) that life takes. Consequently, the plot is the shape of events over time as they get better or worse (Gergen & Gergen, 1988; Jonsson, Kielhofner, & Borell, 1997; Keponen & Kielhofner, 2006).

A narrative's plot reveals its overall meaning because it sums up where life has been and is going. For example, the tragic plot is found when some event results in a steep downward turn in a previously good or improving life. It signifies a life ruined. The melodramatic plot involves a series of upward and downward turns. It reveals a life of struggle. In this way, emplotting life events links them together in a way that makes sense of the life as a whole. Consequently, the various life episodes derive their meaning from the overall shape of the plot. One way of understanding narrative plots that has been used in occupational therapy research and practice is to characterize them as regressive, progressive, or stability narratives (Jonsson, Kielhofner, & Borell, 1997; Kielhofner, Braveman, Finlayson, Paul-Ward, Goldbaum, & Goldstein, 2004). As shown in *Figure 9.1*, a progressive narrative is headed upward; a regressive narrative heads downward; and a stability narrative continues life in a constant direction. People seek to evaluate life events in terms of their significance or impact on the unfolding life story. Most events represent a continuation of the basic direction of life. Others positively change or threaten where life is headed. In evaluating ongoing events of life, the underlying plot (the direction for better or worse that life will take) is always at stake.

People evaluate each new unfolding circumstance of life in terms of how such things have gone before and in terms of where it might lead. For example, Jonsson, Kielhofner, & Borell (1997) studied how older persons anticipated their retirement. Expectations of retirement were always intimately tied to how past and present occupational life, especially work, were experienced. If work was negative, then retirement could be seen as an escape. In this case, life after retirement could be expected to get better. If work was positive, then retirement could continue a good life by providing opportunities to do other valued things; or it could be a loss that would make life worse.

How past and future are linked depends on and reveals the plot. If for example, one is living a tragic narrative, past successes do not portend that things will go well in the future. On the other hand, if one is in a story where things are getting better, past failures will become lessons that provide the person with new strengths or obstacles that were overcome. The significance of the past for the present and the fu-

FIGURE 9.1 The slopes of progressive, regressive, and stable narratives.

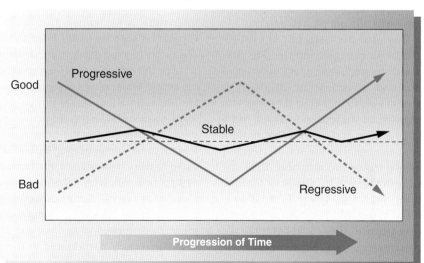

ture depends on and reflects the narrative's plot. In a similar fashion, inevitable or likely events in the future take on their significance with reference to the past and present. How they are seen to relate to past or present also depends on and reflects the underlying plot.

Metaphor

Stories are also given meaning by metaphors (Ganzer, 1993). Metaphor is the use of a familiar object or phenomenon to stand in the place of the less well understood event or situation (Ortony, 1979). Metaphors succinctly characterize complex or emotionally difficult circumstances by evoking something familiar or readily understood to stand in the place of that which is difficult to grasp and/or face. Metaphors also provide a way of dealing with difficult circumstances. For example, when faced with serious or life-threatening illness, people often evoke the metaphor of battle. This metaphor casts the disease as "a threatening" enemy that must be fought and expelled or destroyed.

People also evoke metaphors to make sense of disabilities. Mallinson, Kielhofner, and Mattingly (1996) identified metaphors of momentum and entrapment in the narratives of persons with mental illness. People hospitalized because of their mental illness often referred to their lives in terms of speed, inertia, impetus, acceleration, and deceleration. When they were summing up or evaluating the events of their lives, they related images such as getting life going again, life slowing down, life passing by, life grinding to a halt, or life going nowhere. They used the metaphor of momentum to characterize their struggles, motives, life junctures, and life events by evaluating them in terms of the progression and direction of their lives. Importantly, the way in which they lived their lives also embodied such slowing down, coming to a halt, heading off in wrong directions, and so on. Other persons with mental illness described their life as being severely restricted or confined by life circumstances. Their stories were imbued with the wish for escape or for finding a way out of the maze. They saw their situation as both intolerable and inexorable. They also acted as individuals who were trapped. They could not make decisions. They sometimes exhibited symptoms of agoraphobia and were literally confined in their rooms or

homes. They stayed in dissatisfying relationships, jobs, and life situations.

How Metaphors Shape Narrative Meaning

Schön (1979) noted that metaphors are a primary vehicle through which people comprehend things that have gone wrong in life. Consequently, when lives are troubled and when people are struggling to comprehend difficult, painful, and incomprehensible events, metaphors are effective ways of assigning meaning to them. Moreover, metaphors sum up "what needs fixing" (Schön, 1979, p. 255). In pinpointing the essential nature of life's problems, struggles, and dilemmas, they also imply how they can be solved or overcome. For example, the metaphors of momentum imply solutions of going in a new direction, getting things going, or slowing down. Metaphors of entrapment suggest that one must escape or be freed.

Narrative, Meaning, and Doing

Narratives, with their plots and metaphors, shape how we perceive ongoing life. They are a way of making meaning as life unfolds and as new circumstances present themselves. Consequently, there is always openness in narrative that can take and make meaning of whatever emerges in an unpredictable life (Bruner, 1990a, b; Ricoeur, 1984). Moreover, what we do continues our stories, sometimes aiming toward a particular turn of events or outcome, sometimes moving things along, and sometimes acquiescing to what seems inevitable (Jonsson, Josephsson, & Kielhofner, 2000; Jonsson et al., 1997). Occupation both emanates from and influences where one's story is going (Clark, 1993; Helfrich et al., 1994).

For this reason, narratives can either impede or focus action. For example, if someone already sees his or her life as a tragedy, there is little reason to work toward goals because the tragic plot pronounces that things are ruined. On the other hand, a person who sees his or her life as getting better is likely to be motivated to work hard toward that outcome. In a study of 129 participants with AIDS, Kielhofner et al. (2004) found that clients' narratives were significant predictors of whether they would remain in or drop out of a program of vocational services and of whether those who successfully participated in the program would achieve employment or other productive outcomes.

Summary

The coherence and meaning people achieve in their lives is facilitated through narratives. The following features of narratives give them this integrating and meaning-making potential:

- Narratives tie together past, present, and future as well as integrate multiple themes of self and the world
- Narratives integrate and impart meaning through the use of plot and metaphor
- Narratives are open ended and thus allow comprehension of emergent events and circumstances of life, tying them to what has gone before and what may come next
- Narratives are not only told but are also done
- What one does continues the unfolding of one's narrative.

Given these considerations, an **occupational narrative**[1] is defined as a story (both told and enacted) that integrates across time one's unfolding volition, habituation, performance capacity, and environments through plots and metaphors that sum up and assign meaning to these elements. Both occupational identity and competence are reflected and enacted in occupational narratives.

Five Occupational Narratives

How occupational narratives figure in ongoing life can best be appreciated by detailed examination of such stories. The following sections present five occupational narratives. Each narrative tells about living with an impairment. Gail's, Leena's, and Lisa's stories are rendered in the third person, because the text was shaped by someone other than the story's character. Kelly's story is in the first person because she authored it. Aaron's story is told by his mother, Roberta Holzmueller, with liberal perspectives from Aaron. It il-

lustrates the extent to which crafting an occupational narrative can involve the collective efforts of parents and child.

Aaron's Story[2]

Aaron is planning his sixth birthday party, to which he plans to invite all of the children in his mainstream kindergarten class and a few friends from last year's preschool class. He has a clearly articulated theme (jungle animals) and place (home) where he'd like to have his party. He also has some ideas for things the guests will do (crafts and games, making or pretending to be jungle animals).

One of the assignments Aaron had recently for kindergarten was to research and present to his class the kind of job he would like to have when he grows up. When I asked him what he would like to be when he grows up, his answer was crystal clear and instantaneous: "A dad." In further probing, I asked him if he would like to do other work besides being a dad. He said, "Sure, I'll do my work." When I asked what kind of work it would be, he said, "Whatever they need me to do, I'll do." In still further probing, we discussed what is his favorite part of school (stories), and when I suggested maybe he'd like to be a teacher, he answered, "or run the library." And so it happened that Aaron was the only one in his kindergarten class to research and report on two jobs: being a father and a librarian!

Aaron had a diffuse brain injury during or before birth, for causes that have never been specified to his family. He has been followed in early intervention since birth and received a diagnosis of cerebral palsy when he was a year old. His cerebral palsy is relatively mild, in that he is able to walk without assistance and to perform or approximate many of the gross motor activities his typically developing friends are doing. However, his gross and fine motor skills are well behind those of his age peers. His lack of motor control over certain muscle groups has not allowed him to predict bladder and bowel movements, so he has not yet learned to use the toilet; this is the aspect of his cerebral palsy which bothers him the most right now. Cognitively, he is at or above his peers in reading and math skills, and his social development is right on target.

---

[1] Previous discussions of narrative in relationship to MOHO referred to the concept of volitional narrative. This concept argued that narratives incorporate the essential themes of volition (ability and control in life, interest and satisfaction, and values). We have linked the concept of narrative to the broader constructs of occupational identity and competence in this chapter. Consequently, narratives are now seen as embracing a larger scope of occupational life and experience than previously thought.

As Aaron's mother, I recall with pain the circumstances surrounding his birth. It was completely unexpected. An ultrasound at 12 or 13 weeks indicated everything was all right; I was so relieved. It never occurred to me that our story would be anything but the happy one most people take into a wanted, cherished pregnancy. When Aaron was born, at first I felt like the hero, since he had stopped moving in utero, I called, went in, and was taken care of. Later that evening, when I called to the Infant Special Care Unit and was not able to talk with anyone, I still wasn't worried. But when my husband and I went down and they told us he had had seizures and needed a ventilator and a series of tests (magnetic resonance imaging, electroencephalography), I became frantic. Suddenly I got an image of my "special needs child" and thought of the many children with serious limitations we see out in the world. I thought, "I am going to be one of those parents." I told one of my dear friends, "This is a life-transforming experience," and it really has been.

During Aaron's birth and his first few weeks of life, a couple of experiences really stand out for me. One was with an occupational therapist who examined Aaron when he was a week old and we were preparing to take him home for the first time. She told us, "You don't compare him to other children. You compare him to himself. If you continue to see progress, you are happy. If you see stalls or stagnation, you seek help." In addition, when we took Aaron for his first visit to our pediatrician, he said, "If you have to injure your brain, the best time in life to do it is in utero or at birth." He followed this up with, "If what happened to Aaron happened to us, the results would be catastrophic. But the infant brain is still developing and very malleable, and you will be amazed at what he can do." And, indeed, we have been and continue to be amazed at what Aaron can do.

Both of these examples set me and my family (including Aaron) on a narrative course which is optimistic and full of possibility. Certainly, repeatedly over the past 6 or so years, we have been given less than sanguine news about Aaron. In some cases that news has proved to be incorrect; in other cases the jury is still out. But in these situations we considered the "bad news" and incorporated it into our overall very positive views of Aaron and his growth.

Aaron will tell you that the hardest thing about having cerebral palsy so far has been "the potty." As early as last year, I suspected that Aaron's delay in toilet

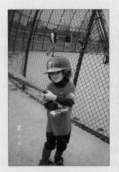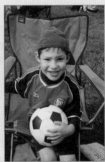

Aaron practices using his muscles by playing sports.

training might be in part muscle and sensation related. On the advice of my wise and thoughtful supervisor in the preschool where I work, I decided to tell Aaron that he had cerebral palsy just about a year ago, when he was about to turn 5. Her theory was that if we start "naming" the disability for him at this young age, it would become a normative part of his narrative, and I believe for the most part we have been successful in this. When I first told him about his cerebral palsy, I asked if he had noticed that sometimes he had more trouble getting his muscles to do things than other kids in his class. He said "yes," and I followed up with, "There's a reason for that. You have something called cerebral palsy, which comes from having hurt your brain when you were a tiny baby." I then pointed out the many, many ways that cerebral palsy does not affect him (e.g., knowing his numbers and letters, making friends, being a good friend, enjoying stories), and highlighted the ways that we think it does (moving his body, especially his fingers, and using the potty).

The other thing that Aaron mentioned as being hard about cerebral palsy is actually a far more universal struggle. He said it is hard when Nathan (his older brother) "beats him up." I was alarmed when he said this, but when I asked further, he said, "Nathan beats me at everything: he dribbles around me, he beats me at basketball, soccer, and chess, and he can bike." Since Nathan is an older brother, it is not hard to explain this as part of having an older brother. However, I do anticipate that as Aaron continues to mature, his ability to compete and participate in sports relative to his age mates may continue to bother him. I have already been thinking about whether to have him continue in mainstream sports activities or to begin thinking about participating in groups like the Special Olympics.

Aaron enjoys school very much. When I asked him what he liked best about it, he said, "the homework." Within school, he likes rug time and calendar and story time. An exciting part of kindergarten for Aaron has been learning to read, and he says he is a "pretty good reader." The topic he likes to learn about most is animals, because "Some of them are wild and some of them are not, but I like them both the same." He is looking forward to first grade, where he hopes he will "read more books."

At home, Aaron enjoys playing all sorts of board games, including "Sorry!," chess, and checkers. He also loves pretend play. Just today, he created an aquarium in our playroom, a day after our visit to the real aquarium. His was far more elaborate, including marine life as well as a zoo! He was particularly delighted to show us his penguin, dolphin, and whale show. Aaron also loves to read books with his family, both books he can read and being read to.

I asked Aaron how he felt about talking about cerebral palsy. He said, "I like talking about cerebral palsy. When I talk about cerebral palsy I learn things." When I asked him about being different from others he said, it felt "good, especially having different hair." As a final question, I asked Aaron what he would say to another child who just found out he had cerebral palsy. His response was, "I have cerebral palsy too."

---

[2]Roberta Holzmueller, Associate Professor at the University of Illinois at Chicago, provided Aaron's Story for this chapter.

As shown in *Figure 9.2*, Aaron's plot shows a positive direction, steadily upward after his birth. As he is a child, his story is still partly located in his mother's memory and formulation. As she realizes and illustrates through his planned adult roles, it will eventually be his story to take over and steer in the direction he chooses.

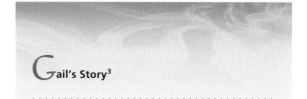

Gail's Story[3]

. . . .

Gail is 49 and lives in a town house in England. Her pet dog, Nutmeg, and her two cats, Comfrey and Woodruff, together with her close friends and family, particularly her mother, form the backbone of her social world. In addition, Gail has five godchildren she adores and spoils, and has recently become a great godmother. Gail has always believed that she can and should contribute to society through her work. However, this belief and unexpected life circumstances took Gail in a direction she would not have anticipated as a young woman.

Experiencing mental illness made Gail recognize the importance of enjoying life and taking responsibility to do so. So Gail went about constructing a full leisure life. Her many leisure interests include playing her clarinet and more recently learning to play the violin. Gail describes great satisfaction from her involvement in music

FIGURE 9.2 Aaron's narrative slope.

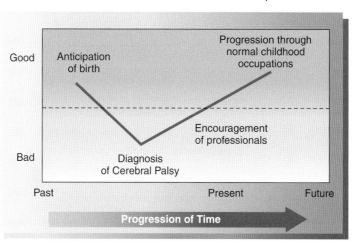

both from the stimulation of the melody and from meeting people with similar interests. In addition Gail satisfies her interest in mathematics by studying a mathematics qualification at a university. She also relaxes through reading and gains a sense of adventure through traveling. Of much less interest to Gail is what she describes as household chores, for example gardening and housework. Though Gail does not enjoy these activities, when she has done them, she finds satisfaction in the end product.

Gail is aware of the capacities and limitations that she has to deal with in her day-to-day life. Her perspective is that her memory fails her regularly, but she com-

pensates for this by writing notes to herself and making lists of tasks to be done. Despite this difficulty Gail is confident in her capacity to undertake the duties of full-time paid employment. She considers this activity more important than routine household chores.

With regard to the rhythms and routines of the day, Gail describes herself as an evening person, finding the mornings a challenge to organize herself. She benefits from a prompt to get up in the morning and finds it helpful to end the day with calming activities which take her mind off the pressures of the day. Her two regular social activities during the week, meeting friends for meal; her responsibility to walk her dog, Nutmeg routinely; and her work schedule construct the pattern of her normal week.

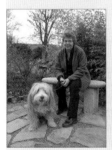 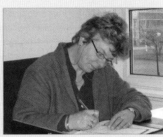

Gail on a daily walk with Nutmeg and Gail at work advocating for others with disabilities.

[3]Jane Melton, Consultant Occupational Therapist in Mental Health at Gloucestershire Partnership NHS Trust in Gloucestershire, United Kingdom, provided Gail's story for this chapter.

Gail's story is one of triumph—an upward movement after a period of illness (*Fig. 9.3*). Her story is one of not only overcoming but capitalizing on adversity to make her life more meaningful and fulfilling.

FIGURE 9.3 Gail's narrative slope.

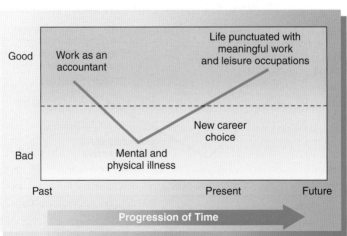

Leena's Story[4]

Leena graduated from high school with top grades and straightaway finished university studies. She always enjoyed the challenge of academic pursuits and thrived when challenged at work. Leena's greatest challenge has been to adapt to chronic pain. At age 35, 10 years ago, she first had surgery on her back. Despite ongoing medical treatment the pain has never fully subsided, and for the past 5 years she has had chronic neurogenic pain. She has come to deal with this pain in the same way she always managed to find a way forward. She uses a metaphor of momentum, noting, "Even if there was a mountain in front of me, I managed to find a route, a canyon—what's my way forward?"

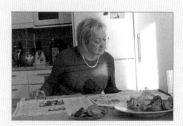

Leena reading the newspaper.

Leena worked as a managing director in a big firm that does international trade. Her work demanded long hours and a lot of traveling. She was a top performer in her field. After the onset of serious chronic pain, Leena knew she would not be able to go back to her old position. Instead, Leena chose to undertake studies in law with the aim of earning a doctoral degree. The following quotation illustrates the extent to which she has had to be flexible in her narrative in order to maintain it: "When I began [university] this time, I decided I wanted a doctoral degree .... Even if it took 20 years, I wanted a doctoral degree. After having studied law for a year, I realize I must be satisfied if I get a bachelor's degree. I think I can do a lot. When I have completed sufficient studies, I can work at home."

Leena's ability to continue the forward momentum of her life is also reflected in the way she has organized her life. She manages everyday tasks with help from her husband and a cleaning lady who takes care of her home a few times a month. (Leena notes that one benefit is that her husband is a better cook than she is.) She attends physical therapy four times a week, which she has scheduled to coincide with when she has to attend lectures at the university.

She reads voraciously both in Finnish and in English; the materials range from scientific articles to novels and detective stories. Even this occupation requires accommodation: "Every now and then I enjoy a newspaper. I like to read the newspaper sitting down but I am always in an awful agony afterwards. Nonetheless, every now and then I want to do it that way. Usually I read lying down and then I easily fall asleep." She used to be such a fast walker that people found it hard to keep up with her pace. Nowadays she requires a cane to make walking bearable. She has found another way to go fast: "You go fast with a bike, and although my leg gets more sore [than from walking], I want to ride a bike, I can't help it. I have learned that I can't ride many days in a row, because if I do that my pain lasts longer and gets worse." By moderating how frequently, how long, or in what way she does what is meaningful, Leena can avoid a level of pain that makes activity impossible. She knows her body well. She ensures that she can do important, enjoyable occupations by respecting the limits that her body sets for her.

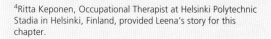

[4]Ritta Keponen, Occupational Therapist at Helsinki Polytechnic Stadia in Helsinki, Finland, provided Leena's story for this chapter.

Leena's story is a stability narrative (*Fig. 9.4*) in which she manages to move forward (her dominant metaphor) facing chronic pain like other life challenges. Notably, her narrative requires her to adapt her plans and routines, and the flexibility to do so makes the narrative possible.

FIGURE 9.4 Leena's narrative slope.

Good

Success in
school and work

Maintaining
meaningful occupations
despite pain

Onset of
chronic pain

New career choice
and adjustment
of life routines

Bad

Past   Present   Future

Progression of Time

Lisa's Story[5]

A visitor has just come to talk with Lisa, who is 54, divorced, and living by herself in her own house near her parents' home in a suburb of Stockholm. After greeting her guest, she sits down but rises immediately, asking, "Do you want a sandwich?"

"No thanks," the guest says.

She fetches some cookies and puts them on the table. She goes to the refrigerator, opens it, and looks inside, saying something to herself about buns. Then she seems to catch herself, embarrassed. Her guest wonders aloud what she said, and Lisa responds, "I was looking for the buns, but I suppose I already ate them." Lisa takes some dark bread from the refrigerator and says, matter-of-factly, "Do you want a sandwich?"

The guest repeats, "No, thanks."

Lisa returns to the table. She looks around. She goes to the sink, saying, "What was I looking for?"

Later, after her lunch, she wipes the wash bowl and then says, "I wonder where I took this from? Where do I keep it? I have no idea!" She looks under the sink. She turns. She looks around more. "No, I think I keep it in the laundry," she says.

In her typically Swedish practical view of the world, it is important to Lisa to remain active and be useful. She announces, "If there is laundry to do, I just start doing it." One of her favorite activities is ironing. When an observer notes that she looks so

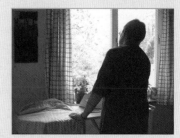

Lisa ironing at home.

peaceful ironing, Lisa explains that when she irons, "It gets nice … and then I like having clean and ironed shirts in the closet … and then you feel useful doing it." Lisa goes on to tell about how on good days she becomes adventuresome and goes into the city to shop for food on sale. Being practical and useful sums up much of how life should be in Lisa's common sense view; however, she has a secret that makes this difficult.

In autumn 1990, Lisa's dementia first showed at work when she developed depression, memory loss, and difficulty concentrating. Her symptoms were interpreted as depression, and she began taking antidepressive medication without any benefit. Her difficulties increased, and she was assigned to less demanding tasks. By the deep winter, she could not handle work at all and had to leave her job with disability benefits. By spring she was hospitalized.

At this time Lisa had severe memory deficits. She could not, for example, recall her own age. As Lisa describes it, she feels "somewhat of a chaos inside." Today, her cognition continues to deteriorate. Lisa is considered to have degeneration of the frontal cortex.

Lisa makes it clear that she must not show her disease to the world, but it is hard work to conceal her difficulties. She wonders, "Perhaps everybody can see I'm this dizzy and crazy," and then she repeats how hard she works to conceal what she is like. Even Lisa's mother, who is the person closest to her, is not entirely aware of her problems. Lisa considers aloud what might happen if her mother knew the facts of her dementia: "Maybe they would take my house away from me, or something like that, and believe I can't manage at all." Then there is the worry about what will happen when her mother is no longer nearby as a source of support. "I worry about the day she dies. Then I will be all by myself with this sticky mess in my head. Then I won't manage and everything will fall apart."

The impending chaos when Lisa's life will come apart hovers relentlessly around her little house. It causes Lisa anxiety over all of the many things that may go wrong and overwhelm her. Thus, "All small things become huge houses. I get a lot of Christmas cards, and I worry about having to find cards to send in return, and then I have to write them out. And find addresses. And then they need stamps and I have to get out to buy stamps. And then I have to mail them

and all." So go Lisa's worries about how she is going to manage.

Lisa reminisces to her guest about the frequent bus trips into Stockholm that were a part of her routine. She is very hesitant to take these trips now. She tells how a few weeks ago she was going to meet her daughter in a large shopping center in the city. When the time came, she could not imagine how to get into the city or return home, so she did not go. Today, she starts to look for her telephone books so she can call the bus company with a question about the schedule. She finds the books in the cleaning cupboard but just stares at them, apparently wondering which one she should consult. Finally, she sighs. "No, today I feel bad. I don't want to do it." Then, as if to explain, Lisa tells her guest, slowly and solemnly, "I'm not that strong anymore. I'm weak and I can't make it. It feels like I just could break down. Before this I was strong, but I'm not anymore."

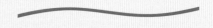

[5]Louise Nygård, Associate Professor and Senior Researcher in the Division of Occupational Therapy at the Karolinska Institutet, Stolkholm, Sweden, provided Lisa's story for this chapter.

The downward slope of Lisa's narrative takes her to the edge of a precipice (*Fig. 9.5*). In any moment she may be found out as incompetent, losing her house and her freedom as she lost her job. One mistake, she believes, could bring her world crashing down on her. Lisa's story is largely lived and is articulated only in sporadic bits. She does not employ a deep overriding metaphor but evokes the household images of a "sticky mess" in her head and the small tasks that become like managing big houses. Nonetheless, her story illustrates that even persons with cognitive limitations manage to emplot their occupational lives.

FIGURE 9.5 Lisa's narrative slope

Working

Good

- -

Depression, memory loss,
difficulty concentrating

At
home

Bad

Left
work

Hospitalization   Incompetence discovered
Loss of home

Past   Present   Future

Progression of Time

Kelly's Story[6]

Walking up the ramp and into the hotel for the Society for Disability Studies (SDS) conference, I can feel a tingling of excitement. As a doctoral student in this burgeoning field, I am surrounded on a daily basis by Disability Studies scholars (both impaired and "temporarily able bodied"), many of whom are among my closest friends. Each new introduction to a disabled scholar at SDS signifies for me a reaffirmation of my involvement in and affection for the disability community. I feel a common bond with these individuals, one that extends far beyond our professional interests and deep into our identity as disabled people.

It wasn't always like this. For the majority of my brief 28 years in this world, I was largely cut off from others with disabilities and therefore often wanted nothing to do with them. Of course, growing up with cerebral palsy, I was exposed to other "handicapped" (still a

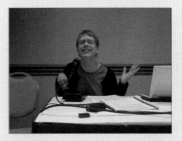

As a doctoral student, Kelly presents a paper at an international conference for Disability Studies scholars.

common and largely acceptable label in the 1980s) children almost every day. At the local rehabilitation center I stretched alongside them on the blue foam physical therapy mats. I played board games with them as my occupational therapist unwaveringly tried to persuade me to use my eternally clenched right hand rather than my relatively dexterous left one. As part of the recreational program I went swimming and even rode horses with other disabled children, all the while feeling removed and distant, even embarrassed to be in their company. Instead, I longed for the "normalcy" of my nondisabled schoolmates. I longed to be integrated into their cliques or just to have someone to eat lunch with; I longed to get into the girls' family Volvos and to play in their bedrooms after school instead of going to therapy. In high school, I longed to get into the boys' cars after school, to hang out with them downtown, to drink beer with them, to be invited to their parties, and to kiss and even to make love to them.

This pressure to be as "normal" as possible seemed to bombard me from all directions. I do not fault my parents, my teachers, or even my therapists for exerting this pressure. In fact, I commend them for it. My mother always says that all she ever wanted was for me to have options. Certainly, my current options are numerous. Graduating with honors from a college prep school where I spent 4 to 5 hours every evening on homework just to keep up with my able-bodied classmates, I was awarded a scholarship at small liberal arts college for women. Here not only did I remain very successful academically, but I developed for the first time a genuine group of friends (with whom I still keep in close touch), and also experienced my first romantic relationship. More important, however, I truly began to explore the personal meaning of my disability.

For the first time in my life, I was living on my own; I was not attending therapy, not wearing orthotics, not depending upon my parents to cook for me, do my laundry, help me with my homework, or tell me when I should go to bed. While I cherished this freedom, it also made me all the more cognizant of my differences. What good was the ability to attend a fraternity party at the nearby men's college if no man would give me the time of day because of my difference? What good was working so hard to prove myself academically as long as I believed that I would still be counted among the 71% of people with disabilities who wanted to work but faced the barrier of discrimination?

I had no choice but to grapple with a harsh realization. Even if I did find a job and a partner, even if I became famous, mothered 10 children, and made a million dollars, I'd never attain the normalcy I once so desperately desired. I simultaneously began to realize that I was not alone in my inability to "fit" into the mainstream. There were millions of us out there! Millions who, because of some kind of physical, mental, or behavioral "deficiency," suffered from unwarranted exclusion and discrimination, who were not afforded the same opportunities as "able-bodied" individuals, and many of whom lived in silence and shame because of it.

Thus began my second vigorous quest as a disabled person. This time I sought not to attain normalcy but rather to discover my history, my culture, and my community of fellow PWDs (people with disabilities). At first I worked in relative isolation. Still the only visibly disabled student in my school, I looked to a still small but ever burgeoning field of knowledge, which I would eventually pinpoint as Disability Studies. Long after finishing my statistics assignment and my Spanish homework, I'd lie awake reading about the passage of the Americans with Disabilities Act and devouring personal narratives written by other disabled individuals. Although their backgrounds and their impairments varied widely, it was utterly amazing how much their experiences of disability seemed to resonate with my own.

Still, my own disability identity was not something I just fell into; acquiring it has been a very gradual process with many bumps along the way. Even as a Disability Studies scholar and disability rights activist, there are still times when I long to be "normal." I want not be stared at when I walk into Starbucks (as if disabled people didn't need coffee too!). I want not be spoken down to or ignored altogether when I try to order a meal or buy a gallon of milk. Sometimes I worry about my ability to find a job, to find a partner, to be a parent. I occasionally still ask my mother the zillion-dollar question: "Will I have a good life?" As if I expect her to look into a crystal ball and provide complete reassurance.

The one thing I have learned, however, is that there are no certainties in life. As trite as such a statement may seem, I cannot think of a more accurate or appropriate way to frame it. Growing up in a small town in Virginia, trying desperately to fit in with my able-bodied peers, I never would have thought that I would be in a doctoral program in Disability Studies in Chicago. Never would I have thought that I would intentionally seek out other adults with disabilities and that some of them would become such wonderful friends. Never would I have thought that I would come to view my disability not as an unwanted appendage but as an integral part of who I am.

I realize that my disability still leaves me much to grapple with, in terms of developing both my professional path and my personal identity. I hope one day I

FIGURE 9.6 Kelly's narrative slope.

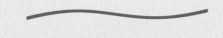

can say I am completely comfortable with myself, but I highly doubt that there are many people in this world, disabled or not, who can honestly make such a claim. To truly understand disability, both professionally and personally, requires a learning curve, and so I have no choice but to do what I've done for my whole life: keep studying. Continuing to listen to others' experiences as well as to my own will, I believe, propel me a long way toward achieving such a goal. Indeed, it already has.

[6]Kelly Munger, a graduate student at the University of Illinois at Chicago, provided her story for this chapter.

Kelly's narrative is one of searching and discovery. Her turning point was when she realized that it was not "normalcy" but identity she was seeking. Her narrative has an upward slope (*Fig. 9.6*) fueled by the quest for that new identity.

The Narratives in Perspective

Each person's story reflects a unique personal journey with its own challenges and accomplishments. Yet woven into these stories are all of the components of occupational identity. That is, each person seeks to make sense of his or her own capacity. Each seeks to find enjoyment and satisfaction in the activities that fill his or her life. Each tries to sort out what is important. Each aims to find and enact roles. Each must deal with the routines of everyday life. Each experiences a body with physical or mental impairments.

These narratives also make comprehensible the things each person does (or does not) do. For example, they reveal why Aaron uses and enjoys his swift imagination, why Gail changed careers, how Leena manages to move forward through life, why Lisa gave up her habit of taking the bus into the city, and why Kelly is pursing a doctorate in disability studies. These decisions and actions all take meaning from and enact the fundamental plot of the narrative to which they belong. As Bruner (1990a) notes, narrative is basic to how we think about our lives. Moreover, how these persons go about life—their occupational competence—is tied to the underlying plots and metaphors of their stories. These persons all clearly conduct their lives in terms of their narratives.

Influences on the Occupational Narrative

Narratives are ultimately shaped by many things. Nonetheless, three factors appear to have an important impact. These are the unfolding events of life, social forces, and the presence or absence of an engaging occupation. The following sections examine each of these factors.

Unfolding Events and Circumstances of Life

Each of the five narratives in this chapter indicates that ongoing events and circumstances of life insert themselves into narratives, having a significant influence on how they unfold. In a longitudinal study, Jonsson et al. (2000) examined how narratives shape and are shaped by what happens as lives unfold. The study began when a group of older persons were anticipating retirement and continued as they continued into their retirement. Over time, the actual direction of the retirees' lives reflected interaction between their original narrative and unfolding events and circumstances. Subjects' narratives readied them to respond in particular ways to ongoing life events and circumstances. Nonetheless, differences in those external circumstances and events could also nudge the narrative in one direction or another. Thus, the stories tended to be resilient, that is, to maintain their own plot. However, whereas life events and circumstances were usually integrated into the existing plot, they sometimes changed. In either case, the narrative had to come to terms with new events and circumstances.

Sociocultural Influences on Narrative

A dynamic tension always exists between how we narrate our lives and what is around the next corner. While each person constructs his or her occupational narrative, the sociocultural context also has important and pervasive influences. First, each person derives a sense of narrative plot and various metaphors from surrounding culture. The themes and images that populate our narratives are those derived from the kinds of discourse we encounter in our everyday worlds. Prevailing plots and metaphors that are part of the language and behavior of any culture serve as templates for how persons can make sense of and enact their lives. Moreover, in the course of socialization and throughout life, societies show to members what kinds of stories can be brought to bear on certain situations or problems.

Each story has borrowed heavily from dominant social themes. To the extent that societies provide prevailing narrative themes, they may influence the kinds of narratives the people in them construct for themselves. Kielhofner and Barrett (1997) document how a

> *In the course of socialization and throughout life, societies show to members what kinds of stories can be brought to bear on certain situations or problems.*

woman living in poverty is located in a narrative of seeking escape and refuge from the ongoing circumstances of her life in the inner city. Such a narrative arises out of social conditions, and it appears common among those who share such conditions.

Because our occupational lives unfold in interaction with others, our narratives are also invariably tied to how others act toward us and how we act toward them. Those who enter and find a place in our lives, and their characteristics and actions, affect our occupational narratives. This feature of narratives was illustrated in the study of retirees when family members were mobilized to do things that avoided the negative turn of events anticipated by their relatives (Jonsson et al., 2000). It is an important feature of social life that we note and seek to influence the occupational narratives of those whose lives intersect with our own. In the end, our stories are tied to theirs.

In sum, social influences on narrative are twofold. First, the content and shape of our narratives are provided by the social context. We invariably construct narratives that draw on socially available plots and metaphors. Second, since we live our occupational narratives in interaction with others, they inevitably affect our stories.

Engaging Occupations

The third phase of the previously noted study of elderly retirees suggests that constructing a positive life story

> *Because our occupational lives unfold in interaction with others, our narratives are also invariably tied to how others act toward us and how we act toward them. Those who enter and find a place in our lives, and their characteristics and actions, affect our occupational narratives.*

> *Engaging occupations evoke a depth of passion or feeling and become a central feature in a narrative.*

requires a person to find and participate in an engaging occupation (Jonsson, Josephsson, & Kielhofner, 2001).

Engaging occupations evoke a depth of passion or feeling and become a central feature in a narrative. They are done with great commitment and perseverance and stand out from the other things a person does. They are infused with positive meaning connected to interest (i.e., pleasure, challenge, enjoyment), personal causation (i.e., challenge, indication of one's competence), and value (i.e., something worth doing, important, contribution to family or society). Thus, the engaging occupation resonates with all aspects of volition. It is typically done with regularity over a long period of involvement and includes several occupational forms that cohere or constitute an interrelated whole. Involvement in an engaging occupation also represents a commitment or sense of duty to the occupation and a connection to a community of people who share a common interest in that occupation. In summary, an **engaging occupation** is a coherent and meaningful set of occupational forms that cohere and evoke deep feeling, a sense of duty, commitment, and perseverance leading to regular involvement over time in relation to a community of people who share the engaging occupation.

The narratives shared in this chapter appear to support the concept of engaging occupations and their potential centrality to achieving a positive occupational narrative. Each person was struggling with the loss of, the challenge of maintaining, or the need to replace an engaging occupation.

Conclusion

This chapter illustrates how people conduct and make meaning out of their occupational lives by locating themselves in an unfolding occupational narrative. As each person lives, he or she develops an occupational identity and occupational competence that represent

ongoing patterns of thinking, feeling, and doing. Occupational identity is reflected in the relative success the person has in formulating a vision of life that carries him or her forward. Occupational competence is reflected in each person's relative success in putting that vision into effect. Occupational identity and competence are reflected in the telling and doing of the occupational narrative.

This is not to suggest that identity and competence are always integrated. Sometimes one is unable to enact the life story one envisions and desires. There is evidence that following onset of disability, many persons initially experience a gap between the identity reflected in their narratives and what they are able to enact (Kielhofner, Mallinson, Forsyth, & Lai, 2001; Mallinson, Mahaffey, & Kielhofner, 1998). These same studies also suggest that one cannot have competence without an intact identity. Crafting life appears to begin with what we imagine when we begin to fashion our occupational narratives. This reflects the fact that narrative is the great mediator between self and life. We always apprehend ourselves and the world around us in terms of our stories. Narrative is both the meaning people assign to occupational life and the medium within which they enact it.

Key Terms

Engaging occupation: A coherent and meaningful set of occupational forms that cohere and evoke deep feeling, a sense of duty, commitment, and perseverance leading to regular involvement over time in relation to a community of people who share the engaging occupation.

Occupational narratives: Stories, both told and enacted, that integrate across time our unfolding volition, habituation, performance capacity, and environments through plots and metaphors that sum up and assign meaning to all these various elements.

References

Bruner, J. (1990a). *Acts of meaning*. Cambridge, MA: Harvard University.

Bruner, J. (1990b). Culture and human development: A new look. *Human Development, 33*, 344–355.

Clark, F. (1993). Occupation embedded in a real life: Interweaving occupational science and occupational therapy. 1993 Eleanor Clarke Slagle lecture. *American Journal of Occupational Therapy, 47,*1067–1078.

Ganzer, C. (1993). Metaphor in narrative inquiry: Using literature as an aid to practice. Paper presented at the 15th Allied Health Research Forum, Chicago.

Geertz, C. (1986). Making experiences, authoring selves. In V. Turner & E. Bruner (Eds.), *The anthropology of experience*. Urbana, IL: University of Illinois.

Gergen, K. J., & Gergen, M. M. (1988). Narrative and the self as relationship. In L. Berkowitz (Ed.), *Advances in experimental social psychology*. San Diego: Academic.

Helfrich, C., Kielhofner, G., & Mattingly. C. (1994). Volition as narrative: Understanding motivation in chronic illness. *American Journal of Occupational Therapy, 48,* 311–317.

Jonsson, H., Josephsson, S., & Kielhofner, G. (2000). Evolving narratives in the course of retirement: A longitudinal study. *American Journal of Occupational Therapy, 54,* 463–470.

Jonsson, H., Josephsson, S., & Kielhofner, G. (2001). Narratives and experience in an occupational transition: A longitudinal study of the retirement process. *American Journal of Occupational Therapy, 55,* 424–432.

Jonsson, H., Kielhofner, G., & Borell, L. (1997). Anticipating retirement: The formation of narratives concerning an occupational transition. *American Journal of Occupational Therapy, 51,* 49–56.

Keponen, R., & Kielhofner, G. (2006). Occupation and meaning in the lives of women with chronic pain. *Scandinavian Journal of Occupational Therapy, 13*(4), 211–220.

Kielhofner G., & Barrett L. (1997). Meaning and misunderstanding in occupational forms: A study of therapeutic goal setting. *American Journal of Occupational Therapy, 52,* 345–353.

Kielhofner, G., Braveman, B., Finlayson, M., Paul-Ward, A., Goldbaum, L., & Goldstein, K. (2004). Outcomes of a vocational program for persons with AIDS. *American Journal of Occupational Therapy, 58,* 64–72.

Kielhofner, G., Mallinson, T., Forsyth, K., & Lai, J-S. (2001). Psychometric properties of the second version of the Occupational Performance History Interview. *American Journal of Occupational Therapy, 55,* 260–267.

Mallinson, T., Kielhofner, G., & Mattingly, C. (1996). Metaphor and meaning in a clinical interview. *American Journal of Occupational Therapy, 50,* 338–346.

Mallinson, T., Mahaffey, L., & Kielhofner, G. (1998). The occupational performance history interview: Evidence for three underlying constructs of occupational adaptation. *Canadian Journal of Occupational Therapy, 65,* 219–228.

Mattingly, C. (1991). The narrative nature of clinical reasoning. *American Journal of Occupational Therapy, 45,* 998–1005.

Ortony, A. (1979). *Metaphor and thought*. Cambridge, MA: Cambridge University.

Ricoeur, P. (1984). *Time and narrative: Vol. 1*. Chicago: University of Chicago.

Schafer, R. (1981). *Narration in the psychoanalytic dialogue*. In W. J. T. Mitchell (Ed.), *On narrative* (pp. 25–49). Chicago: University of Chicago.

Schön, D. (1979). Generative metaphor: A perspective on problem-setting in social policy. In A. Ortony (Ed.), *Metaphor and thought*. Cambridge, MA: Cambridge University.

Spence, D. P. (1982). *Narrative truth and historical truth: Meaning and interpretation in psychoanalysis*. New York: WW Norton.

Taylor, C. (1989). *Sources of the self: The making of the modern identity*. Cambridge, MA: Harvard University.

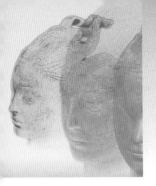

10

Doing and Becoming: Occupational Change and Development

● Gary Kielhofner

What people do propels them through a trajectory of lifelong change. Fidler and Fidler (1983) referred to this process as 'doing and becoming', underscoring how the course of life is shaped by occupation.

When people work, play, and perform activities of daily living, they shape their capacities, patterns of acting, self-perceptions, and comprehension of our world. To a large extent, people author their own development through what they do.

Change Processes Underlying Development

Occupational development involves complex processes of change in volition, habituation, and performance capacity. Chapter 3 identifies three elements involved in any permanent change (*Fig. 10.1*). First, an alteration of some internal or external component contributes something new to the total dynamic, out of which new thoughts, feelings, and actions emerge. Second, when these conditions are repeated sufficiently, volition, habituation, and/or performance capacity coalesce toward a new internal organization. Third, ongoing interaction of the new internal organization with

> *When people work, play, and perform activities of daily living, they shape their capacities, patterns of acting, self-perceptions, and comprehension of our world. To a large extent, people author their own development through what they do.*

consistent environmental conditions maintains a new stable pattern of thinking, feeling, and acting.

Ordinarily, volition, habituation, and performance capacity change in concert. During change, they resonate with and sometimes amplify each other. For example, increases in capacity tend to be accompanied by stronger personal causation. The latter leads to choices to do things that further develop that capacity. The process can also go in the other direction. For instance, older persons whose diminished capacities increase the risk of falling may develop, as part of personal causation, a fear of falling that leads to choices to curtail action. However, by curtailing action, elders may further reduce their capacity and increase the actual risk of falling (Peterson et al., 1999).

Changes in environmental impact are also an important part of any change trajectory. The environment may initiate change. Moreover, change usually involves interacting with different aspects of the environment, modifying surroundings, seeking out new settings, or avoiding past contexts. The influence of these altered person-environment interactions is essential to the change process and, eventually, to the maintenance of new patterns of thinking, feeling, and doing that are the result of change.

In any process of change multiple factors intersect, contributing both synergistic and divergent forces. For example, adolescents discover new capacities and begin to see themselves as more autonomous. Such volitional changes lead adolescents to interpret what they do differently (refusals and defiance, previously viewed as transgressions, now become assertions of autonomy) and to select new action that tests limits and explores risk. Parents and others in the environment may not consistently agree with the adolescent's desires for autonomy and risk taking. Moreover, the adolescent's own habituation may assert old patterns such

FIGURE 10.1 Necessary elements for permanent change.

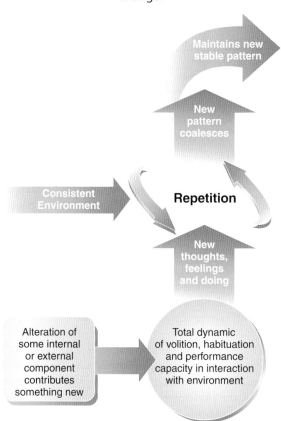

as childhood habits of reliance on parents. Accordingly, change can sometimes be characterized by disorganization, alterations in the pace of change, and backsliding. Change is seldom neat and orderly.

Stages of Change

Change ordinarily occurs across a continuum from exploration to competence to achievement (Reilly, 1974). This continuum is usually involved in **transformational** and **catastrophic change**. That is, people typically progress through these levels of function when they move into new roles, encounter new environments, make lifestyle changes, or reorganize their lives in response to a major disruptive circumstance or event.

This continuum of development may involve all areas of one's occupational life, as when persons who have acquired a major disability must reorganize how they view themselves and their abilities, how they achieve satisfaction and meaning in life, and how they go about their work, leisure, and activities of daily living. The continuum may also apply to only one aspect of a person's occupational life. The person who is retiring, the mother who decides to return to work after her children have left home, and the person who takes up a new serious hobby may develop new occupational participation through the stages discussed in this chapter.

Exploration is the first stage of change, in which persons try out new things and consequently learn about their own capacities, preferences, and values. Persons explore when they are learning to do new occupational forms/tasks, making role changes, or searching for new sources of meaning. Exploration provides the opportunity for learning, discovering new modes of doing, and discovering new ways of expressing ability and apprehending life. It yields a sense of how well one performs, how enjoyable the task is, and what meaning it can have for one's life. Exploration requires a relatively safe and undemanding environment. Since a person who is exploring is still unsure about capacity or desire, the resources and opportunities in the environment are critical.

Competency is the stage of change when persons begin to solidify new ways of doing that were discovered through exploration. During this stage of change persons strive to be adequate to the demands of a situation by improving themselves or adjusting to environmental demands and expectations. Individuals at a competence level of change focus on consistent, adequate performance. The process of striving for competence leads to the development of new skills, the refinement of old skills, and the organization of these skills into habits that support occupational performance. Competency affords an individual a growing sense of personal control. As persons strive to organize their performances into routines of competent behavior that are relevant to their environment, they immerse themselves in a process of becoming, growing, and arriving at a greater sense of efficacy.

Achievement is the stage of change when persons have sufficient skills and habits that allow them to participate fully in some new work, leisure activity, or activity of daily living. During the achievement stage of change, the person integrates a new area of occupational participation into his or her total life. Occupational identity is reshaped to incorporate the new area of occupational participation. Other roles and routines must be altered to accommodate the new overall pattern to sustain occupational competence.

In the case in which all areas of a person's occupational participation are changing, some areas may attain achievement before others. For example, following a traumatic spinal cord injury, a person may first concentrate on redeveloping ways to manage activities of daily living that include moving to independent living from a rehabilitation or institutional setting. Developing patterns of leisure in the new context and returning to work may come later.

Progression Through the Stages of Change

It should also be recognized that persons might move back and forth between stages. For example, having explored various career options and made a choice to enter an educational program, students sometimes find that the choice was not right and return to exploration. Also, Hammel (1999) observed that persons with spinal cord injury often moved back and forth between these stages.

The three stages of change broadly describe the trajectory that occupational change is likely to take. The actual pattern of events, actions, thoughts, and feelings that transpires when someone goes through change is unique for each person and for each episode of change.

Readiness for Change

The three stages of change describe a typical pathway once a person has embarked on the process of change. This presumes that a person is ready to begin making a change. For a variety of reasons this may not be the case. Even persons whose occupational participation is not adaptive are sometimes reluctant to make a change or do not believe a change is possible for their lives. Another factor limiting readiness to change may be proximity to a catastrophic event. Hammel (1999) found that following spinal cord injury, people went through a process of adjustment that preceded concrete steps toward change. At first people were dominated by the sense of loss and a disruption of previous life. Following this, she observed,

persons entered a period of reaction marked by strong feelings of anger, frustration, fear, and/or depression. Next they began to acknowledge going on with life and to formulate intentions to make change. Following this, they begin the exploratory stage of change. Such research suggests that catastrophic change may be marked by a period between the initial event and circumstance that precipitates or necessitates change and the beginning of making the change.

Centrality of the Environment in Change

As already noted, the environment has a pervasive influence in any process of change. The environment can be the source of alterations that precipitate change. Many of the changes that occur in the course of development occur according to socially defined timetables and expectations for change.

The environment can also be a barrier to change. Social definitions of a person's identity or expected behaviors can conflict with personal desires and attempts to change. Realizing change is difficult when the environment fails to support or reward the alterations a person is trying to make. The stages of change also suggest that appropriate environments exist for persons to advance through the stages. For example, for a person to engage in the exploration or competency stage of change, the environment must allow trying out and/or strengthening new action.

Contributions of Change to the Course of Development

As noted previously, the course of development is characterized by an ongoing process of change. The course of any life involves ongoing **incremental** and transformational change. Most lives are affected by one or more periods of catastrophic change.

A cross-sectional view of development will show that at any point in the life cycle aspects of one's occupational life will be at different stages. For example, the older child who has mastered self-care and has integrated it into daily routines (achievement) is at the beginning of exploring vocational interests in play and school. Achievement in work will follow years later. Underlying development, then, is a complex collection of change processes that follow one another, overlap, and interweave.

Transformation of Work, Play, and Activities of Daily Living

Discussions of development often emphasize that particular courses or processes of development are normal. For example, most discussions of childhood development describe various attainments that on average have occurred by a particular age. However, great variation in the course of development occurs across persons. Too much emphasis on norms can distract from the more important change processes that underlie development. Development is first and foremost a change process through which the individual is transformed throughout life.

The most obvious outward manifestation of occupational development is that persons engage in different occupations over the course of their lives. For example, younger children play, older children and adolescents attend school, and adults work. The transformation of occupation across the life span reflects an underlying order realized in the individual but sustained by the sociocultural environment. Socially established and culturally defined patterns of work, play, and self-care over the life span influence the sequence of occupational participation reflected in development.

The following sections provide an overview of the course of occupational development using the typical divisions of childhood, adolescence, adulthood, and later adulthood. The discussions are not meant to be exhaustive or detailed accounts of occupational development. Rather, they offer a perspective from which to consider how volition, habituation, performance capacity, and environment contribute to and undergo change throughout the life course.

Ongoing Tasks of Occupational Adaptation: Identity and Competence

During each stage of development, as internal changes occur and as the environments in which we do things change, we face two fundamental tasks. These are:

- Constructing an occupational identity by which we know ourselves and our lives
- Establishing occupational competence in our patterns of doing.

In each culture the pattern of development is narratively structured. That is, the culture carries a domi-

nant narrative describing the life course (Luborsky, 1993). Nonetheless, these dominant narratives are, to varying degrees, ill suited to define the individual life course (Luborsky, 1993). For example, dropping out of school, changing careers, getting divorced, being widowed, and being fired or laid off from a job all present variations in the life course story that people grapple with in forming their identity. More dramatically, being homosexual, having or acquiring a disability, or wanting to live outside the culturally defined narrative present major challenges for achieving an occupational identity. Consequently, dominant cultural narratives can be sources of constraint that hinder adaptation.

How each person constructs an occupational identity and realizes it in everyday patterns of doing varies from person to person. Some more or less readily accept the dominant narratives shared by the group to which they belong. Others choose a more individualistic course. Still others are thrust by circumstances into charting a different path for themselves. Nonetheless, the challenge of adaptation remains the same: to identify and enact a self and a way of living that is experienced as good, yields a sense of accomplishment, provides grounding in familiar routines, and allows one to realize one's unique potentials, limitations, and desires.

Childhood

Through the course of childhood, extensive transformation of volition, habituation, and performance capacity takes place. These changes allow the child to emerge as an occupational being with personal ways of doing, thinking, and feeling. Childhood occupation both is unique in its own character and serves as a foundation for later competence (Case-Smith & Shortridge, 1996; Hurt, 1980).

Volition

As children experience themselves doing things, their personal causation, interests, and values emerge. The

> *How each person constructs an occupational identity and realizes it in everyday patterns of doing varies from person to person.*

volitional choices of early childhood are mainly activity choices. Later, children begin to make occupational choices to take on personal projects (e.g., learning to play a musical instrument) or discretionary roles (e.g., joining Scouts, a club in school, or a sports team). Occupational choices may at first be assisted or coached by parents, who supply for children the rationale for projects, habits, and roles.

Play is a major vehicle through which the child first develops a sense of personal causation (Bundy, 1997). As noted in Chapter 4, personal causation begins with children's awareness that they can cause things to happen. The desire to have effects in the environment becomes a strong motive and manifests itself in the child's play (Bundy, 1997; Ferland, 1997). Children's awareness of their capacities is gained through engaging with the environment in play, in social interaction, and eventually in other occupational spheres (Lindquist, Mack, & Parham, 1982). At first, children's sense of their abilities is very general (e.g., effort and capacity are not distinguished and not always accurate) (Nicholls, 1984). Through the child's experiences of failure and success, the child's knowledge of capacity and feelings of efficacy become more complex and accurate.

Cultural messages about values influence the child early in life. Adult approval and disapproval of actions guide the child's understanding of the social value of doing certain things. Growing awareness of what parents, siblings, and others value increasingly influences activity and occupational choices. As children learn the value of being productive in occupations (e.g., chores and schoolwork), they increasingly assume responsibility for such behaviors and in turn experience the approval of others that solidifies the commitment to behave accordingly.

Childhood interests reflect expanding capacities. Children are attracted to activities that allow exercise of capacity and yield new experiences. Much of childhood's pleasure comes from the mastery of new actions (Mailloux & Burke, 1997). As new capacities emerge, interest turns toward their use and expansion. For example, increased hand dexterity invites and results from the child engaging in play requiring fine motor control, such as constructing simple projects. Linguistic competence leads to interest in verbal humor and rhymes. Children find particular interest in activities that provide optimal arousal by challenging capacity (Burke, 1977, 1993; Ferland, 1997).

Overcoming Difficulties with Occupational Adaptation in Childhood[1]

Typical childhood development brings with it all kinds of challenges. Some children face additional challenges that make the course of development unique. Consider Hubert, a 7-year-old who has attention deficit disorder and epilepsy with seizures that are only partly controlled. He has been hospitalized repeatedly for lengths of time varying from a few days to weeks. His impairments, hospitalization, and medication side effects have all contributed to his global developmental delay. In particular his motor, process, and communication interaction skills are not those of a typical child his age. While the term *delay* is used to describe Hubert's development, it is not its defining characteristic.

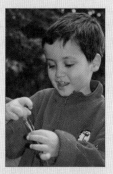

Hubert explores his environment while playing outside.

Despite the challenges he faces, Hubert has been able to attend school and with support from his parents maintains a routine that supports his new role as a first grader. His attention span and concentration are improving, and along with this, his interests have widened to include newfound enjoyment of table games, puzzles, and the computer. He has begun to feel competent at a wider range of occupational forms/tasks and is more aware of and assertive in pursing the things that he enjoys. Hubert is developing his own sense of occupational identity and enacting it in a satisfying way with support from those in his home and school environments. His is a unique but nonetheless adaptive occupational development.

[1] Geneviève Pépin, professor in the Faculty of Medicine Rehabilitation Department at Laval University in Quebec, Canada, provided the case of Hubert for this chapter.

Habituation

The young child's major occupational roles are player and family member (Florey, 1998; Hinojosa & Kramer, 1993). Parents and others see play as the normal business of the child. The player role has its own expectations, as when parents specify where and with what objects children may play. In addition, play is a means of trying out roles in sociodramatic play and games.

The family member role emerges as parents expect and value productive contributions of the child to the routines of family life by engaging in such occupational forms/tasks as picking up toys, doing small chores, and carrying out self-care. As childhood progresses, the range of roles increases to include student, friend, and membership in various childhood groups.

Biologic rhythms provide the child's first consistent patterns. Environmental rhythms allow the child to internalize routines such as sleeping, waking, bathing, eating, playing, and self-care. In time, the child becomes more and more able to organize behaviors to accomplish chores and routines of self-care. Moreover, children find repetition a source of security, predictability, and comfort. Many habits that will be resources throughout life are acquired in childhood. Whereas the major influence on habits is the family routine, the child is affected by each new occupational setting, such as day care and school.

Performance Capacity

Performance capacity undergoes dramatic transformation as the child gains experience, especially from play (Pierce, 1997; Robinson, 1977). Throughout childhood, increasing competence for interacting with the environment leads to the desire and capacity to seek out novel experiences. As children's capacities increase, their world expands (e.g., entering formal education). This process results in exposure to new environments that further impact on the development of capacity.

Occupational Identity and Competence

Occupational identity emerges in childhood. As children acquire the ability to integrate past, present, and future and to imagine themselves in an unfolding story, they begin to narrate parts of their lives and to sort out meanings through stories (Burke & Schaaf, 1997). By late childhood, children have a fairly well developed sense of who they are. The occupational competence developed during childhood similarly tends to follow social norms and expectations. Nonetheless, each child begins to discover and pursue unique interests and aptitudes that individualize identity and competence.

Adolescence

Adolescence is typically a period of stress and turmoil due to both intrapersonal and sociocultural factors (Hendry, 1983). In addition to being a time of accelerated and dramatic biologic change, adolescence can also be an uncertain social transition from childhood to adulthood. The beginning of adolescence is associated with both biologic (puberty) and institutional (junior high school) changes. The end of adolescence was traditionally associated with entry into the worker role, but the timing of work entry can differ radically depending on whether one works directly after high school, attends college, or obtains postgraduate education. Consequently, adolescence has no firm boundaries.

Volition

Adolescence is characterized by an increasing drive for autonomy (Mitchell, 1975; Santrock, 1981). Adolescents must successfully learn to make activity and occupational choices that bring personal satisfaction and meaning while meeting expanding environmental expectations. The most pressing occupational choice of adolescence is selecting a type of work (Allport, 1961).

Adolescents are challenged to maintain a sense of efficacy while facing new social expectations for responsibility and having to acquire an expanding repertoire of occupational forms/tasks. Adolescents also begin to assess their capacity in terms of expected performance in future roles. During adolescence, belief in one's ability to control life outcomes ordinarily increases (Hendry, 1983). Increased freedom of choice challenges adolescents to clarify and establish their values. Rejection of some previous or parental values leads to a more personalized worldview and confirms for adolescents that their values are their own. Establishing values is challenging, since the sources of values in society are many and sometimes contradictory. Not surprisingly, many adolescents experiment and struggle in the process of value formation, often moving between ideal values and the realities of life (Florey, 1998).

Interests also undergo substantial transformation during adolescence. What interests emerge depends very much on the social context. One of the primary influences on interest change is movement out of the family setting where interests are often family centered, into a peer group, where new interests are espoused. Interests also change because the adolescent can do new things, such as dating and driving a car. Adolescents' interests also become more of an expression of identity (Csikszentmihalyi & Rochberg-Halton, 1981). What one enjoys becomes a kind of statement about what kind of person one is.

Habituation

Adolescence is a period of transformation in the roles and habits that regulate everyday behavior. Adolescents try out many of the roles they will hold as adults. Such role experimentation fills several needs for adolescents. It helps them to consolidate their identity, to satisfy the desire for status and independence, and to recognize their abilities for particular roles.

Although some roles continue from childhood into adolescence, the nature of those roles and the expectations associated with them begin to change. In the family context adolescents become more responsible for taking care of themselves (e.g., buying their own clothes, cooking for themselves) and contributing to household (e.g., through part-time work). While there are increasing opportunities to try on a variety of roles, adolescents may be frustrated because certain adult roles are not yet available to them (Hendry, 1983).

For the adolescent, the peer group is a source of information about the world outside the family and is a testing ground for new ideas and behaviors. The role of friend is increasingly important and may undergo several changes during adolescence. Part-time jobs and volunteer work expose many adolescents to the work world and afford opportunity to develop skill in getting and keeping jobs, budgeting time and money, and taking pride in accomplishments. Volunteer work can also serve as a means for exploring future vocations.

New habits are required for the changing circumstances of adolescence and for the world of work. Adolescent habits take over much routine behavior that was previously externally regulated in the family and by the other social contexts. A major impact on the habits of the adolescent is the movement from grammar school to junior high and high school. No longer in a single classroom with a series of daily activities for the entire class, students have individual schedules and must be responsible for being in the right place at the right time. More of adolescents' time is at their personal discretion. They must use time to establish a routine for the student and other roles.

Performance Capacity

Physical growth and change are central to the transformation of performance capacity in adolescence. Adolescents reach or approximate their adult size and begin bodily processes that characterize adulthood. Intellectual, cognitive, and emotional capacities expand in adolescence, allowing greater depths of awareness and comprehension of the world (Mitchell, 1975; Santrock, 1981). The adolescent also expands capacities for communication and interaction.

Occupational Identity and Competence

Adolescents begin to seriously see themselves as the authors of their own lives and to connect present actions with future outcomes and possibilities (Case-Smith & Shortridge, 1996). Adolescents' need to craft their own occupational identity and competence culminates in several important occupational choices, such as selecting a career and finding a partner.

The early adolescent's identity is more concerned with issues of enjoyment. Later, the adolescent gives increasing consideration to sense of capacity and feelings of efficacy and chooses occupations according to internalized values. By late adolescence occupational identity is much more sophisticated and centers on the occupational choices necessary to enter adult life. Nonetheless, this process is highly variable and proceeds at different paces for different persons (Ginzberg, 1971). In fact, because identity and competence are continually evolving and changing with growth and experience, the process of occupational choice is continuous and dynamic.

Struggling to Achieve Occupational Identity in Adolescence[2]

In adolescence, development of one's unique values, interests, and self-efficacy is a central and challenging task to crafting one's occupational identity. For adolescents with a history of abuse, this process is even more difficult, as beliefs about low self-worth and inefficacy can interfere with generating positive experiences in doing. Such adolescents can have difficulty recognizing, enjoying, and finding meaning in their own abilities.

This struggle is illustrated by Amy, a 16-year-old with a history of physical and sexual abuse. At age 12, she became a ward of the state and since that time has had inconsistent contact with her biological parents and siblings. Amy was first hospitalized for severe depression and injury to herself beginning when she was 13.

During her hospitalization, Amy demonstrated a strong talent for and interest in drawing and writing; her creative products were precocious. However, despite her exceptional skills, Amy's volitional characteristics (a sense of inefficacy and self-devaluation, coupled with a tendency to dissociate from her own experience) prevented her from enjoying and investing in her innate talents.

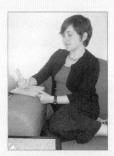

Amy expresses herself through writing.

With persistent verbal encouragement, she would reluctantly engage in writing and drawing to express her feelings and to connect to others. In occupational therapy, she was encouraged to practice and expand her unique expressive capacity. Initially, Amy was very self-deprecating, even when she received praise from both adults and her peers. Over the course of several hospitalizations in the next 3 years, a slow shift took place in her volition. She developed a growing and stable sense that she did have abilities she could enjoy. She

found a sense of meaning in expressing herself through drawing and writing. In time, Amy became empowered to take risks in what she showed others. Her poetry reflected insights into her past and revealed her dreams for the future. By the end of her last hospitalization at age 16, she was actively engaged in drawing and writing; she expressed confidence in herself, and her view of the future was considerably brighter and more positive. She had begun to develop a blooming sense of herself as an artist. This change was even evident in how Amy consistently presented herself. She held her head higher and her voice was stronger. She had achieved critical changes in volition that would support her future development.

[2] Stephanie McCammon, occupational therapist at University of Illinois Medical Center in Chicago, provided the case of Amy for this chapter.

Adulthood

The boundaries of adulthood are closely tied to one's working life. Adulthood typically begins with the assumption of a more or less permanent full-time job or other productive occupation and ends with retirement (Hasselkus, 1998). Adulthood is the longest period of life. Contrary to popular views of adulthood as a period of stability or a state of maturity that is achieved and sustained, adults undergo considerable change. Some of these changes are externally recognizable, as the person passes through a series of steps, crises, or transitions: marriage or divorce, starting a family, changing jobs, and bidding farewell to grown children. Other changes are internal, as the individual sorts out the various meanings, goals, and purposes that guide choice and self-evaluation in adult life.

Volition

Diverse factors, such as economic constraints and obligations of parenthood, affect adult decisions, but for most people adulthood is the time when one truly begins to live one's own life. Adulthood ordinarily is accomplished by an increasing desire to achieve and to work autonomously. For most people, this is accompanied by an increased sense of efficacy.

Early adulthood is generally a period of acquiring and refining abilities for one's line of work. Young workers see themselves as learning and increasing their efficacy. By middle adulthood, individuals have generally realized their peak performance. While the sense of efficacy is often dominated by work, other adult experiences, such as rearing a family and maintaining a household, are also areas that evoke strong feelings about one's effectiveness. Parents often find themselves facing great responsibilities with minimal preparation, such as the challenge of a newborn or confronting an adolescent's rebelliousness. Similarly, such adult responsibilities as maintaining a household and managing personal finances can be sources of stress, accomplishment, and failure.

During adulthood, values usually become increasingly important as a motivating force and a source of self-evaluation. Although personal values related to occupation tend to remain relatively stable throughout adulthood, a general shift does often occur. The goals of early adulthood are focused on instrumental and material values, such as getting ahead at work and earning a satisfactory living. Middle-aged workers may begin to focus more on humanitarian concerns and on themes of legacy (e.g., what one will leave to the future or how one will be remembered by children). Although this particular pattern of value change does not characterize all adults, some shift in values in the course of adult life is likely.

Leisure and work interests are relatively stable. Many adults entered their work because it embodied the opportunity to channel and develop personal interests. However, it is not a universal phenomenon that adults find their work interesting. Many adults pursue their interests avidly and seriously during their leisure time. Other adults use interests as a means of relaxing and regenerating themselves for work.

Habituation

Adulthood is characterized by a variety of socially prescribed and individually chosen roles that structure the adult's daily life and provide identity. Apart from family roles, most of these roles are enacted in community settings (Hasselkus, 1998). Typical adult role transitions include the initiation or end of partnerships, parenthood, changes in work roles, and joining civic and social organizations.

The one pervasive feature of adult life is work. Working requires learning new behaviors, forming new interpersonal relationships, reapportioning one's use of time, and frequently, developing a new identity. The work role also influences other adult roles, especially friendship and leisure roles. Workers often share confidences and decision making with coworkers and may develop strong friendships with colleagues.

Most adults have to divide their time among work, family, community, and leisure roles. Participation in organizational and social roles, volunteering, and participating in religious organizations are other roles that many adults pursue. Because each of these roles can involve substantial investments of energy and time, a large number of people find inevitable conflicts in their use of time. Despite the potential for conflicts in time use, having a combination of roles appears to enhance well-being (Baruch, Barnett, & Rivers, 1980).

Habits of adulthood are necessarily concerned with the efficient allocation of time to various roles and the occupational forms/tasks they require. The division of the weekly routine into time for work, play, rest, self-care, and family is to some extent contingent on the norms of society (e.g., the typical 9-to-5, Monday-through-Friday work week). Adult habits are influenced by their context in other ways as well. For example, factory and hospital work requires a rather rigid adherence to schedules, whereas farmers and university professors must develop their own routines around seasonal variations in work. Marriage, purchasing a home, and the arrival of children also place demands on persons to develop habits for home maintenance and caretaking. Previously accustomed to a routine organized around personal needs and desires, adults typically find themselves having to orient their routines to a broader set of concerns.

Challenges to Occupational Adaptation in Adulthood[3]

Adapting to an impairment can pose a variety of challenges to the ordinary course of adult development. Richard, who contracted polio at age 15, illustrates how one person navigated the course of adulthood. He had significant paralysis of his right leg, as well as severe scoliosis that required major surgery in his teenage years. In his late 40s, Richard developed post polio syndrome, which affected his walking but not his determination and zest for living. With the use of a long leg brace, he has maintained his ability to walk.

Despite being bedridden during most of his adolescence, he independently pursued a job as a dispatcher at the local sheriff's office. This experience increased his sense of efficacy, and he enrolled in college, becoming a medical technologist. Early in his career, he accepted a position as laboratory director in a new rural community hospital, a worker role he held for 37 years. He married before accepting this position and raised three children.

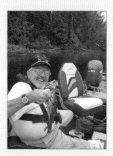

Richard proudly displays his most recent catch.

Having grown up on a farm in the Midwest, Richard values being outdoors and being able to connect with nature. Throughout his life he has enjoyed fishing, hunting, camping, snowmobiling, and traveling. He and his wife of 46 years travel frequently, spending summers in a cabin on a lake. He spends his time fishing, boating, and enjoying the outdoors, interests he has pursued throughout his life. Despite physical challenges, his strong volition has helped him to maintain a rich diversity of occupational participation that brings meaning and purpose to his life.

[3] Christine Raber, assistant professor in the Department of Occupational Therapy at Shawnee State University in Portsmouth, Ohio, provided the case of Richard for this chapter.

Performance Capacity

Adulthood represents both the peaking and declining of abilities. Young adults are still acquiring new abilities, whereas middle and later adulthood is characterized by some waning in capacity (Bonder, 1994). Physical changes affect the occupational performance of adults. Over time, adults experience a decrease in energy and strength, and they have some decrement in sensory perception. It is in adulthood that many people first need glasses or bifocals or a hearing aid. Others find that they must cut back on some vigorous activities.

Identity and Competence

Adults assess and reassess their unfolding life stories (Handel, 1987; Kimmel, 1980). Narrative reassessment typically reflects a transformation from an early concern with competence and achievement to a later concern with value and personal satisfaction. This transformation, sometimes referred to as a mid-life crisis, may lead persons to remake their stories, change careers, or enact similarly drastic alterations in their occupational lifestyles. Whatever life course they choose or life events they must grapple with, adults continue the narrative process of knowing themselves, exploring the worth and meaning of their lives, and seeking to control the circumstances and direction of their lives. For some adults this struggle results in a high level of well-being. Others fail to find a satisfactory and meaningful life course and instead live a life characterized by compromise, conflict, or catastrophe.

Later Adulthood

Later adulthood is defined both by biologic changes and social convention. Retirement and eligibility for social benefits demarcates entry into this period of later adulthood (Bonder, 1994). It is difficult to define later adulthood by chronologic age alone. Rather, it is useful to think of later adulthood as demarked by changes in lifestyle as determined by waning capacity, personal choice, and social convention.

Volition

Older adults' volition is important to help direct the many choices that drive or are in response to necessary changes in lifestyle. Old age is generally accompanied by losses of capacity, and lack of opportunities to use abilities can lead elderly persons to experience diminution of personal causation. Since the loss of capacity may have important implications for independence and lifestyle, some older adults may be especially inventive in sustaining a sense of efficacy, while others may hold unrealistic views of their abilities.

Values typically undergo some transformation and have a pervasive influence on occupational choices in old age. One view holds that older adults shift from instrumental values such as being ambitious, intellectual, capable, and responsible toward terminal values, such as a sense of accomplishment, freedom, equality, and comfort. Whereas this pattern may be true of many older adults, it is most accurate to say that the nature and direction of any value change depend on past and current life circumstances. Nonetheless, for most older adults the importance of work and achievement wanes while other values concerning family, community, and leisure become more significant (Antonovsky & Sagy, 1990). As abilities decline, elderly persons must redefine their standards and revise the way in which values are satisfied. Nonetheless, value commitments are important to maintaining morale in later life.

For many older adults, the relative freedom from obligations in old age provides opportunity to pursue a variety of interests more seriously or fully than before. However, constrained capacity and resources in later life can prevent some persons from pursuing interests. For example, some older adults are involved in solitary and passive occupations, although they would prefer to be involved in social and more active occupations (McGuire, 1980). Older adults can be constrained in their activity choices by a lack of transportation, facilities, money, and companions; by fears of injury, learning new things, or disapproval; and by no longer feeling a sense of satisfaction (McAvoy, 1979; McGuire, 1983).

The Quest for a New Occupational Identity in Later Adulthood[4]

. . . .

One of the most challenging aspects of aging for many older adults is the transition to retirement. As documented in a series of studies (Jonsson et al., 1997; Jonsson, Josephsson, & Kielhofner, 2000, 2001), retirement is an occupational transition that requires considerable reorganization of a person's occupational identity, restructure of roles and habits, and adjustment to changes in the kinds of environments in which one does things. The following case is but one example of the many ways that people manage this occupational transition.

"It took a long time to get used to doing nothing."

Gordon is 78 years old and married. Since retirement Gordon and his wife have divided their time in the summer between Ohio and Maine, where they enjoy family activities and spending time with their nine grandchildren. He grew up in a large family during the Depression, started working as a truck driver at 16, and served in the U.S. army in Korea. Although Gordon only obtained an eighth grade education, his natural talent for efficiency and perseverance served him well in business ventures. He owned and operated a successful store, apartment building, and trucking business and made real estate investments. Known as someone "to get the job done," Gordon is not the type of person to stop until the task is completed.

The transition to retirement was difficult for Gordon, whose values focused on hard work and a steady income and who possessed few hobbies. Additionally, he has physical limitations, the consequence of two strokes, injuries from two falls (one from a ladder and

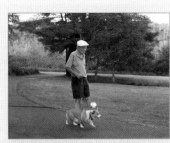

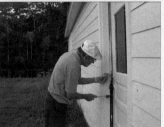

Gordon walks his dog Rascal and helps out around the house.

another from a roof), along with substantial hearing loss.

Over the first years of retirement Gordon had to develop new ways to occupy himself and feel useful. He and his wife now live in a beach house most of the year. Gordon takes regular walks on the beach. Although unsteady on his feet, he walks 2 miles a day with his dog, Rascal. He goes to the senior citizens center, works out at the gym, and frequents the local Veterans of Foreign Wars facility. He spends time with his grandchildren. Finally, Gordon enjoys helping out with household projects at home and in his children and grandchildren's homes. These in particular make him feel valuable.

[4] Jane Clifford O'Brien, associate professor in the Occupational Therapy Department at the University of New England, provided the case of Gordon for this chapter.

Habituation

Role changes in later life sometimes are involuntary and unpleasant. For example, elderly persons may lose the spouse and friend roles through death. Many lost roles are not easily replaced. Older adults who cannot replace lost or diminished roles may experience boredom, loneliness, and depression. Many older adults rely on family, community, or other institutions to provide roles. For example, Elliot and Barris (1987) found that

older adults' role identification was greater in nursing homes that provided more opportunities for activity.

Some persons continue to work beyond ordinary retirement age for income; to feel satisfied, useful, and respected; and/or to have a major role in organizing their lives (Sterns, Laier, & Dorsett, 1994). When it does occur, retirement can be a far-reaching event, because so much of life is geared toward preparation for, entry into, and advancement in work and because work structures a great deal of time and activity. Consequently, the transition from work to retirement is full of both possibilities and pitfalls. Retirement is an entirely individual process (Jonsson, Kielhofner, & Borell, 1997). For one individual it may mean escape from arduous labor and an opportunity to devote time to occupations of a higher priority, such as family involvement, a second career, or hobbies. For another, it may mean loss of social contact and severance from a primary source of self-worth and meaning. Whatever the implications, retirement is a major life event that reshapes an individual's occupational life.

Family roles and relationships are important and often change dramatically in the lives of older adults (Cutler-Louis, 1989). Older adults often spend significant time with adult children and grandchildren. Relationships with adult children can be an important source of gratification sustained by a reciprocal exchange in the form of affection, gifts, and services. Older adults often act as babysitters, confidantes and advisors, house sitters, and providers of income. As older adults become frail, disabled, or chronically ill, adult children may assume responsibility for the care of their aging parents. This role reversal is often complicated and challenging for all involved.

Friendship is another important role of older adults. Although having extensive friendships is not necessary, the person who has a number of friendships is less vulnerable to loss of friends through death. Loss of one's partner in old age may severely disrupt life. One may lose a friend, homemaker, financial supporter, and caretaker, depending on the nature of the relationship. Other role changes may accompany the loss of a partner. The surviving partner may have to take over many things previously done by the spouse.

Elderly persons often possess habits developed over a long period in a stable environment. Changes in underlying capacity and in environment can challenge these habits. At the same time, changing circumstances, such as widowhood or retirement, often impose demands for acquiring new habits. Moreover, as capacities decline, habits become increasingly important to sustain functional performance and quality of life.

Performance Capacity

Aging involves a natural decline in performance capacity and is associated with a high frequency of health conditions that affect capacity (Kauffman, 1994; Riley, 1994). However, substantial losses of ability are not inevitable and may be forestalled if the elderly person remains active. Consequently, age-related changes are unique to each person. Moreover, the impact of such decrements may be mitigated by adapting one's habits and environment.

Occupational Identity and Competence

With aging, the composition and telling of one's life story seems to gain importance. As older adults approach the end of life, both the need to make the most of the time one has and to make sense of the life one has lived become important (Ebersole & Hess, 1981; Hasselkus, 1998). The sense of whether one's life story has fulfilled the cultural ideal can be a source of comfort and fulfillment or of distress (Luborsky, 1993).

For most older adults the central fixture in the life narrative is the transition to retirement, which can mean vastly different things to retirees (Jonsson et al., 1997; Jonsson, Josephsson, & Kielhofner, 2000, 2001). As discussed in the previous chapter, a major factor affecting the extent to which occupational identity and competence are positive for the elderly person appears to be whether the person has an engaging occupation (Jonsson et al., 2001).

Conclusion

This chapter identified some of the major transformations and patterns that characterize the course of occupational development. In attempting to portray what may be typical or ordinary in the developmental course, individual differences are necessarily ignored. However, these differences are critical to development.

> *Indeed, the most remarkable characteristics of any individual journey through life are the singular incidents, the crises, the personal transformations, the setbacks, and other features that deviate from any neat or normative portrayal of development.*

Indeed, the most remarkable characteristics of any individual journey through life are the singular incidents, the crises, the personal transformations, the setbacks, and other features that deviate from any neat or normative portrayal of development.

Moreover, these unique events, struggles, and transformations give each life its special direction, pace, and meaning and hold the key to understanding that particular life.

Key Terms

Achievement: The stage of change when persons have sufficient skills and habits that allow them to participate fully in some new work, leisure activity, or activity of daily living.

Catastrophic change: Stage of change that occurs when internal or external circumstances dramatically alter one's occupational life situation, requiring a fundamental reorganization.

Competency: Stage of change when persons begin to solidify new ways of doing that were discovered through exploration.

Exploration: First stage of change in which persons try out new things and, consequently, learn about their own capacities, preferences, and values.

Incremental change: A gradual alteration such as change in amount, intensity, or degree.

Transformational change: Change that occurs when one fundamentally or qualitatively alters an established pattern of thinking, feeling, and doing.

References

Allport, G. (1961). *Pattern and growth in personality*. New York: Holt, Rinehart & Winston.

Antonovsky, A., & Sagy, S. (1990). Confronting developmental tasks in the retirement transition. *Gerontologist, 30*, 362–368.

Baruch, G., Barnett, R., & Rivers, C. (1980, December 7). A new start for women at midlife. *New York Times Sunday Magazine*, pp. 196–200.

Bonder, B. R. (1994). Growing old in the United States. In B. R. Bonder & M. B. Wagner (Eds.), *Functional performance in older adults* (pp. 4–14). Philadelphia: FA Davis.

Bundy, A. C. (1997). Play and playfulness: What to look for. In L. D. Parham & L. S. Fazio (Eds.), *Play in occupational therapy for children* (pp. 52–66). St. Louis: Mosby.

Burke, J. P. (1977). A clinical perspective on motivation: Pawn versus origin. *American Journal of Occupational Therapy, 31*, 254–258.

Burke, J. P. (1993). Play: The life role of the infant and young child. In J. Case-Smith (Ed.), *Pediatric occupational therapy and early intervention* (pp. 198–224). Stoneham, MA: Andover Medical.

Burke, J. P., & Schaaf, R. C. (1997). Family narratives and play assessment. In L. D. Parham & L. S. Fazio (Eds.), *Play in occupational therapy for children* (pp. 67–84). St. Louis: Mosby.

Case-Smith, J., & Shortridge, S. D. (1996). The developmental process: Prenatal to adolescence. In J. Case-Smith, A. S. Allen, & P. N. Pratt (Eds.), *Occupational therapy for children* (pp. 46–66). St. Louis: Mosby.

Csikszentmihalyi, M., & Rochberg-Halton, E. (1981). *The meaning of things*. Cambridge, MA: Cambridge University.

Cutler-Lewis, S. (1989). *Elder care*. New York: McGraw-Hill.

Ebersole, P., & Hess, P. (1981). *Toward healthy aging: Human needs and nursing response*. St. Louis: Mosby.

Elliot, M. S., & Barris, R. (1987). Occupational role performance and life satisfaction in elderly persons. *Occupational Therapy Journal of Research, 7*, 215–224.

Ferland, F. (1997). *Play, children with physical disabilities and occupational therapy: The ludic model*. Ottawa: University of Ottawa.

Fidler, G., & Fidler, J. (1983). Doing and becoming: The occupational therapy experience. In G. Kielhofner (Ed.), *Health through occupation: Theory and practice in occupational therapy*. Philadelphia: FA Davis.

Florey, L. (1998). Psychosocial dysfunction in childhood and adolescence. In M. E. Neistadt & E. B. Crepeau (Eds.), *Occupational therapy* (pp. 622–635). Philadelphia: Lippincott.

Ginzberg, E. (1971). Toward a theory of occupational choice. In H. J. Peters & J. C. Hansen (Eds.), *Vocational guidance and career development* (2nd ed.). New York: Macmillan.

Hammel, J. (1999). The life rope: A transactional approach to exploring worker and life role development. *Work: A Journal of Prevention, Assessment and Rehabilitation, 12*, 47–60.

Handel, A. (1987). Personal theories about the life-span development of one's self in autobiographical self-presentations of adults. *Human Development, 30*, 83–98.

Hasselkus, B. R. (1998). Introduction to adult and older adult populations. In M. E. Neistadt & E. B. Crepeau (Eds.), *Occupational therapy* (pp. 651–659). Philadelphia: Lippincott.

Hendry, L. B. (1983). *Growing up and going out: Adolescents and leisure*. Aberdeen: Aberdeen University.

Hinojosa, J., & Kramer, P. (1993). Developmental perspective: Fundamentals of developmental theory. In P. Kramer & J. Hinojosa (Eds.), *Pediatric occupational therapy* (pp. 3–8). Philadelphia: Lippincott Williams & Wilkins.

Hurt, J. M. (1980). A play skills inventory: A competency monitoring tool for the 10-year-old. *American Journal of Occupational Therapy, 34*, 651–656.

Jonsson, H., Josephsson, S., & Kielhofner, G. (2000). Evolving narratives in the course of retirement: A longitudinal study. *American Journal of Occupational Therapy, 54*, 463–470.

Jonsson, H., Josephsson, S., & Kielhofner, G. (2001). Narratives and experience in an occupational transition: A longitudinal study of the retirement process. *American Journal of Occupational Therapy, 55*, 424–432.

Jonsson, H., Kielhofner, G., & Borell, L. (1997). Anticipating retirement: The formation of narratives concerning an occupational transition. *American Journal of Occupational Therapy, 51*, 49–56.

Kauffman, T. (1994). Mobility. In B. R. Bonder & M. B. Wagner (Eds.), *Functional performance in older adults* (pp. 42–61). Philadelphia: FA Davis.

Kimmel, D. C. (1980). *Adulthood and aging* (2nd ed.). New York: Wiley.

Lindquist, J. E., Mack, W., & Parham, L. D. (1982). A synthesis of occupational behavior and sensory integration concepts in theory and practice, part 1. Theoretical foundations. *American Journal of Occupational Therapy, 36*, 365–374.

Luborsky, M. (1993). The romance with personal meaning: Gerontology, cultural aspects of life themes. *The Gerontologist, 33*, 445–452.

Mailloux, Z., & Burke, J. P. (1997). Play and the sensory integrative approach. In L. D. Parham & L. S. Fazio (Eds.), *Play in occupational therapy for children* (pp. 112–125). St. Louis: Mosby.

McAvoy, L. L. (1979). The leisure preferences, problems, and needs of the elderly. *Journal of Leisure Resources, 11*, 40–47.

McGuire, F. (1980). The incongruence between actual and desired leisure involvement in advanced adulthood. *Active Adaptive Aging, 1,* 77–89.

McGuire, F. (1983). Constraints on leisure involvement in the later years. *Active Adaptive Aging, 3,* 17–24.

Mitchell, J. J. (1975). *The adolescent predicament.* Toronto: Holt, Rinehart & Winston.

Nicholls, J. G. (1984). Achievement motivation: Conceptions of ability, subjective experience, task choice, and performance. *Psychological Review, 3,* 328–346.

Peterson, E., Howland, J., Kielhofner, G., Lachman, M. E., Assmann, S., Cote, J., & Jette, A. (1999). Falls self-efficacy and occupational adaptation among elders. *Physical & Occupational Therapy in Geriatrics, 16,* 1–16.

Pierce, D. (1997) The power of object play for infants and toddlers at risk for developmental delays. In L. D. Parham & L. S. Fazio (Eds.), *Play in occupational therapy for children* (pp. 86–111). St. Louis: Mosby.

Reilly, M. (1974). *Play as exploratory learning.* Beverly Hills: Sage.

Riley, K. P. (1994). Cognitive development. In B. R. Bonder & M. B. Wagner (Eds.), *Functional performance in older adults* (pp. 4–14). Philadelphia: FA Davis.

Robinson, A. L. (1977). Play, the arena for acquisition of rules for competent behavior. *American Journal of Occupational Therapy, 31,* 248–253.

Santrock, J. W. (1981). *Adolescence: An introduction.* Dubuque, IA: Brown.

Sterns, H. L., Laier, M. P., & Dorsett, J. G. (1994). Work and retirement. In B. R. Bonder & M. B. Wagner (Eds.), *Functional performance in older adults* (pp. 148–164). Philadelphia: FA Davis.

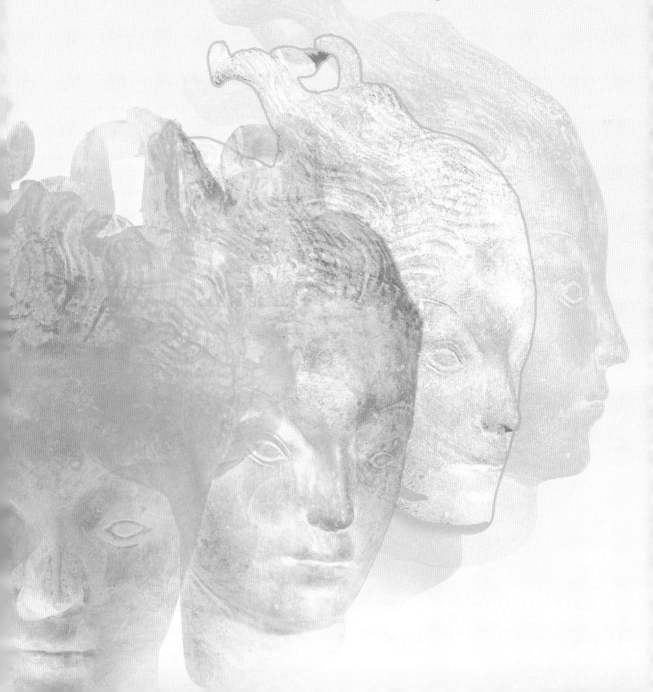

II

Applying MOHO: The Therapy Process and Therapeutic Reasoning

Introduction to Section II

Chapter 11 examines the process of therapeutic reasoning, examining how a therapist, in collaboration with the client, uses theory in getting to know the client and deciding a course of therapy. Chapter 12 discusses the use of unstructured and structured methods of gathering client information for assessment. Chapter 13 examines the process of change in therapy and focuses on actions clients can take to facilitate change. Chapter 14 continues the discussion of change, focusing on what therapists do to support client change.

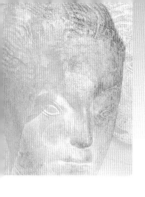

11

Therapeutic Reasoning: Planning, Implementing, and Evaluating the Outcomes of Therapy

- Gary Kielhofner
- Kirsty Forsyth

hapters 2 to 10 present MOHO theory. This chapter begins by describing how that theory is put into practice. It discusses therapeutic reasoning[1], that is how therapists use the theory to understand a client and to develop, implement, and monitor a plan of therapy with a client. Therapeutic reasoning using MOHO should be client centered, theory driven, and evidence based. This chapter emphasizes the client-centered and theoretical aspects of this process. Chapter 27 in Section 5 discusses the evidence base of MOHO that should always be considered in therapeutic reasoning.

Client Centeredness in Therapeutic Reasoning with MOHO

MOHO is inherently a client-centered model in two important ways:

- It views each client as a unique individual whose characteristics determine the rationale for and nature of the therapy goals and strategies
- It views what the client does, thinks, and feels as the central mechanism of change.

Therapeutic reasoning with MOHO focuses on understanding clients in terms of their own values, interests, sense of capacity and efficacy, roles, habits, and performance-related experiences within the relevant environments.

Therefore, the concepts of the theory call attention to the importance of knowing the details of a client's beliefs, perspectives, lifestyle, experience, and context. Moreover, since the logic of therapy emanates from a conceptual understanding informed by the client's characteristics in combination with the theory, the client's unique characteristics always define the goals and strategies of therapy.

As it will be elaborated in Chapter 13, the client's occupational engagement (i.e., what the client does, thinks, and feels) is the central dynamic of therapy. MOHO-based intervention supports the client's doing, thinking, and feeling to achieve change desired by the client and/or indicated by the client's situation. As will be discussed in Chapter 14, MOHO-based practice requires a client-therapist relationship in which the therapist must understand, respect, and support client choices, actions, and experiences. The therapist must communicate with the client, seeking input and valida-

---

[1] The term clinical reasoning is used by authors to refer to the process by which therapists generate an understanding of clients and make decisions in therapy (e.g., Mattingly, 1991; Mattingly & Fleming, 1993). The term therapeutic reasoning is used here instead to avoid medical model connotations of the term clinical and to highlight the client-focused collaborative nature of the proposed reasoning process.

> *Therapeutic reasoning with MOHO focuses on understanding clients in terms of their own values, interests, sense of capacity and efficacy, roles, habits, and performance-related experiences within the relevant environments.*

tion and engaging the client to collaborate in planning, implementing, and evaluating therapy.

Client-centeredness should extend to clients who are unable to verbalize and/or be active in collaboration. The therapist must work to understand the client's view of the world, what matters to the client, what the client enjoys, and how the client feels about his or her abilities. The therapist can also collaborate with family members or others who care about and can serve as advocates for the client.

Theory-Driven Therapeutic Reasoning

Using MOHO as a practice model requires an understanding of its underlying theory. Learning to think with theory evolves over time as the therapist uses it in practice. Importantly, engaging in therapeutic reasoning also enriches the therapist's understanding of the theory. Reasoning involves moving between theory and the circumstances of clients. Thus one's knowledge of theory grows as one sees it represented in different

clients' circumstances. For example, each client reveals a unique instance of personal causation. By seeing how numerous clients conceive of, understand, and feel about their capacity and efficacy, a therapist's understanding of personal causation is enriched.

Therapists' growth in knowledge of MOHO theory will also include a deepened appreciation of its implications in practice. For example, experience will reveal what therapeutic processes and strategies are generally most helpful for particular kinds of client problems. Notably, having a consistent set of theoretical concepts allows the therapist to think more systematically about clients and therapy, thereby enhancing what the therapist learns from experience.

The Six Steps of Therapeutic Reasoning

As illustrated in *Figure 11.1*, therapeutic reasoning involves six steps:

FIGURE 11.1 The six steps of the therapeutic reasoning process.

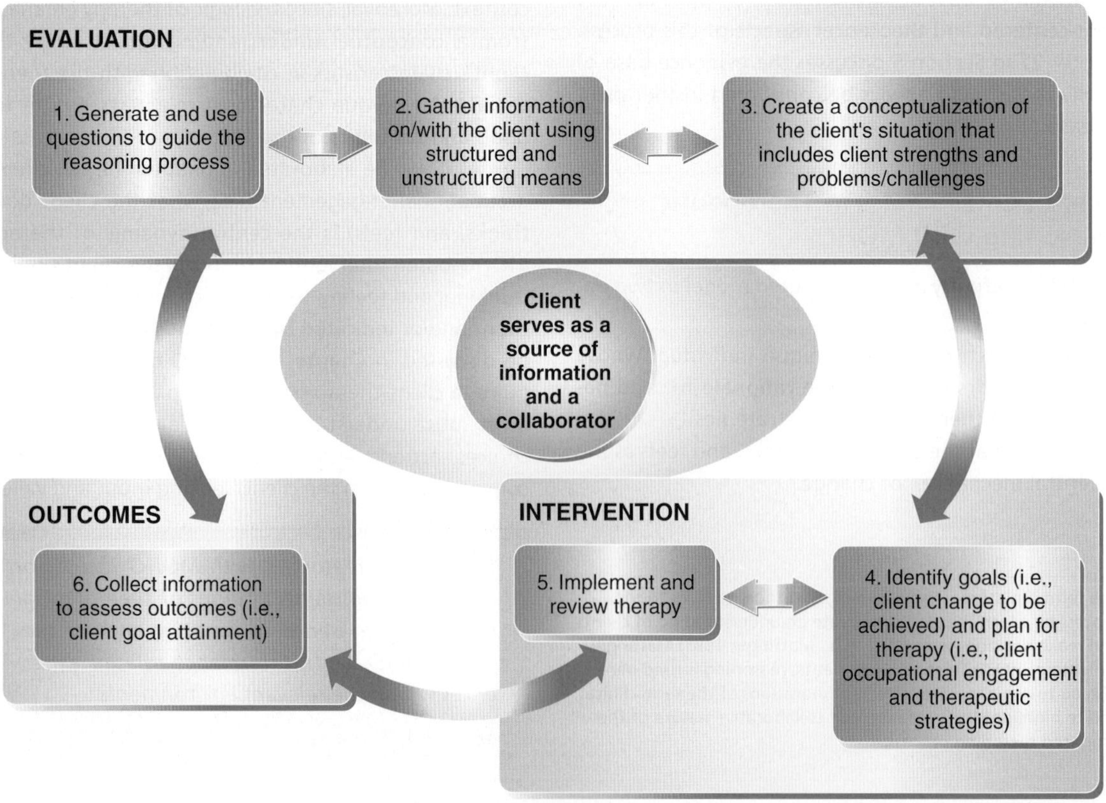

EVALUATION

1. Generate and use questions to guide the reasoning process

2. Gather information on/with the client using structured and unstructured means

3. Create a conceptualization of the client's situation that includes client strengths and problems/challenges

Client serves as a source of information and a collaborator

OUTCOMES

6. Collect information to assess outcomes (i.e., client goal attainment)

INTERVENTION

5. Implement and review therapy

4. Identify goals (i.e., client change to be achieved) and plan for therapy (i.e., client occupational engagement and therapeutic strategies)

- Generating questions on the client. The questions should reflect both what is initially known about the client and what MOHO theory calls attention to about the client. These questions constitute a structured approach to learning about a client.
- Collecting information on and from the client to answer the questions one has generated.
- Using the information gathered to create an explanation of the client's situation.
- Generating goals and strategies for therapy.
- Implementing and monitoring therapy.
- Determining outcomes of therapy.

These steps are not strictly sequential. Therapists generally move back and forth between the first five steps over the course of therapy.

Step 1: Generating Questions to Guide Information Gathering

Therapists must get to know their clients. Getting to know clients is facilitated when one systematically asks questions about the client. MOHO theory allows one to systematically generate these questions. That is, the major concepts of the theory (environmental impact, volition, habituation, performance capacity, participation, performance, skills, occupational identity, and occupational competence) orient the therapist to be concerned about certain things when getting to know a client.

As shown in *Figure 11.2*, these concepts can be used to raise broad questions about clients. The depth with which a therapist will seek to answer these questions and whether all of them will be addressed depends on the client and the circumstances of therapy. The Therapeutic Reasoning Table at the end of Section 2 lists a wide range of questions that might be asked about any given client. Thus, therapists are encouraged to use this table as a resource when first learning how to translate MOHO theory into client questions. It is important to note, however, that these questions are not exhaustive and must be tailored to each client.

As one goes about getting answers to questions, more specific questions are likely to emerge. For example, in response to the first of several detailed questions about interests (i.e., can this person identify personal interests?), a therapist may find that a client cannot identify any interests. In this instance, one would want to know why. Thus, the following questions might be relevant to ask depending on the client:

- Has the client lacked opportunity to develop interests?
- Has the client lost interests because of the interference of an impairment?

On the other hand, if a client identifies several interests, the therapist may wish to go on to ask whether the client participates in these interests and what common themes, if any, exist in the interests. How one proceeds with a line of questioning is always informed by the answers to previous questions.

$\mathcal{G}$eneral **Therapeutic Reasoning Questions for Pediatric Practice**[1]

As this chapter emphasizes, therapists should generate questions to guide their therapeutic reasoning, that reflect the particular circumstances of their client or client population. Therapists often find it useful to have an explicit set of questions for their client population that they follow or draw upon (even if informally) when doing clinical reasoning. The set of questions that follows is an example. These questions were developed for therapists using MOHO to gather unstructured information when working with children and youth and their families.

MOHO Concept	Corresponding Questions
Occupational Identity	• What is the child's sense of who he/she has been, is, and wishes to become in relation to family life, school, friendships, hobbies, and interests? • What is the family's sense of who this child has been, is, and what do they wish him/her to become? How does this affect the child's occupational identity?

MOHO Concept	Corresponding Questions
Occupational Competence	• To what extent has this child sustained a pattern of satisfying occupational participation over time? • Does this child feel he/she can do the things he/she needs to do in school, with friends, and in the community? • To what extent have important people in this child's life sustained patterns of occupational participation over time that reflect their occupational identity in relation to this child (e.g., caregiving, playmate)?
Participation	• Does the child currently engage in work, play, and ADLs that are part of his/her sociocultural context and that are desired and/or necessary for his/her well-being?
Performance	• Can this child do the occupational forms that are part of the work, play, and ADL activities that make up or should make up the child's life? • Can the child do the occupational forms that the family expects the child to do as part of work, play, and ADL activities?
Skill	• Does the child exhibit the necessary communication/interaction, motor, and process skills to perform what the child needs and wants to do?
Environment	• What work, play, and ADL activities does the family consider to be desired and/or necessary for the well-being of this child? • Does the family support the child in developing the necessary volition, habituation, as well as communication/interaction, motor, and process skills needed for participation and development? • What impact do the opportunities, resources, constraints, and demands (or lack of demands) of the environment have on how this child thinks, feels, and acts? • How do the opportunities, resources, constraints, or demands provided by spaces, objects, occupational forms/tasks, and social groups affect the child's skill, performance, and participation?
Volition	• What is this child's view of his/her personal capacity and effectiveness? • What convictions and sense of obligations does this child have? What does the child think is important? • What are this child's interests? What does this child enjoy doing?
Habituation	• What routines does this child participate in and how do routines influence what the child does? • What are the roles with which this child identifies and how do they influence what the child routinely does?

[1]This feature box was provided by Jessica M. Kramer, MS, OTR/L, MOHO Clearinghouse, and Patricia Bowyer, EdD, OTR/L, BCN, postdoctoral fellow, both in the Department of Occupational Therapy at the College of Applied Health Sciences, University of Illinois at Chicago.

General Therapeutic Reasoning Questions for Older Adult Practice

As this chapter emphasizes, therapists should generate questions to guide their therapeutic reasoning that reflect the particular circumstances of their client or client population. Therapists often find it useful to have an explicit set of questions for their client population that they follow or draw upon (even if informally) when doing clinical reasoning. The set of questions that follows is an example. These questions were developed for therapists using MOHO to gather unstructured information when working with older adults and their families.

MOHO Concept	Corresponding Questions
Occupational Identity	• How does this older adult view himself/herself—? Do they perceive themselves to be a grandparent, mother, volunteer, church member, activist? Does the person view himself/herself as not contributing to society or friends and family? As failing to remain active and engaged with life?

MOHO Concept	Corresponding Questions
Occupational Identity	• What is the family's sense of who this older adult is? How does this affect the older adult's view of himself/herself?
Occupational Competence	• Has the older adult been able to meet their responsibilities over time? • Does the older adult perceive himself/herself to be able to do the occupations that they need and/or want to be able to do? • Does the older adult feel competent within their occupational life?
Participation	• Does the older adult currently routinely engage in productive activities, leisure, and self-care activities that he/she needs and/or wants to be able to do?
Performance	• Can this older adult do the self-care, productivity, and leisure that make up his/her life? • Can the older adult perform daily activities to a standard he/she is happy with?
Skill	• Does the older adult exhibit the necessary communication/interaction, motor, and process skills to perform what he/she needs and wants to do?
Environment	• What daily activities does the family consider to be desired and/or necessary for the well-being of this older adult? • Does the family support the older adult in efforts to engage in daily activities? • What impact do the opportunities, resources, constraints, and demands (or lack of demands) of the environment have on how this older adult views himself/herself and his/her abilities? • How do the opportunities, resources, constraints, or demands provided by spaces, objects, occupational forms/tasks, and social groups affect the older adult's participation in daily life?
Volition	• Does this older adult have appropriate confidence in his/her abilities? • What is the set of driving principles this older adult lives by? What is important to him/her, and how does this affect choices to engage in daily activities? • Does the older adult do activities he/she finds enjoyable and satisfying?
Habituation	• What is the daily routine of this older adult and how do routines influence what he/she does? • How does the older adult feel about the routine? • What are the responsibilities the older adult holds, and how do they affect daily routines?

Step 2: Gathering Information on or with the Client

To answer the questions generated in the first step, therapists must gather information on and with the client. Therapists can gather information using both structured assessments and unstructured approaches.

A therapist using structured assessments follows a set protocol that has been developed and tested through research. A therapist using an unstructured approach takes advantage of naturally occurring opportunities to gather information. Structured assessments guard against bias and provide information that is readily interpretable. Unstructured approaches capitalize on opportunities for obtaining useful information in informal, spontaneous, and creative ways. Ordinarily therapists use both means to gather information.

One should approach data gathering systematically and thoughtfully with these concerns:

• The kind of information that is needed to answer the questions one has generated
• The best method to gather that information given the circumstances.

As discussed in Chapters 15 to 18, a wide range of MOHO-based structured assessments have been developed and are available to therapists for information gathering. Therapists using MOHO also use other structured assessments because:

• They use MOHO in association with other conceptual practice models that have their own assessments.
• They choose other assessments that specifically target occupational performance in ways that MOHO-based assessments do not. Such assessments include

FIGURE 11.2 Seven general questions generated from the theory.

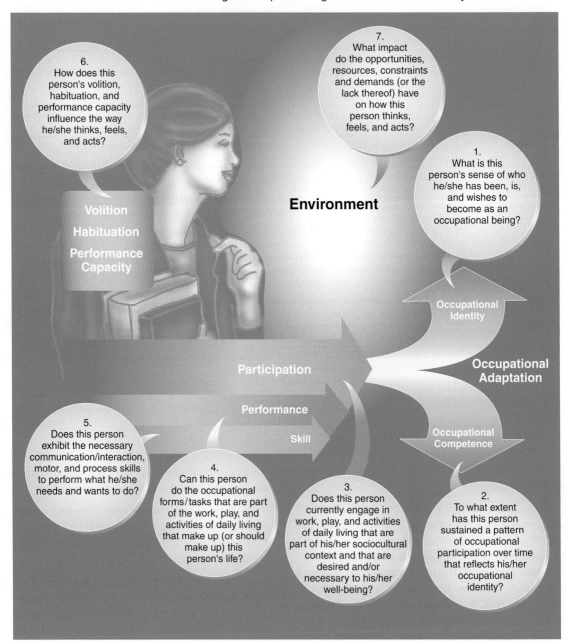

activities of daily living assessments, standardized development assessments, and formal work evaluations. These kinds of assessments are used when the therapist needs information on the client's capacity to do specific occupational forms/tasks, such as dressing, bathing, or driving. Although such assessments were not developed specifically for use with MOHO, they are certainly compatible with it.

- They choose assessments that gather information directly or partly related to constructs in MOHO. An example is the use of structured interest inventories. Since the MOHO-based interest assessments focus mainly on leisure interests, therapists wishing to gather information on work-related interests ordinarily use one of a number of standardized vocational interest assessments.

As noted previously, unstructured approaches to gathering information take advantage of natural circumstances that arise for learning about a client. Unstructured information collection simply involves observing and/or talking with the client. Unstructured methods are used not only as part of initial assessment but also as an important means of continuing the information gathering process throughout the course of therapy. Every opportunity the therapist has to observe and/or talk with a client may yield potentially useful information. If therapists use such opportunities wisely, they can gather a wealth of information efficiently and effectively.

Step 3: Creating a Conceptualization of the Client That Includes Strengths and Challenges

The information gathered to answer questions about a client should be used to create a theory-based understanding of that client. This conceptualization of the client's situation represents a synthesis of the general concepts of the theory with the particular information about the client. The aim of this step is to create an understanding of the client's situation. In this step one uses MOHO theory as a framework for creating a conceptualization or explanation of that particular client's situation. This conceptualization will guide the next step of generating goals and strategies for therapy. Thus, one must identify the problems and challenges to be addressed in therapy as well as strengths that can be drawn on in therapy.

In creating a conceptualization of one's client, it is important to get it right (i.e., to accurately understand the client's situation). For this reason, therapists should involve clients to the extent possible. By working together, the therapist and client can often generate insights into a client's situation that neither had at the outset. Clients know their own experiences. However, clients do not always have a clear picture of all of the factors contributing to that experience. The aim of this step, then, is to generate new insights that will form the basis for a course of action to achieve desired change.

Step 4: Identifying Goals and Plans for Client Engagement and Therapeutic Strategies

The next step is to plan the therapy process. This includes:

- Creating therapy goals with the client
- Deciding what kinds of occupational engagement will enable the client to change
- Determining what kind of therapeutic strategies will be needed to support the client to change.

Goals indicate the kinds of changes that therapy will aim to achieve. Change is required when the client's characteristics and/or environment is contributing to occupational problems or challenges. For instance, if a client feels ineffective, therapy would seek to enable the client to feel more effective. If a client has too few roles, therapy would seek to enable the client to choose and enact new roles. If the environment is hindering the client's performance, therapy would seek to modify that environment. In this way identifying challenges and problems in the third step allows one to select the goals in the fourth step.

The Therapeutic Reasoning Table (at the end of section 2) lists changes that correspond to clients' problems and challenges (see the fourth column of this table). These changes correspond to the kinds of problems and challenges identified in the third column of the table. For example, the table lists the following changes related to personal causation:

- Enhance understanding of performance capacities (strengths and weaknesses)
- Focus attention to more accurately understand how limitations and assets affect occupational performance

- Develop emotional acceptance of limitations and pride in occupational abilities
- Reduce unnecessary feelings of dependence, resentment, or guilt associated with reduced participation
- Increase facility in choosing to do occupational forms/tasks consistent with performance capacity
- Build up confidence to approach occupational forms/tasks within performance capacity
- Increase knowledge and acceptance of using adaptive aids and/or environmental modifications to augment capacity
- Increase willingness to ask for help when needed
- Reduce anxiety and fear of failure in occupational performance
- Build up confidence to face occupational performance demands
- Improve facility to sustain effort for attaining goals and/or completing performance
- Widen expectation of success in performance
- Extend readiness to take on occupational challenges and responsibilities
- Increase sense of control in occupational outcomes.

These changes reflect the concepts of self-efficacy and sense of personal capacity. Therapists should find this list of changes to be useful guides for generating goals when clients are having difficulty with these aspects of personal causation. Similar lists of changes can be found in the table for all the other major MOHO concepts.

Of course, the table is only a beginning point. With experience, therapists will develop facility in identifying what changes are indicated by their clients' typical problems and challenges.

Setting goals (and thereby identifying the types of change that will be targeted in therapy) is only the first part of this step. Next the therapist must plan what will take place in therapy to achieve the goals. As will be discussed in Chapter 13, the central mechanism of change in occupational therapy is the client's occupational engagement (i.e., what the client does, thinks, and feels). Thus, a therapy plan must always specify what the client's occupational engagement will be. Therapists employ a variety of strategies that support clients' occupational engagement and thus facilitate achieving therapy goals. These strategies will be discussed in Chapter 14.

Building on the discussions in Chapters 13 and 14, the Therapeutic Reasoning Table (at the end of section 2) identifies types of client engagement and therapist strategies that may help to achieve the types of changes listed in the table. Therapists will find this table a useful resource for thinking about what will be the client's occupational engagement and what strategies they can use to enable the client's occupational engagement. Both of these aspects of the therapy plan must be monitored and modified in step 5 as therapy unfolds. Nonetheless, it is important to begin with a plan for therapy to support goal attainment.

Successful therapy depends on a client's willingness to accept its goals and strategies. Therefore, the therapist must communicate and collaborate with the client to identify the therapy plan. How this is done depends on the client and must be built around the client's perceptions and desires. The case of Elsie provides an example to illustrate this point.

Elsie

Collaborative goal setting requires a strong respect for the client's perspective. The following example illustrates a collaborative approach to establishing goals.

Elsie was a 45-year-old client in a mental health setting. When she discussed what she saw as her major problem with the therapist, she referred to it as lacking the "oomph" to do what she wanted and needed to do. The client's concept of "oomph" was clearly how she thought about her problem. In fact, she expressed it in a poem entitled "My Get-up-and-go Has Got up and Gone." Because this is how she saw the problem, she saw therapy as a way to get her "oomph" back.

Elsie's occupational therapist collaborated with her in setting goals for therapy, one of which they agreed would be: "Improve Elsie's oomph." What the therapist appreciated was the necessity of validating and reflecting in the goal how her client perceived her own difficulty. Moreover, because Elsie's perspectives were validated, she was much more motivated to engage in therapy.

Step 5: Implementing and Reviewing Therapy

Implementing therapy involves not only following the plan of action set out in the previous step but also being vigilant to monitor how therapy is unfolding. When the therapist reviews therapy, new information may emerge, and which can result in one or more of the following:

- Confirmation of the therapist's conceptualization of the client's situation
- Changes in the therapist's conceptualization of the client's situation
- Confirmation of the utility of the planned client occupational engagement and therapist strategies
- Modification of goals and/or planned client occupational engagement and therapist strategies.

To the extent that therapy unfolds as anticipated, the therapist's conceptualization of the client's situation was most likely accurate and the goals and plan of therapy were appropriate. However, therapists should always expect that at least part of what happens in therapy will be unexpected. When things do not turn out as expected, the therapist returns to earlier steps of generating questions, selecting methods to gather information, conceptualizing the client's situation, setting goals, and establishing plans.

It is important to continue communication with the client as therapy unfolds. Feedback to the clients concerning their progress helps to solidify commitment to therapy. When clients have attained goals, it is important to recognize their accomplishment and to reinforce the efforts they have put forward to accomplish them. Honest discussion with the client about new problems or lack of progress is equally important to maintain trust in the therapeutic relationship. When clients fail to reach goals, the information should be shared in a supportive context that examines the reasons for failure and facilitates the problem solving necessary to formulate attainable goals or to ensure future goal attainment.

Step 6: Collecting Information to Assess Outcomes

Determining therapy outcomes is an important final step in the therapy process. Typically therapy outcomes are documented by:

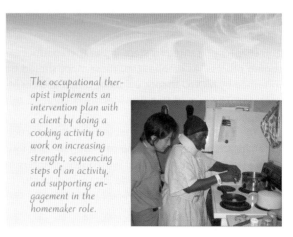

The occupational therapist implements an intervention plan with a client by doing a cooking activity to work on increasing strength, sequencing steps of an activity, and supporting engagement in the homemaker role.

- Examining the extent to which goals have been achieved
- Readministering structured assessments.

Both approaches are valuable in documenting outcomes. Assessing outcomes by examining goal attainment is helpful in reflecting on the extent to which the therapeutic reasoning process resulted in good decisions for therapy. Since goals are formulated in collaboration with clients, examining the extent to which goals have been attained allows a determination of how much the client's desires were achieved.

Structured assessments can provide useful measures of change. Structured assessments are typically given at the beginning and the end of therapy, and differences in the client's score or measure are used as indication of how much change was achieved. MOHO-based assessments are designed to capture one or more of the concepts from the theory (e.g., volition, skill, or participation). Using these assessments is particularly useful when the concept was a target of therapy. Thus for example, if an aim of therapy was to improve volition, skill, or participation, assessments that measure these constructs can be used to demonstrate whether there was improvement. Using structured assessments also allows one to compare change across different clients or when different strategies are used. In this way, they can contribute to evidence-based therapy.

Conclusion

This chapter presented six steps in the therapeutic reasoning process. As emphasized, these steps should be informed by MOHO theory, evidence-based and client-centered. The case of Dan provides an example of this therapeutic reasoning process.

The therapeutic reasoning table that follows Section 2 is an important resource to implementing the first four steps discussed in this chapter. Subsequent chapters in this section and Section 3 provide information useful to implementing the therapeutic reasoning process.

*D*an: An Illustration of Therapeutic Reasoning

Dan was a client in a long-term treatment facility for adolescents with psychiatric disabilities. Dan had had school performance problems and family difficulties related to depression. He also had a history of substance abuse. Dan appeared nervous and uneasy most of the time. The concept of volition naturally led the therapist to wonder about several things about Dan:

- What are Dan's thoughts and feelings about his capacity and efficacy, and do they account for his anxious demeanor?

- Does Dan have interests and act on them, and does he enjoy the things he does?

- What are Dan's values, and is he able to realize them in what he does?

- What kinds of decisions does Dan make about doing things, and how do his personal causation, values, and interests influence these decisions?

These and related questions arose as the therapist came to know Dan. Moreover, they guided the collection of information about him.

The therapist observed Dan in several situations. The therapist also interviewed Dan about the things he did in his life, his experiences at home, in school, and with friends. Finally, Dan filled out some paper-and-pencil as-

sessments that allowed him to tell the therapist about his interests and values. Guided by the MOHO theory of volition, the therapist was able to use the information to construct the following understanding of Dan (*Fig. 11-3*).

At this point in Dan's life, his personal causation was dominated by a sense of incapacity and inefficacy. He felt very little control over most aspects of his life. He showed little interest in most of the things other adolescents enjoyed, and even when doing something that he felt some attraction to, Dan's experience was dominated by anxiety over his performance. His anxiety was fueled at home by an extremely critical parent who constantly anticipated and pointed out Dan's failures. Moreover, because Dan had gained a reputation in school as a difficult student, he faced a similar judgmental attitude from several teachers. Dan felt very pressured by these attitudes because he disliked very much feeling that others perceived him as "bad." Finally, Dan's peers tended to view him as different and did not readily include him in the things they did.

Because of his anxiety over performance, Dan was unable to feel a sense of enjoyment or satisfaction in doing most things. His few interests were solitary, since he was fearful of performing around peers. He very much valued and wanted to be able to do the same things as other adolescents and to be included by them. Because he viewed himself as lacking capacity for these things, he devalued himself, often making disparaging comments about his own performance. This, briefly, was the therapist's conceptualization of Dan's volition and the environmental factors that impacted upon it.

According to MOHO theory, volition—in combination with environmental conditions—influences activity choices. The therapist observed the following characteristics of Dan's choices that emanated from his volition and environment. He consistently avoided doing anything new or facing any kinds of performance demands. When allowed to make his own choices, he always chose to do things that were familiar, safe, and solitary. He was extremely uncomfortable around peers and put forth a great deal of effort to avoid situations in which peers could judge his performance. For example, he would sometimes privately admit his lack of confidence about performance to the therapist, but in a group therapy session with peers present, he insisted that all the things available to do were "stupid," thereby avoiding having to perform in front of his peers.

With this additional information, the therapist could

FIGURE 11.3 A theory-based understanding of a client's volition.

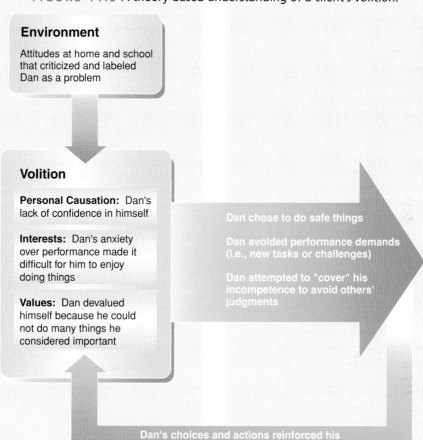

recognize how Dan's volition, along with corresponding environmental conditions, was sustaining him in a maladaptive pattern. That is, his choices to do things were designed to avoid failure and judgment of others, but these choices also ensured that he would neither learn new skills nor develop a stronger sense of capacity and efficacy.

Using lay terms that Dan could understand, the therapist shared his understanding of Dan's situation with Dan to determine whether he agreed. This served not only to make sure that the therapist had accurately comprehended Dan but also to inform Dan in terms he could understand of the theoretical ideas the therapist was using. Dan reluctantly agreed with what the therapist proposed and added some of his own concerns and interpretations. This discussion gave the therapist further insights into Dan and helped Dan learn more about himself. As they came to a shared understanding of Dan's situation, they discussed some ideas for goals for therapy. This discussion informed Dan of how the therapist was conceptualizing his therapy and what it was designed to achieve for him.

Using the theory to make sense of Dan's situation and sharing the therapist's formulation with Dan helped them arrive at mutually agreeable goals for his therapy. Dan's long-term volition-related goals included:

- Increasing Dan's belief in skill and sense of efficacy so that he could make choices to do things he valued and that would lead to improving his performance

- Increasing his range of interests and ability to enjoy doing things, both alone and with peers

- Enabling him to gain competence and thereby a feeling of efficacy in doing what he most valued.

These long-term goals were translated into short-term measurable goals in language Dan understood. For example, one short-term goal was that at the end of every session Dan would be able to report at least one thing he enjoyed about the activity he did.

Next, the therapist and Dan had to decide how to go about achieving these goals. MOHO theory indicates that these volitional changes require the following process. First, environmental conditions outside Dan needed to change to allow a new dynamic out of which new volitional thoughts, feelings, and actions could emerge for Dan. Second, the therapist needed to repeat this situation sufficiently so that Dan's volition could begin to reorganize around a sense of capacity, a desire and enjoyment of doing things, and a positive valuation of himself.

Consequently, the therapist began with the therapeutic strategy of advising and supporting Dan to choose projects in which he could readily succeed and that he saw as valuable. Dan decided to engage in leather work and woodwork. Both occupational forms/tasks involved the use of tools—something important to Dan. Handling the tools symbolized competence to him. Moreover, they allowed Dan to create products that would tangibly affirm his competence. During therapy the therapist gave him constant feedback on his successes and invited Dan to review each session, identifying what he had enjoyed, accomplished, and learned. They dealt with problems and challenges that arose by working together to see how he could achieve good outcomes by problem solving and/or asking for help. This meant redefining help seeking from being a sign of failure to being yet another method Dan could choose and use to accomplish what he wanted. Dan's therapy began with individual sessions in which he could be free of the worry about what his peers would think about his performance. He progressed to doing things in parallel groups when he had developed sufficient capacity and belief in his own abilities to demonstrate his newfound competence in front of peers.

The therapist's understanding of Dan's volition also guided the therapist in the details of his intervention. The therapist knew that when Dan was reluctant to engage in activities, it was because they were too threatening. The therapist observed Dan carefully for signs of anxiety in performance and consistently reoriented him to simply enjoy the activity and use the opportunity to develop some skills (exploration stage of change).

Later, when he had gained some sense of capacity and efficacy, Dan was able to choose and succeed at greater (competence level) challenges, requiring a role within cooperative groups and a routine of performance. For instance, he became part of an adolescent woodworking team that met daily in the wood shop to work on fabricating a game table for their common recreation room.

As they began to plan for Dan's discharge from therapy, the therapist also knew that maintaining the volitional changes he had gained in therapy would require consistent, supportive environmental conditions to allow him to continue his new pattern of thinking, feeling, and acting. Consequently, the therapist made recommendations for Dan's parents and teachers, which were shared with them by the psychologist who managed Dan's case and conducted family therapy with Dan and his parents.

This case example illustrated how:

- MOHO theory can be used to construct a particular conceptualization of a client's situation

- The unique characteristics of the client are combined with MOHO theory to arrive at this conceptualization

- The conceptualization guides selection of therapy goals and the therapy process.

The case also illustrated that the therapeutic reasoning process can be shared actively with the client, who becomes a partner in each step. To the extent that they are capable and willing, clients should always be given an opportunity to participate in the process of thinking with theory. When this happens, the theory not only enriches the therapist's view but enhances the client's self-understanding.

References

Mattingly, C. (1991). The narrative nature of clinical reasoning. *American Journal of Occupational Therapy, 45,* 998–1005.

Mattingly, C., & Fleming, M. (1993). *Clinical reasoning: Forms of inquiry in a therapeutic practice.* Philadelphia: FA Davis.

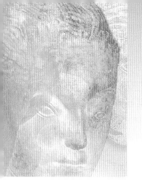

12

Assessment: Choosing and Using Structured and Unstructured Means of Gathering Information

- Gary Kielhofner
- Kirsty Forsyth

As noted in Chapter 11, therapists gather information to answer key questions about the client and to create a conceptualization of the client's situation. Good assessment is critical to understanding clients and their needs. Moreover, assessment is a prerequisite to making good decisions about the goals and strategies of therapy. As Trombly (1993) notes, "we cannot ethically treat what we do not measure" (p. 256). Good practice requires therapists to gather enough information to understand the client and to make sound judgments about the course of therapy.

From the perspective of MOHO theory, comprehensive assessment means that a therapist will at minimum raise and seek answers to questions pertaining to the client's occupational adaptation, volition, habituation, performance capacity, and environmental impact. The questions that the therapist raises will indicate the kind of information that need to be gathered to generate an adequate understanding of the client's situation. The following case illustrates the importance of this point.

Henrietta

Henrietta was 75 years old and had osteoarthritis. The second author of this chapter received a referral to see Henrietta for occupational therapy. The referral stated that Henrietta had recently been hospitalized after sustaining a fractured femur. At our first meeting, Henrietta indicated that she was familiar with occupational therapy. Several months ago, she first received occupational therapy as an inpatient following a mild stroke. She remembered that the therapist asked her about her physical limitations and then recommended that Henrietta receive bathing equipment. Henrietta recalled that initially she was extremely excited at the prospect of being able to bathe again.

Henrietta then came to the occupational therapy department, where the therapist demonstrated how to use the bathing equipment. She then asked Henrietta to try using the equipment to get in and out of the bath. Henrietta remembered that she managed this simulation well, and she never saw the occupational therapist again. In fact, the therapist documented in Henrietta's file that she was able to "transfer in and out of the bath using the bath board and seat." After Henrietta was discharged, another community-based occupational therapist visited her home once to install the equipment.

When asked where the bathing equipment was now, Henrietta answered, "in the closet . . . I never use it." Instead, Henrietta had been washing herself at the bathroom sink. The following is why Henrietta had abandoned the bathroom equipment and begun washing at the sink. First, Henrietta's bathroom at home was much smaller than the one in the hospital. Consequently, she had difficulty maneuvering into position while using her walker. Second, she could not gather and organize all the needed bathing objects within reach, which frustrated her. Third, Henrietta attempted to bathe in the morning, as had always been her habit. However, because this was before her pain medication took effect, she was in pain. Fourth, Henrietta found it very anxiety-provoking to do the routine she had simulated in the hospital with the bath full of hot water and steam.

Despite these factors and because bathing was so important to her, Henrietta chose to continue with the bath. As she proceeded, she realized that she had forgotten some of the therapist's instructions for how to use the bath board and seat. Consequently, she was only able to maneuver part way onto the bath equipment. After several attempts, her skin became sore and she decided she could not manage and gave up.

Henrietta was so flustered by this negative experience and so unsure of her capacity to use the bathing equipment that she resolved never to try bathing with the equipment again. So she asked a neighbor to remove the bathing equipment. Then she put it permanently in the closet.

Following this, Henrietta chose to bathe in the best way she could: washing at the bathroom sink. However, her endurance was severely taxed by this process. It was during this morning wash at the bathroom sink that Henrietta, exhausted, slipped and fractured the neck of her femur.

While it was obviously not intended, the two occupational therapists' failure to do adequate assessment contributed to Henrietta's fall and fracture.

The therapists needed more information about Henrietta than they gathered. They might have recognized the need to gather more information had they generated the following MOHO-based questions:

- Did Henrietta have adequate motor and process skills to manage bathing at home with the prescribed equipment?
- What was Henrietta's daily habit of bathing? How would this habit influence her success in bathing?
- When the new equipment (objects) are put into the physical space of Henrietta's bathroom along with

other objects (e.g., her walker, soap, shampoo, towels, robe), how will the overall bathroom space and objects collectively affect her performance?

- How will Henrietta experience her first attempt to bathe at home?
- Will she feel an adequate sense of efficacy to continue using the equipment?

Gathering adequate information to answer these questions would have pointed to the utility of:

- Helping Henrietta find a way to transport and arrange her bathing objects in reach of the bathing seat
- Solving problems of dealing with limited maneuvering space
- Providing further training and practice in the use of the adaptive equipment under real-life conditions
- Giving her verbal encouragement and reassurance to reduce her anxiety
- Altering daily habits so that she could bathe in the afternoon or evening, when she had less pain.

Even if Henrietta had not been able to bathe with these interventions, the therapist could have worked with her to establish a different, safe way of getting washed. Certainly, the additional time and cost of doing adequate assessment would have been substantially less than the expense of Henrietta's hospitalization for the hip fracture. As this case illustrates, taking time to do adequate assessment can be very cost effective. Failing to gather adequate information can have high human and economic costs.

Making Decisions About Information Gathering

Given that most occupational therapy contexts require one to be as efficient as possible in assessment, it is important to make sound decisions about what information to gather and how to gather it. Therapists must always balance limitations on available time and other practical constraints with the need to learn as much as possible about the client. Decisions about information gathering focus one three interwoven issues:

- Getting the most important information
- Ensuring that the information is complete and accurate
- Choosing the best means of gathering the information.

The best way to ensure that one is gathering the most important information is to generate clear questions that will be answered by assessment. Chapter 11 discussed generating questions using MOHO theory. Generating these questions is a necessary prelude to gathering information. Ensuring that the information is complete and accurate requires therapists to be aware of the client's characteristics, the circumstances of the therapeutic relationship, and the particular strengths and weaknesses of approaches to information gathering. Choosing the best means of gathering information takes the therapist back to the first two issues. Selection of means for gathering information should be guided by the questions the therapist wants answered and by considerations of what means of information gathering will provide the most accurate and complete information given the client and other circumstances. As noted in Chapter 11, therapists ordinarily draw upon both unstructured and structured means of assessment. Both are considered below.

Deciding When and How to Use Unstructured Information Gathering

Therapists should routinely use unstructured approaches to gathering information (i.e., informally observing or talking with a client). Unstructured approaches to gathering information are useful as supplements to structured approaches, for taking advantage of unexpected opportunities to obtain useful information and for monitoring the process of therapy. Sometimes, unstructured approaches are the only option available to the therapist.

As noted previously, unstructured approaches to gathering information take advantage of natural circumstances that arise for learning about a client. The following are some common circumstances in which therapists will decide to make use of unstructured information gathering methods:

- There is no appropriate structured assessment for the question one wants to answer or for the type of client one has
- The client is uncomfortable with or unable to complete a structured assessment
- The therapist wishes to augment information collected by structured assessments

- An unexpected opportunity to obtain useful information arises.

Unstructured information collection can occur in a wide range of circumstances, such as:

- Having a conversation with a client while beginning a therapy session
- Observing a student's performance when visiting the classroom
- Listening to a client's comments about the workplace where he was injured
- Noting the affect of a client during a group session
- Listening to a client's occasional stories about what happened since the last therapy session.

Unstructured methods are an important means of continuing the information gathering process throughout the course of therapy. Every opportunity the therapist has to observe and/or talk with a client potentially yields useful information. If therapists use such opportunities consistently and wisely they can gather a wealth of information.

Unstructured methods of information gathering are particularly dependent on having identified questions that one wants answered. When guided by such questions, therapists can be more vigilant to look for opportunities to find information, and they can more appropriately undertake unstructured methods. For instance, if a therapist has questions about a client's volition, then any informal conversation with that client can be directed to answering those specific questions. On the other hand, if a therapist has not consciously generated questions about the client, opportunities to learn critical things about the client are likely to be lost. Generating theory-based questions is an important step to going about unstructured information gathering in a systematic and disciplined way.

Gathering Information on the Lived Body

Since no structured assessments exist for gathering information on the lived body experience, therapists must always use unstructured methods for this purpose. As discussed and illustrated in Chapter 6, understanding a person's performance experience can be extremely important. However, because disability can radically alter experience from what is ordinary, therapists must take special care in gathering such information. Grasping what the client is experiencing is complicated by the fact that it might differ radically from the therapist's own experience. The suggestions offered here are based on methods developed in a study of unilateral neglect (Tham, Borell, & Gustavsson, 2000).

A combination of observation and informal interviewing appears to be the most effective approach. Because it is often very difficult for clients to describe their lived body experiences, therapists should begin by explaining that such information will help the therapist and client better plan therapy and by reminding clients that they are experts on their own experience.

It is also helpful to talk to clients while they are performing tasks or immediately thereafter. This strategy both calls clients' attention to their experience and allows them to tell about it while the memory of the experience is fresh. Another useful strategy is to ask clients to describe how performing in the present differs from how it used to feel before the onset of the disability. Sometimes it is helpful to share what other clients have previously described to see if clients recognize it as similar to their own experiences. The kind of description given in Chapter 6 can also be a good starting point for asking clients about their own experiences. Finally, the therapist should refine what is asked as clients are able to begin talking about their experiences. Using phrases that the client used and asking for their meaning can help focus discussion.

Proper Use of Unstructured Methods to Ensure Dependability

When using unstructured methods to gather information, therapists use much the same kind of logic and safeguards that qualitative researchers use when they gather information from field observation and interviews (Denzin & Lincoln, 1994; Hagner & Helm, 1994; Hammersly, 1992; Krefting, 1989; Miles & Huberman, 1994; Wolcott, 1990). Although it is not possible to review here all of the kinds of concerns and practices that qualitative researchers have in mind when collecting

and interpreting information, three important strategies for ensuring dependability of information gathered by unstructured methods will be discussed:

- Evaluating context
- Triangulation
- Validity checks.

Evaluating Context

Circumstances have an important influence on the information one receives. For example, a client struggling with some problem suddenly confides in a therapist about his fears for the future. From such an encounter, the therapist may have much more honest and useful information than the information previously gathered in a formal interview. On the other hand, circumstance may make the information suspect. For example, if a client is reporting on her performance in a group and it is clear she is trying to impress another group member, the therapist may have reasons to suspect that the report is exaggerated. Circumstances often tell the therapist how much confidence to place in the information and how to interpret it.

Triangulation

Triangulation is a method of helping to ensure that information is accurate by comparing it with information from another source (Denzin & Lincoln, 1994). Thus, for example, one may compare what clients say they can do with observation of their performance or with what a spouse or caretaker says the person can do. Another method of triangulation is to compare the same type of information collected over time. Observing performance or asking about a client's view of the future more than once is a way of checking whether one observation or response was truly representative of how the person performs or feels.

Validity Checks

When using unstructured methods, therapists should be vigilant to ensure that their interpretation of the meaning of the information is valid. First, a therapist should ask whether an interpretation corresponds logically and structurally with the general picture obtained from earlier information. If it does, then one has a stronger basis to consider the interpretation. The therapist may also ask whether the interpretation corresponds with case examples and other discussions offered by the theory that guided the information gathering.

Another important method of checking the validity of one's interpretations is to continue to collect information that will either support or refute the interpretation of the previous information's meaning. Finally and importantly, one can and should check interpretations of information by asking the client if the interpretations are valid. For example, observation of a client's behavior in a task situation suggests that the client was anxious and the therapist interprets this information as meaning the client's sense of efficacy in a particular task is poor. The therapist can check the validity of this interpretation by sharing it with the client to ask whether he or she agrees. In sum, a therapist using unstructured methods can ensure validity by employing a careful and reflective attitude and by checking up on information and its interpretation.

*U*sing Unstructured Assessment in the Course of Therapy[1]

. . . .

Jennifer is a patient in rehabilitation following a cerebrovascular accident. She was originally assessed by the occupational therapist using the Model of Human Occupational Screening Tool (MOHOST), since she had such emotional difficulty talking about her life situation and was not considered a candidate for a full interview. Another reason the therapist chose to use the MOHOST with this client was that it allowed the therapist to gather a broad range of information, including motor, process, and communication skills as well as information about Jennifer's environment, habituation, and volition. In doing the assessment, the therapist identified that she wanted to gather more information on Jennifer's volition.

During a therapy session, when Jennifer was folding laundry, she spontaneously shared her concern that she would no longer be able to contribute to her family. While reassuring Jennifer, the therapist also asked further questions to better understand Jennifer's sense of efficacy and her values around her family role. This be-

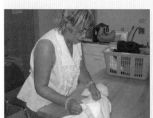

gan an informal conversation that continued into another session when Jennifer was practicing a cooking activity. During their time in the kitchen the therapist was able to further explore Jennifer's volition.

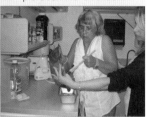

Jennifer provides valuable information to her occupational therapist while folding laundry and baking a cake.

The information gathered using unstructured methods during these two therapy sessions provided valuable information that the therapist was able to incorporate with other information to construct a better conceptualization of Jennifer's circumstances and to develop treatment goals in collaboration with Jennifer that better met her needs. This kind of unstructured information gathering is an invaluable part of the therapist's usual assessment strategy, and as in this case, it routinely augments the information gathered with structured assessments.

────────

[1] The case of Jennifer was provided by Lisa Castle, Director of Occupational Therapy, and Tunde Koncz, Occupational Therapist, both of the University of Illinois Medical Center at Chicago.

Selecting Structured Assessments

Chapters 15 to 18 present and discuss 20 structured assessments that have been developed for use with MOHO. These assessments are designed to provide therapists with the best possible means of gathering relevant, sound, and thorough information. *Table 12.1* lists these assessments and the MOHO concept on which they provide information. Each of these assessments reflect years of development and have been studied and refined to enhance their dependability and practical value. These assessments range from a few minutes to over an hour to complete. The amount of time and effort each assessment takes is generally proportional to the amount of information it gathers. Thus, in selecting which of these as-

TABLE 12.1 MOHO-Based Assessments, Concepts on Which They Provide Data, Methods They Use, Populations for Which They are Designed, and Where They Are Discussed in this Text

Assessment (Chapter)	Occupational Adaptation		Volition			Habituation		Skills			Performance	Participation	Environment		Method of Data Gathering			Population			
	Identity	Competence	Personal Causation	Values	Interests	Roles	Habits	Motor	Process	Communication/ Interaction	Performance	Participation	Physical	Social	Observation	Self-report	Interview	Children	Adolescents	Adults	Elderly
Assessment of Communication and Interaction Skills (15)										X					X			X	X	X	X
Assessment of Motor and Process Skills (15)								X	X						X			X	X	X	X
Assessment of Occupational Functioning (18)			X	X	X	X	X	X	X	X							X		X	X	X
Child Occupational Self Assessment (16)		X	X	X	X	X	X	X	X	X		X				X		X	X		
Interest Checklist (16)					X											X					
Model of Human Occupation Screening Tool (18)			X	X	X	X	X	X	X	X	X	X	X	X	X		X		X	X	X
NIH Activity Record (16)			X	X	X	X	X				X	X	X			X			X	X	X
Occupational Circumstances Assessment- Interview and Rating Scale (17)			X	X	X	X	X				X	X	X	X			X			X	X
Occupational Performance History Interview-II (17)	X	X	X	X	X	X	X				X	X	X	X			X		X	X	X
Occupational Questionnaire (16)			X	X	X	X	X					X				X			X	X	X

Assessment																						
Occupational Self Assessment (16)	X	X	X	X	X	X	X	X	X	X	X	X	X	X	X	X				X	X	X
Occupational Therapy Psychosocial Assessment of Learning (18)		X	X	X	X	X	X	X	X	X	X	X	X	X	X		X			X	X	
Pediatric Interest Profile (16)	X	X		X	X				X				X		X			X		X		
Pediatric Volitional Questionnaire (15)		X	X	X						X	X	X		X			X			X		
Role Checklist (16)		X	X		X								X		X				X	X	X	X
School Setting Interview (17)							X	X	X	X	X		X	X	X	X	X	X	X	X		
Short Child Occupational Profile (18)		X	X	X	X	X	X	X	X	X	X	X	X	X	X		X	X	X	X	X	
Volitional Questionnaire (15)		X	X	X	X	X								X	X			X	X	X	X	X
Worker Role Interview (17)		X	X	X						X	X	X	X			X		X		X	X	
Work Environment Impact Scale (17)										X	X	X	X	X	X	X	X	X		X		

sessments to use for a given client, therapists will need to carefully think about the kind and depth of information needed and the time available for assessment.

Table 12.1 also indicates the age groups with which the assessments are used. More specific information on the age-appropriateness of each assessment will ordinarily be covered in the manuals or texts that accompany the assessments. In the end, appropriate use of the assessments in terms of age depends on a therapist's judgment. For example, the appropriateness of some assessments that require abstract thought and self reflection will depend less on chronologic age than on intellectual development and personal maturity of the client. Therapists should always be vigilant to consider a client's developmental readiness and ability to participate in any assessment process.

Another important consideration is the client's capability to participate in the assessment. MOHO-based assessments range from those that require clients to ac-

tively participate in self-assessment to those that require minimal or no action on the part of the client. In a number of instances, the administration of assessments can be altered to accommodate the client's limitations. For example, a client whose motor abilities impair speech could respond to an interview using augmented communication, or a client with motor limitations that prevent writing can respond to self-reports verbally. Most manuals for MOHO-based assessments provide guidelines for whether and how the administration can be accommodated and still maintain psychometric properties of the assessment. If the client's limitations are of the kind that such an accommodation of the assessment cannot be made, there are often still alternatives. For instance, therapists have often found it useful to ask family members to respond to assessments on behalf of the client.

Table 12.2 indicates the minimal type of effort and time required of the therapists and the requirements

TABLE 12.2 Therapist and Client Requirements for MOHO Assessment Administration

Assessment	Therapists' Requirements for Administration	Client Requirements to Participate	Estimated Total Therapists Time[a]
Assessment of Communication and Interaction Skills	Observe client in a goal–oriented activity that involves social interaction, complete scale[b]	Engage in some social interaction	20–60 minutes
Assessment of Motor and Process Skills	Observe client in a goal–oriented activity that involves social interaction, complete motor and process scales	Perform an occupational form (simple to complex)	30–60 minutes
Assessment of Occupational Functioning	Administer interview or explain self-report format to client	Answer interview questions (interview format) Read and write (self-report format)	20–30 minutes as interview 12 minutes as self-report
Child Occupational Self-Assessment	Introduce assessment, give directions, provide support to complete self-report, review ratings with client	Concentrate, read, write	35–45 minutes
Interest Checklist	Explain instructions, discuss client responses	Read and write	15–30 minutes
Model of Human Occupational Screening Tool	Collect information via chart review, interview, observation, from surrogates, and complete scale[c]	Minimally interact with the environment	10–40 minutes
NIH Activity Record	Explain instructions, discuss client responses	Concentrate, read, write	15–30 minutes

TABLE 12.2 Therapist and Client Requirements for MOHO Assessment Administration *continued*

Assessment	Therapists' Requirements for Administration	Client Requirements to Participate	Estimated Total Therapists Time[a]
Occupational Circumstances Assessment—Interview and Rating Scale	Conduct semi-structured interview, and complete scale	Answer questions	25–50 minutes
Occupational Performance History Interview—II	Conduct a semi-structured interview; complete three scales and complete life history narrative slope	Answer questions	45 minutes–1 hour
Occupational Questionnaire	Explain instructions, discuss client responses	Concentrate, read, write	15–30 minutes
Occupational Self Assessment	Explain instructions and discuss client responses	Concentrate, read, write	15–35 minutes
Occupational Therapy Psychosocial Assessment of Learning	Observe student; interview student, parents, teacher; complete scale	Participate in school, and answer questions	45 minutes–1 hour
Pediatric Interest Profiles	Explain instructions, provide support to complete self-report as needed, discuss client responses	Look at pictures or read, use a crayon or write (depending on which profile is used)	15–30 minutes
Pediatric Volitional Questionnaire	Observe client across 1or 2 settings; complete scale	Minimally interact with environment	15–30 minutes each observation 5–10 minutes for rating scale
Role Checklist	Explain instructions, discuss client responses	Concentrate, read, write	10–15 minutes
Short Child Occupational Profile	Collect information via chart review, interview, observation, from surrogates; and complete scale	Minimally interact with environment	10–40 minutes
School Setting Interview	Interview student	Answer questions	40 minutes–1 hour
Volitional Questionnaire	Observe client across 1 or 2 settings: complete scale	Minimally interact with environment	15–30 minutes each observation 5–10 minutes for rating scale
Worker Role Interview	Conduct semi-structured interview, complete scale[c]	Answer questions	30 minutes–1 hour
Work Environment Impact Scale	Conduct semi-structured interview and complete scale	Answer questions	30 minutes–1 hour

[a]Does not include time for clients to complete self-administered assessments.
[b]Completing MOHO instrument scales ordinarily involves using a 4-point rating scale and entering clarifying/qualifying comments.
[c]There are interview formats available that allow the MOHOST or WRI to be combined with the OCAIRS, saving administration time.

for client participation of the MOHO-based structured assessments. In thinking about which structured assessments to choose, this table can be a helpful guide.

Ensuring Client-Centered Assessment

Client-centered practice requires that therapists chose the form of assessment that maximizes client involvement to the extent possible. Where direct involvement of the client in the assessment is not possible, then therapists should make every effort to construct an understanding of the client's perspective. Clients who are least able to self-describe and self-advocate deserve the most careful assessment of their volition. There are ways to gain insight into the volition of lower-functioning clients. The Volitional Questionnaire (VQ) and the Pediatric Volitional Questionnaire (PVQ) (Chapter 15), and the Model of Human Occupation Screening Tool (MOHOST) and the Short Child Occupational Profile (Chapter 18) work well with such clients. Additionally, therapists can make good use of unstructured means of assessment for such clients.

Enhancing the Efficiency of Assessment Administration

Whatever structured or unstructured assessment(s) therapists choose, there are a number of additional strategies can make assessment more efficient. Some assessments are designed so that they can be administered simultaneously. For example, some of the interviews can be combined into a single interview. Similarly, a therapist doing an observation can complete more than one assessment based on a single observation. Another strategy to achieve more efficiency is to complete an assessment while engaging in therapy. Also, one can accomplish therapeutic aims during assessment. The following are examples of overlapping assessment and therapy:

- An interview can be done while making a splint or helping a client practice a skill
- Observation of volition or skill can be done during a therapy session in which the client is performing
- Self-administered assessments can be incorporated into group interventions aimed at helping clients solve problems or set goals related to their occupational adaptation.

The following are examples of how therapists accomplish therapeutic aims during assessment:

- During an interview, the therapist builds rapport with a client
- As part of assessment, the therapist provides feedback to a client or shares information about the client's situation
- Engaging in an assessment helps a client clarify values
- Participating in an assessment process gives a client a more realistic view of personal capacity
- The occasion of completing an assessment and discussing results can be used to collaborate on treatment goals and strategies.

In the best therapy, assessment and intervention are interwoven. The therapist's use of both structured assessments and informal methods of information gathering can be readily woven into the process of therapy. Therapists who are creative in how they integrate assessment and intervention make time for more comprehensive assessment.

Incorporating Assessments Other Than Those Based on MOHO

Therapists often use MOHO in combination with other practice models or with theories borrowed from other disciplines or professions. When this is the case, assessments that correspond to those models and theories may be used. Occupational therapists also use assessments other than those based on MOHO because they are part of an interdisciplinary approach or because administrative or regulatory bodies require their use. A third reason for using assessments with different origins is that no MOHO-based assessments available for a given client group or situation or that the chosen assessment provides critical information not provided by existing MOHO-based assessments (e.g., detailed examination of activities of daily living).

For a variety of reasons, then, therapists basing practice on MOHO will use assessments other than those presented in Chapters 15 to 18. When this is the case, it is important to consider why one is using the assessment, what kinds of information it provides, and how it can best be used in relation to the model and the MOHO-based assessments that are being used.

The Role of Diagnosis in Choosing Assessments

None of the MOHO-based assessments are designed for use with clients from a specific diagnostic group. MOHO focuses on understanding the impact of a disease or impairment on the person's occupational life, not on the disease or impairment itself. Therefore, most of the assessments will work with clients who have a wide range of diagnoses. This is not to say that the therapist should ignore the diagnosis or impairment in selecting assessments. Two important considerations in selecting assessments that do emanate from the client's diagnosis or impairments are:

- Whether the diagnosis or nature of the impairment has implications that are better addressed by certain assessments
- Whether the impairment limits the client's ability to do what is necessary to participate in the assessment.

Some MOHO-based assessments are particularly relevant to a given population. For example, the NIH Activity Record (ACTRE) (Chapter 16) gathers information on pain and fatigue. Therefore, for clients who are likely to experience pain and fatigue that impacts occupational performance, the ACTRE would be the better choice.

When a diagnosis is known to routinely produce certain kinds of occupational consequences, it may warrant use of particular assessments. For example, chronic, severe depression typically results in severe volitional problems. For this reason, the Volitional Questionnaire (Chapter 15) is frequently an assessment of choice for these types of clients. Also, traumatic injuries or catastrophic illnesses that significantly alter a person's life (e.g., persons with spinal cord injury or AIDS) often produce changes in interests and participation in interests, changes in roles, and changes in occupational identity and occupational competence. For this reason, such clients are good candidates for use of the Modified Interest Checklist (Chapter 16), the Role Checklist (Chapter 16), and the Occupational Performance History Interview (Chapter 17), since all three assessments provide information on changes that occur as the result of diseases or impairments that change a person's life.

Knowing what implications for assessment emanate from a client's diagnosis or impairment, requires that the therapist must have two kinds of information. First, the therapist needs some knowledge of how the diagnosis or impairment is likely to impact the client occupationally. Second, the therapist must know the content and organization of the MOHO-based assessments. When these two factors are known, the therapist can make intelligent matches.

Cultural Considerations in Using MOHO-Based Assessments

Most MOHO-based assessments were developed in collaboration with persons representing multiple cultures and languages. Research indicates that many MOHO-based assessments do not reflect cultural biases. For example, studies of the Assessment of Motor and Process Skills (AMPS) (Fisher, 1999) indicate that it is free of cultural bias (Fisher, Liu, Velozo, & Pan, 1992; Goto, Fisher, & Mayberry, 1996). Studies of these assessments are valid cross-culturally and when administered in different languages according to the work cited with them:

- Worker Role Interview (WRI) (Haglund, Karlsson, Kielhofner, & Lai, 1997)
- Worker Environment Impact Scale (WEIS) (Kielhofner, Lai, Olson, Haglund, Ekbladh, & Hedlund, 1999)
- Occupational Performance History Interview—II (OPHI-II) (Kielhofner, Mallinson, Forsyth, & Lai, 2001)
- Assessment of Communication and Interaction Skills (ACIS) (Kjellberg, Haglund, Forsyth. & Kielhofner, 2003)
- Occupational Self-Assessment (OSA) (Kielhofner & Forsyth, 2001).

Ensuring that assessments are relevant and valid with persons from diverse cultural backgrounds requires ongoing development and research. Such work is being undertaken across the MOHO-based assessments. Nonetheless, therapists should always be vigilant to consider whether an assessment is valid for clients based on their cultural background.

A further point should be made about MOHO-based assessments in relation to culture. Because the theory of this model incorporates culture into its concepts (e.g., volition and social environment), many of the assessments are specifically designed to capture a client's unique cultural perspective. For example, the OPHI-II elicits and considers culturally influenced values, interests, roles, and occupational narratives. For this reason, such assessments are particularly useful when therapists desire to gather information about the client's culturally influenced thoughts, feelings, and actions.

Using MOHO-Based Assessments To Demonstrate Client Change And Therapy Outcomes

A number of MOHO-based assessments can be used to document change in clients and to evaluate the impact or outcomes of therapy. *Table 12.3* lists the assessments that provide data relevant to evaluating client change and demonstrating impact. It also indicates the type of change that the assessment would capture. Which assessment one chooses for capturing change or demonstrating program outcomes depends on what changes services are designed to achieve. Outcome measures should be targeted to the aspects of clients that the services aim to achieve.

How to Choose Assessments

Choosing which assessments to use routinely is one of the most important decisions therapists make about their practice. The following steps are helpful in making an informed decision:

● Become familiar with all potentially relevant MOHO assessments and identify those that appear most suitable for use
● Pilot these assessments in practice to evaluate their utility

TABLE 12.3 MOHO Assessments Suitable for Indicating Client Change and Program Outcomes

Assessment (Chapter)	Type of Change Captured by Assessment
Assessment of Communication and Interaction Skills (15)	Change in skill
Assessment of Motor and Process Skills (15)	Change in skill
Child Occupational Self-Assessment (16)	Change in values and competence
Model of Human Occupational Screening Tool (18)	Change in how volition, habituation, skill, and environment support participation
NIH Activity Record (16)	Change in participation and fatigue, pain, perceived competence, interest, value in what one routinely does
Occupational Questionnaire (16)	Change in participation; in competence, interest, value in what one routinely does
Occupational Case Analysis Interview and Rating Scale (17)	Change in how volition, habituation, skill, environment, and goal setting support participation
Occupational Self-Assessment (16)	Change in values, competence, environmental impact
Occupational Therapy Psychosocial Assessment of Learning (18)	Change in student's adaptation to student role and its demands
Pediatric Interest Profiles (16)	Change in children's and adolescents' interests, perceived competence, participation
Pediatric Volitional Questionnaire (15)	Change in children's volition (motivation to do things)
Role Checklist (16)	Change in roles and value assigned to roles
Short Child Occupational Profile (18)	Change in how children's volition, habituation, skill, environment support participation
School Setting Interview (17)	Change in student-environment fit to support participation
Volitional Questionnaire (15)	Change in volition (motivation to do things)
Worker Role Interview (17)	Change in psychosocial readiness for work

• Develop an assessment strategy that allows flexibility to meet individual client needs.

Identifying and Examining Potentially Relevant Assessments

This first step involves simply becoming familiar with the range of assessments developed for use with MOHO. *Table 12.1* provides an overview of the assessments, and *Table 12.2* indicates the time, effort, and client participation required for each assessment. These tables help to identify assessments that are potentially most suitable to one's population and context. Another resource for identifying potentially relevant assessments is *Figure 12.1*. The figure categorizes MOHO-based assessments according to whether they are general (providing data on many MOHO concepts and designed for use across practice settings) or specific (focused on one or a few concepts and/or designed for specific practice settings).

When there is time only for a single evaluation or for doing an initial evaluation, it is recommended that therapists select an assessment from the first row that will provide more comprehensive information (i.e., cover most or all of the MOHO concepts). If one's clients tend to have specific weaknesses or challenges, you may choose an assessment that focuses on that specific area (see middle of *Fig. 12.1*). Such assessments are often completed after an initial more comprehensive assessment but may be used alone if appropriate to the focus of the intervention. If working in a specialized setting, such as a school or a work rehabilitation program, consider the assessments listed at the bottom of *Figure 12.1*. These assessments may be used either alone or in combination with comprehensive assessments.

Once one has selected potentially relevant assessments, the next step is to become familiar with them. Chapters 15 to 18 provide descriptions and case examples for each assessment. Examining copies of the assessments and reading articles that discuss the assessment's development and/or use in practice are also recommended. Finally, since one should be aware of the evidence behind assessments, tables in Chapter 27 provide a summary of the evidence associated with each assessment at the time of completing this text. Additional information may be obtained at the MOHO

Clearinghouse website (www.moho.uic.edu). An evidence-based search engine at the website provides access to comprehensive bibliographies for each assessment. The site also provides access to listserve discussions about practitioners' experiences with the assessments.

Piloting Assessments in Practice to Evaluate Their Utility

With the exception of the AMPS (Chapter 15), therapists can learn to administer MOHO-based assessments from manuals developed for each assessment or from available guidelines. (Information on purchasing manuals and accessing guidelines can be found at www.moho.uic.edu.) After accessing the relevant information for administration, one should try out an assessment. This allows one to determine how an assessment works in one's context. Piloting a few potentially relevant assessments provides an opportunity to test out which assessments best meet one's working style and are best suited to one's clients.

Developing an Assessment Strategy

A single MOHO-based assessment may meet all one's needs. However, most therapists find it helpful to create an information-gathering strategy with optional assessments and a means to decide which to use for specific clients. For example, an occupational therapist working in a psychiatric rehabilitation setting uses the assessment strategy shown in *Figure 12.2*. Because most of the clients coming into the setting are initially functioning at too low a level for an interview, the therapist has chosen the Model of Human Occupation Screening Tool (MOHOST) (Chapter 18) as the overall assessment to be used with all clients. If a client does initially have the ability to engage in an interview, the therapist uses the Occupational Circumstances Assessment—Interview and Rating Scale (OCAIRS) (Chapter 17) as the primary interview. This interview may be done on only a small number of clients as an initial assessment. It may be done later with some clients when they progress to the point of being able to participate. Other clients who progress and identify the goal of returning to work or achieving employment may be interviewed with the Worker Role Interview (WRI) (Chapter 17) or the Worker Environment Impact

FIGURE 12.1 A decision tree for selecting MOHO assessments.

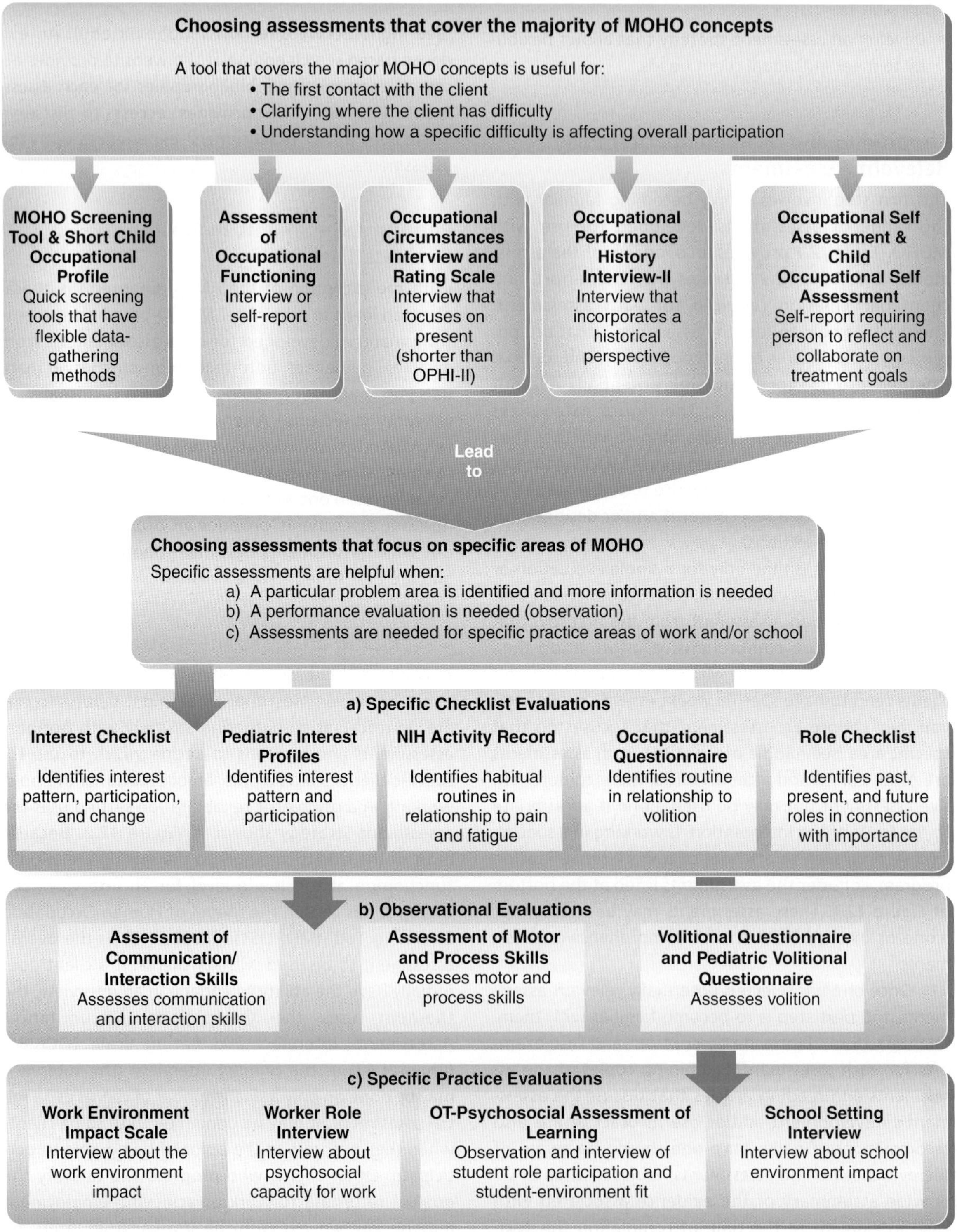

Choosing assessments that cover the majority of MOHO concepts

A tool that covers the major MOHO concepts is useful for:
- The first contact with the client
- Clarifying where the client has difficulty
- Understanding how a specific difficulty is affecting overall participation

MOHO Screening Tool & Short Child Occupational Profile
Quick screening tools that have flexible data-gathering methods

Assessment of Occupational Functioning
Interview or self-report

Occupational Circumstances Interview and Rating Scale
Interview that focuses on present (shorter than OPHI-II)

Occupational Performance History Interview-II
Interview that incorporates a historical perspective

Occupational Self Assessment & Child Occupational Self Assessment
Self-report requiring person to reflect and collaborate on treatment goals

Lead to

Choosing assessments that focus on specific areas of MOHO

Specific assessments are helpful when:
- a) A particular problem area is identified and more information is needed
- b) A performance evaluation is needed (observation)
- c) Assessments are needed for specific practice areas of work and/or school

a) Specific Checklist Evaluations

Interest Checklist
Identifies interest pattern, participation, and change

Pediatric Interest Profiles
Identifies interest pattern and participation

NIH Activity Record
Identifies habitual routines in relationship to pain and fatigue

Occupational Questionnaire
Identifies routine in relationship to volition

Role Checklist
Identifies past, present, and future roles in connection with importance

b) Observational Evaluations

Assessment of Communication/ Interaction Skills
Assesses communication and interaction skills

Assessment of Motor and Process Skills
Assesses motor and process skills

Volitional Questionnaire and Pediatric Volitional Questionnaire
Assesses volition

c) Specific Practice Evaluations

Work Environment Impact Scale
Interview about the work environment impact

Worker Role Interview
Interview about psychosocial capacity for work

OT-Psychosocial Assessment of Learning
Observation and interview of student role participation and student-environment fit

School Setting Interview
Interview about school environment impact

FIGURE 12.2 Example of an assessment strategy for a psychiatric rehabilitation setting.

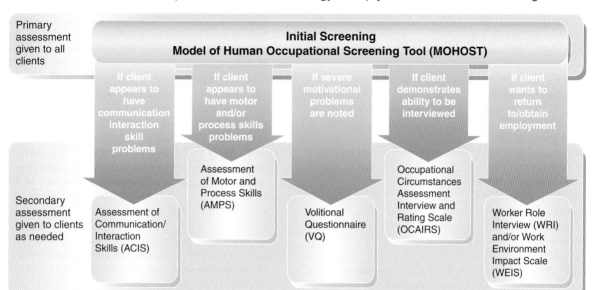

Scale (WEIS) (Chapter 17). Since the latter is designed to interview clients concerning a specific job setting or type of job setting, ordinarily only clients with previous employment are candidates for this assessment.

The assessment strategy shown in *Figure 12.2* also indicates that when the MOHOST identifies problems in skills, the Assessment of Motor and Process Skills (AMPS) or the Assessment of Communication and Interaction Skills (ACIS) (Chapter 15) may be done. Finally, when clients show more extreme problems in motivation, the Volitional Questionnaire (VQ) (Chapter 15) may be used. Since these are observational assessments, they can be used with clients who are at a lower level of functioning than is required for the interviews.

A strategy of assessment, such as the one just described, allows for many different configurations of assessments according to clients' needs and characteristics. One client may be assessed only through repeated applications of the MOHOST to monitor progress and identify intervention needs. Another client, who showed clear problems in communication and interaction, may be assessed with the ACIS following the MO-HOST. Repeated use of the ACIS may be used to monitor the client's response to social skills training and need for further intervention or support. Still another client who shows some cognitive impairment that af-

fects occupational performance but wants to live in the community may be assessed (following the MOHOST) with the OCAIRS and the AMPS to gather critical information for intervention and discharge planning.

As this example illustrates, having a strategy of assessment allows the therapist to be:

- Efficient, avoiding assessments that are unnecessary or unsuitable
- Client-centered, by choosing assessments that reflect client needs and characteristics
- Comprehensive, by getting information that is necessary to understand the client's specific occupational problems and challenges to design the best intervention.

Developing an assessment strategy takes some time and experimentation, but it is the surest means of doing optimal assessment for clients.

References

Denzin, N.K., & Lincoln, Y.S. (Eds.) (1994). *Handbook of Qualitative Research.* Thousand Oaks, CA: Sage.

Fisher, A. G. (1999). *Assessment of Motor and Process Skills,* 3rd Ed. Ft. Collins, CO: Three Star.

Fisher, A. G., Liu, Y., Velozo, C. A., & Pan, A. W. (1992). Cross-cultural assessment of process skills. *American Journal of Occupational Therapy, 46,* 876–885.

Goto, S., Fisher, A. G., & Mayberry, W. L. (1996). The assessment of motor and process skills applied cross-culturally to the Japanese. *American Journal of Occupational Therapy, 50,* 798–806.

Haglund, L., Karlsson, G., Kielhofner, G., & Lai, J. S. (1997). Validity of the Swedish version of the Worker Role Interview. *Scandinavian Journal of Occupational Therapy, 4,* 23–29.

Hagner, D.C., & Helm, D.T. (1994).Qualitative methods in rehabilitation research. *Rehabilitation Counseling Bulletin, 37,* 290–303.

Hammersly, M. (1992). Some reflections on ethnography and validity. *Internal Journal of Qualitative Studies in Education, 5,* 195-203.

Kjellberg,A., Haglund, L., Forsyth. K., & Kielhofner, G. (2003). The measurement properties of the Swedish version of the Assessment of Communication and Interaction Skills. *Scandinavian Journal of Caring Sciences, 17(3),* 271–277.

Kielhofner, G., & Forsyth, K. (2001). Development of a client self-report for treatment planning and documenting therapy outcomes. *Scandinavian Journal of Occupational Therapy, 8 (3),* 131–139.

Kielhofner, G., Lai, J. S., Olson, L., Haglund, L., Ekbadh, E., & Hedlund, M. (1999). Psychometric properties of the work environment impact scale: A cross-cultural study. *Work, 12,* 71–78.

Kielhofner, G., Mallinson, T., Forsyth, K., & Lai, J. S. (2001). Psychometric properties of the second version of the occupational performance history interview (OPHI-II). *American Journal of Occupational Therapy, 55,* 260–267.

Krefting, L. (1989). Disability ethnography: A methodological approach for occupational therapy research. *Canadian Journal of Occupational Therapy, 56,* 61–66.

Miles, M.B., & Huberman, A.M. (Eds.) (1994). Qualitative data analysis. Thousand Oaks, CA: Sage.

Tham, K., Borell L., Gustavsson A. (2000). The discovery of disability: A phenomenological study of unilateral neglect. *American Journal of Occupational Therapy, 54,* 98-106.

Trombly, C. (1993). The issue is—anticipating the future: Assessment of occupational functioning. *American Journal of Occupational Therapy, 47,* 253–257.

Wolcott, H. F. (1990). On Seeking and Rejecting Validity in Qualitative Research. In E.W. Eisner & A. Peshkin (Eds.), *Qualitative Inquiry in Education: The Continuing Debate* (pp. 121–152). New York: Teachers College.

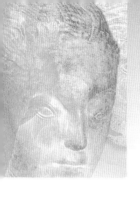

13

Occupational Engagement: How Clients Achieve Change

- Gary Kielhofner

- Kirsty Forsyth

The purpose of this chapter is to examine how clients achieve change in therapy. Volition, habituation, and performance capacity are fashioned, maintained, and altered by what people do and how they think and feel about their doing. Moreover, the environmental conditions in which people engage in occupation are also key determinants of whether and how change takes place.

The premise of this chapter, then, is that all change in occupational therapy is driven by clients' occupational engagement.

The term **occupational engagement**[1] refers to clients' doing, thinking, and feeling under certain environmental conditions in the midst of or as a planned consequence of therapy.

... all change in occupational therapy is driven by clients' occupational engagement.

Key Dimensions of Occupational Engagement

When clients engage in occupational forms/tasks in therapy or as a result of therapy, volitional, habituation, and performance capacity are all involved in some way. For example, in any moment of therapy a client may do any of the following:

- Draw on performance capacity to exercise skill in occupational performance
- Evoke old habits that shape how the occupational performance is done
- Enact or work toward a role
- Feel a level of satisfaction/enjoyment (or dissatisfaction/displeasure) with occupational performance
- Assign meaning and significance to what is done (i.e., what this means for the client's life)
- Feel able (or unable) in doing the occupational form/task.

Each of these aspects of what the client does, thinks, and feels shapes the change process. For this reason, therapists should always be mindful of their clients' volition, habituation, and performance capacity as well as environmental conditions in the midst of therapy and how these elements are interacting as the therapy unfolds. Therapeutic reasoning involves carefully monitoring the client's process of occupational engagement.

---

[1]The term *engagement* is used in the American Occupational Therapy Association Practice Framework to connote not only client doing, but also to imply choice, motivation, and meaning (American Occupational Therapy Association, 2002). Consistent with the argument made here, the framework also views engagement as a key element of therapy. The Occupational Therapy Practice Framework also identifies the use of enabling activities and adjunctive methods as legitimate components of therapy. Enabling activities are designed to improve specific performance capacities and skills and can include contrived activities designed to exercise capacity. Adjunctive methods prepare the client for performance by affecting performance capacity; they include such things as exercise, physical modalities, and splinting. The rationale for enabling activities and adjunctive methods is provided by other models of practice. Their rationale derives from concepts other than those proposed by MOHO, which focuses specifically on the role of occupational engagement to facilitate change.

One way in which therapists can be especially attentive to the dynamics of occupational engagement is to consider the major efforts clients make during occupational engagement that can be important contributors to change. In the following sections we consider nine important dimensions of occupational engagement that contribute to change. These include when clients:

- Choose or make decisions
- Commit
- Explore
- Identify
- Negotiate
- Plan
- Practice
- Reexamine
- Sustain.

In the sections that follow, we will define, examine, and provide examples of these important dimensions of occupational engagement.

Choose/Decide

Client choices and decisions are central to effective therapy. As discussed in Chapter 2, activity choices shape what we do in the immediate future. Such choices and decisions are often the first step toward change. Such things as selecting what to do, how to do it, and what to aim for are also central to therapy as they represent the client's volitional involvement in the therapy process. Persons **choose** or **decide** when they anticipate and select from alternatives for action. A wide range of choices and decisions may take place in the therapy context. The following are examples:

- A child in therapy chooses to play with a new toy that previously seemed too challenging.
- A client decides to focus on a particular short-term goal in therapy.
- A client selects a particular piece of adaptive equipment for activities of daily living.
- A client chooses to engage in a valued occupational form despite some anxiety and fear of failure.
- A client chooses to indulge a particular interest by selecting what to do in a leisure group.

> *Therapeutic reasoning involves carefully monitoring the client's process of occupational engagement.*

- After being shown alternative ways of performing, a client decides on a particular technique.
- A client chooses whether to have a personal care attendant for self-care to have more energy and time to devote to work.

By making such choices and decisions, clients can shape the nature of their own therapy and what that therapy aims to accomplish. The very process of making choices can help clients feel more in control of their lives. Often, when the client has limited performance capacity, making choices and decisions is one of the most empowering things the client can do. Finally, choices and decisions are critical, since they influence what will change, what will remain the same, and how the change will unfold.

Commit

For long-term change to occur in therapy, clients must **commit** themselves to undertake a course of action for accomplishing a goal or personal project, fulfilling a role, or establishing a new habit. As discussed in Chapter 2, occupational choice always involves commitment because it requires one to sustain action over time. Committing to a course of action is also an act of hope, since the client's intention is to achieve some goal, occupy a place in the social world, or modify his or her lifestyle in anticipation of improving life. Some examples of committing in therapy are:

- After a period in a supported living facility, a client concludes that it is time to work toward living independently in an apartment and commits to that goal.
- A client in a rehabilitation program who has been out of work for years following onset of chronic disability resolves to work again.
- After examining their daily routines, a group of clients agree together to develop long-range plans for achieving more productive lifestyles. They all agree to set weekly goals and report their goal accomplishment to each other.

As the examples indicate, commitment ordinarily follows a process of information gathering and reflection, so that clients have an idea of the obligations they are assuming. The process of commitment is closely tied to development of occupational identity and competence, since it involves decisions about how the occupational narrative will be continued or changed.

𝒰wabunkonye: Committing to a New Worker Role[2]

. . . .

Uwabunkonye, a 63-year-old Nigerian man, sustained an ischemic stroke in 2003 but made an excellent recovery. He now has only a stiff gait and minimal difficulty with fine motor control of the left hand. He has been on medical disability for 2 years, since his stroke. Uwabunkonye was a high school teacher prior to his stroke but could not go back to that job, as left-sided weakness and dizziness meant he could not stand or look up to write on the chalk board.

He is the primary caregiver to his wife, who has Alzheimer's, and takes an active role in the lives of his four children, two of whom still live at home. Uwabunkonye did not want to relinquish his role as a 'worker.' With assistance from his occupational therapist he was able to *reexamine* his abilities, which have changed as a result of his stroke. Together, they evaluated his process skills, motor skills, ability to work in certain environments, his motivation for a different occupation, and his physical capacity. The outcome of the evaluation helped Uwabunkonye *identify* "Medical Transcriptionist" as the most suitable vocational choice. It would allow him to continue working but also maintain his involvement with his family and his interests. He *committed* himself to this goal, *sustained* his on-line studies, and successfully obtained a certification on line. He is looking for a permanent job as a Medical Transcriptionist.

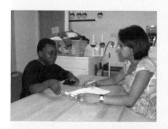

Uwabunkonye works with the occupational therapists to reexamine his work capacity and identify a new vocation.

[2]*The case of Uwabunkonye was provided by Supriya Sen, MS, OTR/L, Occupational Therapist, University of Illinois Medical Center of Chicago and Adjunct Faculty Member, Department of Occupational Therapy, University of Illinois at Chicago.*

Explore

As discussed in Chapter 10, the first stage of change is exploration. **Exploration** includes investigating new objects, spaces, and/or social groups and occupational forms; doing things with altered performance capacity; trying out new ways of doing things; and examining possibilities for occupational participation in one's context. The following are some examples of exploration:

- A client with hemiplegia explores different techniques for putting on clothes.
- A client with a recently acquired cognitive disability tries to do a familiar occupational form/task, exploring how altered capacities impact performance.
- A client recently discharged from an institutional setting to a group home walks in the neighborhood to see what is in it and joins a leisure activity in the evening to see what the other residents are like.
- A child tries out a new communication device to see how it works.
- An older person, who gave up a hobby because of fading vision, tries using larger materials and tools to see if doing it is still enjoyable with the modifications.
- An adolescent in a work program tries out different occupational forms/tasks to see what kind of productive activity is most satisfying to do.

Exploring options, feelings, and experiences is central to making informed decisions in therapy. Successful exploration is especially important with individuals who have a newly acquired disability.

Identify

Identifying refers to locating novel information, alternatives for action, new attitudes, and new feelings that provide solutions for and/or give meaning to occupational performance and participation. Locating this information can result from such processes as discussion with therapists, self-reflection, examining alternatives, or hearing feedback. Some examples of identifying are:

- After hearing feedback on performance and discussing it with the therapist, a client identifies that the interpersonal difficulties he experiences are related to skill problems in the physical domain.
- During the Occupational Performance History Interview a client identifies with therapist feedback

that the occupational narrative underlying her life story is a tragedy, something she would like to change.

- A client who is anxious identifies the specific occupational forms/tasks and performance contexts that cause the most anxiety.
- Following a therapy session, a client reflects and identifies that her fear of failure gets in the way of her finishing things.

As the examples indicate, identification involves insight into something of which the client previously lacked awareness. Such insight supports change because it gives the person critical information to know what to do or to guide decisions.

Eva: Reconstructing Occupational Identity by Identifying New Occupations[3]

At age 27, Eva found herself in a psychiatric center in Spain. She was married to a professional man of considerable wealth and had become accustomed to a life among those in high society. During an interview with an occupational therapist, Eva was asked about her values. She summed up her view of the world in the following words: "What you have is all that you are." Eva's materialistic values had contributed to a shopping addiction. To cover her mounting debts and keep her husband from knowing about her addiction, she stole money from the bank where she worked.

Shocked to learn about her theft, her husband agreed to give her another chance. However, she soon returned to her compulsive shopping and ran up new debts. When he realized what was happening, her husband decided to seek a divorce. After the divorce, Eva had no resources and returned to living with her parents, who had to mortgage their house to pay Eva's debts.

At this point Eva was referred again to an occupational therapist. With feedback from her therapist Eva *identified* that her only way of feeling good about herself was to buy clothes, jewelry, cosmetics, massages, and beauty treatments. The therapist helped Eva to *explore* other ways she could feel good about herself and

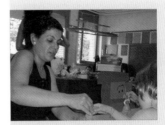

*Eva helps a child complete a craft project as part of her **commitment** to her new volunteer role.*

to enjoy doing things other than shopping. Since she now had no financial resources, Eva *identified* that she had to learn to control her compulsive conduct while also giving up occupations she had previously enjoyed such as sailing, eating in expensive restaurants, and skiing. She had lost all of her roles. Eva was faced with reconstructing her occupational identity.

Eventually Eva decided to return to her unfinished university studies in labor relations because she had determined that it was important for her to have a degree. Because of financial constraints, she had to work and study at the same time. Eva also decided to volunteer every weekend in a social center for children to give something back to society, another discovered value. She **committed** herself to both roles. Her responsibilities include **planning** and carrying out activities for children every weekend. Eva finds a great deal of meaning in working with children. She is very conscious of educating them in values of friendship and equality values instead of focusing on material things. She has developed new friends among the volunteers with whom she shares the free time. Lisa credits her successful reconstruction of her occupational identify to her experiences in occupational therapy.

[3]*The case of Eva was provided by Laura Vidaña Moya, Occupational Therapist, Barcelonian Association of Compulsive Gambling and Addictions, Barcelona, Spain.*

Negotiate

When possible, the client should be involved in a process of negotiation throughout therapy. The onset of disability often results in new situations and experiences that create a gap between disabled persons' and others' perspectives, desires, and expectations. Moreover, the client will sometimes differ with the opinion of the therapist concerning the nature of impairments and their consequences. **Negotiation** involves give-and-take with others that creates mutually agreed-upon perspectives and/or finds a middle ground between different expectations, plans, or desires. The following are examples:

- A client's therapist recommends that the client use a certain piece of bathing equipment. The client prefers not to depend on the equipment and agrees to try alternative methods of bathing first.
- On advice from the therapist, a client negotiates with the supervisor at work for accommodations that could enhance work performance.
- After attending an energy conservation program, a client negotiates with family members for ways household chores can be fairly redistributed in the family.
- Clients in a leisure-planning group have differing ideas about what to do on the next outing. They agree to plan for two outings so that both ideas can be accommodated.

Negotiation can be difficult for clients, given the power differential that often exists between health care providers and clients. By giving clients clear messages that they can negotiate, the therapist creates a more collaborative context. By creating a vision of therapy goals and procedures, negotiation can positively affect a client's willingness to cooperate in therapy. Moreover, negotiation with others in one's environment is critical to filling roles effectively and otherwise participating in the social context.

Plan

Because impairments can impose new conditions that invalidate habitual ways of doing things, it is often critical for clients to think through how they will go about doing something before they attempt it. Moreover, persons who are attempting a new performance or a new pattern of participating in occupations are more likely to be successful if they have created an agenda for doing so. **Planning** refers to establishing an action agenda for performance and/or participation. The following are examples:

- A client who wants to start exercising regularly by swimming finds out where the nearest swimming pool is, calls and ascertains the hours it is open, and locates a bus route for getting there.

- Clients in a work program are getting ready to go on job interviews. With the guidance of the therapist they consider what to do if the interviewer asks about gaps in their employment history and whether and how to disclose the nature of their disabilities.
- Clients in a cooking group plan the content of the meal, make up a grocery list, decide where to go for the groceries, and anticipate how much money they will need to make the purchase.

By focusing on the steps required for doing something, planning helps to ensure success. Also, because planning makes the process of accomplishing something concrete, it can allay a client's anxiety about performance.

*A*hmad: **Planning New Family Roles and Routines**[4]

. . . .

Ahmad is a 22-year-old Arab Jordanian university student. He lives with his four siblings in suburban Amma. Ahmad's mother died when he was 17. His father passed away 4 months ago.

Ahmad was always socially active with classmates and many friends. Moreover, he was a serious student who studied long hours. After his father's death, Ahmad had to take over managing family affairs while his older sister managed domestic duties. Ahmad also faced the prospect that his older sister, who was to marry in 2 months, would leave him with all family and domestic responsibilities.

Ahmad met with an occupational therapist, complaining of inability to function both at home and at university. He had lost interest in things that he used to enjoy. He often felt hopeless or anxious, worrying about a range of imagined future troubles. He had problems concentrating and making decisions. Ahmad also complained of insomnia, severe headaches, and dizziness, which were not responding to medical treatment. These symptoms started when Ahmad's father was hospitalized and became more serious after his death.

He was deeply conflicted about the responsibilities of being a guardian for his younger siblings. He was overwhelmed with his responsibilities for managing the household finances, his younger siblings' needs and activities, and the household tasks he would inherit once his older sister left. Despite these difficult emotions, Ahmad tried to hide his worries from his siblings.

First, the occupational therapist validated Ahmad's experiences and helped him to see how his physical symptoms were a reaction to the overwhelming nature of the responsibilities he had inherited due to his family circumstance. With the help of this therapist, Ahmad examined how his personal values were leading him to take on the worries and tasks associated with his and his siblings' situation. With guidance, he was able to **reexamine** his situation and **identify** a new strategy for managing his family's needs. Ahmad **decided** that he would ask his siblings to take on some new roles and patterns. Consistent with cultural expectations that he would be in charge as the oldest male sibling, Ahmad would take on a role as family supervisor. However, completion of necessary tasks for managing the household would be distributed among all members of the family.

Ahmad related to the therapist he didn't know how to approach sharing this new plan with his siblings. After **exploring** options he **identified** the following strategy. He arranged that one of his father's friends whom his siblings greatly respected would gather the family, propose this new arrangement, and introduce Ahmad's new position at home. When asked, the family friend readily agreed to do this, which gave Ahmad a renewed sense of confidence and relief. After the family friend met with the siblings, they all agreed to the **plan** and started **prac-**

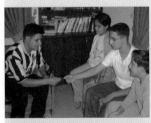

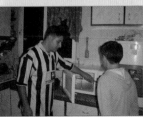

Ahmad and his siblings plan and practice the division of family tasks, including money management and cooking.

ticing their new responsibilities and daily life patterns.

Freed from his heavy burden, Ahmad began to **explore** how he could reschedule his daily life, allowing time and energy for his interests as well as his university studies, while at the same time managing his new family responsibilities. For instance, he started to go for a walk early in the morning as a way to relax himself. He **committed** himself to focus on what he valued most: helping and supporting. There were still challenges, since his new family role and responsibilities still restricted him from doing many things he would otherwise choose to do. Nonetheless, he was able to accept the reality of his present situation and find the best way achieve a sense of meaning and control in his life.

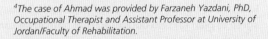

[4]The case of Ahmad was provided by Farzaneh Yazdani, PhD, Occupational Therapist and Assistant Professor at University of Jordan/Faculty of Rehabilitation.

Practice

Clients **practice** in therapy when they repeat a certain performance or consistently participate in an occupation with the effect of increasing skill, ease, and effectiveness of performance. Practice aims to enhance effectiveness on doing an occupational form and/or participating in an area of occupation, such as self-care, work, school, or leisure. The following are some examples of practicing:

- A client participates in a daily leisure group, doing a variety of social occupational forms, and in the course uses and refines communication/interaction skills while building a sense of efficacy in being able to interact with others.
- A student with problems in process skills practices doing his school tasks using a set of visual cues that help develop habits for better organizing and sequencing actions to meet the expectations of the student role. In the course of this process, the client also identifies more strongly with the student role and more clearly internalizes its expectations.
- A client in a vocational program role-plays a job interview twice before actually going on the interview to internalize the attitudes and behaviors that are appropriate to someone applying for a job.

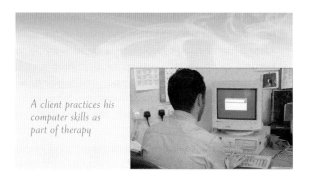

A client practices his computer skills as part of therapy

mands and current capacity and begins to think about what other types of work might be possible.

Letting go of thoughts, habits, responsibilities, and ways of doing things is not always easy, but unless the client is able to recognize the problems associated with them and also see alternatives, change cannot occur.

- A client does her daily routine of hygiene using adaptive equipment, learning how to handle and adjust the equipment and forming a habit of going through the self-care routine and developing a sense of efficacy in doing it.
- A child plays several times a day with an adapted toy, developing a sense of how it feels to do the action and experience a sense of pleasure in being able to manage it effectively.

The key element in practice is that a client has the opportunity to repeat something to consolidate the volition, habituation, performance capacity, and environmental factors shaping an effective and satisfying way to perform and/or participate.

Reexamine

Therapy is often a time when clients must leave behind perceptions, feelings, beliefs, and patterns of acting that are no longer valid or that have led to difficulties. **Reexamination**, then, involves critically appraising and considering alternatives to previous beliefs, attitudes, feelings, habits, or roles. The following are examples:

- A client whose habits have contributed to dissatisfaction with everyday life considers alternative ways of organizing the daily routine to include more enjoyable things.
- A client whose sense of capacity has always underestimated strengths reflects with the therapist on successes achieved in therapy and what they say about the client's abilities.
- A client who has had the goal of returning to a particular job considers the gap between the job de-

*B*en: **Sustaining Participation in New Occupations[5]**

Ben is in his late 20s. He is a pleasant, mild-mannered man who for 5 years has experienced paranoid symptoms leading to multiple admissions to an acute hospital. His family has a strong history of schizophrenia, and various family members have committed suicide in the past, including his grandfather, an uncle, and his older sister.

He has lived all his life in a small rural community and is the youngest of three brothers. He lives with his elderly mother, having found it too difficult to live independently. He has also found it too difficult to find work in the open job market, although he once worked regularly for one of his brothers in the building trade.

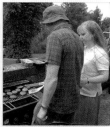

Ben chooses barbecuing and gardening as activities to explore in therapy, and he commits to sustain engagement in those activities.

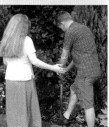

Ben now has very little contact with any of his three brothers; he explains this by saying, "I suppose we've just grown apart." He has also lost contact with all of his friends. Meanwhile, his mother continues to support him and to visit him regularly when he is in hospital. She appears to be very understanding.

Ben is struggling to find a meaningful routine within the community and feel this would be supportive of his mental health. He states that he feels useless and a failure, and he feels "down" because he feels bored. Although he tries to engage in occupations, he often fails and can't complete the activities. Ben has **committed** to working with the community mental health occupational therapist. He has **identified** a range of potential interests to explore with the therapists. He has **decided** to engage in these activities and is motivated to **sustain** effort to complete the activities with the therapists' support. He **negotiated** aspects of the activities he felt he needed therapist support with. He **reexamined** his performance on completion of the activity with the therapists and **committed** to continue **practice** these activities.

[5]The case of Ben was provided by the second author of this chapter.

Sustain

One of the challenging aspects of therapy is sustaining effort over time despite such things as difficult barriers, pain, failures, and slow progress. By its nature, therapy can be taxing for clients. However, as noted earlier in this chapter, change requires repeated action over time. **Sustain** refers, then, to persisting in occupational performance or participation despite uncertainty or difficulty. The following are examples:

- Despite feeling anxious, a client completes all of the steps required of an occupational form/task. This reinforces for her that, despite her doubts, she did have adequate capacity.
- A child whose distractibility makes focusing difficult manages to stay focused throughout a classroom exercise. Afterward, he has a sense of accomplishment.
- A client who has returned to work after an accident goes to work each day despite experiencing mild pain and concerns over re-injury. With the thera-

pist's reassurance that there is no serious risk, in time the client feels less pain and more secure.
- After a long period of isolation, a client is trying to become more socially active. After joining a club that meets weekly, the client persists in going, although feeling socially inadequate and tempted to stay home. Each time, however, the client enjoys it and feels more confidence.

As the examples indicate, persistence takes effort but has its rewards in feelings of accomplishment, new learning, and development of a sense of efficacy.

Considering Client Occupational Engagement in Therapeutic Reasoning

The first part of the chapter identifies nine key processes that characterize client occupational engagement and that contribute to change. These do not exhaust the possibilities for what clients do to achieve change; however, they provide a starting point for thinking about how clients achieve change. As such they help therapists plan for how therapy goals will be achieved. That is, they provide a framework for thinking about what clients will do to achieve change in the direction specified by a given therapy goal. The Therapeutic Reasoning Table (at the end of Section 2) provides examples of these types of occupational engagement that correspond to types of client change (see the fifth column of this table). The table shows what kinds of occupational engagement may contribute to different types of change.

Yolanda: How Occupational Engagement Facilitated Change for a Child

Yolanda is 4 years old and lives with her mother, father, and 6-year-old brother in a small town. She has severe cerebral palsy resulting from anoxia at birth. She has fluctuations in tone (i.e., she is very "floppy" much of the time but also has a marked extensor thrust). She has limited head control and disconjugate eye movements. She cannot talk and has other oral motor problems. Yolanda can make her preferences clear, and she is generally cheerful and interested in things going on around her. For example, Yolanda is passionate about computer games and single-switch toys.

Despite her communication impairments, Yolanda very much values interacting with other children. Her mother notes that it is important to her to wear clothes and have her hair done like other children, and Yolanda very much wants to do things that she sees other children do. Recently, her mother has observed that Yolanda becomes upset and irritable when her brother goes out to play in the street with other children. Yolanda spends most of the day in an adapted chair or buggy, both of which are difficult to get out of the house. Therefore, she cannot readily go out and join the other children. Instead, she watches the children play in the street from the front windows of the house. Yolanda's sense of inefficacy in achieving something about which she cares deeply is clear in the frustration she shows while watching the other children. Consequently, the therapist and Yolanda's mother together decided it was essential to enable Yolanda to play with other children. As a first step the therapist recommended that a ramp be installed at the front door of the home.

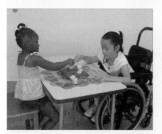

By playing a board game with a friend, Yolanda *practices* doing activities from her wheelchair. (Photo courtesy of Erin Boodey, Occupational Therapist, University of Illinois Medical Center at Chicago.)

Yolanda is unable to propel a chair herself and would benefit from a powered chair. However, Yolanda has been quite fearful of being in a powered chair. The therapist previously gave Yolanda opportunities to try out such chairs. When she did so, Yolanda had difficulty controlling her body and the chair. She clearly felt out of control in the chair and was too anxious to be able to learn to use it. Yolanda instead used a buggy, in which

she felt safe but had to be propelled by others.

Now that Yolanda wanted to play with other children, the buggy posed a constraint because it did not allow her to play. Therefore, the therapist tried out a number of seats and wheelchairs with Yolanda, finally settling on one with small wheels that had to be pushed by another child or attendant and from which Yolanda could safely play in the street.

To use the new chair Yolanda had to **practice** doing things in it. Consequently, she improved her head control and concentration and increased her sense of efficacy to the point at which she could use the chair without fear. The neighborhood children welcomed Yolanda and willingly propelled her chair along as they engaged in play. Soon she was routinely part of the group of children, was confident in joining them, had developed a friend role, and was learning to communicate with them in simple ways. Bolstered by a growing success in joining and interacting with friends at play, Yolanda became ready to try out in occupational therapy a variety of self-powered go-carts. After some **exploration** she found one with which she was comfortable and selected it. She became very motivated to master navigation with the chair. After a period of practice she developed the necessary motor and process skills for effective maneuvering of the chair. When Yolanda went to school a year later, she was using her own motorized chair.

As the case illustrates and *Figure 13.1* shows, the changes in Yolanda over time represent a complex resonating process driven by her occupational engagement. Certainly Yolanda went from being afraid and unable to use a powered chair to feeling efficacious and being skilled at using one, but the process of change underlying it involved interacting changes in her volition, habituation, performance capacity, and environment. She simultaneously increased confidence for interacting with children, assumed the player role, and developed new communication and interaction skills for socializing with the children in play.

Therapy influenced the process at key points, as shown by the dark arrows in *Figure 13.1*. Other environmental factors, such as the children's acceptance of and willingness to play with Yolanda, are also important. Yolanda's own thoughts, feelings, and actions were cen-

FIGURE 13.1 How occupational engagement facilitated the process of Yolanda's change.

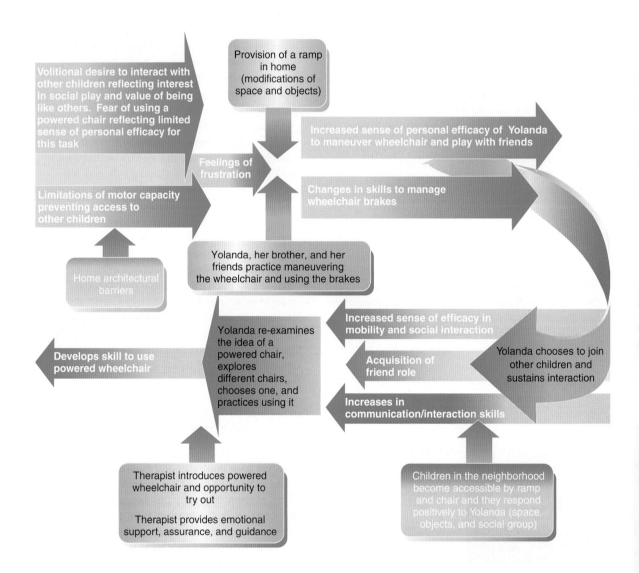

tral to her change. Her efforts to **practice** doing things from her new chair led to an increased sense of efficacy and changes in her performance capacity. Her **choice** to interact with the children was necessary to the change. By **sustaining** social play with the children, she developed new skill and confidence. Finally, she **reexamined** whether she wanted a powered chair, explored different chairs and selected one, and then practiced with the selected chair. Therapy could only remove constraints and provide opportunities and resources that enabled Yolanda to undertake the change process herself through her own occupational engagement.

Nancy: How Occupational Engagement Facilitated Change for an Older Adult [6]

. . . .

Nancy is 78 years old. She lives alone in a sheltered house where she has lived for 5 years, since her husband died. She lives in a small town where she has lived all her married life. Nancy has a son and daughter who live locally and visit daily. Nancy was admitted to hospital following a fall outside while shopping at her local grocery store. She sustained a fractured right clavicle as a result of her fall. She was transferred from acute hospital to a rehabilitation ward for therapy. On admission into the ward, pain restricted Nancy's use of her right arm. She was wearing a collar and cuff, a short-term provision for 2 weeks.

Nancy is an active lady who identifies strongly with her homemaker role. She prides herself on being independent and self-sufficient, looking after herself and her home. She feels it is highly important to retain her previous level of independence and values independence equally with her family and her home. Nancy's homemaker responsibilities structure her daily routine in conjunction with self-care routines and pursuit of leisure activities. Nancy reports a strong network of friends and family and visits friends and meets them in a local café on a regular basis. She also regularly speaks with family and friends on the telephone.

Nancy feels a loss of confidence since her fall, and she is unsure of her sense of efficacy with daily tasks. She reports being anxious about attempting to engage in daily tasks due to fear of falling, as well as a loss in motor skill and stamina with daily tasks since her hospital admission. Nancy would like to return back to being active, independent, and confident with daily tasks as she was previously. She particularly highlights her lack of control with regard to her self-care routine and how this is deeply troubling her. It was clear that Nancy had particular values regarding her self-care routine. Before her fall, she liked to have a shower every morning and always wore a skirt and makeup irrespective of her daily plans. Nancy shared that this is a longstanding and important routine that she identifies with.

Nancy felt she had lost control over her morning self-care routine, as the norm on the ward was for patients to wash from a basin at the bedside and wear a nightdress during the day. Therefore, she felt she lacked daily structure. Additional to this change in routine, Nancy required assistance to attend to self-care activities because of her reduced motor skills and confidence. As a result Nancy felt she had lost her sense of control, privacy, and routine with morning self-care tasks that she reported previously "set her up for the day."

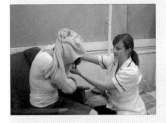

Nancy practices an alternative dressing technique to regain independence in self-care.

Nancy said that she wished to have a shower within the ward; however, she was anxious about standing on a wet floor because of her reduced motor skills and her fear of falling. Options were explored with Nancy as to how to gradually facilitate independence with showering within the ward environment. It was decided that a shower chair would be suitable to support a shower with the occupational therapist's assistance.

Nancy **negotiated** with her daughter to bring in day clothes to provide Nancy with a "sense of normality." The therapist also successfully negotiated with ward staff for Nancy to get dressed in day clothes on a daily basis. Because of her restricted right arm function, alternative dressing techniques were **explored** and tried with Nancy to support independent dressing. She selected particular techniques and reported these to be helpful in her achieving independence. Nancy reported she always used to stand to get dressed, but because of her reduced confidence and fear of falling, she identified that sitting would be a preferable option to allow her to complete tasks independently.

Nancy **committed** to engaging in practicing self-care tasks on a daily basis and received positive feedback and physical assistance from the occupational therapist. Gradually, Nancy improved her stamina and sense of efficacy with showering and dressing. Nancy **negotiated** to withdraw the shower chair and engaged in showering while standing with supervision of the occupational therapist. She then progressed to independent use of the shower within the ward. Nancy **practiced** alternative techniques to dressing, and reported confidence in completing dressing in a seated position using the alternative dressing techniques that she incorporated into her new morning self-care routine within the ward. Nancy reported satisfaction with morning self-care routine after a period of rehabilitation. Nancy was able to **identify** regained confidence and a sense of efficacy with tasks of self-care and dressing. She reported she "felt like her old self," and her family also reinforced how well she looked.

---

[6]The case of Nancy was provided by Emma Dobson, Senior Occupational Therapist at SWITCH Partnership, Lanarkshire, UK.

Nancy engaged in reestablishing independence with a valued occupation (her morning routine), and this involved a process of interacting changes involving her physical capacity, volition, and habituation within the context of the physical and social environment.

Nancy played a pivotal role in facilitating her process of change to achieve occupational engagement

(*Fig. 13.2*). Her ability to **decide** and **identify** her occupational goal through her value structure led Nancy to be able to actively engage in **negotiating** and **committing** to rehabilitation and to develop a meaningful **plan** despite her own anxieties and confidence issues following her fall. Nancy's **commitment** to **practicing** on a daily basis and being receptive to **exploring** and using alternative techniques and equipment within the ward to achieve goals led to her ability to regain independence with self-care tasks. This independence was **sustained** through positive feedback from occupational therapy staff and also, more importantly, by Nancy **reexamining** her progress and **identifying** improvement and change. This resulted in Nancy experiencing feelings of success about her situation and regain confidence and physical skill. Ultimately, Nancy was able to achieve independence with her morning self-care routine.

Nancy sustained her regained independence in self-care and developed growing confidence to engage in other valued routine activities that she identified as significant and meaningful to support her to return home. After **negotiating** with the therapist to identify strategies to achieve a successful discharge home and reintegration into the community, Nancy was discharged home after a period of rehabilitation.

Conclusion

This chapter examines the process of change in therapy, focusing on two key points. First, change involves complex reorganization in which multiple simultaneous alterations in volition, habituation, performance capacity, and environmental conditions resonate with each other. Second, the process of change is always driven by the client's occupational engagement. The true dynamic of change is what the client does, thinks, and feels. This chapter offers nine key aspects of occupational engagement that represent important contributors to change. Any therapist who seeks to facilitate a client's change process will do well to pay attention to the unfolding dynamics of change and to the client occupational engagement that fuels that change process.

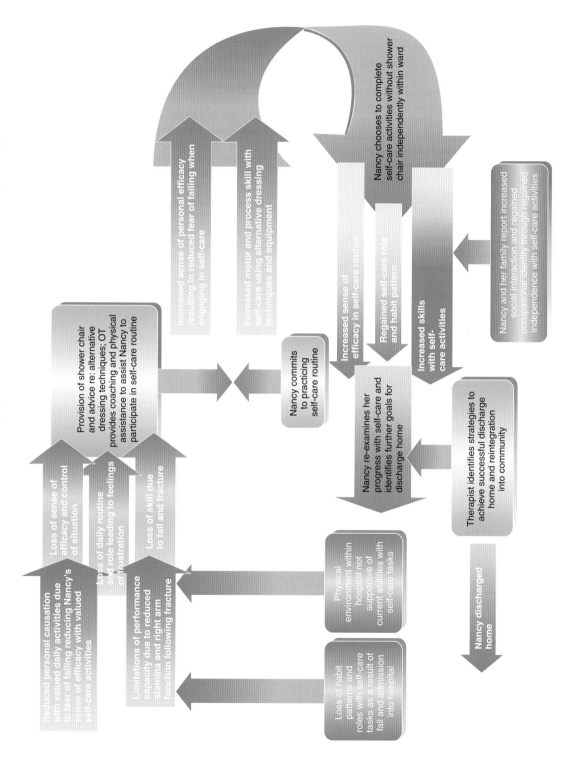

FIGURE 13.2 How occupational engagement facilitated the process of Nancy's change.

Reduced personal causation with valued daily activities due to fear of falling reducing Nancy's sense of efficacy with valued self-care activities

Loss of sense of efficacy and control of situation

Loss of daily routine and role leading to feelings of frustration

Loss of skill due to fall and fracture

Limitations of performance capacity due to reduced stamina and right arm function following fracture

Loss of habit patterns and roles with self-care tasks as a result of fall and admission into hospital

Physical environment within hospital not supportive of current abilities with self-care tasks

Provision of shower chair and advice re: alternative dressing techniques; OT provides coaching and physical assistance to assist Nancy to participate in self-care routine

Nancy commits to practicing self-care routine

Nancy re-examines her progress with self-care and identifies further goals for discharge home

Therapist identifies strategies to achieve successful discharge home and reintegration into community

Nancy discharged home

Increased sense of personal efficacy resulting in reduced fear of falling when engaging in self-care

Increased motor and process skill with self-care using alternative dressing techniques and equipment

Increased sense of efficacy in self-care routine

Regained self-care role and habit pattern

Increased skills with self-care activities

Nancy chooses to complete self-care activities without shower chair independently within ward

Nancy and her family report increased social interaction and regained occupational identity through regained independence with self-care activities

183

Key Terms

Choose/decide: To anticipate and select from alternatives for action (e.g., choose an occupational form or select goals).

Commit: To obligate one's self to a course of action for accomplishing a goal or a personal project or fulfilling a role or establishing a new routine.

Explore: To investigate new objects, spaces, and/or social groups and occupational forms; do things with altered performance capacity; try out new ways of doing things; and examine possibilities for occupational participation in one's context.

Identify: To locate novel information, alternatives for action, and new attitudes and feelings that provide solutions for and/or give meaning to occupational performance and participation.

Negotiate: To engage in give-and-take with others that creates mutually agreed perspectives and/or finds a middle ground between different expectations, plans, or desires.

Occupational engagement: clients' doing, thinking, and feeling under certain environmental conditions in the midst of or as a planned consequence of therapy.

Plan: To establish an action agenda for performance and/or participation.

Practice: To repeat a certain performance or consistently participate in an occupation with the effect of increasing skill, ease, and effectiveness of performance.

Reexamine: To critically appraise and consider alternatives to previous beliefs, attitudes, feelings, habits, or roles.

Sustain: To persist in occupational performance or participation despite uncertainty or difficulty.

Reference

American Occupational Therapy Association (2002). Occupational Therapy Framework: Domain and process. *American Journal of Occupational Therapy, 56,* 609–639.

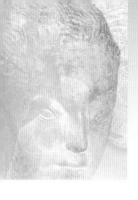

14

Therapeutic Strategies for Enabling Change

- Gary Kielhofner
- Kirsty Forsyth

Chapter 13 examined client change in therapy. It emphasizes the role of the client's occupational engagement in change. This chapter examines how occupational therapists can interact with clients to support their occupational engagement and facilitate desired change. It discusses specific therapeutic strategies derived from MOHO.

Therapeutic Use of Self and Therapeutic Strategies

The relationship between therapist and client is always an important determinant of the success or failure of occupational therapy (Hopkins & Tiffany, 1983; Peloquin, 1990). Therapeutic use of self mainly focuses on maintaining a good working relationship between the client and therapist and addresses various interpersonal issues that naturally arise in the context of this relationship. A new conceptual practice model, the *Intentional Relationship*, introduced by Taylor (in press) provides an excellent and detailed map of the theoretical and practical elements of maintaining a therapeutic relationship. Therapeutic strategies are those actions of the therapist that are directed specifically to supporting client occupational engagement as shown in *Figure 14.1*. In this chapter we discuss the therapeutic strategies that emanate from MOHO.

Nature of Therapeutic Strategies

A **therapeutic strategy** is a therapist's action that influences a client's doing, feeling, and/or thinking to fa-

cilitate desired change. Therapeutic strategies should always be based on a conceptualization of the client's circumstances as discussed in Chapter 11. Moreover, therapeutic strategies should be used reflectively, so that the therapist can adjust their use in the course of therapy to meet the client's needs. This chapter discusses the following therapeutic strategies:

- Validating
- Identifying
- Giving feedback
- Advising
- Negotiating
- Structuring
- Coaching
- Encouraging
- Providing physical support.

They are the kinds of strategies that therapists using MOHO undertake to support client occupational engagement.

Validating

To **validate** is to convey respect for the client's experience or perspective. Service providers often overlook or fail to take seriously the experience of people with disabilities (Toombs, 1992; Wendel, 1996). Therapists must carefully attend to and acknowledge the client's experience, whether it is the lived body experience, the experiences associated with volition (enjoyment, painful loss of capacity, anxiety), or experiences stemming from societal reaction to the disability. Negative experiences such as pain, anxiety, hallucinations, shame,

FIGURE 14.1 Therapeutic strategies support client occupational engagement.

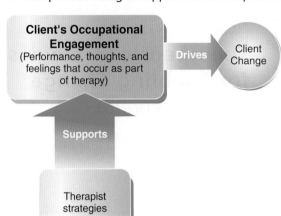

and/or anger may interfere with the client's occupational engagement.

Each moment of therapy is potentially charged with thoughts and feelings that accompany what a client does. Consequently, a client's experiences resonate outward to larger implications, intentions, worries, hopes, and disappointments. Validating these experiences is essential to effective therapy. Validation is also important for very low functioning clients with limited communication abilities. In these circumstances, validation may involve things as simple as acknowledging the presence and unique identity of a client. Such validation can serve to scaffold the volition of persons who lack sufficient internal volitional motives. Some examples of validation:

- A client diagnosed with schizophrenia is severely withdrawn. Each day the therapist visits the client briefly at the same two times. The therapist greets the person by name, reintroduces herself, and makes comments related to the client's past interests. After a week the client makes eye contact.
- A child becomes very flustered in therapy. The therapist offers the opportunity to take a break and acknowledges that therapy is sometimes hard work.
- A client with recent spinal cord injury is planning a first weekend home since being in rehabilitation. In the midst of the process the client becomes tearful and shares his fears about managing everything

and facing neighbors and old friends from a wheelchair. The therapist acknowledges that this is a challenging situation and that most clients are very anxious on their first trip home.

- A student who has been struggling to master use of a computer achieves something she has never done before. She lets out a shriek of pleasure. The therapist rushes over and gives her a round of applause and congratulations.
- A client begins participating in the Occupational Circumstances Assessment—Interview and Rating Scale (OCAIRS). As the client talks about her life, she stops suddenly and indicates that she does not feel able to go on answering questions. The therapist acknowledges that the client was talking about an extremely difficult topic and that her life experiences must have been very hard to bear. The therapist also points out how useful the information was and how grateful the therapist is for the client's honesty and willingness to share her experiences. She offers to continue the interview at a later point if the client prefers.

As the examples illustrate, therapists must first attend to clients' experiences before they can validate them. This means taking care to observe how the clients act and react in therapy, looking for signs of enjoyment, anxiety, boredom, investment, outrage, shame, excitement, and so forth. Finally, simply asking the client about and demonstrating an active interest in the client's thoughts and feelings are also important.

*N*ino: Using Validation to Elicit Participation in Therapy[1]

Nino is a 70-year-old Georgian woman who has struggled with cancer for decades. When referred to a palliative home care team, she was fatigued and in extreme pain from the metastasis. Her ability to perform was severely limited by her symptoms and the high dose of antidepressants and sedatives she was taking. Nino felt desperate and that she was "closing her eyes" on all of the important things she used to do. She lived with her husband, who had become her main caregiver, and her daughter, who had returned home to support her mother and help with housework.

For some time Nino vacillated between being a "fighting spirit" and in a state of helplessness and hopelessness. During the first session with the occupational therapist, her husband reported that Nino was refusing to eat or engage in conversation. Given the client's withdrawal, the therapist knew it would be important to build a strong alliance and find some way to rekindle some of Nino's fighting spirit.

The therapist began by ***encouraging*** Nino to retell her own life story, starting from early childhood. She used the Occupational Performance History Interview (discussed in Chapter 17) as a framework for interviewing Nino. Throughout the interview the therapist ***validated*** Nino's feelings. Bolstered by the encouragement, questions, and validation, Nino began to tell her story.

She lost her parents in early childhood and was brought up by an aunt, who allowed her to read books the whole day. Nino found a love of art and as a young woman visited operas, theaters, and art galleries. She also discovered a love of science, went on to earn a university degree in microbiology, and eventually headed a research laboratory. She married when she was 35 and soon became a mother. Shortly after the birth of her

child she was operated on for cancerous fibroma and fell into a depressive state due to hormonal changes. While struggling with her own illness, she lost her brother. Despite this and other difficult times, Nino felt that she had accomplished a great deal in her career and had been a good mother. She felt that she had now reached a low point in her life, not only because of her prognosis, but importantly because she was forced to "do nothing during the day."

During the interview, Nino also revealed a desire to attempt embroidering again, although she expressed fear that it might not be possible because of trembling in her hands. She also expressed a wish to be involved in kitchen activities to free up the family. She expressed her deepest desire as "I just want to do something myself."

The therapist observed Nino in her daily routine and ***gave her feedback*** that she was overtiring herself in the mornings when doing self-care independently. The therapist ***advised*** Nino that by practicing energy conservation and by ***structuring*** her day according to priorities she could achieve her goals. The therapist arranged therapy sessions in which Nino's family was also present so she could instruct them on how to support Nino. She ***coached*** Nino on visualization and relaxation techniques for pain management and on how to conserve her energy. Nino was able to engage in the activities she wanted and reported feeling alive and competent again. (Along with this, she was able to get by with less medication.) She started to routinely demonstrate to her family that she could still do "simple but dignified" things. Recently she made the decision to join family and friends in the country for what she knew would be a last summer holiday, one like so many she had enjoyed before.

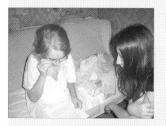

The therapist validates Nino's feelings as she shares her life story.

[1]*The case of Nino was provided by Maria Kapanadze, occupational therapy student, Georgian Occupational Therapists Association, Tbilisi, Georgia.*

Identifying

Therapists need to be able to **identify** for clients a range of personal procedures and/or environmental factors that can facilitate occupational performance and participation. For example:

- A therapist becomes aware that a client is very anxious and flustered about using public transportation. The therapist suggests a number of ways the client can manage the anxiety, including some ways she can ask for assistance if she is not sure what to do.
- A client with AIDS has been out of work for 3 years because of complications of the illness. He now wants to return to work but is worried about how he can manage the medications he must take several times a day. The therapist uses her understanding of his legal rights for workplace accommodation to suggest the kinds of possible reasonable accommodations that he can request.
- The therapist shares a range of strategies that a client with unilateral neglect can use to help notice things on the neglected side of her body.
- Through observation, the therapist comes to understand and notes occupational forms/tasks a person with a stroke is able to do with and without assistance.
- A client has stated that he wants to go to a day center. The therapist compiles a list of possible day centers for the client within a reasonable traveling distance.

In sum, the therapeutic strategy of identifying provides the client an understanding of the personal and environmental opportunities and resources. It can also provide the client information about options for enhancing occupational performance and participation in work, play/leisure, and activities of daily living that clients want and need to do.

Jane: Working with Clients to Identify New Possibilities[2]

. . . .

Jane is a 25-year-old Scottish woman who has Multiple Sclerosis and has been admitted to an inpatient unit because her physical decline was leading to an inability to

manage within the community. This is Jane's first stay in an inpatient unit. Jane works in a financial organization, and this environment demands very long working hours. Jane lives alone and is keen to be able to return to independent community living. Jane is also a caregiver to her 52-year-old mother, who has depression. Although Jane had a large group of friends when she went through university, she can't identify current friends or interests outside of her working life. She has no other family members and feels "very responsible" for the care of her mother, whose health has been declining in recent months.

During therapeutic encounters, the occupational therapist *validated* Jane's feelings about her reduced physical capacities and her worry about being able to return to independent community living. The therapist provided Jane with *feedback* on her current abilities and limitations through *encouraging* engagement in everyday occupations, such as making a hot drink. The therapist also *advised* Jane to review her previous occupational lifestyle within the context of reduced physical capacity. The therapist supported Jane by starting to *identify* alternative roles, habits, and values. They discussed the occupational issues together and *identified* a range of options that could be targeted for change. These included the consideration of alternative techniques to complete occupations that required less physical effort, reducing her hours of employment, *identifying* a range of additional supports that could help with the care of her mother, *identifying* a range of interests that she would find recreational, and building a new habit *structure* that would allow her to have time for her own relaxation. The therapist *negotiated* a plan of action with Jane to ensure they both had the same vision for how therapy would unfold.

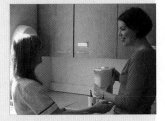

The therapist provides Jane with feedback and encouragement as she makes a hot drink.

Giving Feedback

Therapists gather information to arrive at a conceptualization of a client's situation. For example, therapists using MOHO draw conclusions about a client's performance capacity, habituation, volition, and environmental impact to understand how these factors influence a client's skill, performance, and participation. Therapists also draw on this conceptualization to form an understanding of ongoing action of the client. When therapists share their overall conceptualization of the client's situation or their understanding of the client's ongoing action, they are **giving feedback**. Some examples:

- A client has agreed to be observed with the Assessment of Motor and Process Skills. After completing the observations, the therapist shares the results of the assessment with the client and explains what it revealed.
- A therapist has observed a client informally during therapy. These observations confirm what the therapist learned in the initial interview—that the client holds impossibly high standards that result in constant self-devaluation. The therapist reminds the client of this conceptualization, since she previously shared it with the client. She now presents her observations of how the client has continued to devalue her own performance over the past two therapy sessions. The therapist also provides an alternative interpretation of the client's performance that emphasizes a number of strengths.
- In a cooking group a client refuses to collaborate with other clients. Afterward, the therapist asks to speak with the client and notes that while he has agreed that his uncooperative behavior gets him into trouble, he still does it.
- A client who has difficulty performing self-care states that she is afraid she will end up in a nursing home. The therapist indicates that while she still has difficulty, she has made significant progress, which bodes well for her return to independent self-care.
- An adolescent with mental retardation participates in an occupational form/task that he initially hesitated to do. After the session the therapist praises him for making a difficult choice and for completing the occupational form/task.

As the examples illustrate, giving feedback can serve a variety of purposes, such as these:

- Helping a client have a more accurate sense of capacity or understand a performance problem
- Letting a client know the value (positive or negative) of a behavior
- Reframing a client's interpretation of something
- Offering a different vision of the future than that held by the client.

Consequently, feedback can provide information that enhances skill and performance. Giving feedback that reframes something can address volition by influencing how clients interpret, experience, or anticipate the future.

Advising

Therapists **advise** clients when they recommend intervention goals and strategies. Thus, advising involves:

- Sharing what outcomes appear feasible and desirable
- Indicating possible options for achieving outcomes in therapy.

Advising should take place as part of a give-and-take process whereby the client and therapist mutually decide on therapy goals and strategies. However, because the therapist has collected information and used it in combination with MOHO concepts to create a conceptualization of the client's situation, the therapist is in a position to make recommendations for the client's consideration. These recommendations ordinarily contain information or insights beyond the client's thoughts and feelings. Therefore, sharing the advice with the client can serve to broaden or alter the client's perspective.

In the process of advising, a therapist may seek to persuade a client to make a particular informed choice or decision. For example, a therapist often provides the rationale for a given option with an eye to influencing the client to agree to select that option or to make a particular commitment. Therapists most often seek to persuade a client when the client hesitates, has difficulty making a choice in therapy, or has problems committing to a particular long-term goal, project, role, or change in lifestyle. For example, a therapist may advise a client on such basic things as which occupational form/task to undertake in a work setting, school, or day center and such complex things as whether it makes sense for a client to commit to a specific living option. Sometimes advice seeks to persuade a client against a particular choice or commitment. This occurs when the therapist's conceptualization of the client indicates that certain choices may produce undesirable consequences or that certain goals are not feasible.

To advise a client effectively, the therapist must seek to understand the client's volition. For example, the therapist may consider what volitional factors are influencing a client's difficulty in making a choice. Alternatively, the therapist may consider what factors contribute to a client's strong preference or commitment to a choice that is not adaptive (e.g., feelings of inefficacy, not seeing the value of doing something). By doing so, the therapist can give honest advice with empathy for the client's perspective and desires.

Whereas advice and the persuasion that often goes with it can be a useful therapeutic strategy, therapists must be careful to advise without coercing the client. Persuasion occurs when the client, in response to information and suggestions, changes his or her own mind freely. Coercion occurs when the client gives in against his or her will. Coercion should never be a part of advising a client.

Some further examples of advising:

- A therapist recommends to a client who is nearing discharge from physical rehabilitation that he should complete a home visit to ascertain environmental changes needed to support performance after discharge.
- A therapist advises a client with a mild cognitive problem about which occupational forms/tasks may pose safety risks. The therapist further recommends that the client practice them in therapy to develop safe habits.
- A therapist advises a client with brain injury that learning to drive is not feasible given the client's visual and perceptual deficits. The therapist also suggests that the client explore use of public transportation to support the client's goal of working.
- A student is having difficulty beginning schoolwork. The therapist advises the student as to which steps to take first and how to approach the schoolwork.

Advising clients is important to client-centered practice because it allows the client to make informed

decisions. It is important that the therapist take the time to explain to the client the rationale behind the advice, so the client can truly make informed decisions.

Emma: Negotiating Client Goals for Occupational Therapy[3]

Emma attends *Steps to Independence*, a home-based course developed by occupational therapists at South Birmingham Primary Care Trust in England. The course is targeted specifically for people with a learning disability. As part of her initial evaluation in this program, Emma was assessed with the Model of Human Occupational Screening Tool (see Chapter 18), the Occupational Self Assessment (OSA) (see Chapter 16) and the Assessment of Motor and Process skills (see Chapter 15). Among other things, the results of these assessments identified that Emma's occupational participation would be enhanced by developing skills in the areas of problem solving, goal setting, and planning. Based on her evaluation of Emma, the occupational therapist also concluded that Emma would greatly benefit from a self-directed learning process and by generating better insight into her capacities, especially her individual learning style.

The occupational therapist **advised** Emma of her thoughts about areas for personal growth that the assessment process suggested. Moreover, as part of the process of discussing Emma's responses on the OSA, the therapist **negotiated** with Emma which goals would be a priority for her. They agreed to identify one goal to work on at a time and then problem-solve the best way to approach the goal.

Emma used a goal-planning software tool, Step Planner. The therapist **coached** Emma in how to use Step Planner on a laptop computer to design a goal in a step-by-step approach to ensure that it was well planned and achievable. Emma took responsibility for completing each step to reach her goal while her therapists **provided feedback** and **encouraged** her. On completion of the course, Emma earned a certificate of achievement that acknowledged her success and accented the feedback her therapists had provided on Emma's growth. Emma continues to use Step Planner to set goals to make changes she wants in her life.

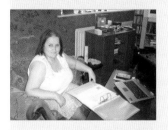

The coaching and feedback Emma receives allows her to continue to use the Step Planner to develop goals.

[3]The case of Emma was provided by Laura White, Dip COT, Advanced Occupational Therapist, South Birmingham Primary Care Trust, Sutton Coldfield, West Midlands, United Kingdom.

Negotiating

Therapists **negotiate** when they engage in give-and-take with the client to achieve a common perspective or agreement about something that the client will or should do in the future. Negotiation occurs when the client and therapist have differing information or viewpoints about some aspect of the client's occupational circumstances. Negotiation may be necessary to resolve disagreement between the therapist and client. Other times the therapist and client are simply comparing and reconciling their different perspectives.

Negotiation implies that the therapist must be careful to be aware of and elicit client views. Without such efforts the client's viewpoint can be obliterated by institutional routines or by the plans of service providers, including the therapist. Thus, negotiation begins with a respectful elicitation of a client's thoughts and feelings throughout the therapy process. Some examples of negotiation:

- A client states uncertainty over whether occupational therapy can do anything for him. The therapist presents a number of changes he could achieve and how they would be achieved in therapy. The therapist then asks for the client's perspective on this information and whether he thinks the changes seem valuable to him. After deliberation they agree on therapy goals that incorporate both the client's ideas and some of what the therapist envisioned.
- A therapist notes that a client is unwilling to work toward a level of independence in self-care that is easily within his reach. The therapist discusses this with the client, asking for the client's perspective. As a result, the therapist comes to understand that the client has different, culturally specific criteria for judging the situation. He views it as a matter of honor that his family take care of him. After learning his perspective, the therapist acknowledges it but points out how it can create difficulties for him and his family. While the client is not able to accept the therapist's viewpoint, he does agree that they can continue to discuss the topic as part of his therapy.
- A student informs the therapist that he plans to drop out of high school because he is so frustrated. The therapist talks with the student to ascertain his sources of frustration. She then offers to convene the school team to talk with the student about what things can be changed. The student agrees to attend the meeting to see if things can be improved enough to persuade him to stay.

As the examples indicate, negotiation always requires respect for and understanding of the client. It often means that the therapist must be willing to compromise, to see things differently, or to depart from usual procedures.

The give-and-take of negotiation can be very important to empower clients. Successful negotiation requires the therapist to understand what the client is being asked to concede and to make sure to offer incentives that are worth it to the client. Furthermore, therapists must model the same openness and flexibility of thinking and acting that they are asking of clients.

Structuring

Therapists must often structure clients' occupational engagement. **Structuring** refers to establishing parameters for choice and performance by offering clients alternatives, setting limits, and establishing ground rules. Structuring can often serve to create reasonable demands for clients to make choices, perform, maintain habits, and fulfill roles. Some examples:

- Stating the importance of mutual respect and collaboration in a goal setting group.

- Offering a child the choice between two toys in a therapy session.
- Letting a client know that if he has too much pain or fatigue during a session of practicing dressing, he can take a break.
- Communicating to clients during a goal-setting exercise that members of the group are expected to set goals, follow through on what they committed to do, and report back to the group.
- Informing a client in a work program that she is expected to arrive on time and stay focused on work responsibilities.
- Organizing a personal care session with a client who has a hip replacement to introduce and practice with a long-handled shoehorn, stocking aid, and elastic laces. Due to the client's lack of mobility, the therapist places the needed objects within the client's reach.

Structuring can give a client a sense of control and safely make opportunities and constraints in the environment clear. Structuring can be used to convey expectations and is useful for helping clients to internalize role scripts and to learn to be effective members of groups. Moreover, external expectations can be a support to volition (Jonsson, Josephsson, & Kielhofner, 2000). That is, persons can find it easier to be motivated to do things when others expect them to do so.

*M*arco: Structuring a Motivating Environment[4]

Marco was a 4-year-old boy with cortical blindness and floppy muscle tone. When he began occupational therapy, his parents' biggest concern was that he was not able to engage in play with peers and his younger brother.

During evaluation, the therapist observed that he could not raise his head for more than 30 seconds while lying prone. However, he appeared interested in his environment and would stop moving to listen to surrounding noises, would gaze at light toys, and attempted to reach and roll toward his parents and brother.

The therapist *identified* for Marco's parents that Marco could achieve his goals of interacting with the environment and improve his motor skills by increasing his trunk strength, muscle tone, and head control. She then *negotiated* with Marco's parents to set occupational therapy goals centered on Marco sustaining upright posture while engaged in play activity. She *structured* his intervention sessions to include the toys and games that Marco most enjoyed. Within that motivating environment, she used neurodevelopment techniques and provided *physical assistance* so Marco could practice moving his body and building strength. Marco's parents were also *coached* and *advised* on techniques and strategies they could use at home to support Marco's skill development.

Within 6 months Marco showed improvement and could sit up and play with other preschoolers and his little brother for almost 45 minutes with physical support. Marco's parents reported that Marco often had increased vocalizations that indicated excitement in the car on the way to therapy, an indicator that he was enjoying his new ability to interact with friends and toys.

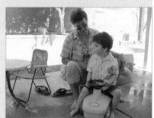

The therapist provides physical support in an environment structured to support Marco's volition.

[4]The case of Marco was provided by Susan Roberts, Occupational Therapist, Changes Occupational Therapy, New York.

Coaching

Therapy involves clients in such things as exploring new ways to perform or practicing performance to increase skills. Therapists **coach** when they instruct, demonstrate, guide, verbally prompt, and/or physically prompt clients. Some examples of coaching:

- During a role-playing exercise designed to help a client with a psychiatric condition learn and exhibit effective communication/interaction skills, the therapist demonstrates assertive behavior and then guides a client through how to assert himself in a simulated interaction.

- While a client with head injury is trying a new occupational form/task, a therapist helps her problem-solve by cueing her to notice what is happening.
- Serving as a job coach for a client with cognitive impairments in a supported employment program, a therapist demonstrates to the client how to greet fellow workers.
- A therapist guides a child with perceptual-motor difficulties as she engages in gross motor play. The therapist demonstrates how to do something, reminding the child to pay attention to bodily experience. Once the client begins, the therapist prompts her on how to move.
- Working with an adolescent whose performance anxiety often gets in the way of enjoyment, the therapist redirects his attention to aspects of the performance that may be enjoyable or satisfying.

As the examples illustrate, coaching is often directed to enabling clients to develop performance capacity and enhance skill. However, coaching also influences a client's volition, in that during a performance it can redirect the client's attention to aspects of the performance to affirm satisfaction and enjoyment. Coaching may also take place in the context of role performance and therefore support the client to engage in roles effectively.

Encouraging

Therapy often involves clients in such things as exploring new situations, choosing to take risks, and sustaining effort when it is difficult. Therapists enable clients to do these things by **encouraging** them. That is, they provide emotional support and reassurance to clients. The following are examples of encouraging:

- A therapist reassures a child who appears anxious that the purpose of a game in therapy is to have fun. She does this through her smile and exaggerated actions, since it is not clear whether the child understands language. The therapist confirms this by laughing and hugging her when the child makes a mistake.
- A client is anxious about the transition to independent living. The therapist indicates to the client that he expects the transition to go well and uses

phrases like "things are going to be OK" and "everything will work out."

- An elderly client is becoming discouraged while practicing a self-care routine. The therapist uses phrases like "you can do it," "you're nearly there," and "you're doing great" to keep her going within the occupational form/task.

As the examples show, encouraging is ordinarily necessitated by clients' personal causation difficulties and/or by gaps between their performance capacity and the things they are attempting to do. Encouragement supports clients' volition, enabling them to feel greater confidence, to relax and enjoy themselves, and/or to recall why something is worth the effort. In short, it serves to elicit positive thoughts and feelings about performance.

*M*ariana: Encouraging Clients to Try to Participate in Occupations[5]

Mariana is a 43-year-old Portuguese woman. She has had psychiatric problems for the past 13 years. In the past year her functioning has dramatically decreased (she managed personal care only with assistance and spent most of her day in bed). She panicked when left alone and needed constant attention. In past several moths, she has been accompanied 24 hours a day by her husband and a friend. Consequently, she was referred by her psychiatrist to a psychiatric rehabilitation program.

The thought of attending the day program and disrupting her comforting routine made her very anxious. She had no hope that she would be able to achieve any change. The occupational therapist began by *validating* Mariana's feelings. Then she informed Mariana about the unit's program and *negotiated* with her and her husband that Mariana would come to the program only 2 days the first week. Moreover, her husband would take her in the morning and her friend would accompany her home in the afternoon. They also agreed that it would be Mariana's choice whether to increase the number of days she attended the program each week. Reassured by this plan, Mariana agreed to give the program a try.

The results of Mariana's assessment showed that her life was dominated by the patient role. Although she saw herself as a wife and a friend, she couldn't fulfill responsibilities associated with these roles. Her low personal causation, especially a very low sense of self-efficacy, prevented her from doing the things she used to do. Moreover, she had lost functional habits and had instead established a pattern of dependence.

The therapist **advised** Mariana of her conclusions, and Mariana agreed. Together they decide to begin by focusing therapy on her role as a homemaker. She was able to identify that she used to be a good homemaker who cooked excellent meals. Consequently the occupational therapist **advised** Mariana that she would likely benefit from joining a cooking group (clients who planned, shopped for, and prepared lunch at the program).

She also **validated** Mariana's anxiety and worries about joining the group and **negotiated** what tasks Mariana would engage in (simple tasks, such as peeling potatoes or washing vegetables). Although Mariana had the skills to perform these tasks competently, she complained about her anxiety and incapacity. She would then forget what she was doing, dropping equipment and ingredients. The therapist accompanied her all the time, doing the same task as Mariana, **encouraging** her and **coaching** her to redirect her attention to the task. During and after the sessions, the therapist **gave feedback** about her performance, pointing out that she could complete the tasks efficiently to help her reformulate her sense of efficacy. The therapist **identified** for Mariana that her anxiety was what most limited her performance and **advised** her to join a relaxation group to learn some relaxation strategies.

After several sessions, Mariana was more confident, performed tasks without coaching, and tried to solve problems, only occasionally needing validation or coaching. Thus the therapist **encouraged** her to cook a recipe of her own. To reduce her anxiety, the therapist **structured** the task by helping Mariana identify and write down the ingredients and procedures. During the cooking session, the occupational therapist gave **encouragement** and **feedback**, reaffirming Mariana's competence.

After several weeks, Mariana was able to cook some recipes all alone and was showing pride in her accomplishment. She had even progressed to the point that she could shop alone in the community for ingredients. Mariana began to cook at home and recently asked the therapist to help her find new, more elaborate recipes.

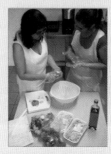

The therapist encourages Marina to cook and coaches her through the occupational form/task.

[5]*The case of Mariana was provided by Ana Cristina Maria de Moura Farinha, occupational therapist, Hospital Miguel Bombarda, Lisbon, Portugal.*

Providing Physical Support

Lack of motor skills may require a therapist to provide physical support. **Physical support** is when the therapist uses his or her body to provide support for a client to complete all or part of an occupational form/task when the client cannot or will not use his or her own motor skills. Occupational therapists who work with clients who have physical disabilities are likely to use this strategy frequently, as this client group often has reduced motor skills. Therapists working in psychiatry may also need to use this strategy, as a lack of motor skills may be associated with members of this client group (e.g., an older person with dementia, side effects of medication, physical deconditioning). Some examples are:

- A client is unable to open a jar while making a meal. The therapist loosens the top on the jar to make it easier for the client to use his weakened grip to open the jar.
- The therapist uses her body to support a client who has had a stroke to get out of bed in the morning and transfer to a chair. The therapist then retrieves the client's clothes from the wardrobe and lays the clothing within reach because the client's mobility skills are impaired.

- Within his morning routine, a client who has Parkinson's disease has difficulty bending to his feet. The therapist helps him to wash his feet, get socks over his toes, and put on his shoes.
- An older client who walks with his walking frame to the kitchen to make breakfast loses his balance, requiring the therapist to gently put her hand on his back to provide stability until he regains his balance.
- A person who has had schizophrenia for many years and has reduced physical flexibility because of side effects of medication needs the therapist to get some woodwork materials for him from a high shelf.
- A child who reaches for a toy requires the therapist to stabilize the child's base of support, which allows her to have a more effective reach skill.

This strategy focuses on the physical aspects of completing occupational forms/tasks and can be used with any client who is experiencing reduced motor skills.

Using Therapeutic Strategies to Support Client Change

The strategies just presented are used by therapists to influence and complement the occupational engagement of a client. They are ultimately aimed at enabling the client to achieve specific kinds of changes. The final column of the Therapeutic Reasoning Table (at the end of Section II) indicates therapeutic strategies that support occupational engagement to achieve changes related to MOHO concepts (see the final column of this table). For example, the following strategies are related to supporting clients' occupational engagement for achieving change in their sense of capacity:

- *Validate* how difficult it can be to have a impaired or altered body
- *Structure* the therapeutic environment to allow the client to use his or her body within meaningful occupational forms/tasks
- *Advise* the alteration of daily habits, using energy conservation techniques and written and verbal cues
- *Coach* the person in the use of new objects and adapted methods of completing occupational forms/tasks
- *Coach* the person with verbal cueing to overcome subjective experiences of the body
- *Provide* physical supports when needed to support lack of performance capacity

- *Encourage* the person who is engaged in occupational forms/tasks. This encouragement should be highly empathic and attentive to understanding the lived body experience
- *Encourage* the client when using adaptive strategies.

As noted earlier, the logic for the strategies follows from the theory. Therefore, the strategies in the table take their logic from the corresponding discussions in the earlier theory chapters. The logic for these strategies and the change that these strategies are meant to support are found in Chapter 4 in the discussion of volition and more specifically of personal causation. Therefore, in considering these strategies, therapists should be mindful of the theoretical concepts behind them. As noted earlier, the strategies discussed in this chapter and presented in the Therapeutic Reasoning Table are not meant to be exhaustive. Rather, they provide a starting point for thinking about what a therapist can and should do to support clients' occupational engagement and change processes.

Therapists will employ a combination of these strategies in each encounter with a client. While these strategies should be used genuinely and naturally as situations arise, it is important that the therapist be reflective about using strategies. This means anticipating, when possible, the kinds of strategies that might benefit a client. It also means carefully monitoring a client's needs throughout therapy to select appropriate strategies. Having an awareness of the strategies discussed above is the first step in being reflective.

Chapter 13 notes that therapeutic change is a dynamic, unfolding process. To effectively use therapeutic strategies, the therapist must monitor the unfolding events that are part of the change process. Changes in personal causation, interests, values, roles, habits, performance capacity, skill, and performance often occur together and influence each other in therapy. Moreover, the therapist will need to consider how the environment affects the change process. Change cannot be fully pre-planned. Rather, by monitoring how things

> *To effectively use therapeutic strategies, the therapist must monitor the unfolding events that are part of the change process.*

are unfolding, therapists can implement useful therapeutic strategies that can support client change.

Putting It All Together: Two Case Examples

The following two case examples illustrate how the therapeutic strategies and principles offered here can be implemented. The first client is from the first author's practice; the second client's therapist is the second author.

Jim

Jim was an adolescent client in a psychiatric setting. He had a history of depression, chronic school truancy, and substance abuse. A few months before, he ran away from home and was living with friends and on the streets of Los Angeles. One of the aims of therapy was to improve Jim's very poor personal causation. During several successive occupational therapy sessions, Jim engaged in woodworking. His sense of capacity and personal efficacy was very low. Jim was initially very reluctant to try woodworking even though it was clear that he was very attracted to doing it when he saw other adolescent clients in the wood shop. The therapist had to carefully advise and encourage Jim to undertake a personal project (making a small table), assuring him that he would **coach** Jim in the necessary skills and help him through each step. Consequently, Jim made the choice to undertake this project.

Despite increasing skill and success in each subsequent session, Jim persisted in downgrading his own capacities. Moreover, he needed **encouragement** to get started and to continue during each therapy session. Unsure of each new step, he required **encouragement** and **coaching** to keep him involved and help him know how to undertake the step. After each session Jim was quick to attribute positive outcomes to the therapist's assistance and difficulties to his own lack of skill. Each time this occurred, the therapist carefully gave Jim **feedback** to reframe how he was interpreting the session, guiding him to think about what he had accomplished during the session. The therapist also pointed out increases in his performance that had occurred across sessions and how much less support he had needed during each successive session.

These strategies seemed to help Jim in the next session. However, over several sessions he seemed to become even more agitated and upset over minor failures, even though his overall skill in performance was increasing. At the end of one therapy session he disavowed interest in the woodworking and pronounced it "a stupid waste of time."

The therapist was able to recognize Jim's struggle with his growing interest in woodworking and his increasing valuation of being good at it. As these two volitional changes took place, they raised the stakes for Jim's personal causation, making any of his lingering thoughts and feelings about not being effective more painful.

The therapist used the following statement that reflected strategies of **feedback**, **validation**, and **encouragement**. "Jim, I don't believe that you think woodworking is stupid. In fact, I think that you really want to do it more than ever, which makes you more concerned over whether you can do it well. That makes you anxious. I know it doesn't feel good. But if you avoid it, you're never going to see how good you can be at doing this. Even though it's hard for you, remember that I'll support you and I have confidence that that you can do it." Jim listened but did not say anything in response before leaving. Jim arrived at his next therapy session to announce that he had been working on a plan to make a piece of furniture and requested additional time in the wood shop to undertake this project.

Let us consider in even more detail what happened across these few therapy sessions. *Figure 14.2* illustrates the key processes involved. Jim entered therapy with a particular stable volitional pattern: a sense that he could not succeed, accompanied by a tendency to disavow interest in things. It became clear in therapy that Jim did see working with the kind of equipment that was in the wood shop (e.g., table and band saws, electric drill press) as symbolizing a world of technology and competence—a world he dared not imagine entering despite his attraction to it. By avoiding it, he could avoid the pain of failure. The therapist had to

FIGURE 14.2 Therapist strategies and dynamics of Jim's change during woodworking.

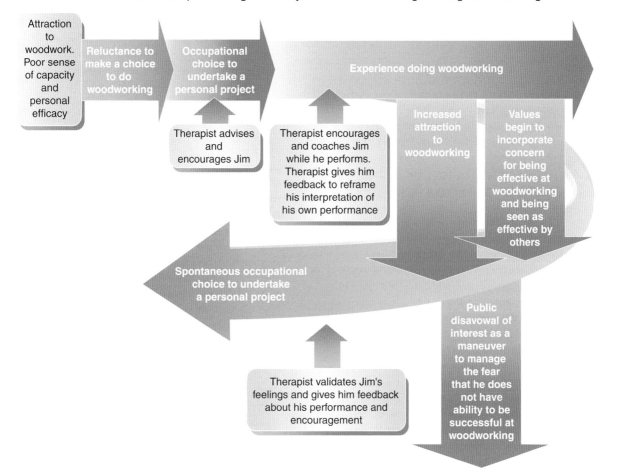

begin by ***advising*** and ***encouraging*** Jim to try to choose a personal project. As Jim worked on this project, it was necessary to provide ongoing ***encouragement***, ***coaching***, and ***feedback*** about what appeared to be going on. Jim was able to progress volitionally so that he enjoyed and increasingly valued woodworking. However, this raised the stakes for him, and given his limited sense of capacity, Jim became overwhelmed with fear of failing. His protestations of disinterest were maneuvers to avoid the possibility of painful failure. The therapist provided Jim further ***feedback*** about his improving performance along with ***validation*** and ***encouragement***. This empowered Jim to understand his own situation and reconsider his own volitional self-understanding. This allowed him to imagine success and allowed his interests and values to

energize him toward an independent occupational choice for a personal project.

Importantly, this choice shifted Jim into a new mode of action. He was soon proudly showing other clients and therapists the progress of his work and insisting that the therapist let him do every step of the project on his own. By the time he was discharged, he had negotiated access to a neighbor's workshop and had several woodworking projects planned to help furnish his quarters in the basement of his parent's home. Of course, the most important transformation in Jim was the development of his personal causation. He achieved and was able to generalize a growing sense of capacity and personal efficacy. He was beginning to see himself as a person effective in realizing values.

Betty

Betty was 71 years old. The therapist joined the inpatient rehabilitation ward when Betty had already been in the ward for 2 weeks. When the therapist first went to see Betty, she was slumped in her chair. She had right hemiplegia with no active range of motion in her right arm. She had some leg movement, although it was restricted. Her mouth drooped slightly and her speech was slurred.

The therapist **identified** that Betty seemed discouraged and gave Betty **feedback** about this. Betty agreed. She indicated that she did not really see the point of therapy given her slow progress and acknowledged that she was overwhelmed by the uncertainty of her future. The therapist **validated** Betty's feelings. Given Betty's despondence and reluctance for therapy, the therapist stopped by Betty's room at the end of each day to see her for a few minutes. This had the advantage of making a daily connection with Betty and gave her the sense she mattered to the therapist.

During one of these brief visits, the therapist advised Betty that the best way to feel more control over her situation was to identify some goals of her own for therapy. The therapist encouraged Betty to complete the OSA, indicating that it would help her think about what was most important to her and what she would want to accomplish in therapy. With some coaching, Betty was able to complete the OSA in her next therapy session, and she selected four OSA items as priorities for change:

- Taking care of myself
- Getting along with others
- Working toward my goals
- Having a satisfying routine.

The therapist asked Betty to discuss her choices. Explaining her first priority, Betty stated that she lived alone and prided herself on being able to take care of herself. She lived in a first-floor rented flat in Edinburgh, Scotland, where she had lived for 51 years. She was very emotionally attached to her home. She had moved there when she married and had raised her child there.

She was also very particular about her self-care. She took a bath and put on makeup every day. She set her hair in curlers every Saturday night so that she would look "presentable" for church on Sunday. She preferred to wear skirts, sweaters, and tights and was very particular about her clothes, as she did not want to be "mutton dressed as lamb."

Betty had an active and structured routine at home. She got up at 7:30 A.M. and would then take a bath and get dressed. She made her bed and opened the curtains. Then she prepared a light breakfast of cereal and toast. Most of her morning consisted of household duties, such as cooking, cleaning, and hand laundry. Betty stated she was very "house proud" and previously managed do all of her own housework. She had a light meal for lunch and a snack at tea time. Afternoons she shopped in her neighborhood, entertained or met friends, walked and sat in the park, or went into the city center using public transportation. She would go out every day and walk to local shops. Weekends were different. On Saturday she prepared soup that she would eat during the week. She went to church on Sunday and visited with her daughter and friends both days. She enjoyed reading and watching a few favorite TV shows in the evening, going to bed by 10:00 P.M. Betty described this routine as full, noting that there was always something to do at home and that she felt always "on the go." Her priority of being able to take care of herself meant getting back to this routine.

When asked about her second priority, getting along with others, Betty furnished the following information. Betty and her husband had managed a pub for most of their working lives. Betty served drinks and meals in the lounge bar for 24 years, until her husband's death 27 years earlier. She was very proud of this job and valued it very much. She regretted having to retire when her husband died, but she was not able to run the pub herself. When asked what she particularly enjoyed about this job, she quickly indicated it was the social aspect.

She considered herself an outgoing person who also led a very active social life at home. For example, she has a friend across from her flat who joined her for a meal once a week. She met another friend in town for coffee a couple of times a week. Several neighbors and their daughters visited her routinely, so she ordinarily entertained one or more guests each day, often for tea. When the therapist asked her why she had asked for no visitors and had chosen a private room in the rehabilitation hospital, since this isolated her, Betty stated that she felt very conscious of her drooping mouth and felt that she could not communicate anymore with others the way she was used to doing.

Betty's OSA priority 3 was "working toward my goals." To Betty this meant "getting home as quickly as possible." Her OSA priority 4 was "having a satisfying routine." Explaining this, Betty shared that she was extremely bored in rehabilitation. She felt that she could not do anything herself, which also made her feel helpless and frustrated. Her perception was that other clients, relatives, or nurses completed everything for her. She still wakes at 7:30, but now lies in bed thinking about how dependent she is until the nurses get to her around 8:30. She says starting her day this way makes her feel especially depressed and useless.

The therapist *validated* Betty's feelings by carefully listening to her and indicating that she realized Betty was in a very difficult emotional situation. She also *advised* Betty that there were things that could be done to help her achieve her goals and to make things more tolerable for her in the hospital. They *negotiated* that she should set therapy goals and discussed the possibilities. Betty indicated that for her, a very important goal was to return home to live alone. Betty and the therapist also agreed that two other, shorter-term goals were that she would have a productive and satisfying routine in the hospital and would feel confident interacting with other clients in occupational therapy.

At the next therapy session the therapist suggested *structuring* the following schedule for Betty in the hospital. During weekdays there would be a specific personal care program that would happen between 7:30 and 8:30 A.M. This would be carried out by a member of the occupational therapy team or a selected nurse. Breakfast would be at 9:00. Then Betty would read the newspaper until the occupational therapy session at 10:00. The occupational therapy session lasted until noon. Lunch on the ward was between noon and 1 P.M. Betty attended physical therapy for an hour after lunch. She then rested for an hour before receiving visitors.

The therapist *negotiated* with Betty's family to arrange a rotation of visitors at this time. The therapist also arranged for a television to be brought into Betty's room so that she had some entertainment at night. Weekends were also scheduled to allow for maximum use of time. Betty's daughter volunteered to support Betty with outdoor occupational forms/tasks on the weekends in the mornings. This required Betty to be issued an attendant-propelled wheelchair. The therapist *coached* the daughter in its use, including car transfers, and gave the daughter and Betty an opportunity to practice these skills. A hairdresser was arranged for Betty for Saturday afternoons. Arrangements were also made for her minister to visit her on Sunday until she felt able to go to church with her daughter. This restructuring of Betty's routine was effective in allowing her to find her ongoing experience personally satisfying.

Betty was highly committed to achieving independence in the area of self-care because of her value of privacy and her pride in her appearance. The therapist structured self-care sessions so that Betty could develop skills in personal care without feeling overwhelmed and concluding that she could not do anything. The Assessment of Motor and Process Skills (AMPS) showed that Betty had deficits in walking, stabilizing, aligning, positioning, reaching, and coordinating. The therapist therefore *coached* Betty to get out of bed safely and obtain objects from the wardrobe by providing verbal instructions and prompts. Betty stated she felt physically unsure when bathing, which made her very anxious. Therefore, the therapist provided *physical support* and *encouragement* to reassure her. The occupational therapist also *advised* Betty to use a bath board and seat to get in and out of the bath. The occupational therapist *structured* the environment to include this equipment. Betty explored the new objects and practiced them with substantial *coaching* and *encouragement* from the therapist.

However, Betty became despondent over the procedure, and an alternative was quickly identified. The occupational therapist *advised* that there was another piece of equipment that would provide more support and require less physical capacity from Betty. Betty explored using this equipment and was able to use it with *encouragement* from the therapist. Practice was arranged so that Betty could generate habits around the use of the equipment.

Betty was very particular about dressing. She insisted on using her clothes and did not wish to explore alternative clothing. The therapist **validated** this desire despite it posing greater functional challenges for Betty. Because of Betty's affected arm and her consequent skill deficit with reaching, coordinating, manipulating, and gripping, the therapist **coached** Betty in one-handed techniques to put on clothes. Betty was very anxious while attempting dressing. Since being in hospital she had failed repeatedly to complete parts of her personal care routine. Consequently, she expected failure again. Betty struggled with positioning garments to allow easier access. She would forget the technique and be unable to sustain performance. The therapist was careful to respond to Betty's anxiety and provide **validation** and **encouragement** that reassured her. She also provided **physical support** and **coaching** to ensure that Betty would be able to succeed and complete the occupational forms/tasks.

Therefore, despite difficulty, Betty sustained her performance. Based on this success, Betty began to practice putting on her jumper while in the ward during the day. Initially, Betty felt exhausted after personal care sessions and required therapist **feedback** to reframe her discouragement by stressing what she had accomplished. The therapist **structured** Betty's social environment by informing the nursing staff of Betty's routine and arranging for both nursing staff and the occupational therapy assistant to support Betty to practice dressing to create habits around these new ways of doing things.

Betty also attended an occupational therapy session in the department daily. The sessions were held in the morning with several other clients who attended at the same time. The therapist was careful to **structure** Betty's experience. In the early sessions Betty was more of an observer and completed an occupational form/task on her own with **coaching** from the therapist. Initially she was self-conscious because of her drooping mouth and did not want to socialize. Therefore, working within a parallel group situation without high demands for interaction was less threatening for her. Gradually she began to interact more. The

therapist then paired her with others to complete occupational forms/tasks in a cooperative group situation. The therapist purposively paired Betty with a talkative client who would stimulate communication. Betty soon made friends and asked to be moved from the side room in the ward to be nearer her friends from occupational therapy in the main ward.

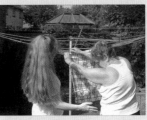

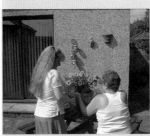

As Betty hangs the wash and plants flowers, the therapist provides coaching and encouragement.

In this parallel group context, the therapist offered Betty increasingly challenging occupational forms/tasks. Since Betty had been a homemaker who routinely entertained people, she was keen to do things that contributed to that role. The therapist identified the kinds of occupational forms that were within Betty's performance capacity, advising Betty on what she might choose to do. First, Betty tried a ready-mix sponge cake that only required stirring in a few ingredients and baking. This provided her with instant success, promoting her sense of capacity. Betty shared the cake with a few other clients. The therapist had previously **coached** these clients to encourage Betty with positive feedback. Similarly, the therapist told nursing staff about Betty's accomplishments and asked them to reinforce this achievement. Subsequently, Betty undertook a range of more challenging occupational forms/tasks, including making sandwiches, cheesecakes (a favorite of her friend who used to visit), simple meals, and soup.

Betty was very particular about soup. When the therapist **advised** Betty to consider using canned soup because it would be more convenient, given that she was now effectively one handed, Betty refused and **negotiated** to try to make her own soup from raw ingredients. She had made soup every week of her married life and used to give it to her visitors when they called. She stated she was known for her soup all over Scotland, and it was a source of pride. In addition, she pointed out that canned soup simply did not have the same nutrients as homemade soup. As Betty and the therapist discussed soup, it became clear that making soup was an important form of leisure participation for Betty. It structured her day and provided enjoyment when shared with her visitors. Therefore, the therapist **validated** Betty's choice to attempt making soup from raw ingredients. She advised Betty about pieces of adaptive equipment she would require for vegetable preparation and coached Betty in proper use. Although it was difficult and took Betty a whole morning to make the soup, she sustained her performance because she found it meaningful and satisfying. The first session made it apparent that once Betty was set up to prepare the vegetables, she could spend all morning engaged in this occupational form with minimal support from occupational therapy staff. Next, the therapist arranged it so that on days Betty made soup it was taken to the ward for lunch. In this way Betty received glowing feedback from the other clients and ward staff.

The occupational forms/tasks were structured to provide the opportunity for Betty to develop and/or compensate for skill deficits. For example, Betty had difficulty with transporting objects. Initially, due to her lack of confidence and motor skills, the therapist organized the needed objects within reach to allow Betty to experience success and enjoyment. As Betty gained a better sense of her own capacities and efficacy, especially her recognition that she could succeed despite her impairments, the therapist decided to introduce more challenge. For example, Betty became responsible for collecting needed objects. To help her, the therapist advised Betty to explore adaptive objects such as different trolleys and/or a pocketed apron. Betty chose to use an upright trolley, and the therapist coached and encouraged her to practice so that it became more habitual. The therapist initially had to closely supervise and provide physical support to reduce the risk of falling. In

addition, Betty was easily fatigued, so that she needed to increase her endurance. Initially, she used a chair with supportive arms; with time, she was able to work from a tall stool that allowed her to maintain a semi-standing position and stand for short periods.

Betty's success inspired several other clients who wanted to be involved. Therefore, a "soup group" was created. Members worked toward their own occupational goals within this common occupational form/task. Betty's role was to organize everyone and welcome new members. At the end of 3 weeks, both the team and Betty's family could see major improvements in Betty's mood, social ability, and performance capacities. For example, one nurse who had been on holiday noted that Betty had become a "completely different person" who was chatty, motivated, and engaged in life again. Another nurse commented, "occupational therapy had given Betty back a sense of who she was." Betty continued to make improvements and was discharged to her home.

Figure 14-3 illustrates the key processes involved in Betty's therapy. Betty initially could not engage in therapy because she was anxious and discouraged by her lack of progress. The therapist had to deal with Betty's anxiety and discouragement by first **validating** Betty's feelings. The therapist also **structured** her environment quickly to show Betty that she was committed to supporting Betty's recovery. As therapy unfolded, other strategies were used to facilitate improvement in communication/interaction skills and Betty's volitional status. These included **encouraging**, **structuring**, **coaching**, **advising**, **giving feedback**, and providing **physical support**.

Conclusion

This chapter presented and discussed a number of strategies that therapists use to facilitate and complement clients' occupational engagement. These and other strategies form an important component of planning and implementing occupational therapy as discussed in Chapter 11. To facilitate therapeutic reasoning about this aspect of therapy, the Therapeutic

FIGURE 14.3 Therapist strategies and dynamics of Betty's change during occupational therapy.

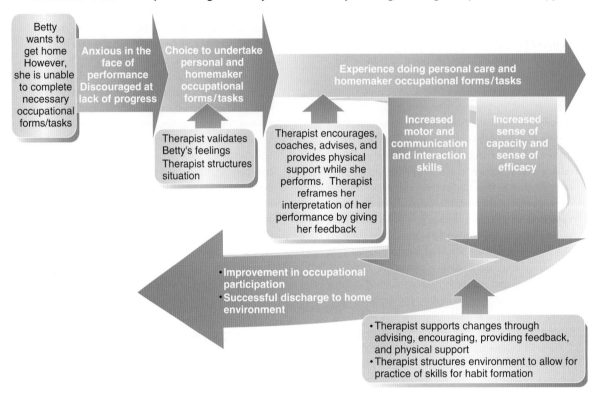

Reasoning Table (at the end of Section 2) contains examples of the therapeutic strategies discussed in this chapter, indicating how they can support different forms of client occupational engagement.

Key Terms

Advise: Recommend intervention goals and strategies to the client.

Coach: Instruct, demonstrate, guide, verbally prompt, and/or physically prompt clients.

Encourage: Provide emotional support and reassurance.

Give feedback: Share an overall conceptualization of the client's situation or an understanding of the client's ongoing action.

Identify: Locate and share a range of personal, procedural, and/or environmental factors that can facilitate occupational performance and participation.

Negotiate: Engage in give-and-take with the client to achieve a common perspective or agreement about something that the client will or should do in the future.

Physically support: To use the physical body to support the completion of an occupational form/task or part of an occupational form/task when clients cannot or will not use their motor skills.

Structure: Establish parameters for choice and performance by offering clients alternatives, setting limits, and establishing ground rules.

Therapeutic strategy: Action that influences a client's doing, feeling, and/or thinking to facilitate desired change.

Validate: Convey respect for the client's experience or perspective.

References

Hopkins, H. L., & Tiffany, E. G. (1983). Occupational therapy: A problem solving process. In H. L. Hopkins & H. D. Smith (Eds.), *Willard and Spackman's occupational therapy* (6th ed., pp. 89–100). Philadelphia: Lippincott.

Jonsson, H., Josephsson, S., & Kielhofner, G. (2000). Evolving narratives in the course of retirement: A longitudinal study. *American Journal of Occupational Therapy, 54* (5), 463–470.

Peloquin, S. M. (1990). The patient-therapist relationship in occupational therapy: Understanding visions and images. *American Journal of Occupational Therapy, 44,* 13–21.

Taylor, R. (in press). *The Intentional Relationship: Use of Self in Occupational Therapy.* Philadelphia: FA Davis

Toombs, K. (1992). *The meaning of illness: A phenomenological account of the different perspectives of physician and patient.* Boston: Kluwer Academic.

Wendel, S. (1996). *The rejected body: Feminist philosophical reflections on disability.* New York: Routledge.

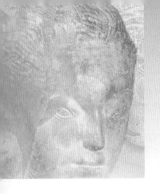

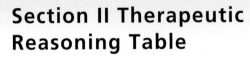

Section II Therapeutic Reasoning Table

- Kirsty Forsyth
- Gary Kielhofner

This therapeutic reasoning table lists information that is designed to serve as exemplars. It should not be used in an inflexible manner and should always be adapted to the unique characteristics of each client. Understanding this table requires that one read the rest of the text. Chapters 11, 12, 13, and 14 refer directly to this table.

Questions	Strengths	Problems/Challenges	Changes	Client Occupational Engagement	Therapist Strategies
PERSONAL CAUSATION					
• What is this person's view of personal capacity and effectiveness and how does it affect the choice, experience, interpretation, and anticipation of doing things? • What abilities or limitations stand out in this person's view of self? • Is the sense of capacity accurate? • Is this person aware of abilities and limitations? • Does this person feel in control of her or his own thoughts, feelings, and actions and the occupational consequences of these? • Does this person expect to achieve desired outcomes? • Does this person have confidence, anxiety, or other feelings in the face of change?	• Aware of capacity (strengths and limitations) • Ability to choose occupational forms/tasks within capacity and take on appropriate challenges and responsibilities • Adequate confidence to make decisions about engagement in occupational forms/tasks • Seeks out appropriate occupational challenges based on an adequate knowledge of capacity • Seeks assistance appropriately and makes use of environmental adaptations • Feels in control of occupational performance • Expects success within occupation • Reasonable expectations of success in occupational performance situations • Confident to face occupational performance demands • Ability to sustain effort to attain occupational goals/complete occupational forms/tasks	• Lack of awareness of capacity (strengths or limitations) • Underestimation of abilities leading to: ∘ unnecessary dependence on others ∘ avoiding occupational forms/tasks commensurate with performance capacity leading to reduced occupational performance ∘ failing to seek out occupational challenges that would promote learning/growth in skill • Overestimation of abilities leading to: ∘ Taking unnecessary risks by seeking challenges that are higher than performance capacity, resulting in poor occupational performance, danger, stress, damage, or injury. • Failure to seek assistance appropriately or make use of needed environmental adaptations • Feelings of lack of control over occupational performance leading to anxiety (fear of failure) within occupations • Poor frustration tolerance leading to disengagement with occupational forms/tasks • Poor concentration leading to difficulty in completing occupational forms/tasks • Expectation of failure in occupational performance • Avoidance of performance, failure to set occupational goals, or lack of adequate effort to complete occupations or lack of follow through on occupations/goals	• Enhance the client's understanding of occupational abilities (strengths and limitations) • Focus attention to more accurately note how strengths and limitations affect occupational performance • Develop emotional acceptance of limitations and pride in occupational abilities • Reduce unnecessary feelings of dependence, resentment, or guilt associated with loss of participation • Increase ability to choose and do occupations that are consistent with capacity • Build up confidence to approach occupational forms/tasks within capacity • Increase knowledge and acceptance of using equipment and/or environmental modifications to augment capacity • Increase willingness to ask for help when needed within an occupational form/task • Reduce client's anxiety and fear of failure in occupational performance • Build up confidence to face occupational performance demands • Improve the client's ability to sustain effort for attaining goals and/or completing occupational performance • Increase expectation of success in occupational performance • Extend a client's readiness to take on occupational challenges and responsibilities • Increase sense of efficacy in occupational life circumstances	• Commit to overcoming fear in occupational performance • Explore alternative ways of doing an occupational form/task that compensates for performance capacity limitations • Re-examine previously held beliefs about effectiveness in achieving occupational outcomes • Re-examine anxieties and fears in the light of new performance experiences • Identify occupational forms/tasks within/beyond performance capacity • Negotiate an appropriate level of risk within occupational performance • Choose to do relevant and meaningful things that are within performance capacity • Choose to engage in occupational forms/tasks that challenge the person • Sustain performance in occupational forms/tasks despite anxiety • Practice asking for and using help appropriately • Practice performance to reinforce sense of efficacy	• Structure environment to allow client to take risks safely • Validate client's thoughts and feelings concerning performance capacities • Validate how difficult it can be to do things that provoke anxiety • Identify client's strengths and weaknesses in occupational performance • Give feedback to client about match/mismatch between choice of occupational forms/tasks and performance capacity • Give feedback to support a positive re-interpretation of their experience of engaging in an occupation • Advise client to do relevant and meaningful things that match performance capacity • Advise client to engage in occupational forms/tasks within performance capacity to assure high degree of success. • Encourage client to sustain effort in difficult occupational circumstances. • Encourage client to use performance capacities in the face of anxiety • Physically support when necessary to ensure success • Coach when appropriate to ensure success

Questions	Strengths	Problems/Challenges	Changes	Client Occupational Engagement	Therapist Strategies
INTERESTS					
• Can this person identify personal interests? • What occupations does this person enjoy doing? • What are the aspects of doing that this person enjoys most (e.g., physical challenge, intellectual stimulation, social contact, and aesthetic experience)? • Does this person do the things he/she enjoys? • Is anything interfering with this person's feeling of pleasure and satisfaction in performance ?	• Able to identify interests • Able to pursue interests	• Inability to identify interests • No/limited feeling of attraction • No/limited pleasure in doing things • Disengagement from occupational forms/tasks • Inability to pursue interests • Feelings of boredom • Feelings of frustration at lack of engagement in interests	• Changes in client's attraction, participation, and enjoyment/satisfaction in occupation • Increase client's ability to identify interests • A client has a greater desire to do things • The client has an increased willingness to chose to engage in interests • The client has an increased participation in things of interest • Generating a greater sense of enjoyment/satisfaction in doing things	• *Commit* to developing interests • *Explore* opportunities to identify interests • *Re-examine* past interests • *Identify* potential interests • *Choose* between potential interests • *Plan* strategies of how to pursue interests • *Perform* interests • *Sustain* performance in interests • *Practice* pursuing interests	• *Structure* the therapeutic environment to offer ongoing opportunities and resources to identify interests and to support engagement in interests • *Negotiate* a client's interests will be the focus of therapy • *Validate* client's attraction to occupational forms/tasks • *Give* feedback as required while the client is engaging in the occupational form/task • *Identify* the essence of the attraction to the old interest through the experience of old interests if the person no longer has the skill to engage in that particular occupational form/task • *Identify* resources in the client's social environment to support identified interest • *Encourage* continued engagement in interests when client gets discouraged • *Advise* client to re-adapt previous interests, exploration of new interests • *Coach* client to attend to pleasure in action

Questions	Strengths	Problems/Challenges	Changes	Client Occupational Engagement	Therapist Strategies
VALUES					

• What is the organising theme in this person's sense of values?
• What things are most important to this person to do?
• What standards or other criteria does this person use to judge his/her own performance?
• Are the values to which this person ascribes really his or her own?
• Can this person prioritise among what is important?
• Is this person clear as to what his or her values are?
• How do this person's values match or conflict with his or her performance capacity?
• Does this person hold values that lead to adaptive occupational choices?
• Does this person's values match or conflict with social & cultural norms?
	• Identifies and engages in personally meaningful and valuable occupations
	• Readily sorts out what is most important in a situation
	• Employs realistic standards to evaluate self and others
	• Identifies values as own
	• Can readily identify and prioritize among goals
	• Can pursue and realize goals
	• Has values/standards consistent with capacity
	• Values lead to positive choices
	• Has values matched to context
		• Difficulty identifying and engaging in personally meaningful and valuable occupational forms/tasks
		• Difficulty sorting out what's most important in an occupational situation
		• Employs unrealistically high or low standards to evaluate self and others
		• Ascribes to values defined by others rather than self
		• Inability/difficulty identifying & prioritising among occupational goals
		• Inability to pursue and realise occupational goals
		• Values/standards inconsistent with performance capacity
		• Values lead to negative occupational choices
		• Values conflict with context
			• Increase client's ability to reflect and acknowledge that they are able to do things that are important to them
			• Increase satisfaction and self-esteem from realizing occupational goals
			• Increase the client's ability to identify what's most important in an occupational situation
			• Develop more realistic values/standards for assessing themselves and others
			• Strengthen sense of what is most personally significant within occupational life
			• Increase client's ability to identify & prioritize among occupational goals
			• Increase ability to pursue and realize occupational goals
			• Increase client's ability to maintain their effort so that they can realize occupational goals
			• Adjust client's values/standards to match performance capacity
			• Develop values that support positive occupational choices
			• Develop values consistent with context (or find context consistent with values)
				• *Explore* occupational forms/tasks /environments embodying different values/standards
				• *Re-examine* current values in light of:
				  • current performance capacities
				  • environmental context
				• *Identify:*
				  • appropriate standards for self and others
				  • values consistent with capacity
				  • realistic long and short term goals
				• *Choose:*
				  • to engage in valued/meaningful occupational forms/tasks
				  • among occupational goals and values
				• *Negotiate* selection/ application of occupational goals/ values/ standards
				• *Commit* to:
				  • realistic occupational goals
				  • attainable standards
				  • Plan for occupational goal attainment
					• *Validate* client's value system as important driver of the therapeutic plan
					• *Identify* conflicts between values and:
					  • performance capacity
					  • environmental values
					• *Give feedback* on how clients values/standards:
					  • do not seem personally cogent
					  • lead to self-devaluation
					  • set up unattainable standards/occupational goals
					• *Identify* realistic long & short term occupational goals with/on behalf of the client
					• *Negotiate* with client concerning:
					  • values and standards to be applied in therapy
					  • priorities of occupational goals
					• *Advise* client to:
					  • select occupational performance and participation that reflects personal meaning
					  • seek out environments consistent with occupational goals
					  • change standards to be more consistent with performance capacities
					• *Structure* therapeutic environment to:
					  • facilitate setting , planning, and realizing occupational goals
					  • allow exposure to appropriate reference groups and role models
					• *Give feedback* on how the client is moving towards occupational goals

Questions	Strengths	Problems/Challenges	Changes	Client Occupational Engagement	Therapist Strategies
ROLES					
• What is the overall pattern of role involvement of this person? • Does this person have roles that impact positively on his/her identity, use of time, and involvement in social groups? • Is the person over or under involved in roles? How important is each role to the person? • Can this person meet the obligations of each role? • Are collective role requirements too few, too demanding, or make conflicting demands on this person?	• Aware of responsibilities associated with success in various roles • Able to meet multiple role expectations • Able to structure day through role involvement • Positively identifies with roles	• Poor awareness of responsibilities associated with success in various roles (poor role scripts) • Difficulty meeting multiple role expectations (role conflict) • Difficulty structuring the day due to lack of roles (role loss) • Doesn't identify with roles	Changes in identification with roles: • The client has an improved awareness of responsibilities associated with success in various roles (poor role scripts) • Increase the client's commitment to assuming specific roles that are necessary and desirable in their life • Increase identification with self-enhancing disability related roles (e.g., self care manager, disability advocate/activist) Changes in enactment of roles: • Increase client's ability to become more effective in order to meet multiple role expectations through negotiation of realistic role responsibilities • Improve routine as a result of role change • Perception of self in a more manageable and fulfilling number of roles • Increase self perception as being able to manage and fulfil a number of roles • Improve routine due to role acquisition	• Commit to altering roles • Commit to behaviours required to make changes in role scripts or role repertoire • Explore potential strategies for altering responsibilities and structure to the day • Explore role responsibilities for identified valued roles • Re-examine role responsibilities • Identify valued roles • Negotiate range and content of roles • Choose to prioritize specific valued roles to allow for reduced role conflict • Perform behaviors consistent to role responsibility • Practice behaviors required for enactment of role	• Structure therapeutic environment to provide opportunities to discuss roles and their related expectations • Structure environment to provide opportunities to engage in the behaviour required by the role to allow for internalising of the role script and development of supportive routine • Validate the challenges around role change and assuming responsibilities • Give feedback on appropriateness of their understanding of role responsibilities • Identify appropriate role behaviors or role conflicts • Advise the client to make choices (volition) around reducing their responsibilities • Advise the person to identify other ways of meeting their responsibilities that doesn't require time from them, discuss/negotiate roles and their related expectations • Advise the client to leave roles behind or to enter into new roles • Coach person in role enactment • Encourage people to make choices to engage in new roles (or old roles in an adapted way e.g. with configuration of new role responsibilities)

Questions	Strengths	Problems/Challenges	Changes	Client Occupational Engagement	Therapist Strategies
HABITS					
• Does this person have well established habits ? • What kind of routine does this person have and is it effective? • What is this person's characteristic style of performance and is it effective? • What quality of life is provided by the habitual routine of this person?	• Has a habitual routine that allows for the completion of specific occupational forms/tasks • Able to internalize the habitual use of a new object or a new way of completing an occupational form/task • Routines are organized and allow for the completion of needed collection of occupations	• Difficulty completing a specific occupation due to lack of habitual structure • Difficulty internalizing the habitual use of a new object or a new way of completing an occupation • Disorganised routines that makes it difficult for the person to complete required occupation	• Changes in client's habits to accommodate an acquired impairment and/or enhance occupational performance and occupational participation • Increase client's effectiveness so that they are able to complete a specific occupation by altering their habitual way of doing it • Acquisition of a new habit pattern that incorporates a new object and/or new way of completing an occupation (e.g., acquiring a habit for using adaptive equipment or acquiring the habit of energy conservation in completing typical daily tasks) • Increase client's organization of daily routines that improve effectiveness in managing role related responsibilities	• Commit to changing habits • Explore ways of organizing self and environment to support habit formation • Re-examine usefulness of previous habits structure • Identify new habitual ways of completing occupational forms/tasks • Negotiate options of altering methods of completing occupational forms/tasks or organising occupational forms/tasks into alternative routine • Choose between different ways of doing or routines of doing • Perform one or more occupational form/task in a consistent manner to support habit formation • Practice actions that make up the intended new habit	• Structure therapeutic environment to support habit training within an occupation and/or routine. Offer repetitive opportunities to engage in the routine • Structure usual environment with structures to support habitual routine e.g., have a person in the social environment reinforce habits • Negotiate options of altering methods of completing occupational forms/tasks or organising occupational forms/tasks into alternative routine • Validate that it is hard to change habits • Identify new habitual ways of completing occupational forms/tasks • Advise new habits around a particular occupational form/task or routine • Coach by giving consistent verbal prompts to reinforce habit • Encourage sustained effort until the person is able to complete the occupational form/task and/or routine

Questions	Strengths	Problems/Challenges	Changes	Client Occupational Engagement	Therapist Strategies
PERFORMANCE CAPACITY					
• Are there underlying impairments of performance capacities? • What is the experience of the impairment and its implications for function being remedied or compensated for? • Do any experiences interfere with this person's occupational performance and how so? • What are the consequences of sensory, motor, or other capacities for this person's experience of performing occupational forms/tasks? • How do experiences (e.g., pain, fatigue, dizziness, confusion, or altered bodily perceptions) influence this person's occupational performance?	• Able to incorporate damaged/estranged parts of the body into occupational forms/tasks • Able to manage altered bodily experiences	• Difficulty incorporating damaged/estranged parts of the body into occupational performance • Negative experiences engaging in occupational forms/tasks due to altered bodily experiences e.g. sensations, hallucinations	• Develop new ways of managing symptoms to allow them to engage in occupation • Incorporate changes to their body and new equipment into occupational performance • Increase feeling of how to do things & confidence when doing things with an altered body or despite symptoms • Increase understanding and better management of such things as altered bodily sensations, hallucinations, pain, fatigue, pain, and altered perception to minimize interference with occupational performance	• *Commit* to changing performance capacity and/or to adapting for loss of performance capacity • *Explore* new ways of incorporating damaged/estranged parts of body • *Identify* strategies of how to manage altered bodily experiences • *Choose* new methods to complete an occupational form/task • *Perform* successfully by engaging in occupations incorporating damaged/estranged parts of body • *Practice* to endure successful ongoing completion of occupational forms/tasks incorporating damaged/estranged parts of body	• *Validate* how difficult it can be to have a damaged or altered body • *Structure* therapeutic environment to allow the client to experience using their body within meaningful occupational forms/tasks • *Advise* the alteration of daily habits, using energy conservation techniques, and written and verbal cues • *Coach* the person in the use of new objects and adapted methods of completing occupational forms/tasks • *Coach* the person by verbal cueing to overcome subjective experiences of their body • *Provide* physical supports when needed to support lack of performance capacity • *Encourage* the person when the client is engaged in occupational forms/tasks. This encouragement should be from a highly empathetic other who is attentive to understanding the lived body experience • *Encourage* when using adaptive strategies

Questions	Strengths	Problems/Challenges	Changes	Client Occupational Engagement	Therapist Strategies
SKILLS					
• Does this person have adequate motor, process, and communication/ interaction skill ability?	• Has adequate motor, process, and/or communication/interaction skills to allow the client to engage in occupational forms/tasks	• Difficulty with motor, process, and/or communication/interaction skills while performing an occupation	• Increase in skill within occupational performance by: ○ Acquiring new information that enhances skill ○ Learning a strategy that results in increased skill • Learning to use more adaptive skills to compensate for weaker skills (e.g., using process skills to make up for lack of motor skills) • Compensation for immutable impairments of performance capacity through learning to capitalize on changes in the environment (space, objects, forms/tasks, and groups)	• *Commit* to improving or compensating for lack of skill • *Explore* possible solution to skill deficit • *Re-examine* previous skill ability • *Identify* new ways of using current skill or adapting for lack of skill effectively that are acceptable and maintain the meaning of the occupational form/task. • *Negotiate* solutions to difficulties with therapist where possible • *Choose* to use alternative methods of supporting skill deficit • *Perform* occupational forms/tasks that challenge the persons current skill level • *Practice* using the skill through repeated engagement in occupational forms/tasks that challenge the person to use the skill in a graded way • *Practice* substitution of certain skills for others (e.g., using process skills to organise occupation to adapt for the lack of motor skill)	• *Structure* environment to challenge skill ability • *Negotiate* with client around treatment strategies of improving skills or adapting for lack of skill • *Validate* how difficult it can be to have skill deficit • *Advise* the client to a) perform particular occupational forms/tasks that will build skill and/or b) introduce new objects to compensate for lack of skill and/or c) change the demands of the occupational form/task to accommodate the skill deficit and/or d) change the social environment to support skill deficit e.g., teach spouse of person how to best support their relative • *Coach* by demonstrating, guiding and/or verbally instructing the person to enable them to show skill or effectively adapt for skill deficit and achieve effective performance • *Provide physical support* due to lack of motor skills • *Encourage* client to sustain performance when they are showing signs of frustration or difficulty when trying to use their skills or learn how to adapt to skill deficit

Questions	Strengths	Problems/Challenges	Changes	Client Occupational Engagement	Therapist Strategies
PHYSICAL ENVIRONMENT					
• Do the spaces in which the person performs/tasks their occupations represent physical barriers or supports that impact on performance ? • Do the objects this person uses support performance? • Do the spaces and objects constitute a physical environment with adequate resources for doing things this person needs and wishes to do ?	• Physical spaces supportive of occupational performance • Objects adequate to support reduced capacity	• Physical space cluttered, unsafe, or otherwise not supporting occupational performance • Naturally occurring objects not supportive of reduced performance capacity	• Change in physical space and objects to facilitate occupational performance and occupational participation through improving ease of access and use, including: ○ Adaptations to naturally occurring objects or new object	• *Commit* to habit training around altered space and new objects • *Explore* new ways of altering physical space and objects • *Re-examine* physical layout of environment • *Negotiate* possibilities for changing space and objects • *Negotiate* solutions to difficulties with therapist where possible • Choose appropriate physical environmental strategies	• *Validate* with the client how difficult and emotional it can be to alter physical spaces and use new objects • *Negotiate* possibilities for changing space and objects • *Advise* about the physical modification of home, school, and/ or work space e.g. moving furniture around to create more physical space • *Identify* the learned habits that are attached to how the physical space has been set up within the person's environment • *Identify* the physical space required for the successful completion of occupational forms/tasks and the consequence of reduction of physical space for any new objects that are placed within the person's environment • *Encourage* person to make changes to physical environment

Questions	Strengths	Problems/Challenges	Changes	Client Occupational Engagement	Therapist Strategies
SOCIAL ENVIRONMENT					

• Does the environment provide appropriate occupational forms/tasks in which this person can engage?
 • Do the occupational forms/tasks sufficiently challenge this person and provide a sense of worth?
 • Do interactions with others support or inhibit this person's performance?
 • Do the social groups of which this person is a member support the assumption of meaningful roles?
 • What are the reactions of others in occupational behavior settings to this person's disability?
	• Family has the knowledge and skills that allows them to appropriately support their relative
	 • Routine ways of completing occupational forms/tasks are in line with the persons capacities
	 • Supportive social attitudes
		• Family/family member do not have enough skill to support their relative's lack of ability
		 • Family member does not have enough knowledge to support their relative's possessive engagement in occupational forms/tasks
		 • The usual way of completing an occupation is no longer supported by the ability of the client
		 • Negative social attitudes, discrimination due to disability
			• Immediate social group (family) are altered in ways to increase performance and/or participation:
			   ◦ Increase in information about client's needs and desires
			   ◦ Change in expectations for performance/ participation
			 • Increase ability of family member to provide support/assistance
			 • Occupational forms/tasks performed in various contexts are altered, made available to allow better performance and greater participation
			 • Social attitudes and behaviors are more conducive to participation
			 • Discrimination and other negative attitudes/practices are reduced
			 • Laws and practices are made more conducive to participation
				• *Commit* to altering social environment
				 • *Explore* new social groups and occupational forms/tasks
				 • *Re-examine* old social groups and occupational forms/tasks
				 • *Identify* altered ways of completing occupational forms/tasks
				 • *Identify* people in social environment who can support occupational performance
				 • *Negotiate* with relatives about social environmental needs
				 • *Choose* to complete occupational forms/tasks in new ways and/or enter into new social groups
				 • *Practise* altered way of completing occupational form/task
					• *Structure* environment to allow for repeated experience (habit training) until the relative has a high sense of personal causation about helping their relative
					 • *Negotiate* with relatives about social environmental needs
					 • *Validate* difficulties of changing social environment
					 • *Identify* altered ways of having the social environment support the client to engage in occupational forms/tasks
					 • *Identify* the relative's volitional process while they are helping the client
					 • *Advise* relatives about the occupational forms/tasks the client requires support with, and the clients abilities and limitations
					 • *Advise* client and relative about available support networks
					 • *Advise* about changing the demands of the occupational form/tasks and subsequent practice required for habit training
					 • *Coach* the relatives how to support their relative. This may require the relative to be involved in the clients treatment sessions

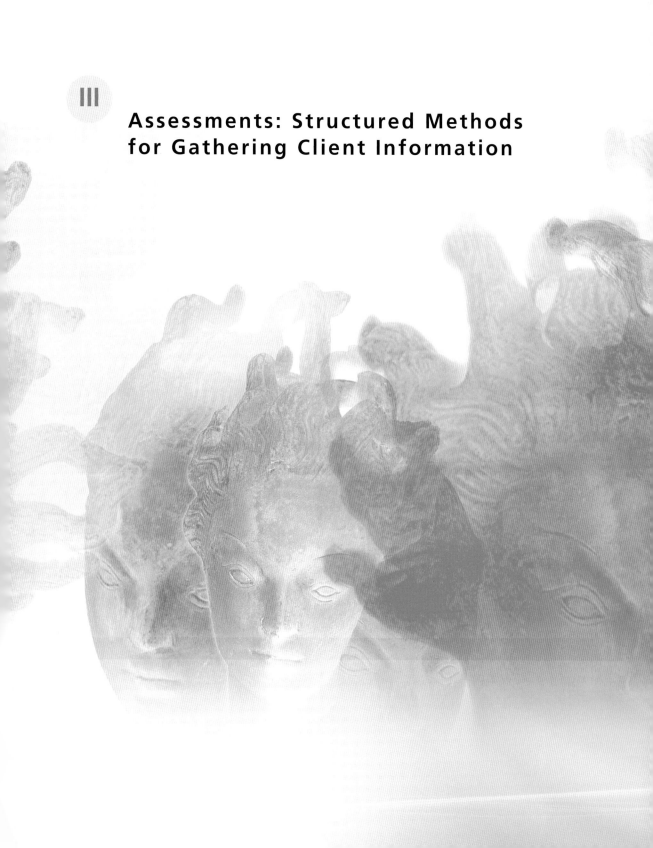

III

Assessments: Structured Methods for Gathering Client Information

Introduction to Section III

This section is divided into four chapters. Each chapter discusses MOHO-based assessments that use a particular method of gathering client information. Chapter 15 discusses assessments that use observation as the method of information gathering. Chapter 16 presents client self-report assessments. Chapter 17 presents interview assessments. Chapter 18 presents assessments that use mixed methods of information gathering. Each chapter discusses the assessment, its administration, and the information it yields. Information on the evidence base underlying the assessments that are discussed in this section can be found in Chapter 25.

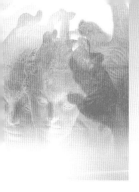

15

Observational Assessments

- ● Gary Kielhofner
- ● Susan M. Cahill
- ● Kirsty Forsyth
- ● Carmen Gloria de las Heras
- ● Jane Melton
- ● Christine Raber
- ● Susan Prior

The four assessments discussed in this chapter gather information from observation of a client's behavior. Two of these assessments provide information on a client's skills:

- The Assessment of Motor and Process Skills (AMPS)
- The Assessment of Communication and Interaction Skills (ACIS)

The other two provide information on a client's volition:

- The Volitional Questionnaire (VQ)
- The Pediatric Volitional Questionnaire (PVQ)

All four assessments are designed to capture qualitative information about the client that is entered as comments on the rating scale forms. The ratings provide profiles of strengths and weaknesses of the client and can be scored to provide measures of skill or volition.

Assessments of Skills

The Assessment of Motor and Process Skills (AMPS) (Fisher, 2003) and the Assessment of Communication and Interaction Skills (ACIS) (Forsyth, Salamy, Simon, & Kielhofner, 1998) have been developed to gather information on skills. Both the AMPS and the ACIS employ observation of clients performing occupational forms/tasks. The AMPS and ACIS provide a unique ap-

proach to assessing a client's ability to perform in everyday occupational forms/tasks. These assessments provide detailed information about actual performance. They identify both strengths and difficulties a person demonstrates in doing a given occupational form/task.

Assessment of Motor and Process Skills

The Assessment of Motor and Process Skills (AMPS) (Fisher, 2003) gathers information on skills by observing the person doing selected activities of daily living, including personal activities of daily living as well as domestic or instrumental activities of daily living. A wide range of internationally and cross-culturally standardized tasks can be drawn on when administering the AMPS. The AMPS can be used with children 3 to 4 years of age and older, adolescents, and adults.

The AMPS consists of two scales that separately measure process and motor skills. The two scales are administered simultaneously, and this allows for direct evaluation of the interactive nature of motor and process skills, such as the use of process skills to compensate for limitations in motor skills.

Each item on the two scales is scored with a four-point rating that considers the effectiveness, efficiency, and safety of a client's performance. The motor skills scale gathers information on the actions done to move oneself or objects. The process skills scale gathers information on the logical sequencing of actions, selection and appropriate use of tools and materials, and adaptation to problems.

The AMPS yields a measure of both process and motor skills that takes into consideration the level of difficulty of the occupational forms/tasks the client was observed doing and that also adjusts for the tendency of the particular rater to be more severe or lenient in assigning ratings. To make these adjustments, the AMPS is scored by a computer. Moreover, raters must first be trained and calibrated as to their severity/leniency. After training, therapists are provided with software for computer scoring of the AMPS.

The AMPS provides detailed and useful information about how a person performs. For persons who have difficulty performing, the AMPS identifies what aspects of performance (i.e., skills) are problematic and how complex an occupational form/task the person can perform. The ratings of the items on both scales indicate areas of skill that are intact and areas in which the person is having difficulty. Through the use of the AMPS the occupational therapy practitioner is able to evaluate the quality of the person's motor and process skills. The results can be interpreted to provide information about the person's motor and process skills ability in relation to community living. For both motor and process skills research has determined cutoff scores below which persons have difficulty with community living.

- Select menu item "MOHO Related Resources"
- Link to "Other Instruments Based on MOHO" to access link to AMPS Project International Web site.

ADMINISTRATION

Administration and scoring of the AMPS takes 30 to 60 minutes. The therapist first interviews the client and/or the client's caregiver to ensure that the client will be observed doing things that he or she has experience with and that are relevant. The therapist then selects four or five of the standardized occupational forms/tasks that are of an appropriate level of difficulty and are relevant to the client. Next, the client chooses two or three that he or she will perform.

After observing the client's performance, the therapist scores the 16 motor and 20 process skill items and enters these scores into the computer. The AMPS computer program is used to generate AMPS instrumental activities of daily living (IADL) motor and process ability measures and a variety of reports that can be used for documentation, treatment planning, and research.

Assessment of Motor and Process Skills (AMPS)

- Gather's information about the motor and process skills that a person displays while engaging in occupation

- Information regarding AMPS training and assessment purchase can be found at AMPS Project International Web site, *http://www.ampsintl.com/*, or
  - Visit *www.moho.uic.edu*

Andrew

Using the AMPS to Generate Environmental Supports for Independence

Andrew is a 50-year-old man with moderate intellectual impairment and chronic back pain that he has experienced since being in a car accident some years ago. Andrew is very tall and obese. He was referred to the occupational therapist and other members of a multidisciplinary team by his family physician because of the concern that he was increasingly becoming unable to manage living independently.

Andrew had been living in a rented house in the countryside outside London for 10 years, since his immediate family members died. During this time, he managed to live in the house, but his living conditions were often marginal. He did not attempt to organize or maintain his home environment. He survived on prepared convenience foods purchased from a local supermarket—a diet that contributed to his obesity. He had no awareness of the value of the money that he had accumulated from his state benefit. He had become increasingly isolated, and his only access to support was via a neighbor who assisted him with financial matters such as paying his rent and other household bills. Andrew was increasingly facing situations he could not manage without help. His hygiene deteriorated. Moreover, he was growing more and more anxious about his situation.

Andrew identified that he had difficulty in carrying out many household chores. Among these were building the coal fire that heated his house and getting into the bath. The latter problem he perceived as due mainly to his back pain. Andrew was unemployed but had formerly worked as a farm and forestry laborer. He expressed a strong desire to learn better control of his environment and to have more social interaction. However, he was unsure as to whether or how this could be possible.

Choice and Use of the AMPS

Because Andrew was having difficulty performing his activities of daily living, the occupational therapist chose to use the AMPS to gather information on Andrew's motor and process skills. This assessment would also highlight his strengths and weaknesses in performing daily living tasks necessary for community living that he desired to improve.

The therapist identified five tasks of appropriate challenge for Andrew from the standard tasks available in the AMPS. From these, Andrew chose to perform three tasks: preparing a cheese sandwich, preparing a fresh fruit salad, and hand-washing dishes. He considered these occupational forms/tasks to be meaningful in his life.

The evaluation was carried out in the occupational therapy kitchen, as Andrew did not have all of the tools and equipment required for these tasks at home. Andrew engaged in a few practice sessions before the formal AMPS administration to allow him to become familiar and practiced in the activities and the environment.

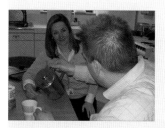

Based on his AMPS results, Andrew and his occupational therapist have tea so he can practice the motor skills stabilizing and gripping objects.

Results of the Evaluation

Andrew scored 2.0 on the motor skill scale and 1.1 on the process scale. Both scores indicate that he is on the borderline, where skill deficits begin to negatively impact on performance of daily living tasks and where the majority of people have difficulty with independent living.

AMPS also identified Andrew's adequate motor and process skills along with specific areas of difficulty during performance, as indicated in *Figure 15.1 A and B*.

Andrew demonstrated ineffective motor skills across all of his performance in the following areas:

- Positioning and bending the body appropriately to the task
- Coordinating two body parts to stabilize task objects
- Maintaining a secure grasp on task objects.

In the area of process skills, Andrew experienced difficulty in these areas:

- Choosing appropriate tools and materials
- Using objects according to their intended purpose
- Heeding (attending to the purpose of) the specific occupational form/task he was doing
- Inquiring about necessary information
- Initiating actions or steps without hesitation
- Organizing tools and materials in an orderly, logical, and spatially appropriate fashion
- Navigating (appropriately moving) his hands and body around objects
- Noticing and responding to nonverbal task-related environmental cues
- Accommodating his actions to overcome problems
- Benefiting from experience to prevent reoccurrence of problems.

Finally, his skill in restoring (i.e., putting away tools and materials or clearing work surfaces) was markedly deficient.

FIGURE 15.1A Andrew's strengths and problems observed during the administration of the AMPS.

Motor Skills			
Posture	**A**	**D**	**MD**
STABILIZING the body for balance	X		
ALIGNING the body in vertical position	X		
POSITIONING the body or arms appropriate to task		X	
Mobility	**A**	**D**	**MD**
WALKING: moving about the task environment (level surface)	X		
REACHING for task objects	X		
BENDING or rotating the body appropriate to the task		X	
Coordination	**A**	**D**	**MD**
COORDINATING two body parts to securely stabilize task objects		X	
MANIPULATING task objects	X		
FLOWS: executing smooth and fluid arm and hand movements	X		
Strength and Effort	**A**	**D**	**MD**
MOVES: pushing and pulling task objects or level surfaces or opening and closing doors or drawers	X		
TRANSPORTING task objects from one place to another	X		
LIFTING objects used during the task	X		
CALIBRATES: regulating the force and extent of movements	X		
GRIPS: maintaining a secure grasp on task objects		X	
Energy	**A**	**D**	**MD**
ENDURING for the duration of the task performance	X		
Maintaining an even and appropriate PACE during task performance	X		
Process Skills			
Energy	**A**	**D**	**MD**
Maintaining an even and appropriate PACE during task performance	X		
Maintaining focused ATTENTION throughout task performance	X		

Key: **A** = Adequate **D** = Difficulty **MD** = Markedly Deficient

FIGURE 15.1B

Process Skills			
Using Knowledge	**A**	**D**	**MD**
CHOOSING appropriate tools and materials needed for task performance		✗	
USING task objects according to their intended purposes		✗	
Knowing when and how to stabilize and support or HANDLE task objects	✗		
HEEDING the goal of the specified task		✗	
INQUIRES: asking for needed information		✗	
Temporal Organization	**A**	**D**	**MD**
INITIATING actions or steps of task without hesitation		✗	
CONTINUING actions through completion	✗		
Logically SEQUENCING the steps of the tasks	✗		
TERMINATING actions or steps at the appropriate time	✗		
Space and Objects	**A**	**D**	**MD**
SEARCHING for AND LOCATING tools and materials	✗		
GATHERING tools and materials into task workforce	✗		
ORGANIZING tools and materials in an orderly, logical, and spatially appropriate fashion		✗	
RESTORES: putting away tools and materials or straightening the workplace			✗
NAVIGATES: maneuvering the hand and body around obstacles	✗		
Adaptation	**A**	**D**	**MD**
NOTICING AND RESPONDING appropriately to nonverbal task-related environmental cues		✗	
ACCOMMODATES: modifying one's actions to overcome problems		✗	
ADJUSTS: changing the workspace to overcome problems	✗		
BENEFITS: preventing problems from recurring or persisting		✗	

Key: **A** = Adequate   **D** = Difficulty   **MD** = Markedly Deficient

Interpretation of the Results

In the area of motor skills, the following qualitative observations also were made during the AMPS assessment. Andrew used inappropriate biomechanical lifting techniques that combined with his old back injury impairment limited his ability to bend or lift from a low height. These problems were exacerbated by the fact that standard work surfaces were not ergonomically suitable for Andrew. Because of his physique, his body and arm positioning in relation to work surfaces and objects made performance difficult for him.

Andrew's problem with gripping objects appears related to his experience. The therapist determined through interviewing Andrew that he had mainly used gross motor skills in most of his lifetime occupations. Thus, his fine motor finger and hand function was not well developed, which limited his performance in occupational forms/tasks that required fine motor skill.

In the area of process skills, it was clear Andrew had problems in performing the newly learned tasks. For example, when preparing the sandwich, he did not incorporate some ingredients he had previously decided to include. When asked about this following the evaluation, Andrew said that he had "forgotten." This exemplifies Andrew's general difficulty with completing all of the steps or components of an occupational form/task. This same problem is echoed within other skill areas, such as restoration of objects to their original condition and location after finishing. Andrew also appeared to misinterpret or misunderstand some information that he received. This was made more problematic by the fact that Andrew did not seek clarification.

Andrew hesitated when beginning and during familiar tasks. He organized his workspace so that it was crammed. He used some tools in such a way that he could have injured himself. He generally had difficulty adapting to his environment and responding to environmental changes.

Despite Andrew's problems in both motor and process skills, he did have many adequate skills. These strengths indicated that he did not require assistance at all times during performance. Identification of Andrew's problem areas pointed to the specific kinds of supports that would allow him the opportunity and confidence to engage safely in routine occupational performance. By examining each area of weakness, the therapist was able to identify and implement corresponding strategies of environmental support.

Usefulness of the Information for Therapeutic Reasoning

With the information provided by the motor scale, the occupational therapist was able to make specific recommendations that Andrew's environment be suitably adapted to accommodate his motor needs. His motor skills problems were linked to two factors:

- His use of poor body mechanics related to his back
- The lack of fit between household objects and his unusually large stature.

Consequently, the following strategies were undertaken to assist him. His kitchen was modified with consideration to his height. Household equipment was purchased and installed to limit difficult bending or lifting. For example, he purchased a front-loading washing machine, and his small refrigerator was elevated to waist height. His bathroom was altered to incorporate a walk-in shower and a raised toilet. His bed was modified to be suitably supportive and at the correct height. A chair to suit his stature was purchased. Finally, a referral was made to physiotherapy to teach him proper techniques and exercises for his back.

By identifying his weaknesses, the process scale highlighted Andrew's need for regular assistance with some tasks and prompting with others, as well as the need for support for problem solving when faced with difficult or novel situations. The following resources were developed to address these ongoing needs. The occupational therapist and community support worker developed protocols for empowering Andrew to carry out tasks as independently as possible but within his skill capacity. For example, they created pictorial shopping lists, recipe cards, and telephone number lists. Methods of carrying out the routine things that Andrew did were developed to consider his process skills. The information generated about process skills identified strengths and weaknesses Andrew would bring to performance and thereby pointed to environmental supports he would need. For example, tending to the fire that heated his home was split into component parts; Andrew does what he safely can, and his care worker completes the other parts.

Andrew also attended a community group run by the occupational therapist and community nurse to address issues of safety at home. Furthermore, with support Andrew enrolled in a basic literacy college course. As Andrew gained awareness of his own capacities, his sense of efficacy improved significantly. With the regular support he received at home, he was able to function safely and with a reasonable degree of independence.

As this case illustrates, the AMPS provides critical objective information concerning occupational performance that guides therapists in making decisions about therapy. It is also useful for documenting the need for resources that enable persons to perform in the community. The comprehensiveness and precision of the AMPS in providing detailed and research-based information makes it an important asset in understanding and meeting a client's performance needs.

Assessment of Communication and Interaction Skills

The Assessment of Communication and Interaction Skills (ACIS) is a formal observational tool designed to measure an individual's performance in an occupational form/task within a social group (Forsyth et al., 1998). The instrument allows occupational therapists to determine a client's strengths and weaknesses in interacting and communicating with others in the course of daily occupations. The ACIS has been developed for use in a wide range of settings.

ACIS observations are carried out in contexts that are meaningful and relevant to the clients' lives. Because social situations cannot be standardized with the same precision as solitary occupational forms/tasks, such as those used in the AMPS, the ACIS does not adjust scores for the type of social group or task in which the person is observed. Rather, a format exists for classifying the context of observation and its degree of approximation to the kind of everyday social situations in which the client wants to or does perform. The therapist seeks to make observations in the client's actual environment or in contexts that resemble the client's environment as much as possible. The group context can range from a dyadic interaction to participation in a large group. A wide range of group contexts can be used for observation. These include task-oriented groups, meetings, work teams, games, and other leisure events.

The ACIS contains a single scale that consists of 20 skill items divided into 3 communication and interaction domains: physicality, information exchange, and relations. The items are rated on a four-point scale similar to that of the AMPS but with a focus on the impact of the skills on both the progression of the social interaction and occupational form/task and on other persons with whom the client interacts. For example, the scale considers whether others are made comfortable, appropriately informed, and helped by the actions of the client. Because the rating of communication and interaction requires judgment about appropriateness to the social context, the therapist using the scale must have social competence to understand the norms and expectations of the context.

Although formal development of the instrument has centered on clients with psychiatric impairments, the instrument has been successfully used with clients who have a wide range of impairments. The ACIS is used when a client appears to have difficulty in communication and interaction or when the client reports such difficulty. Research to date has focused on adolescents and adults, but the scale appears to be appropriate for children who are at the age when the full range of basic communication and interaction skills are ordinarily developed (i.e., older than 3–4 years).

Administration

The ACIS is supported by a detailed manual designed to instruct and guide the therapist in its use (Forsyth et al., 1998). The manual provides criteria for applying the rating to each item, supported by examples. The therapist begins by interviewing the client (or a significant other) to ascertain what types of contexts would be appropriate and meaningful for observing the client. To administer the ACIS, the occupational therapist observes clients' communication and social interaction while they engage with others as part of completing an occupational form/task. The observing therapist can be the group leader or a participant. Therefore, the ACIS can be administered during a therapeutic group.

The total administration time for the ACIS varies from 20 to 60 minutes. Observation time ranges from 15 to 45 minutes. The rating is completed after conclusion of the session. Rating time ranges from 5 to 20 minutes depending on the amount of qualitative comment the therapist wishes to enter into the form. It may be possible to observe more than one person during an observation session; however, the dependability of doing so has not yet been examined in research.

In its current state of development, the ACIS is most effectively used to generate a profile of strengths and weaknesses and qualitative details about any client's problems. This profile is the most important source of information for deciding what skills to target for change. In addition, the qualitative information gained in the course of administering the ACIS is often helpful for understanding why a particular client is having difficulty with some communication or interaction skills. A final use of the ACIS is to identify social environments with the most positive impact on the client's communication and interaction. ACIS scores vary with the environmental context, and the more supportive contexts will produce higher scores. Such information can be useful in deciding what kinds of group assignment or living placement is best for a client.

Assessment of Communication and Interaction Skills (ACIS)

- Gathers information about the communication skills that a person displays while engaged in occupation
- Can be ordered through the MOHO Clearinghouse e-store *http://ascendant.cas.uic.edu/retail/*, or
  - Visit *www.moho.uic.edu*
  - Select menu item "MOHO Products"
  - Link to ACIS assessment for more information about the assessment and for example assessment forms. To link to the MOHO Clearinghouse e-store, left-click on the "Buy Now" button.

Stephen

Stephen is a 19-year-old British university student. He has Asperger's syndrome and has difficulties in communication and interaction skills. He did well in his studies at school, particularly in science and mathematics. He has an interest in computers and was proud of being allowed into an information technology course. However, he struggled with being away from home for the first time, and he found the changes both in routine and in peer students challenging. He did not do as well as expected in his first semester examinations. Stephen gradually withdrew from classes and returned home. His parents, worried by Stephen's low mood and his increased anxiety and obsessive behaviors, sought support from a local community mental health team.

Selecting the ACIS

Following initial assessment, the occupational therapist set goals with Stephen, who very much wanted to return to university to study. He decided to transfer to the university in his home city. In the interim, he agreed to pursue some voluntary work to maintain an active routine and a productive role, both of which he identified as important. Because Stephen identified socializing with peers as an area of difficulty, the occupational therapist completed the ACIS with him. Results are detailed in *Figure 15.2*.

Interpretation of the ACIS

The occupational therapist rated in the ACIS in two environmental contexts (i.e., making lunch with peers in an unfamiliar environment and eating lunch with peers in a familiar context). The ACIS observations revealed that Stephen tended to become distracted from the occupation at hand when he focused on socializing, and conversely, his communication skills deteriorated when he focused on the occupation. He had difficulty maintaining a dual orientation to what he and the others were doing while also communicating and interacting effectively with his peers. For example, while engaging in the collaborative task of preparing a meal, Stephen moved away from the other group members to work on the sidelines with his back to others. Thus, collaborative

FIGURE 15.2 Results of two ACIS observations with Stephen.

	Observation while working in collaborative group preparing lunch in an unfamiliar environment.				Observation while in familiar environment eating lunch with peers.			
Physicality								
Contacts	1	2	3	**4**	1	2	3	**4**
Gazes	**1**	2	3	4	1	**2**	3	4
Gestures	1	**2**	3	4	1	**2**	3	4
Maneuvers	**1**	2	3	4	1	2	**3**	4
Orients	**1**	2	3	4	1	2	3	**4**
Postures	1	**2**	3	4	1	2	3	**4**
Information Exchange								
Articulates	1	2	3	**4**	1	2	3	**4**
Asserts	1	2	3	**4**	1	2	3	**4**
Asks	1	**2**	3	4	1	**2**	3	4
Engages	**1**	2	3	4	**1**	2	3	4
Expresses	**1**	2	3	4	**1**	2	3	4
Modulates	1	**2**	3	4	1	**2**	3	4
Shares	1	**2**	3	4	1	**2**	3	4
Speaks	1	2	3	**4**	1	2	3	**4**
Sustains	**1**	2	3	4	**1**	2	3	4
Relations								
Collaborates	**1**	2	3	4	1	**2**	3	4
Conforms	**1**	2	3	4	1	**2**	3	4
Focuses	**1**	2	3	4	1	**2**	3	4
Relates	**1**	2	3	4	1	**2**	3	4
Respects	**1**	2	3	4	1	**2**	3	4

Key: 4 = Competent   3 = Questionable   2 = Ineffective   1 = Deficit

group activities were more challenging for him than parallel activities such as eating.

Stephen also showed difficulties in the following areas independent of the type of environment. He lacked non-verbal communication and had difficulty initiating and sustaining conversations. He appeared unaware of the expectations of others in conversations. The occupational therapist also noticed that others appeared un- comfortable in Stephen's company. In part this reflected his tendency to be very direct in his criticisms of others and to divulge personal information beyond what was normative.

Using the ACIS Results

After receiving feedback on these findings from the ACIS assessment, Stephen agreed to join a social skills program. He focused on learning strategies for engaging and sustaining appropriate conversations and being more aware of subtle social norms. In order to try out and practice the skills he is learning in a supportive environment Stephen also joined two groups organized by the occupational therapist; a football group and a gym group. Stephen and the occupational therapist review the groups each week to discuss skills he has used during the sessions from each of their perspectives.

As his confidence grew, Stephen felt ready to progress toward his goal of volunteering. The local volunteer coordinator met with Stephen and the occupational therapist to discuss opportunities. They identified a local charity that needed support with office administration and typing. The post involved routine tasks of photocopying and filing, as well as setting up a database. Stephen felt confident that his skills would be useful in this setting and agreed to begin volunteer work there.

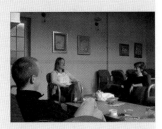

Stephen chats with other volunteers in the break room.

At his next appointment with the occupational therapist, Stephen remarked that the volunteer placement was not suiting him and he was thinking of leaving. The occupational therapist asked if she could visit him at work to observe his problems. On the visit the occupational therapist identified that the job was different from the profile provided by the volunteer coordinator. Stephen was expected to carry out duties as required, and these were often tasks done in cooperation with other volunteers. Stephen and the occupational therapist decided to speak with the office manager. The occupational therapist used the ACIS results to explain to the manager how Stephen can be supported to function at his best, highlighting that Stephen finds it difficult to socialize while working on tasks. The manager was apologetic, explaining that the team had been involving Stephen in team tasks intending to make him feel welcome. They agreed to revert to the original plan.

Stephen, the manager, and the occupational therapist worked out a variety of tasks and routines for the volunteer work. At their next meeting, Stephen advised the occupational therapist that he was much happier in his placement. In addition to feeling that he was contributing to the work of the charity, he reported that he was getting along well with his colleagues at break times.

A few months before the next academic term started the occupational therapist and Stephen visited the university support services. They discovered that an introduction to study course was being offered in the summer. Stephen felt that this course would be of benefit, allowing him to become familiar with the university campus before the semester started. He was also hopeful that he would get to meet other students. Thus, he chose to enroll in it.

As this case illustrates, the ACIS can be helpful in providing detailed information about the kinds of challenges clients face in interaction and communication. This information is useful to the therapist in planning intervention. It can also be used to provide feedback to clients and to consult with others who may need to accommodate or support the client's communication and interaction skills.

Volitional Questionnaire and Pediatric Volitional Questionnaire

Volitional Questionnaire

The Volitional Questionnaire (VQ) is appropriate for any individual for whom self-report assessment of volition is not readily feasible (e.g., individuals with dementia or brain damage or persons with extreme volitional problems due to environmental stresses or social traumas). The VQ is based on the recognition that clients who have difficulty formulating goals or expressing their interests and values verbally routinely communicate them through actions. For example, persons indicate interest by how much energy they direct to doing something or the affect they display while doing it. Thus, the VQ scale is composed of 14 items that describe behaviors reflecting values, interests, and personal causation. The items are scored using a four-point rating (passive, hesitant, involved, and spontaneous). The rating indicates the extent to which the client readily exhibits volitional behaviors versus the amount of support, encouragement, and structure that is necessary to elicit them. The scale reflects the fact that persons with higher volition choose action and demonstrate positive affect more readily, whereas persons with more limited volition need additional environmental resources and supports.

The VQ recognizes that a client's motivation may vary in different environments according to how much the features of each environment match the client's interests, values, and personal causation. Consequently, clients are often observed in more than a single context. An environmental form can be used to record information about relevant features of the environment that influence volition.

Research on the VQ (Chern, Kielhofner, de las Heras, & Magalhaes, 1996) shows that the items on the scale are ordered in a particular sequence from less to more volition. This sequence indicates a volitional continuum that begins with basic behaviors such as being able to indicate preferences and initiate action. Higher levels of volition are indicated by the client's willingness to try to solve problems or correct mistakes and in the display of pride. The highest level of volition is indicated by such behaviors as seeking challenges and new responsibilities. Practical experience with the VQ indicates that a client's improvement in volition ordinarily reflects the sequence of lower to higher volition. A specific intervention protocol, the remotivation process, has been developed for persons with volitional problems (de las Heras, Llerena, & Kielhofner, 2003). This protocol involves constant use of the VQ to guide intervention and monitor the client's progress.

ADMINISTRATION

The VQ is supported by a detailed manual that discusses the purpose and uses of the VQ and describes the administration protocol in detail (de las Heras, Geist, Kielhofner, & Li, 2003). Each of the items on the VQ scale is explained in terms of what it is intended to capture. Guidelines for rating each item are supported by multiple examples. The manual is designed for therapists who wish to learn administration of the VQ through self study.

Occupational therapists administer this scale by observing and rating patients while they engage in work, leisure, or daily living tasks. As noted above, the four-point rating indicates the amount of volitional spontaneity (versus passivity or need for support and encouragement) the individual demonstrates. Because of the nature of the rating scale, the observing therapist can provide support and structure if it is necessary to elicit volition. This feature of the VQ means that it can be administered as part of a therapy session and that it can be used to explore what kind of environmental supports enhance a given client's volition.

The therapist may make more than a single observation. The strategies for selecting the context(s) of observation vary with each client, but the underlying goals are to identify these factors:

- Those factors in the social and physical environment that most affect volition both positively and negatively
- How stable or variable volition is across environments
- The level of motivation a client typically displays
- The kinds of environmental supports that enhance the individual's volition
- The client's interests and values.

This kind of information allows the therapist to determine the environmental contexts and strategies that will facilitate positive development of the individual's volition.

In addition to completing the environmental form and the rating scale, therapists can conclude by writing a brief narrative that describes these factors:

- The client's interests and values
- The amount and kind of support required for the client to accomplish a behavior
- The influence of values, interests, and personal causation on the client's motivation to engage in activities
- The influence of different environments on the client's volition.

Observation periods ordinarily last approximately 15 to 30 minutes. The scale and the environmental form can be completed in less than 10 minutes. Because the assessment can be administered as part of a therapy session in which the environment is systematically varied, it can be used efficiently to explore how different environmental factors influence volition. The VQ is useful for monitoring volitional change over time, and it can be taught to clients, when appropriate, to monitor their own motivational level.

Grace

Grace is 89. She has lived in the American Midwest in a continuing care retirement community for the past 5 years. She moved to the retirement community approximately 5 years after her husband died. It is in the hometown where Grace grew up and close to one of her younger sisters. This was a major move, since she had lived for 30 years in Arizona. Grace is the second eldest of 12 children, and the age difference between Grace and the sister who now lives nearby is nearly 17 years.

Grace was unable to have children. Having a family was important to her, and she talked regularly about the loss she felt with not being able to have children. She has been married three times. Her first husband died unexpectedly after 5 years of marriage, and her second marriage ended in divorce after 3 years. Her third marriage, to a psychiatrist, lasted over 30 years. Her third husband had Alzheimer's disease, and Grace served as his primary caregiver for 5 years. Grace was a psychiatric nurse for nearly 40 years, and she met her third husband in the veterans hospital where they worked. She expressed great satisfaction with her work role and was very proud of the fact that she returned to school in her 40s to obtain a bachelor of science in nursing degree.

Although she initiated the move to the retirement community, Grace's adjustment was not easy. She had a great deal of distress, frequently calling and berating her sister, claiming inaccurately that the sister had made Grace move. Initially perplexed by Grace's behavior, the sister slowly began to recognize signs of cognitive deterioration in Grace. Grace was diagnosed with dementia by her primary care practitioner after nearly 4 years of living in her own apartment at the retirement commu-

nity. Following a second major fall (the first resulting in a right hip fracture and the second causing a left humeral fracture), it was determined that Grace would benefit from living in the secure assisted-living section for residents with memory impairments. She had been on this unit for nearly a year when consultation with occupational therapy was requested to assist Grace to better adjust to the unit. She was often isolative, depressed, suspicious, and argumentative with staff.

Grace was independently mobile on unit, using a wheeled walker while being able to walk short distances safely without it. However, she would often park her walker, walk away, and then be unable to find it. Grace was able to complete all of her self-care with reminders and verbal cues to identify and correct errors. Grace used the phone in her room to call her sister independently but often made mistakes with dialing out and asked staff for assistance with placing calls to her sister. Grace often called her sister in the middle of the night, particularly when she was distressed or angry.

Her adjustment to the unit was difficult. Grace kept to herself mostly, isolating from other residents and staying in her room much of the time. She came to meals with reminders and coaxing and rarely participated in any of the activities on the unit. When she was out of her room, she tended to pace, and often went outside to the enclosed patio. Her mood varied from depressed to angry and suspicious. Grace previously received short-term rehabilitation services for her two fractures. Her sister reported that Grace did not participate well in therapy either time. She became increasingly upset and suspicious each time, refusing treatment and requiring discharge from services.

Just before the request for occupational therapy consultation, Grace expressed suicidal thoughts when her sister and brother-in-law went out of town on a short vacation. Staff reported that since this incident, Grace's mood was still depressed but not suicidal. Just after Grace's suicidal episode, a nurse obtained a 6-week-old kitten for Grace, hoping this would help Grace "take her mind off her troubles." Grace had been caring for the kitten approximately a month when the occupational therapist completed the Volitional Questionnaire (VQ) as part of the consultation.

Administration of the VQ

The VQ was done during a 30-minute visit in which the therapist visited with Grace and the kitten in Grace's room. This activity was chosen to build trust with Grace. Also, by using an environment where Grace was comfortable, the therapist hoped to discover Grace's volitional strengths. To supplement information gathered with the VQ, the occupational therapist also gathered information on Grace's current behavior and past history using unstructured interviews with unit staff and Grace's sister and by informally observing Grace on the unit. It was noted in the VQ and other interactions with Grace that although her verbal skills were better preserved than those of many other residents on the unit, she often repeated herself and retold several recurring stories about her past. These communications provided to be helpful insights about her values, as the themes in her stories were consistent, focused on the importance of family relationships, independence, and her desire to be her "own person." When interacting with her kitten, Grace repeatedly stated she liked cats because "They are their own person. No one owns them."

Interpretation of the VQ

In the VQ (*Fig. 15.3*), all of Grace's involved and spontaneous scores occurred as Grace interacted with her kitten. It was apparent that Grace readily adopted the role of caring for the kitten, always referring to herself as "mommy." She could not recall the name that staff initially gave to the kitten, and instead called her kitten "baby" or "sweetie." Her motivation to care for the kitten was strong and spontaneous. For instance, she always brought food from her meals back to the kitten. Grace's memory deficits caused her anxiety over caring for the kitten. She worried that the kitten had no food or that it had escaped from her room. She demonstrated motivation to solve problems and always sought help from the staff when she perceived the kitten needed something that she could not provide. Grace often attempted to care for the kitten's litter box, resulting frequently in a clogged toilet and the box being moved around her room. Nonetheless, this behavior also showed her desire to provide care and her engagement with the kitten. The kitten's spontaneity and playfulness created a natural motivator for Grace and provided a new meaningful occupation for her.

Because of her sensory and cognitive impairments, Grace had little volitional continuity from her previous interests in games (cards, bingo, and going to casinos) and traveling. While her sister stated that Grace was always well dressed and that she loved to be pampered with manicures and doing her makeup, Grace said that she "did not like to be fussed over." The therapist wondered whether this comment indicated a change in her interests. Through using the VQ and other observation, it became apparent that Grace's social discomfort drove this comment. Soon, participating in manicures became the main activity that Grace was willing to engage in with the therapist. This insight highlights how behavioral observations and using the VQ can sort out the difference between expressed preferences and willingness to engage in and try new things. Through the VQ, additional observations, and interviews with her sister and staff, the following volitional strengths were noted for Grace:

- Grace was motivated by her values of independence and being in relationships, and the kitten provided a natural opportunity to exercise these values through developing her parenting relationship with the kitten.
- Grace responded well to having her feelings validated in a trusting relationship.
- Grace's volition was enhanced when the social environment supported her sense of efficacy and honored her values.

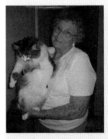

Grace affectionately cuddles with her kitten.

Grace's volitional weaknesses were seen in her lowered sense of capacity, her beliefs that she was unable to participate in past interests, and her loss of control and sense of despair in coping with the changes in her physical environment. While Grace verbally expressed a lack of attraction to some occupa-

FIGURE 15.3 Results of Grace's Volitional Questionnaire observation.

Client: Grace					Therapist:	
Age: 89		Gender: M (F)			Date:	
Diagnosis: Dementia					Facility:	
Visiting: Sharing magazine & playing with kitten					**Comments**	
Shows curiosity	P	H	(I)	S	Actively watched kitten play, followed kitten's spontaneous movements when pointed out to her	
Initiates actions/tasks	P	H	(I)	S	Reached for magazine when offered and encouraged	
Tries new things	P	(H)	I	S	Declined looking at magazine pictures when offered	
Shows pride	P	H	I	(S)	Expressed pride in her ownership and care of the kitten	
Seeks challenges	(P)	H	I	S	Did not attempt to create play with kitten even after a demonstration	
Seeks additional responsibilities	(P)	H	I	S	No effort to show therapist kitten's arrangement in her room (even after... see above)	
Tries to correct mistakes/failures	(P)	H	I	S	Did not try to clean up kitten's water bowl after she accidentally kicked it	
Tries to solve problems	P	H	I	(S)	Moved kitten from nightstand to prevent knocking over lamp	
Shows preferences	P	(H)	I	S	With prompts, chose one picture over another in magazine	
Pursues an activity to completion/ accomplishment	(P)	H	I	S	No effort to review contents of magazine with therapist, even with prompts and invitations	
Stays engaged	P	H	(I)	S	Interacted with kitten each time it approached her	
Invests additional energy/emotion/attention	(P)	H	I	S	Did not make an effort to keep up with kitten as it explored	
Indicates goals	(P)	H	I	S	Unable to indicate any goals even when encouraged and instead made negative comments about growing old	
Shows that an activity is special or significant	P	H	I	(S)	Laughing and smiling when playing with kitten, concerned that kitten "behave"	

Key: P = Passive   H = Hesitant   I = Involved   S = Spontaneous

tions, these comments were driven by her depression and cognitive impairments and contradicted some things that she still was interested in pursuing. Behavioral observations as captured in the VQ helped

identify these remaining interests. When Grace did not feel supported, she became more suspicious and at times paranoid and therefore had great difficulty directing and showing interest and investment in doing things, resulting in her isolating herself in her room. The staff often interpreted this behavior as her choice, and if Grace declined encouragement from staff to come out of her room, and join in, staff would leave her alone. The staff's perception was that pushing her made her feel more paranoid.

Use of the VQ in Consultation

The therapist shared the findings of the VQ with staff and recommended changing their approach with Grace. Instead of encouraging her to come out of her room, staff were directed to talk with Grace about her major life interests, current and past. They were also guided in how to build trust with Grace more effectively by supporting her sense of efficacy and honoring her values in their interactions. Staff found that these strategies of interaction proved much more effective in drawing Grace out and reducing her negative behaviors. Moreover, as the kitten grew, its desire to explore the environment beyond their room created opportunities for Grace to connect more with others and decreased her isolative behavior. Her depression and suspiciousness gradually faded, and Grace began to increase her interactions with residents and staff spontaneously, and she appeared to feel more in control of her choices for doing things. Caring for her kitten and visiting remain her valued occupations.

Volitional Questionnaire (VQ) and Pediatric Volitional Questionnaire (PVQ)

- Gather information about volition (motivation) and about the effect of the environment on volition
- Can be ordered through the MOHO Clearinghouse e-store *http://ascendant.cas.uic.edu/retail/*, or
  - Visit www.moho.uic.edu
  - Select menu item "MOHO Products"
  - Link to VQ or PVQ assessment links for more information about each assessment and example assessment forms. To link to the MOHO Clearinghouse e-store, left-click on the "Buy Now" button.

Pediatric Volitional Questionnaire

The Pediatric Volitional Questionnaire (PVQ) (Basu, Kafkes, Geist, & Kielhofner, 2002) is an observational assessment similar to the VQ. It intends to capture a younger child's volition. The PVQ was originally developed for and studied on children aged 2 to 6 years. In practice, many clinicians find it useful for older children and even adolescents who have significant developmental delays.

The items on the PVQ parallel many of those on the VQ, but the items are designed to be developmentally appropriate to younger children. This accounts for the practical relevance of the tool to clients who are chronologically older than 6 years but developmentally suited for the assessment. Like the VQ, the items are rated on a four-point scale (passive, hesitant, involved, and spontaneous). By systematically capturing how children react to and act within their environments, the PVQ provides both insight into the child's motivation and information about how the environment supports or constrains the child's volition.

Children with cognitive or motor problems that limit their ability to act on the world need support in the development of their volition. However, their volition is ordinarily the most difficult to understand. When children are unable to express their likes, dislikes, confidence, or fears, there is a greater challenge to understand how they are motivated. Nonetheless, a great deal can be learned about children's motives by observing how they go about doing things. Withdrawal, enthusiasm, hesitation, and persistence are all examples of observable behavior patterns that reveal important things about a child's volition. By providing a means of systematically observing such behavior patterns, the PVQ yields a picture of a child's volition.

The PVQ is also designed to gather information on how the environment influences the child's volition. An environmental form is used to systematically record information on the environments in which the child is observed. Use of the PVQ ordinarily involves observation of the child in different contexts to determine environmental impacts on volition. Alternatively, the therapist may create different conditions within therapy to examine how different conditions in the environment affect the child's volition. With such information, the therapist can alter or make recommendations for altering the physical and social environment to maximize the child's desire for action and his or her feeling of accomplishment and enjoyment. The PVQ also provides qualitative information that can be used in designing treatment programs and interventions as well as for providing feedback and suggestions to parents, teachers, and other caregivers.

ADMINISTRATION

The PVQ is explained in a detailed manual that discusses its purpose, uses, and administration protocol (Basu et al., 2002). Each of the items on the PVQ scale is explained in terms of what it is intended to capture. Guidelines for rating each item are supported by examples. Notably, the examples in this manual include children with a wide range of function. Therefore, the PVQ can readily be applied to children with a wide array of impairments. The manual is designed for therapists who wish to learn administration of the PVQ through self study. A videotape is also available for therapists to observe and practice the rating procedure.

The PVQ consists of a 14-item rating scale that systematically captures information about the child's volition. In addition to the rating scale, there are forms for collecting information on features of the environment that affect volition and on the child's volitionally influenced style of interacting with the environment.

The therapist begins application of the assessment with observation of the child in play and/or self-care. It is recommended that the therapist observe the child in various contexts to determine how differing environmental factors affect the child's volition. Appropriate settings include the classroom, home, playroom, playground, and clinic. The therapist ordinarily observes the child for 15 to 30 minutes in each context.

After the observation, the therapist completes the rating scale and if desired adds qualitative comments to this scale. These comments ordinarily explain the rationale for or elaborate the ratings that were assigned to the child. At the bottom of the PVQ scale, the therapist summarizes main issues relevant to the child's volition. The PVQ includes forms for systematic consideration of how different contexts influence the child's volition.

Freddie

Freddie is a boy aged 5 years 3 months who will be moving from early childhood (EC) special education services to elementary school. Freddie has been receiving occupational therapy since birth to address functional limitations due a brain infection and resulting cognitive impairments. He is in good health. He wears an ankle–foot orthosis on his right leg and receives gastronomy feedings with supplemental oral feedings. Freddie shows little desire to accept spoon feedings, participate in dressing, play with toys, or work at the table. He prefers to interact with adults and peers and explore his environment by climbing on furniture, walking, and attempting to run. Freddie's teacher reports that he rarely sits down. In addition, he doesn't tolerate coloring at the table or being read to. Freddie's expressive and receptive language is delayed. However, he is able to say, "ma ma ma" when he is upset and responds when his name is called. Freddie is a happy boy who is always smiling and enjoys music.

Rationale for Using the PVQ

The elementary school special education team reviewed reports provided by the EC providers. Although these reports provided information regarding Freddie's developmental skills and abilities, they did little to shed light on Freddie as an individual or as an occupational being. The team thought, given his complex medical history and the breadth of his needs, that more information was warranted to make the transition to elementary school an easy one for Freddie. The team was especially curious to learn more about Freddie's participation in activities that have been problematic for other new students in the past, such as snack or lunch time and circle time. In an effort to develop a child-centered and truly individualized educational plan, the special education program supervisor recommended that a member of the team observe Freddie in his EC classroom. The occupational therapist volunteered and recommended that she complete the PVQ to gain insight into Freddie's volition and to identify the best ways to support him in his school program.

Administration of the PVQ

The occupational therapist visited Freddie's classroom twice to complete the PVQ. She watched as Freddie interacted with his teacher and the classroom assistant. During the observation session, Freddie smiled, attempted to engage the occupational therapist in interactions on numerous occasions, and did not appear bothered by her presence.

Snack Time Observation

The first observation took place in Freddie's classroom during snack time. During the 20-minute observation, Freddie struggled to remain seated at the child-sized table and was frequently redirected back to his seat. Approximately 5 minutes into the observation, the teacher requested that the classroom assistant help Freddie to sit in a chair with a seat belt. When directed to this chair, Freddie sat down independently and waited as the belt was fastened as if this was routine for him. After the belt was fastened, Freddie tapped the table, swung his feet, and made vocalizations directed to the other children.

Throughout the session, the teacher encouraged Freddie to drink juice out of a paper cup and eat a cookie. Freddie happily smiled at the other children and tried to grab for their snack items, which were out of reach. He turned his head away from items that were presented to him by the teacher. On one occasion he appeared to gag. When the teacher turned her attention away from Freddie to address another student, he grabbed at a plate of nearby cheese crackers and attempted to place a handful in his mouth. The teacher turned her attention back to Freddie before he was able to actually put the crackers in his mouth. She removed the cheese crackers from his hand and placed them on the table. The teacher then picked up one cracker and tried to feed it to Freddie. Freddie again turned his head away from the teacher and did not accept the food.

When presented with juice in a paper cup, Freddie became excited, picked it up, and crushed it. Freddie laughed as the juice spilled onto the table and his arm. He licked the juice off his arm as the teacher tried to clean up the mess as quickly as possible. The second time Freddie was given juice, the teacher held the paper cup and presented it to him. Freddie turned away from

the teacher. After this attempt, the teacher told Freddie that he was "all done" and turned her attention to another student. Freddie continued to sit at the table in the seat belt chair and smile and vocalize to his classmates.

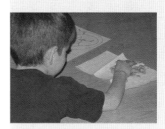

Once his teacher is pre-occupied, Freddie reaches for some nearby cheese crackers.

Circle Time Observation

The second observation took place in Freddie's classroom during circle time. The children were cued that circle time was starting when the teacher rang a bell. When Freddie heard the bell he immediately stopped playing at the water table and ran to his place on the carpet. The classroom assistant chased after Freddie with a towel to wipe his hands and provided him with assistance in removing his smock. Freddie rocked back and forth and clapped his hands rhythmically while waiting for the rest of the students to get to their places so that circle time could begin. Once all of the children arrived, the teacher led the class through a routine consisting of calendar activities and songs.

Freddie attended to the teacher as she led the class through the days of the week. During the observation Freddie stood up in his spot, jumped up and down, and began rocking side to side. The classroom assistant patted the ground and Freddie returned to a seated position. This occurred on two occasions. Freddie made eye contact and smiled at peers and adults alike. He vocalized during the songs and tapped a student sitting next to him as if to share his excitement. He required hand over hand assistance to hold a tambourine and shake it during a song. During this time Freddie made eye contact and smiled at the classroom assistant who was assisting him.

When the teacher began to read a book, Freddie again stood up. He walked over to the book and attempted to turn the pages. The classroom assistant brought him back to his area on the carpet and encouraged him to look at the book. Freddie again got up and

FIGURE 15.4 Freddie's PVQ ratings and summary.

Session I   Date: 1-5-06   Setting: Classroom-Snack time

Shows curiosity	Initiates actions	Task directed	Shows preferences	Tries new things	Stays engaged	Expresses mastery pleasure	Tries to solve problems	Tries to produce effects	Practices skill	Seeks challenges	Modifies environment	Pursues activity to completion	Uses imagination
(S)	**(S)**	S	**(S)**	**(S)**	S	S	S	S	S	S	S	S	S
I	I	I	I	I	I	I	**(I)**	**(I)**	**(I)**	**(I)**	I	I	I
H	H	**(H)**	H	H	**(H)**	**(H)**	H	H	H	H	H	**(H)**	H
P	P	P	P	P	P	P	P	P	P	P	**(P)**	P	**(P)**

Session II   Date: 1-9-06   Setting: Classroom-Circle time

Shows curiosity	Initiates actions	Task directed	Shows preferences	Tries new things	Stays engaged	Expresses mastery pleasure	Tries to solve problems	Tries to produce effects	Practices skill	Seeks challenges	Modifies environment	Pursues activity to completion	Uses imagination
(S)	**(S)**	**(S)**	**(S)**	**(S)**	**(S)**	S	S	S	S	S	S	S	S
I	I	I	I	I	I	**(I)**	I	**(I)**	**(I)**	I	I	**(I)**	I
H	H	H	H	H	H	H	**(H)**	H	H	**(H)**	H	H	H
P	P	P	P	P	P	P	P	P	P	P	**(P)**	P	**(P)**

Key: P = Passive   H = Hesitant   I = Involved   S = Spontaneous

Summary:

 Strengths:
  Shows curiosity
  Initiates actions
  Shows preferences
  Tries new things

 Needs support:
  Remain task directed (snack time)
  Stay engaged (snack time)
  Practice skills (snack time and circle time)

 Other notes:
  Freddie did not appear to engage in any behavior that would suggest that he
  intended to modify the environment or use imagination

moved toward the book. This time the teacher told the classroom assistant to take Freddie back to the water table so that he could play there.

Interpretation of PVQ Findings and Recommendations

After the two observations, the occupational therapist shared her findings (*Fig. 15.4*) with the elementary school special education team. She indicated that two primary differences were noted between the observations. First was the manner in which Freddie accepted assistance from the classroom staff and practiced skills. Over the course of the observation, Freddie demonstrated the ability to show preferences and practice skills. He was not given the opportunity to feed himself during snack time. The behavior he exhibited, such as turning his head away from food that was presented to him by the teacher and grabbing at the snack items of his peers, suggested that he was interested in feeding himself and not in being fed. Other observations, such as Freddie's desire to hold the cup himself and take a drink, support this notion as well. Freddie's reaction may be due in part to the fact that he is primarily fed through a gastronomy tube. Based on his history, it may be assumed that Freddie might have had negative experiences related to oral feeding, as well as invasive medical procedures that might lead to aversion. Despite a possible aversion to orally presented nutrition, Freddie tried to practice self-feeding skills but was not supported. He was stopped from feeding himself crackers. Further, he was not given an additional chance to drink from a cup independently.

The therapist concluded that Freddie would benefit from the opportunity to practice self-feeding skills with preferred food items. The teacher could present two food items, such as cheese crackers and cookies, and allow Freddie to choose by reaching toward a particular item. Because the teacher is concerned about Freddie putting too much food in his mouth at a time, she could place one food item in front of him at a time. This would control his intake, but also support his desire to feed himself. The therapist also recommended that the team should explore a sturdy plastic cup, perhaps with a straw or sippy lid, to support Freddie's desire to drink independently.

The second difference between the two observations was Freddie's ability to remain task directed and engaged. Freddie required external support, the seat belt chair, to do this during snack time. However, he was able to remain in the carpet area during calendar time without external support and only needed a few reminders to sit down. It is possible that his desire to stay engaged and task directed is a result of the degree to which the individuals in his context support his preferences and his desire to practice and master skills.

The therapist recommended that Freddie be allowed to feed himself in a typical classroom chair before requiring that he use a seat belt chair. He has demonstrated the ability to remain engaged and task directed previously without such a constraint. In addition, she recommended that classroom staff alter their expectations of Freddie during snack time or lunchtime and that they consider affording Freddie the opportunity to stand up, move around, and return to the table with a verbal or visual cue, as observed in circle time.

The therapist predicted that Freddie would choose continued participation if allowed to practice skills. She recommended that besides letting him feed himself, the team should further support his participation during circle time. Freddie's attempts to turn the pages of the teacher's book demonstrate his innate curiosity, initiative, and willingness to be engaged in listening to the story. Given his limited language skills, this level of participation might be the most appropriate for him at this time. Thus the therapist recommended that Freddie be given an opportunity to act as the teacher's helper and perhaps turn the pages of the book.

As this case illustrates, the PVQ framed the occupational therapist's observations and allowed her to gain a richer understanding of Freddie's participation in school occupations. By using this assessment, the occupational therapist was able to contribute to the team's knowledge of Freddie. Data from the PVQ, combined with information related to skill development, supported the team in developing a unique and child-centered educational plan.

Conclusion

This chapter presented four assessments that use observation as a means of collecting information about clients. Two assessments provide important information about clients' motor, process, communication, and interaction skills. The two volitional assessments provide information about the client's motivation. All four assessments use rating scales to record the observations and allow qualitative information to be gathered as well. Although they do so in different ways, each of the assessments also takes into consideration the effects of the environment on the observed skill or volition.

References

Basu, S., & Kafkes, A., Geist, R., & Kielhofner, G. (2002). *The Pediatric Volitional Questionnaire (PVQ) (Version 2.0).* Chicago: Model of Human Occupation Clearinghouse, Department of Occupational Therapy, College of Applied Health Sciences, University of Illinois at Chicago.

Chern, J., Kielhofner, G., de las Heras, C. G., & Magalhaer, L. C. (1996). The Volitional Questionnaire: Psychometric development and practical use. *American Journal of Occupational Therapy, 50* (7), 515–525.

de las Heras, C. G., Geist, R., Kielhofner, G., & Li, Y. (2003). *The Volitional Questionnaire (VQ) (Version 4.0).* Chicago: Model of Human Occupation Clearinghouse, Department of Occupational Therapy, College of Applied Health Sciences, University of Illinois at Chicago.

de las Heras, C. G., Llerena, V., & Kielhofner, G. (2003). *Remotivation process: Progressive intervention for individuals with severe volitional challenges. (Version 1.0)* Chicago: Department of Occupational Therapy, University of Illinois at Chicago.

Fisher A. G. (2003). *Assessment of motor and process skills* (5th ed.). Ft. Collins, CO: Three Star.

Forsyth, K., Salamy, M., Simon, S., & Kielhofner, G. (1998). *The Assessment of Communication and Interaction Skills (version 4.0).* Chicago: Department of Occupational Therapy, University of Illinois at Chicago.

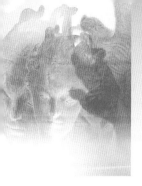

16

Self-Reports: Eliciting Clients' Perspectives

- Gary Kielhofner
- Kirsty Forsyth
- Meghan Suman
- Jessica Kramer
- Hiromi Nakamura-Thomas
- Takashi Yamada
- Júnia Rjeille Cordeiro
- Riitta Keponen
- Ay Woan Pan
- Alexis Henry

Clients are experts on their own lives. The assessments discussed in this chapter have been designed to capture this expertise, allowing clients to record information about themselves, their life circumstances, and their environments. These assessments give clients a voice in characterizing their lives and their desires. The very process of filling out these assessments often helps clients clarify their thoughts and feelings about their circumstances. Moreover, the use of client self-report actively engages clients in generating information that can influence the therapeutic process and support a client-driven approach to practice (Restall, Ripart, & Stern, 2003).

These self-report assessments are designed to be user friendly, and much focus has been placed on clarity of language, directions, and form design during the development of these assessments. The goal has been to make the self-reports accessible and meaningful across a variety of intervention contexts for clients with a range of abilities and needs. The use of self-report assessments has two benefits. First, clients often see re-

vealing patterns in their own responses that augment insight and support problem solving and planning. Second, the assessments are designed to be used as part of a dialogue between therapist and client that aims to generate a deeper understanding of the client's circumstances and to determine directions and strategies for therapy. Consequently, therapists should always discuss self report responses with the client to clarify both their meaning for the client and their significance for the direction therapy should take.

While these assessments are ordinarily administered as forms to be filled out independently by the client, therapists do administer them in different ways to accommodate needs of clients. For example, they are sometimes given verbally when clients have difficulty reading or writing. Sometimes they are used as part of a group planning or problem-solving exercise. Family members may report the information on the client's behalf if the client is incapable of reporting it.

The self-report instruments discussed in this chapter:

- The Modified Interest Checklist
- The Occupational Questionnaire (OQ) and NIH Activity Record (ACTRE)
- The Occupational Self-Assessment (OSA) and Child Occupational Self-Assessment (COSA)
- The Pediatric Interest Profiles (PIP)
- The Role Checklist.

With the exception of the Interest Checklist, which existed prior to the introduction of the model MOHO and was later modified, these assessments were developed as part of efforts to apply MOHO concepts in practice and research.

Modified Interest Checklist

The Interest Checklist was originally developed by Matsutsuyu (1969). Later, when the checklist was being used routinely in association with MOHO, it was modified by Scaffa (1981) and then by Kielhofner and Neville (1983). They retained its 68 interests but altered

how clients responded to them to gather more detailed information. The Modified Interest Checklist (Kielhofner & Neville, 1983) also includes the opportunity to indicate what current interests are, how interests have changed, and whether one participates or wishes to participate in an interest in the future.

The Modified Interest Checklist is a leisure interest inventory appropriate for adults and adolescents. Although it can be used to gather information relevant to a person's overall occupational interests, its main focus is on avocational interests that influence activity choices. This checklist is interpreted by examining each client's unique pattern of interests. Therapists and researchers have also made numerous modifications to the Interest Checklist to reflect local customs and cultures. One example is a British Activity Checklist that uses a modified rating scale and alternative method of interpreting results. Another example is the Japanese Elderly Version of the Interest Checklist (Yamada, Ishii, & Nagatani, 2002), illustrated in the Akira case.

FIGURE 16.1 Format of the Modified Interest Checklist.

Activity:	What has been your level of interest?						Do you currently participate in this activity?		Would you like to pursue this in the future?	
	In the past ten years			In the past year						
	Strong	Some	No	Strong	Some	No	Yes	No	Yes	No
Gardening/Yardwork										
Sewing/Needle work										
Playing cards										
Foreign languages										
Church activities										
Radio										
Walking										
Car repair										
Writing										
Dancing										
Golf										
Football										
Listening to popular music										

Administration

As shown in *Figure 16.1*, clients indicate their level of interest in each of the items over the past 10 years and the past 1 year. Further, clients indicate whether they actively participate in and would like to pursue each potential interest in the future. After completion of the checklist, the occupational therapist and client discuss the responses. This is particularly useful for appreciating the impact that disability has had on how the client is experiencing an activity or the significance of disability in altering a client's attraction to particular kinds of activities. Giving directions to clients and discussing their responses takes at least 15 minutes, and clients who need support to complete the assessment may require more time.

Modified Interest Checklist

. . . .

- Gathers information on strength of interest, present, and future engagement in 68 activities
- Can be downloaded from the MOHO Clearinghouse Web site at *www.moho.uic.edu/mohorelatedrsrcs. html#OtherInstrumentsBasedonMOHO,* or
  - Visit *www.moho.uic.edu*
  - Select menu item "MOHO Related Resources"
  - Link to "Other Instruments Based on MOHO"

Akira: An Illustration of Use of the Interest Checklist Japanese Elderly Version (ICJEV)

. . . .

Akira is a married elderly man living in a nursing care facility in Tokyo due to onset of dementia. Before retirement he worked as a carpenter. Upon moving to the nursing care facility, he seemed depressed and refused to join group programs such as chorus and handicrafts. In order to meet Japanese laws and regulations related to older adults living in nursing care facilities, group programs are common services provided to residents.

Akira's occupational therapist used the ICJEV to better understand Akira and his interests and to provide him with pleasurable experiences in the context of group intervention.

Using the ICJEV, Akira indicated two strong interests, gardening/vegetables and taking care of pets or animals. He explained to the therapist why he was so strongly interested in those activities. Prior to institutionalization, he had a small yard and grew vegetables for many years. He also had a dog, and he said, "Somehow my dog understands me." However, he could not take his dog into the nursing care facility, and he expressed his difficulty making the transition to his new living situation by saying, "I had to give up my yard and dog." He also indicated casual interest for listening to the music and singing songs, but he preferred listening to his favorite singers and singing his favorite songs to listening to new music (*Fig. 16.2*).

Akira's responses on the ICJEV confirmed that he was not satisfied with his environment in the institution. Upon moving to the nursing care facility, he had felt forced to give up his favorite interests. The occupational therapist sought to provide Akira with opportunities to continue his previous interests in his new living situation. The occupational therapist asked Akira to teach her how to grow vegetables. Akira told the occupational therapist that he would like to grow baby tomatoes because he was familiar with the plant. The occupational therapist and Akira worked together to prepare the soil and planters. Since Akira's planters were set in a hallway of the facility, Akira started watering the planters without any help from his occupational therapist. When his tomatoes started blooming, Akira noted in his notebook how many flowers bloomed. Then, when his tomatoes stated fruiting, he carefully counted each day which tomatoes were ripe enough for picking. Akira still refused to join group programs, but he liked growing his tomatoes, and his daily routine was organized around maintenance and supervision of them. Akira didn't voluntarily initiate conversation with the occupational therapist about his tomatoes, but he would engage in some discussion when she asked him about them.

Through this interaction, Akira began to develop trust for the occupational therapist. As their relationship grew, Akira and his occupational therapist started

FIGURE 16.2 Akira's responses on the ICJEV.

Occupational Forms	Interest		
	Strong	Casual	No
1. Gardening/Growing vegetables	✗		
2. Sewing			✗
3. Radio			✗
4. Going for a walk			✗
5. Haiku/Senryu (Japanese poetry)			✗
6. Dancing			✗
7. Listening to music		✗	
8. Singing		✗	
9. Taking care of pets or animals	✗		
10. Lectures			✗
11. TV/Movies			✗
12. Visiting acquaintances			✗
13. Reading			✗
14. Traveling			✗
15. Enkai (Japanese style parties)			✗
16. Sumo			✗
17. Dusting/Laundry			✗
18. Politics			✗
19. Clubs for women/elderly people			✗
20. Clothes/Hair style/Makeup			✗
21. Picking wild plants			✗
22. Socialization with the opposite sex			✗
23. Driving			✗
24. Gate ball (Japanese croquet)			✗
25. Cooking			✗
26. Collection			✗
27. Fishing			✗
28. Shopping			✗
29. Ground golf (Japanese style par three hole)			✗
Other special interests: (none indicated)			

discussing how he could expand his activity of growing vegetables within the facility. The occupational therapist also encouraged Akira to explore new or related interests.

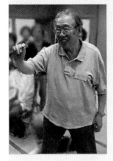

Akira explores new interests, here a game of darts, along with other residents in the nursing care facility.

Occupational Questionnaire and the National Institutes of Health Activity Record

The NIH Activity Record (ACTRE) (Furst, Gerber, Smith, Fisher, & Shulman, 1987; Gerber & Furst, 1992) and the Occupational Questionnaire (OQ) (Smith, Kielhofner, & Watts, 1986) are self-report forms that ask the client to indicate what activity he or she engages in over the course of a weekday and weekend day. The OQ and AC-TRE are appropriate for use with adolescents and adults.

The OQ, on which the ACTRE is based, is the simpler form. It asks respondents to report what they are doing during each half-hour waking period of their day. Then they indicate the following:

- Whether they consider it to be work, leisure, a daily living task, or rest
- How much they enjoy it
- How important it is
- How well they do it.

The last three questions give insight into the volitional characteristics of the activity pattern. That is, they reveal the personal causation, interest, and value of the activity. The questionnaire also provides information about the person's habit patterns (i.e., the typical use of time) and about occupational participation (i.e., the kind of work, leisure, and self-care that make up a person's current life).

The ACTRE, developed for use with persons who have physical disabilities, asks additional questions pertaining to pain, fatigue, difficulty of performance, and whether one rests during the activity (*Fig. 16.3*). Consequently, in addition to the information provided by the OQ, the ACTRE provides detailed information about how a disability influences performance of everyday activities (e.g., it asks about the level of energy required, the amount of pain and fatigue, and whether rest was taken during the activity). The ACTRE is designed to be used primarily as a 24-hour time log completed at three points during each day. This method helps improve the accuracy of the instrument, since recall is of a very recent past.

Although both forms are designed to be used as self-reports, they can be administered as semi-structured interviews. The forms are ordinarily used to report on an actual period of time, being filled out as diaries during the reporting period. However, it is sometimes more practical to ask clients to use the forms to describe a typical day. Each of these methods has its advantages (e.g., diaries tend to be more accurate but may reflect an unusual day). Actual use depends on the purpose and circumstances of therapy. Ordinarily, therapists minimally ask clients to report on a weekday and a weekend day, but this also depends on circumstances in which the instruments are being used.

In addition to providing details about a client's use and experience of time, these instruments may give the occupational therapist important information about the following kinds of problems:

- Particularly troublesome times or activities in the daily schedule
- Disorganization in the person's use of time
- Lack of balance in time use
- Problems such as a lack of feeling competent, a lack of interest, or a lack of value in daily activities.

The instruments can be used to produce scores that represent the amount of value, interest, personal causation, pain, and fatigue experienced in a day. In addition to the possibility of generating such numbers from the instruments, the results of the instruments can be graphically portrayed for or by the client. For example, the time spent in any area (e.g., work, play, or rest) can be portrayed as the portion of the day devoted to each of these life spaces, the portion spent doing things not valued, and so on. This can be done as an

FIGURE 16.3 Format of the NIH Activity Record.

					Question 1	Question 2	Question 3	Question 4	Question 5	Question 6	Question 7	Question 8
Name			Age			Day/Date			I.D.#			
Day 1			Afternoon		During This Time I Felt Pain	At the Beginning Of This Half-Hour I Felt Fatigue	I Think That I Do This	I Find This Activity To Be	For Me This Activity is	This Activity Causes Fatigue	I Enjoy This Activity	I Stopped To Rest During The Activity
Key	Half-Hour Beginning At		C a t e g o r y*	Activity	1=Not at All 2=Very Little 3=Some 4=A Lot	1=Not at All 2=Very Little 3=Some 4=A Lot	1=Very Poorly 2=Poorly 3=Average 4=Well	1=Very Difficult 2=Difficult 3=Slightly Difficult 4=Not Difficult	1=Not Meaningful 2=Slightly Meaningful 3=Meaningful 4=Very Meaningful	1=Not at All 2=Very Little 3=Some 4=A Lot	1=Not at All 2=Very Little 3=Some 4=A Lot	1=Yes 2=No
	12:30 PM				1 2 3 4	1 2 3 4	1 2 3 4	1 2 3 4	1 2 3 4	1 2 3 4	1 2 3 4	1 2
	1:00 PM				1 2 3 4	1 2 3 4	1 2 3 4	1 2 3 4	1 2 3 4	1 2 3 4	1 2 3 4	1 2
	1:30 PM				1 2 3 4	1 2 3 4	1 2 3 4	1 2 3 4	1 2 3 4	1 2 3 4	1 2 3 4	1 2
	2:00 PM				1 2 3 4	1 2 3 4	1 2 3 4	1 2 3 4	1 2 3 4	1 2 3 4	1 2 3 4	1 2

*Key to Category:

Rest (RE) - rest periods taking one-half hour or longer

Self-Care (SC) - personal care activities including dressing, grooming, exercises, normal meals, showering, or other similar activities

Preparation or Planning (PP) - time spent preparing to do an activity or planning when and how to do your daily or weekly activities

Household Activities (HA) - cooking, cleaning, mending, shopping for or putting away groceries, gardening, or other similar activities

Work (WK) - paid or volunteer activities in or out of the home, school work, writing papers, attending classes, studying, or other similar activities

Recreation or Leisure (RL) - hobbies, TV, games, reading (unless done during short rest breaks), sports, out-for-meals, movies, adult education classes, shopping, gardening, talking with friends, or other similar activities

Transportation (TR) - traveling to and from activities

Treatment (RX) - doctor or therapy appointments, home exercise, etc.

Sleep (SL) - when you go to bed for the night

individual or group exercise. It provides clients with a new way to examine their patterns of doing things and identify changes they would like to make. Used in this way, these instruments can help to establish therapeutic goals in collaboration with the client. Like all self-report assessments, they are best supplemented with an in-depth discussion with the client. Giving directions to clients and discussing their responses takes at least 15 minutes, and clients who need support to complete the assessment may require more time.

Occupational Questionnaire (OQ)

- Records information in half-hour intervals throughout the day. Information includes a person's perception of competence, value of activity, and enjoyment of activity.
- Can be downloaded from the MOHO Clearinghouse Web site at *www.moho.uic.edu/mohorelatedrsrcs.html#Other InstrumentsBasedonMOHO*, or
  - Visit www.moho.uic.edu
  - Select menu item "MOHO Related Resources"
  - Link to "Other Instruments Based on MOHO."

NIH Activity Record (ACTRE)

- Records information in half-hour intervals throughout the day. Information includes a person's perception of competence, value of activity, enjoyment of activity, difficulty, pain, and rest.
- Copies of the NIH ACTRE and a method of scoring with a computer spreadsheet can be obtained directly by writing or e-mailing Gloria Furst, OTR/L MPH, Department of Health and Human Services, National Institutes of Health, Rehabilitation Medicine Department, Building 10, CRC, Room 1-1469, 10 Center Drive, MSC 1604, Bethesda, Maryland 20892-1604. Phone 301-402-3012; fax 301-480-0669; e-mail *gfurst@nih.gov*

- Or visit *www.moho.uic.edu/mohorelatedrsrcs. html#OtherInstrumentsBasedonMOHO* to obtain e-mail address to request NIH Activity Record.

Lin: An Illustration of the Use of the OQ

Lin is a 25-year-old man who lives in Taipei. He was diagnosed as having obsessive-compulsive disorder with a suspected schizoid personality. Lin was admitted to a psychiatric ward because of emotional difficulties that stemmed from his army training. He displayed compulsive behaviors since his first year in college. Lin spent a great amount of time washing himself, washing his hands, and folding his clothes. However, he was able to adjust to the requirements of college life and to graduate with a bachelor's degree in accounting.

After graduation, he enlisted in the Taiwanese army. However, he was unable to cope with the army routines. He spent too much time washing himself and his hands, and he was disciplined for these behaviors. He was sent to the army-affiliated hospital for screening and was diagnosed as having an adjustment disorder. Eventually, he was dismissed from the army because he was unable to cope with army life. Since that time, he has been living alone in an apartment in Taipei, relatively isolated from others and without employment.

Lin was referred to occupational therapy for evaluation of his communication and interaction skills, roles, and habits. In addition to other assessments, the occupational therapist asked Lin to complete the OQ to assess his daily routines and role performance. Lin was very serious about filling out the questionnaire and took a great deal of time deciding how to respond, making several corrections.

The OQ (*Fig. 16.4*) highlighted that Lin spent about 10.5 hours in mainly passive and solitary leisure

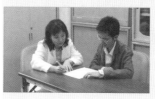

The occupational therapist shows Lin how to complete the OQ.

FIGURE 16.4A Lin's Responses on the Occupational Questionnaire.

Time	Typical Activities	Question 1 I consider this activity to be: W: Work D: Daily living task R: Recreation RT: Rest	Question 2 I think that I do this: VW: Very well W: Well AA: About average P: Poorly VP: Very poorly	Question 3 For me this activity is: EI: Extremely important I: Important TL: Take it or leave it RN: Rather not do it TW: Total waste of time	Question 4 How much do you enjoy this activity? LVM: Like it much L: Like it NLD: Neither like nor dislike D: Dislike it SD: Strongly dislike
06:30–07:00	Sleep	W D R **RT**	VW **W** AA P VP	**EI** I TL RN TW	**LVM** L NLD D SD
07:00–07:30	Breakfast	W **D** R RT	**VW** W AA P VP	**EI** I TL RN TW	**LVM** L NLD D SD
07:30–08:00	Computer	**W** D R RT	VW **W** AA P VP	EI **I** TL RN TW	**LVM** L NLD D SD
08:00–08:30	Computer	**W** D R RT	VW **W** AA P VP	EI **I** TL RN TW	**LVM** L NLD D SD
08:30–09:00	Read Newspaper	**W** D R RT	VW **W** AA P VP	EI **I** TL RN TW	**LVM** L NLD D SD
09:00–09:30	Reading	**W** D R RT	VW **W** AA P VP	**EI** I TL RN TW	**LVM** L NLD D SD
09:30–10:00	Reading	**W** D R RT	VW **W** AA P VP	**EI** I TL RN TW	**LVM** L NLD D SD
10:00–10:30	Listen to Music	**W** D R RT	**VW** W AA P VP	**EI** I TL RN TW	**LVM** L NLD D SD
10:30–11:00	Music	**W** D R RT	VW **W** AA P VP	EI **I** TL RN TW	**LVM** L NLD D SD
11:00–11:30	Music	**W** D R RT	VW **W** AA P VP	EI **I** TL RN TW	**LVM** L NLD D SD
11:30–12:00	Lunch	W **D** R RT	**VW** W AA P VP	**EI** **I** TL RN TW	**LVM** L NLD D SD
12:00–12:30	Lunch	W **D** R RT	**VW** W AA P VP	**EI** **I** TL RN TW	**LVM** L NLD D SD
12:30–01:00	Computer	W D **R** RT	VW **W** AA P VP	EI **I** **TL** RN TW	**LVM** L **NLD** D SD
01:00–01:30	Computer	W D **R** RT	VW **W** AA P VP	EI **I** **TL** RN TW	**LVM** L **NLD** D SD
01:30–02:00	Go to Library	W D **R** RT	VW **W** AA P VP	EI **I** **TL** RN TW	**LVM** L **NLD** D SD
02:00–02:30	Library	W D **R** RT	VW **W** AA P VP	EI **I** **TL** RN TW	**LVM** L **NLD** D SD
02:30–03:00	Exercise	W D **R** RT	VW **W** AA P VP	EI **I** **TL** RN TW	**LVM** L **NLD** D SD
03:00–03:30	Exercise	W D **R** RT	VW **W** AA P VP	EI **I** **TL** RN TW	**LVM** L **NLD** D SD
03:30–04:00	Play ball	W D **R** RT	VW **W** AA P VP	EI **I** **TL** RN TW	**LVM** L **NLD** D SD
04:00–04:30	Play ball	W D **R** RT	VW **W** AA P VP	EI **I** **TL** RN TW	**LVM** L **NLD** D SD
04:30–05:00	Play ball	W D **R** RT	VW **W** AA P VP	EI **I** **TL** RN TW	**LVM** L **NLD** D SD
05:00–05:30	Dinner	W **D** R RT	**VW** W AA P VP	**EI** **I** TL RN TW	**LVM** L NLD D SD
05:30–06:00	Dinner	W **D** R RT	**VW** W AA P VP	**EI** I TL RN TW	**LVM** L NLD D SD

FIGURE 16.4B Lin's Responses on the Occupational Questionnaire. (*continued*)

Time	Typical Activities	Question 1 — I consider this activity to be: W: Work, D: Daily living task, R: Recreation, RT: Rest	Question 2 — I think that I do this: VW: Very well, W: Well, AA: About average, P: Poorly, VP: Very poorly	Question 3 — For me this activity is: EI: Extremely important, I: Important, TL: Take it or leave it, RN: Rather not do it, TW: Total waste of time	Question 4 — How much do you enjoy this activity? LVM: Like it much, L: Like it, NLD: Neither like nor dislike, D: Dislike it, SD: Strongly dislike
06:00–06:30	Watching	W D **R** RT	VW **W** AA P VP	EI I TL **RN** TW	LVM **L** NLD D SD
06:30–07:00	TV	W D **R** RT	VW **W** AA P VP	EI I TL **RN** TW	LVM **L** NLD D SD
07:00–07:30	&	W D **R** RT	VW **W** AA P VP	EI I TL **RN** TW	LVM **L** NLD D SD
07:30–08:00	Phone	W D **R** RT	VW **W** AA P VP	EI I TL **RN** TW	LVM **L** NLD D SD
08:00–08:30	Call to	W D **R** RT	VW **W** AA P VP	EI I TL **RN** TW	LVM **L** NLD D SD
08:30–09:00	Friend	W D **R** RT	VW **W** AA P VP	EI I TL **RN** TW	LVM **L** NLD D SD
09:00–09:30	Bathing	W D **R** RT	VW **W** AA P VP	EI I TL **RN** TW	LVM **L** NLD D SD
09:30–10:00	Bathing	W D **R** RT	VW **W** AA P VP	EI I TL **RN** TW	LVM **L** NLD D SD
10:00–10:30	Bathing	W D **R** RT	VW **W** AA P VP	EI I TL **RN** TW	LVM **L** NLD D SD
10:30–11:00	Clean up room	W D **R** RT	VW **W** AA P VP	EI I TL **RN** TW	LVM **L** NLD D SD
11:00–11:30	Clean up room	W D **R** RT	VW **W** AA P VP	EI I TL **RN** TW	LVM **L** NLD D SD
11:30–12:00	Clean up room	W D **R** RT	VW **W** AA P VP	EI I TL **RN** TW	LVM **L** NLD D SD
12:00–12:30	Go to sleep	W D R **RT**	VW **W** AA P VP	**EI** I TL RN TW	**LVM** L NLD D SD

activities, 3.5 hours in activities of daily living, and 4 hours doing work-related things. The way in which he rated activities was revealing for both the therapist and Lin. Together they identified the following patterns. The only thing Lin indicated doing very well was eating meals, which along with sleep, were the only things that he rated as extremely important. Similarly, these and mainly passive leisure things were what he indicated liking most. While he did not see himself as having a problem doing anything or find anything he did to be a waste of time or distasteful, he also did not indicate that he valued or derived a high level of competence or enjoyment from anything productive. Moreover, his response to activities sometimes appeared to be as closely related to the time of day as to what he was doing, suggesting that he was not deriving a specific sense of value, competence, or interest from what he did.

Lin found the information derived from the OQ to be very revealing. It made him more aware of features of his daily routine. He indicated that his routine "just sort of happened." He did not actively choose it. Moreover, he indicated that it was a sad thing that the highlight of his day was when he ate meals. Thus, he was strongly motivated to try to improve his daily life.

After the evaluation, Lin collaborated with the therapist to identify goals for himself. Since his length of hospital stay was anticipated to be only a few days, Lin and his therapist decided to focus on goals and plans that he could work on in his community life. Using information from the OQ, Lin identified the goals of redesigning his lifestyle according to the major roles he wanted in his life. He planned how to reduce the time he spent in leisure and self-care to have more time to engage in productive things. He systematically examined each of the things he did in the course of the day, deciding what kinds of changes he would like to make to feel more productive and involved. He was then able to choose things he wanted to do and plan for how to integrate these into his daily routines. This planning process of itself helped Lin feel that he could control and improve his daily life.

Occupational Self Assessment and Child Occupational Self Assessment

The Occupational Self Assessment (OSA) (Baron, Kielhofner, Iyenger, Goldhammer, & Wolenski, 2006) and the Child Occupational Self Assessment (COSA) (Keller, Kafkas, Basu, Federico & Kielhofner, 2005) are designed to capture clients' occupational competence for doing everyday occupations. They also allow clients to indicate personal values and to set priorities for change by assessing the importance of those everyday occupations. Thus, the OSA and COSA are designed to give voice to the client's perspective and to give the client a role in determining the goals and strategies of therapy.

The OSA and COSA are also designed to be outcomes measures that capture self-reported client change. To be used as outcomes measures, the OSA and COSA are administered at the beginning and end of therapy. The OSA also includes a key form that translates a client's responses into overall measures of competence and values.

Administration

The OSA consists of a self-rating form, as shown in *Figure 16.5*. The OSA includes a series of statements about everyday occupational activities, to which clients respond by labeling each in terms of how well they do the activity on a four-point scale. Clients then respond to these same statements, indicating the importance of each on a four-point scale. During the administration of the initial OSA, once clients have completed the ratings, they establish priorities for change. There is a column on the form in which the client selects and ranks the areas for change. When completing the OSA, some clients independently determine their priorities for change and then discuss them with the therapist. Other clients, who need or want more structure, do this with the therapist while reviewing their responses to the OSA. The OSA also includes a form on which the therapist and client together may formally record and review therapy goals and strategies. The OSA manual also includes a paper keyform for each rating scale, competence and value, that allows one to add up responses and generate a measure, or score, and error.

FIGURE 16.5 Sample Portion from the OSA.

						Step 2: Next, for each statement, circle how important this is to you.				Step 3: Choose up to 4 things about yourself that you would like to change (You can also write comments in this space)
Step 1: Below are statements about things you do in everyday life. For each statement, circle how well you do it. If an item does not apply to you, cross it out and move on to the next item.	I have a lot of problem doing this	I have some difficulty doing this	I do this well	I do this extremely well		This is not so important to me	This is important to me	This is more important to me	This is most important to me	I would like to change
Concentrating on my tasks	Lot of problem	Some difficulty	Well	Extremely well		Not so important	Important	More important	Most important	
Physically doing what I need to do	Lot of problem	Some difficulty	Well	Extremely well		Not so important	Important	More important	Most important	

247

Therapists should plan at least 15 minutes to give directions to clients and to discuss their responses after the assessment is complete. Clients who need support to complete the assessment may require more time. Therapists using the key forms should put aside another 5 minutes to derive client measures.

The COSA is similar to the OSA in that it assesses occupational competence in and value of everyday activities. However, to facilitate children's responses, the COSA uses faces and stars to describe the rating choices as shown in *Figure 16.6*. Children can complete the COSA by using a paper and pencil form or by doing a card sort. After responding to the COSA items, children have an opportunity to talk about any additional concerns and strengths that were not addressed in the COSA items by responding to a series of open ended followup questions. The COSA does not include a step of selecting areas of priorities for change. Instead, the therapist structures the process, helping the child review the items and select priorities for change. Most young clients take 20 to 30 minutes to complete the COSA with support, and discussion of results can usually be completed in 15 minutes.

When therapy is terminated (or when progress or followup information is desired), the OSA or COSA followup forms can be administered. Comparing the initial OSA and COSA responses with followup responses provides a visual representation of how the client has changed on each item, as is illustrated in Kerri's case. In addition to qualitatively comparing changes in OSA responses to assess outcomes, the OSA client measure and error term generated by the keyform can also be compared to document change over time.

The Occupational Self Assessment (OSA)

- Assesses a client's sense of occupational competence for performing everyday occupations. The OSA also allows clients to indicate the importance of everyday occupations and set priorities for change.

- Can be ordered through the MOHO Clearinghouse e-store *http://ascendant.cas.uic.edu/retail/*, or
  - Visit *www.moho.uic.edu*
  - Select menu item "MOHO Products"
  - Link to OSA assessment for more information about the assessment and example assessment forms. To link to the MOHO Clearinghouse e-store, left-click on the "Buy Now" button.

The Child Occupational Self Assessment (COSA)

- Assesses a young client's sense of occupational competence for performing everyday occupations. The COSA also allows clients to indicate the importance of everyday occupations. Visual cues and two administration versions of the COSA facilitate children's understanding of the self-report.
- Can be ordered through the MOHO Clearinghouse e-store *http://ascendant.cas.uic.edu/retail/*, or
  - Visit *www.moho.uic.edu*
  - Select menu item "MOHO Products"
  - Link to COSA assessment for more information about the assessment and example assessment forms. To link to the MOHO Clearinghouse e-store, left-click on the "Buy Now" button.

Sinikka: Using the OSA to Support Client Collaboration in Therapy

Sinikka is a 30-year-old catering worker who lives in Helsinki. She has had complex regional pain syndrome for the past 2.5 years, since a workplace accident in which she sustained an electrical shock from a food processor to her right, dominant hand. Sinikka sought a variety of interventions to no avail. These included previous occupational therapy that emphasized assessment of her hand function and learning to use a wrist support.

FIGURE 16.6 Sample Portion from the COSA

Myself	I have a big problem doing this	I have a little problem doing this	I do this ok	I am really good at doing this	Not really important to me	Important to me	Really important to me	Most important of all to me
Keep my mind on what I am doing	☹☹	☹	☺	☺☺	★	★ ★	★ ★ ★	★ ★ ★ ★
Do things with my family	☹☹	☹	☺	☺☺	★	★ ★	★ ★ ★	★ ★ ★ ★

Sinikka recently began a pain rehabilitation program consisting of group treatment followed by outpatient, individualized therapy. Sinikka is anxious about her condition and symptoms and angry about the lack of efficacy of the previous care she received. She indicates that she feels like her hand and arm are living a life of their own over which she has little control.

She feels that everything seems to be closing down on her. To maintain some measure of control, she has organized a structured daily routine aimed at minimizing her chronic pain. For example, at home she uses electronic equipment to reduce work demands, spaces her workload, and uses her left hand whenever possible. She frequently wakes up during the night because of pain. When she tries activities that are not part of her routine, she is hesitant and fearful of evoking pain, and she has difficulty making decisions. She was very dependent on the therapist to guide her in doing anything new. Still, Sinikka expressed doubt over whether therapy would help her in the long run.

The therapist introduced the OSA to Sinikka as a means of giving her an opportunity to take more control over her life and the therapeutic process. Sinikka's initial responses on the OSA are shown in *Figure 16.7*. The therapist discussed the responses with Sinikka. Sinikka indicated that the chronic pain had made many negative changes in her ability to do things she valued. These included difficulties in her roles as daughter-in-law, spouse, sister, home maintainer, caregiver, and worker. She explained that before her injury, she saw herself as a woman who was able to do anything she undertook and was recognized by others as resourceful and self-reliant. Now even the people closest to her could not comprehend her situation. She had very high standards for

to use her dominant hand effectively left her feeling ineffective and helpless at times. Also, asking for help was not something Sinikka felt comfortable doing. She summed up her experience as being like floating paralyzed in a big lake, unable to move or swim.

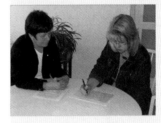

Sinikka contemplates her current life circumstances while completing the OSA.

During the next therapy session, the therapist asked Sinikka about their previous session, thinking that she might want to add something or continue the conversation they had begun after Sinikka completed the assessment. Sinikka told the therapist that doing the OSA had a profound effect on her. She found herself many times during the day just sitting deep in her thoughts. She told the therapist that she had started to think about what she really wanted in her life and what kind of options she would have in the future.

At this point she decided to choose the following priorities from the OSA statements to work on in therapy:

- Being involved as a student, worker, volunteer, and/or family member

- Handling my responsibilities

- Making decisions based on what I think is important.

Consequently, therapy sessions were organized to address these goals. The therapist supported Sinikka in

FIGURE 16.7 Sinikka's initial responses on the Myself Section of the OSA.

Myself	Competence				Values			
	Lot of problem	Some difficulty	Well	Extremely well	Not so important	Important	More important	Most important
Concentrating on my tasks		X				X		
Physically doing what I need to do		X					X	
Taking care of the place where I live	X							X
Taking care of myself			X				X	
Taking care of others for whom I am responsible		X						X
Getting where I need to go		X				X		
Managing my finances			X					X
Managing my basic needs (food, medicine)			X				X	
Expressing myself to others			X			X		
Getting along with others			X					X
Identifying and solving problems				X		X		
Relaxing and enjoying myself		X						X
Getting done what I need to do		X				X		
Having a satisfying routine		X			X			
Handling my responsibilities		X						X
Being involved as a student, worker, volunteer, and/or family member		X						X
Doing activities I like		X						X
Working towards my goals			X				X	
Making decisions based on what I think is important		X						X
Accomplishing what I set out to do			X				X	
Effectively using my abilities			X			X		

choosing occupational forms/tasks for therapy that were linked to her roles and habits. Her ability to make decisions both for what to do and how to proceed in doing things quickly progressed. She resumed cooking, because this was an important part of her homemaker role. She worked at the computer to be productive by doing some of the bookkeeping for her husband's business. Lastly, she reengaged in an old hobby of silk painting. She did these things in therapy to get support for any adaptation and problem solving. She then carried them out at home routinely.

Sinikka had to drive her car quite a distance to go to therapy. This was hard because the rough road near her house made driving a challenge and precipitated pain. The therapist discussed with her the possibility of looking into a car with an armrest, wondering if the support for the arm would make any difference. Sinikka responded by renting such a car from a dealer to try it out and went on to trade cars. She managed to get her personal insurance to pay for aids she found useful in kitchen tasks as well as for a movable armrest for the computer she used at home.

She gave one of the silk scarves she decorated to her mother-in-law, which was very symbolic for Sinikka. Then, when her mother-in-law became ill, Sinikka took responsibility for driving her to appointments at the hospital. During therapy, Sinikka also spent time discussing plans to work in the future. She decided to explore how she might build on her experience in catering by finding a job in the hotel industry. A few months after therapy ended, the therapist received an e-mail message from Sinikka. She was excited because she had secured a work training position in a high-class hotel.

Kerri: Using the COSA to Facilitate Engagement in Inpatient Intervention

Kerri was 11 years old and had Klippel Trenaunay Weber syndrome, which is characterized by varicose veins, arteriovenous malformation, and bone and soft tissue hypertrophy. In Kerri's case, this syndrome caused multiple hemangiomas on her body, excessive bleeding,

and pain. She was transferred from inpatient rehabilitation to a pediatric intensive care unit (PICU) 2 hours from her home on account of uncontrolled bleeding following the resection of a hemangioma on her vulva. She had been on bedrest in the PICU for 32 days when she was referred to occupational therapy due to concerns about depression and deconditioning.

Upon discussing Kerri's case with other members of the health care team, the occupational therapist learned that Kerri refused to speak to the doctors when they examined her during daily rounds. The nurses said that they had trouble getting Kerri to cooperate for bed mobility as needed to complete hygiene and change her bandages. The physical therapist had been attempting to see Kerri for 2 weeks but reported that she consistently refused therapy.

At first Kerri was reluctant to speak with the occupational therapist. The therapist explained that she wanted to learn more about how Kerri wanted to spend her time. Kerri demonstrated a hesitant interest in talking to the therapist about this. Kerri made general statements such as, "I don't like it when the people bother me" and "I feel tired," but she had difficulty articulating her feelings more specifically. The occupational therapist decided to administer the COSA to help guide Kerri's communication and to get a more detailed picture of Kerri's perception of her occupational performance.

Kerri took her time and thoughtfully filled out the COSA (*Fig. 16.8*). When she was done, the therapist asked Kerri if they could discuss her answers. First, they discussed Kerri's perceived strengths. Kerri identified herself as being really good at doing things with her family, keeping her mind on what she was doing, and taking care of her things. The therapist asked additional questions to determine what made Kerri feel successful in these areas. The therapist learned that Kerri felt successful in her interactions with her family because they listened to her and because she was able to help decide what they would do together. Kerri felt she was able to keep her mind on what she was doing because she was "smart" and "good at figuring things out." Kerri also told the therapist that she needed to be good at taking care of her things in the hospital because if someone moved one of her possessions, she might not be able to

FIGURE 16.8 Kerri's COSA responses that changed from initial administration to follow-up administration after several months in therapy.

COSA ITEMS	Initial COSA competence response	Follow-up COSA competence response	Initial COSA value response	Follow-up COSA value response
Dress myself	I have a big problem doing this	I have a little problem doing this	Really important to me	Really important to me
Get around from one place to another	I have a little problem doing this	I have a big problem doing this	Most important of all to me	Most important of all to me
Do things with my friends	I have a little problem doing this	I have a big problem doing this	Really important to me	Most important of all to me
Make others understand my ideas	I do this OK	I am really good at doing this	Important to me	Really important to me
Keep working on something even when it gets hard	I do this OK	I am really good at doing this	Important to me	Really important to me
Calm myself down when I am upset	I do this OK	I am really good at doing this	Important to me	Really important to me
Make my body do what I want it to do	I have a big problem doing this	I have a little problem doing this	Most important of all to me	Most important of all to me
Finish what I am doing without getting tired too soon	I have a little problem doing this	I have a big problem doing this	Really important to me	Really important to me

reach it and if something got lost, she was not able to get up and look for it.

Next, they discussed the problem areas that Kerri also identified as being important to her. The results of the COSA indicated that Kerri perceived herself as having a big problem with several activities that she felt were important, including dressing, making her body to do what she wanted it to do, and getting around from one place to another. Kerri stated that dressing was a problem because it hurt when the nurses moved her body around. She reported that pain also limited her ability to get her body to do what she wanted. Kerri explained that she was unable to do things with her friends because they were all several hours away in her hometown and because phone calls from the hospital were too expensive. Kerri received orders to be on mandatory bedrest, but she reported difficulty with bed mobility, such as rolling onto her side to reach an item on her night stand.

On the COSA qualitative follow-up questions, Kerri reported that her movement was limited by weakness and pain. She said that the most painful part of her day was when the nurses and doctors moved her body during examinations and routine care. She also identified watching TV as her only leisure activity. Additional things she felt she was good at included art and playing with animals, although she had not done either of those activities during her hospital stay.

The occupational therapist thought that using Kerri's answers on the COSA to create her goals for therapy could improve her feelings of autonomy and self-efficacy and motivate her to participate in therapy. Kerri worked with the therapist to develop goals based her responses on the COSA. These were her initial goals:

- Kerri will identify three leisure activities she can participate in while maintaining her movement precautions.
- Kerri will participate in an upper extremity exercise program four or five times per week to improve independence in bed mobility.
- Kerri will don a pullover shirt with moderate assistance while seated in bed.

Kerri participated in occupational therapy twice or three times each week to address these goals. Kerri worked together with the occupational therapist to form a "Rehab Plan" and posted it in her room so she and the therapist would know what activities they would do during each session to meet her goals. Although Kerri resisted exercise at first, the therapist explained how strengthening her arms would help her perform her own bed mobility so the nurses wouldn't have to lift her and roll her. Kerri and the occupational therapist worked together to find ways to make exercise fun, such as combining it with art activities (e.g. painting while wearing wrist weights).

With time, Kerri became independent in her exercise program and was able to roll to and from side-lying independently and with reduced pain. With her improved strength and endurance, she demonstrated an improved tolerance for caregiving. Over the next 2 months, Kerri's health improved and her bedrest order was canceled. Her doctors encouraged her to get up into her wheelchair each day. Although Kerri had previously identified getting around from one place to another as something that was important to her, she refused to get out of bed with therapy or nursing. The occupational therapist chose to administer the COSA again. She explained to Kerri that she wanted to learn how her perceived performance and priorities had changed and make new goals for her "Rehab Plan."

Kerri's responses on the second administration of the COSA showed that she still perceived herself as having a problem with dressing, making her body do what

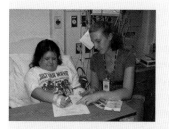

Kerri completes a follow-up COSA after several months of therapy with her occupational therapist to check on her progress toward goals and to identify new goals for intervention.

she wanted it to do, and getting around from one place to another, but she no longer identified these as big problems (*Fig. 16.8*). She also identified two new problem areas, finishing what she was doing without getting tired too soon and doing things with friends. She identified herself as being really good at more areas, including calming herself when she was upset, working on something even when it got hard, and making others understand her ideas.

Kerri and the therapist went over her responses together. Kerri explained to the occupational therapist that she was afraid of being in pain if she tried to sit up to dress herself. Although Kerri was now allowed to get up into her wheelchair, she reported that she was scared to transfer out of the wheelchair because it was painful and only wanted her parents to transfer her because she felt they would be more gentle than the nurses. However, she agreed to try to transfer with her parents to get out of bed. She also reported that she was only able to stay up for about 30 minutes before she became tired and had to return to bed.

Based on her responses, Kerri and the occupational therapist worked together to establish new goals:

- Kerri will spend time in her wheelchair at least 5 days each week.
- Kerri will participate in three social activities with children her age each week.
- Kerri will complete upper body dressing independently.

Kerri and the occupational therapist again came up with strategies to meet her goals. The therapist told Kerri that there were many ways to get to and from her wheelchair. The therapist explained to Kerri how she could use the things she was good at, especially making others understand her ideas and working on something even when it gets hard, to help her achieve this goal. They agreed that the occupational therapist should see how Kerri's parents were transferring Kerri and work together identify what strategies they could use to make it less painful. Kerri also agreed to tell her parents and the therapist which parts of the transfer were painful so they could make the transfer more tolerable. Although they were unable to arrange for Kerri's friends from home to come see her, the occupational therapist suggested that Kerri meet some new people by participating in social activities with other children in the hospital. Kerri was reluctant at first, but she agreed to try participating in social activities with the Child Life program for a week. Kerri and the occupational therapist agreed to try several techniques for dressing, and Kerri could choose the one she liked the best. To help Kerri choose a technique, they decided to keep track of how tiring each technique was, how long the technique took, and the amount of pain it caused.

Kerri remained hospitalized in the PICU for 112 days before she was stable enough to be transferred to an inpatient rehabilitation facility closer to her home. Following the second administration on the COSA, the occupational therapist made recommendations to improve Kerri's transfers to her wheelchair. By incorporating Kerri's feedback and following the therapist's recommendations, Kerri's parents were able to increase her independence in transferring, reduce her pain, and decrease the physical demands on themselves. By the time of discharge, she was able to transfer to her wheelchair with minimal assistance and complete her upper body dressing with assistance only for setup. Because she was able to get out of her room each day for activities, she was able to build friendships with two other clients her age in the hospital. Overall, she responded well to the use of the COSA to give her more control over her occupational therapy treatment in an inpatient setting.

As these two cases illustrate, the OSA and COSA provide an excellent means of giving clients a voice about their own problems, strengths, and desires. The instruments also begin a process that can empower and enable clients to achieve more control over their situations and over the objectives and course of their

therapy. Finally, as Kerri's case illustrates, the instruments can serve as a concrete means to demonstrate change achieved in therapy. This is helpful not only to document change but also for clients to objectively see and be reinforced by the changes they accomplish.

The Pediatric Interest Profiles

The Pediatric Interest Profiles (PIP) (Henry, 2000) are three age-appropriate profiles of play and leisure interests and participation that can be used with children and adolescents. The 3 profiles are:

- The Kid Play Profile designed for use with children 6 to 9 years of age
- The Preteen Play Profile for children aged 9 to 12 years
- The Adolescent Leisure Interest Profile for adolescents aged 12 to 21.

The items, the questions about them, and the response formats of each version of the PIP have been designed to be appropriate for and easily understood by clients within the targeted age range.

In the Kid Play Profile, the child answers up to 3 questions about each of 50 activity items. For each activity item, the child is asked, "Do you do this activity?" If the answer is yes, the child is also asked, "Do you like this activity?" and "Who do you do this activity with?" The child answers the questions by circling or coloring in a response. As shown in *Figure 16.9*, simple stick figure drawings and words are used to depict each item. In addition, simple drawings and words are used to represent each possible response. The Kid Play Profile activity items are grouped into eight categories: sports, outside activities, summer activities, winter activities, indoor activities, creative activities, lessons and classes, and socializing.

In the Preteen Play Profile, the child answers up to 5 questions about each of 59 activity items. For each activity item, the child is asked, "Do you do this activity?" If the answer is yes, the child is also asked:

- How often do you do this activity?
- How much do you like this activity?
- How good are you at this activity?
- Who do you do this activity with?

The child answers the questions by circling a response. As with the Kid Play Profile, stick figure drawings are used to depict each activity. The Preteen Play Profile items are grouped into eight categories: sports, outside

FIGURE 16.9 Sample items from the Kid Play Profile.

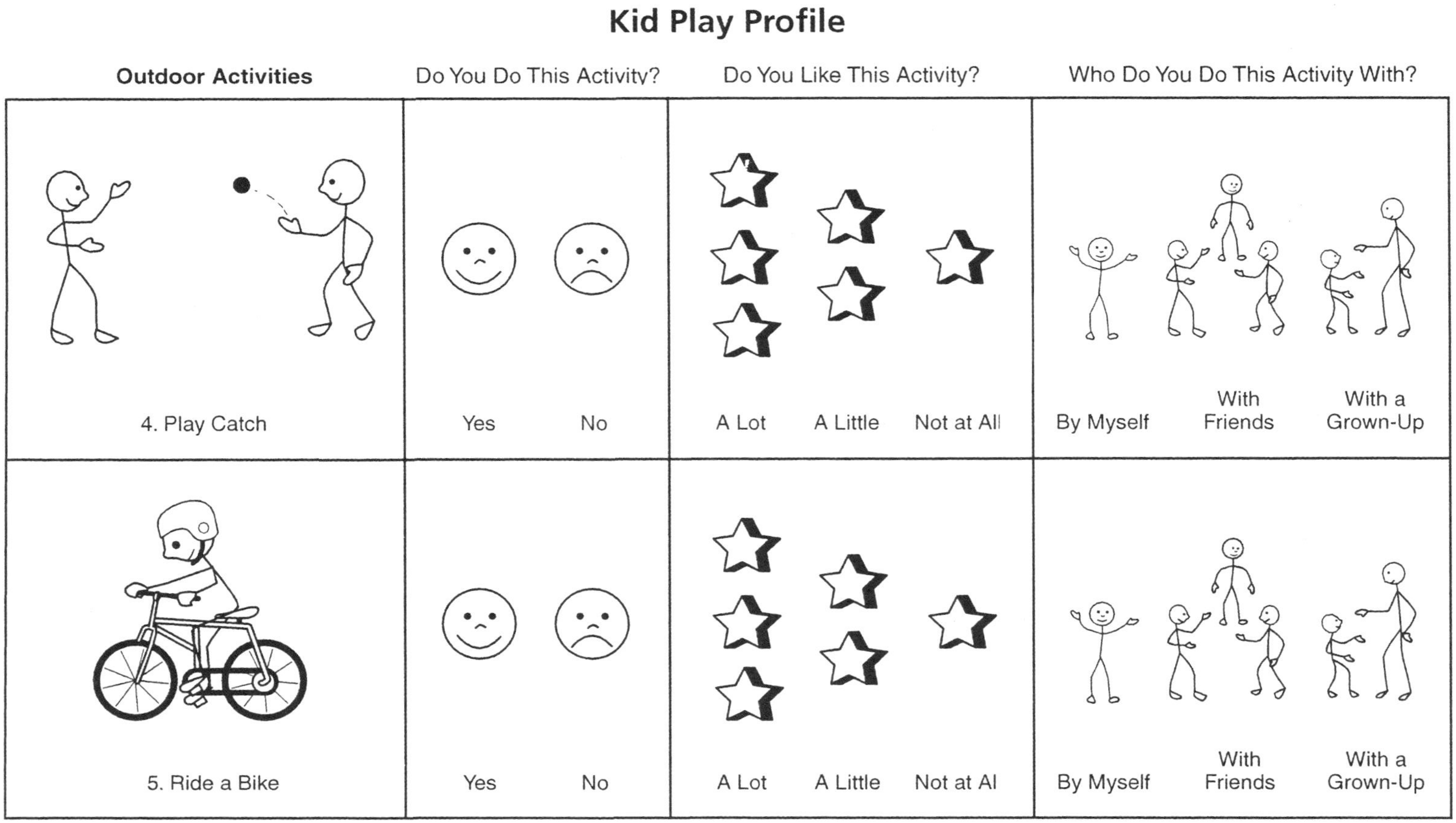

Kid Play Profile

Outdoor Activities	Do You Do This Activity?	Do You Like This Activity?	Who Do You Do This Activity With?
4. Play Catch	Yes No	A Lot A Little Not at All	By Myself With Friends With a Grown-Up
5. Ride a Bike	Yes No	A Lot A Little Not at Al	By Myself With Friends With a Grown-Up

activities, summer activities, winter activities, indoor activities, creative activities, lessons/classes, and socializing.

In the Adolescent Leisure Interest Profile, the adolescent answers up to 5 questions about each of 83 activity items. For each activity item, the adolescent is asked, "How interested are you in this activity?" and "How often do you do this activity?" If the adolescent does the activity, he or she is also asked:

- How well do you do this activity?
- How much do you enjoy this activity?
- Who do you do this activity with?

The adolescent is instructed to place a check mark beside one of the responses to each question. No drawings are used in the adolescent profile. The Adolescent Leisure Interest Profile activity items are grouped into eight categories: sports, outside activities, exercise, relaxation, intellectual activities, creative activities, socializing, and club/community organizations.

Therapists can use the information gathered with the PIP to identify children or adolescents who may be at risk for play-related problems and/or who have a limited repertoire of play activities. The PIP can also be used to identify specific play activities that are of interest to an individual child or adolescent so that those activities can be used to engage the child in therapeutic or educational interventions.

Administration

These three paper-and-pencil self-report assessments are quick and easy to administer. Each profile lists and/or depicts via pictures a variety of play and leisure activities and asks the child or adolescent to respond to multiple questions about the activities. These questions focus on the child's participation in the activities, feelings of enjoyment and/or competence in the activities, and whether the activities are done alone or with others. The Kid Play Profile takes children about 15 minutes to complete, the Preteen Play Profile approximately 20 minutes, and the Adolescent Leisure Interest Profile about 30 minutes.

It is recommended that the PIP be used to facilitate a conversation between the therapist and the child or adolescent. The PIP can provide a means to engage children or adolescents in a more detailed interview about their play experiences. Children, in particular, seem to enjoy telling stories about their play. Such interviews can enhance rapport between the client and therapist and can give a more detailed picture of any play or leisure-related problems.

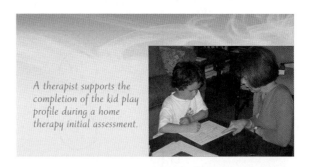

A therapist supports the completion of the kid play profile during a home therapy initial assessment.

℘ediatric Interest Profiles

- Includes three age-appropriate profiles of play and leisure interests and participation:
    - Kid Play Profile (ages 6–9 years)
    - The Preteen Play Profile (ages 9–12 years)
    - The Adolescent Leisure Interest Profile (Ages 12–21)
- Can be downloaded from the MOHO Clearinghouse Web site at *www.moho.uic.edu/mohorelatedrsrcs. html#OtherInstrumentsBasedonMOHO*, or
    - Visit *www.moho.uic.edu*
    - Select menu item "MOHO Related Resources"
    - Link to "Other Instruments Based on MOHO."

ℐerome: An Illustration of Use of the Kid Play Profile

Jerome was 6 years old and attended first grade at an urban public elementary school in Maryland. He lived with his mother, maternal grandmother, and 8-year-old brother, Joe. Jerome's mother worked full time in a manufacturing plant and attended school one evening a week. Jerome's parents were divorced. Jerome and his brother visited their father in Pennsylvania one weekend each month and for three week-long vacations each year. Jerome's grandmother provided child care for Jerome and his brother when their mother was working or at school.

His mother reported that Jerome had always been more difficult than her other son. As a baby he was not easily soothed, was a picky eater, and rarely slept through the night. She felt that she had to carry him all the time. As a toddler, he was very physically active and frequently got bumps and bruises. His high level of physical activity continued as he grew older and entered school. At the end of the day, Jerome's mother noted, he was "literally bouncing off the walls." In addition, since toddlerhood, he had been very particular about his clothing, disliking most types of underwear, socks, turtleneck shirts, and jeans. His mother reported, "Sometimes we go through five shirts in the morning before he is ready for school."

Jerome enjoyed kindergarten, but his progress in developing preacademic skills such as letter recognition and writing was slower than for most of his classmates. First grade was more difficult. Jerome had trouble attending in class, was often disruptive because he could not sit still, and was falling further behind in developing reading readiness skills. He was having difficulty with handwriting and other fine motor tasks. While his teacher was very supportive and patient, she was beginning to feel frustrated with her inability to manage his behavior in the classroom and worried about his ability to keep up with the pace of classroom activities. He interacted only minimally with classmates and on the playground spent most of his time on the swings or running in circles. Since the middle of the school year, Jerome had been receiving resource room help for language arts and classroom-based occupational therapy for fine motor activities and handwriting.

At a recent parent meeting, Jerome's mother expressed concern about his increasing social isolation. She was concerned because Jerome told her that he ate lunch alone, usually played by himself during recess, and did not get included in most social activities. Jerome's classroom teacher confirmed this.

The occupational therapist administered the Kid Play Profile to gain Jerome's perspective on his play participation and interviewed Jerome's mother and teacher about his behavior at home and school. Jerome was able to complete the Kid Play Profile with considerable assistance from the occupational therapist. His responses on the Kid Play Profile indicated that he primarily enjoyed outdoor gross motor activities such as biking, roller-blading, swimming, sledding, going to the playground, and playing superheroes. He seemed to enjoy few indoor or fine motor activities but indicated that he liked to build things. He told the occupational therapist that his favorite play activities were riding his bike and climbing on the jungle gym at the playground. He reported that he most often played by himself or sometimes with his older brother but said that his brother "doesn't always like to do stuff with me." He indicated that he had a few friends at school but could name only one boy in his class (Andrew) with whom he played during recess. When asked if he had any other friends, he said, "Well, they don't really like me." He reported that there were no kids in the neighborhood with whom he could play. His mother confirmed that Jerome and his older brother did not always play together. She indicated that Jerome was actually more skilled at gross motor activities, such as biking and roller-blading, than his older brother and that the older brother preferred more creative or indoor activities such as drawing, listening to music, reading, or watching TV. She noted, "They are like night and day." Her biggest concern about Jerome was his academic performance and the fact that he did not seem to know how to make friends.

The classroom teacher confirmed that Jerome did not seem to be making friends in school. She was concerned that his disruptive behavior was causing him to be marginalized by other classmates. On the playground, she had observed that he had difficulty following the rules of organized games such as soccer and kickball and was often not invited to play by the other children.

The interventions recommended by the occupational therapist primarily addressed Jerome's social skills and his actions in the classroom. She referred Jerome to the Friendship Group, jointly run by herself and the school psychologist. The goals of this group were to help referred children develop appropriate social interaction skills in the context of structured play with one other child. Jerome was encouraged to invite one classmate to participate in the Friendship Group with him. The play activities used in the group required cooperation, taking turns, and negotiation. The group taught skills in communication and self-regulation. The occupational therapist suggested that the group have a superhero theme on Jerome's first day to capture his interest and provide motivation for engagement.

The occupational therapist also encouraged Jerome's mother to foster more play between Jerome and his brother. She suggested that Joe might be encouraged to share with Jerome his interest in drawing or building things with construction toys such as Lego or K-Nex. Such activities would also help the development of Jerome's fine motor skills. Because Jerome enjoyed and was good at a variety of gross motor activities, the occupational therapist encouraged his mother to help him build friendships based on these interests. The occupational therapist suggested that participating in recreational programs at the local community center might help Jerome find friends with similar interests and that his mother could help Jerome arrange occasional play dates with one other child.

The Role Checklist

The Role Checklist (Oakley, Kielhofner, & Barris, 1985) was developed to obtain information on clients' perceptions of their participation in occupational roles throughout their life and on the value they place on those occupational roles. The checklist can be used with adolescents or adults. Respondents indicate for each of the 10 occupational roles listed:

- Whether they have held the role in the past
- Whether they are currently in the role
- Whether they expect to be in the role in the future
- How much they value the role.

Brief definitions of each role are provided, followed by examples of that particular role.

Since MOHO is concerned with how roles structure occupational participation, the definitions employ the criterion of at least weekly involvement in each role. Thus, for example, being a family member is defined

not merely as a kinship but as doing something with a family member such as a child, parent, spouse, or other relative at least once a week. In this way, when persons indicate they are in a role, it also means that the role influences what the person does.

The Role Checklist can be filled out in a few minutes either independently or with the assistance of the therapist. Occupational therapists have reported that it is important to discuss the pattern of responses with clients to obtain more detailed information about their role pattern and its meaning for occupational participation, and this process may take about 15 minutes. Some therapists have clients fill it out along with several other members of a group, so that discussion can be used to search for the meaning of each person's responses. In this context, the checklist can facilitate planning future role behavior.

The Role Checklist is interpreted by examining the pattern of responses; a summary sheet aids in the visual examination and interpretation of the response pattern. For example, it may reveal the following kinds of patterns:

- Loss of many or all occupational roles
- Lack of involvement in roles that are valued
- Overcommitment and difficulty discriminating between the importance of roles
- Desires for future roles that are incompatible with capacities or other role responsibilities.

Occupational therapists find that sharing such interpretations of the Role Checklist with clients is critical both to give information to the client and to validate whether the therapist's interpretation fits with the client's experience.

Administration

The therapist begins by explaining the purpose of the checklist and informing the client that they will discuss responses together. The checklist is relatively simple in format and ordinarily easy for clients to complete. The client considers each of 10 occupational roles described on the checklist, which is divided into 2 parts. In part 1, clients check roles they have performed in the past, are currently performing, and/or plan to perform in the future. For example, a client who volunteered in the past, does not volunteer at present, but anticipates volunteering in the future, the client would check the role *volunteer* in both the past and future columns. *Past* refers to anytime up to the preceding week. *Present* includes the week prior, up to and including the day of administration of the checklist. *Future* refers to tomorrow onward. These instructions are on the checklist, and the therapist can review them at the beginning of administration if it is deemed useful to the client.

In part 2 of the checklist, the client rates each role as to whether he or she finds it not at all valuable, somewhat valuable, or very valuable. Value refers to the personal worth or importance of the role.

The occupational therapist ordinarily remains with the client to answer or clarify questions. When followed up with an interview, the Role Checklist further helps the occupational therapist and client identify patterns in role selection, preference, and performance. For example, they can examine the following:

- The kinds of roles persons have been successful at over the course of their lives
- The kinds of roles they have avoided or given up
- Whether roles focus on particular kinds of occupational forms/tasks (e.g., social relationships, service delivery)
- Whether they have a balance among roles
- If they are performing roles they consider not at all valuable.

Such discussions are helpful to both the client and therapist in providing insights into the client's life.

Role Checklist

- The Role Checklist provides information on what roles a person values and perceived participation in roles in past, present, and future
- Copies of the Role Checklist can be obtained directly by e-mailing or writing Frances Oakley, MS, OTR/L, BCN, BCG, FAOTA, National Institutes of Health, Building 10, CRC, Room 1-1469, 10 Center Drive MSC 1604, Bethesda, MD 20892-1604; e-mail: *foakley@nih.gov*
  - Or visit *www.moho.uic.edu/mohorelatedrsrcs. html@OtherInstrumentsBasedonMOHO* to obtain an e-mail address to request the Role Checklist.

Alexandro: Using the Role Checklist to Explore Future Roles

Alexandro retired when he was 60 years old, and 2 years later he was diagnosed with emphysema. At that time he was a smoker and carried out an active daily routine, including some hobbies such as cooking and playing tennis. During his initial admittance to a pulmonary rehabilitation program he was introduced to the Brazilian Portuguese version of the Role Checklist (Cordeiro, Camelier, Oakley, & Jardim, 2007) to identify his current pattern of role engagement and future roles. After completing the assessment, Alexandro and the occupational therapist discussed his responses to gain a clearer picture of his occupational role history and the activities and values encompassed in each role. This discussion of his responses, shown in *Figure 16.10*, revealed the following relevant information.

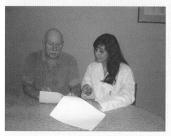

Alexandro talks about his past engagement in hobbies, including tennis and sculpting.

Although Alexandro kept the hobbyist/amateur role throughout his life, sculpting was one specific activity he wished to resume in the future. Although Alexandro also wanted to continue his involvement in tennis, he also wanted a quieter activity he could do on days that he did not feel well. Alexandro had some experience with clay sculpting when he was a young man, but had not participated in this artistic role for many years. Alexandro also identified the volunteer role as very valuable but did not report holding it in the present and did not indicate that he planned to perform it in the future. The therapist talked with Alexandro about the possibility of resuming the volunteer role. Alexandro seemed interested in acquiring volunteer work but was concerned, as he had experienced an interruption of this role in the past and felt badly when his volunteer work ended.

FIGURE 16.10 Alexandro's responses on the Role Checklist.

Role	Role Identity			Value Designation		
	Past	Present	Future	Not at all valuable	Somewhat valuable	Very valuable
Student	X				X	
Worker	X				X	
Volunteer	X					X
Care giver	X	X	X			X
Home maintainer	X	X	X			X
Friend	X	X	X			X
Family member	X	X	X			X
Religious participant	X			X		
Hobbyist/Amateur	X	X	X			X
Participant in organizations	X				X	
Other: NA						

Using the information provided by the Role Checklist, the occupational therapist worked with Alexandro to plan his intervention. First, the occupational therapist arranged for Alexandro to attend the clay class held by the rehabilitation program. He was initially scheduled to attend a soapstone class, which he found to be a less interesting medium for sculpture. As Alexandro had expressed his desire to improve his routine with new roles, the therapist and Alexandro agreed to find a temporary volunteer role that Alexandro could try out before committing to long-term involvement. Alexandro was introduced to a school of art that provided instruction to disabled and nondisabled students. In this setting, Alexandro could choose to develop new skills for clay modeling or to act as a volunteer, helping other pulmonary rehabilitation patients. After attending several classes and getting to know the students at the school and the classes offered there, Alexandro began to encourage students to resume or broaden their hobbyist/amateur roles, and he soon signed up as an official volunteer with the school.

As with this case, the Role Checklist often serves as a catalyst for discussion of realistic priorities with clients. Also, clients often find the checklist to be affirming, since it gives them a concrete representation of their life pattern. For example, one depressed patient, having filled out the form, noted his several past roles. He reflected that he had been feeling very incompetent, but when he saw how many roles he was able to fill in the past, he felt better about his abilities and more hopeful for the future. Finally, as with Alexandro and his very specific ideas about role engagement, discussing responses on the checklist is always important for understanding what clients mean when filling out the form.

Conclusion: Self-Report Assessments in Perspective

This chapter presented self-report assessments and illustrated their use through case examples. The cases demonstrated that clients of various ages and in various contexts can use self-report assessments to identify concerns and participate in intervention planning. All of these assessments allow clients to provide information about themselves by completing paper and pencil forms, or when necessary, the assessments can be administered as an interview. As noted throughout the chapter, these assessments should always be used in the context of a discussion between the therapist and client to clarify responses and validate interpretations, as well as to achieve mutual agreement about their implications for therapy.

References

Baron, K., Kielhofner, G., Iyenger, A., Goldhammer, V., & Wolenski, J. (2006). *The Occupational Self Assessment (OSA) (Version 2.2)*. Model of Human Occupation Clearinghouse, Department of Occupational Therapy, College of Applied Health Sciences, University of Illinois at Chicago.

Cordeiro, J. R., Camelier, A., Oakley, F., & Jardim, J. R. (2007). Cross-cultural reproducibility of the Brazilian Portuguese version of the Role Checklist for Persons with Chronic Obstructive Pulmonary Disease. *American Journal of Occupational Therapy*, 61, 33–40.

Furst, G., Gerber, L., Smith, C., Fisher, S., & Shulman, B. (1987). A program for improving energy conservation behaviors in adults with rheumatoid arthritis. *American Journal of Occupational Therapy*, 41, 102–111.

Gerber, L., & Furst, G. (1992). Scoring methods and application of the Activity Record (ACTRE) for patients with musculoskeletal disorders. *Arthritis Care and Research*, 5, 151–156.

Henry, A. D. (2000). *The Pediatric Interest Profiles: Surveys of play for children and adolescents*. Unpublished manuscript, Model of Human Occupation Clearinghouse, Department of Occupational Therapy, University of Illinois at Chicago.

Keller, J., Kafkes, A., Basu, S., Federico, J., & Kielhofner, G. (2005). *The Child Occupational Self Assessment (version 2.1)*. Model of Human Occupation Clearinghouse, Department of Occupational Therapy, College of Applied Health Sciences, University of Illinois at Chicago.

Kielhofner, G., & Neville, A. (1983). *The modified interest checklist*. Unpublished manuscript, Model of Human Occupation Clearinghouse, Department of Occupational Therapy, University of Illinois at Chicago.

Matsutsuyu, J. (1969). The Interest Check List. *American Journal of Occupational Therapy*, 23, 323–328.

Oakley, F., Kielhofner, G., & Barris, R. (1985). An occupational therapy approach to assessing psychiatric patients' adaptive functioning. *American Journal of Occupational Therapy*, 39, 147–154.

Restall, G., Ripart, J., & Stern, M. (2003). A framework of strategies for client centred practice. *The Canadian Journal of Occupational Therapy, 70* (2), 103-112.

Scaffa, M. (1981). *Temporal adaptations and alcoholism*. Unpublished master's thesis, Virginia Commonwealth University, Richmond.

Smith, N. R., Kielhofner, G., & Watts, J. (1986). The relationship between volition, activity pattern, and life satisfaction in the elderly. *American Journal of Occupational Therapy*, 40, 278–283.

Yamada, T., Ishii, Y., & Nagatani, R. (2002). Establishing the activities for the Interest Checklist of Japanese Elderly Version. *Japanese Journal of Occupational Behavior, 6(1)*, 25–35.

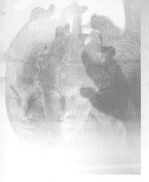

17

Talking With Clients: Assessments That Collect Information Through Interviews

- Gary Kielhofner
- Kirsty Forsyth
- Christine Clay
- Elin Ekbladh
- Lena Haglund
- Helena Hemmingsson
- Riitta Keponen
- Linda Olson

Whether formal or informal, client interviews provide a large portion of the information through which therapists come to know their clients. Five interview assessments have been developed for use with MOHO:

- Occupational Circumstances Assessment—Interview and Rating Scale (OCAIRS)
- Occupational Performance History Interview— Second Version (OPHI-II)
- School Setting Interview (SSI)
- Worker Role Interview (WRI)
- Work Environment Impact Scale (WEIS).

Each of these assessments has a distinct format and purpose. The Occupational Circumstances Assessment— Interview and Rating Scale (OCAIRS) focuses primarily on the client's current occupational participation. The Occupational Performance History Interview-Second Version (OPHI-II) is a life history interview. The Worker Role Interview (WRI) is designed for use with injured or disabled workers. The Work Environment Impact Scale (WEIS) was developed to examine the impact of the work environment on the worker. The School Setting Interview (SSI) is designed to assess school environment impact and identify the need for accommodations for students with disabilities.

These assessments all have some common features. Each has a semi-structured interview that the therapist adapts to fit the circumstances of the client. After the interview is conducted, the therapist must have some means of analyzing the information. Each assessment has a rating scale or checklist that, when completed, represents what was learned in the interview. Each of these assessments also has a means of recording qualitative information gathered during the interview.

Occupational Circumstances Assessment—Interview and Rating Scale

The Occupational Circumstances Assessment— Interview and Rating Scale (OCAIRS) (Forsyth et al., 2005) is based the Occupational Case Analysis Interview and Rating Scale (Kaplan, 1984; Kaplan & Kielhofner,

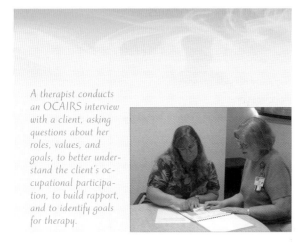

A therapist conducts an OCAIRS interview with a client, asking questions about her roles, values, and goals, to better understand the client's occupational participation, to build rapport, and to identify goals for therapy.

1989). The OCAIRS provides a structure for gathering, analyzing, and reporting data on the extent and nature of an individual's occupational participation. The OCAIRS is designed to be relevant to adolescent and adult clients with a wide range of backgrounds and impairments.

Administration

A manual details the OCAIRS, providing information on conducting the interview and completing the scale (Forsyth et al., 2005). The OCAIRS consists of a semistructured interview that can be adapted to each unique client. The assessment manual details interview formats for mental health, forensic, and physical rehabilitation practice contexts. After conducting one of these interviews, the therapist completes a rating scale and records comments regarding the client's occupational functioning. The interview can be conducted in about 20 to 30 minutes with practice, and completion of the scale takes between 5 and 20 minutes, depending on the therapist's familiarity with the assessment and the level of detail in the comment sections. In addition, the Worker Role Interview (Chapter 17) assessment manual and the Model of Human Occupation Screening Tool (MOHOST) (Chapter 18) assessment manual outline how the OCAIRS can be simultaneously administered to save administration time.

The rating scale is completed by checking off criteria that best describe the client and then using them as a guide to selecting the appropriate rating. A sample item is shown in *Figure 17.1*. When all ratings are transferred to one of the assessment summary forms, the OCAIRS rating scale provides a profile of strengths and challenges, which is useful for therapy and discharge planning.

Occupational Circumstances Assessment— Interview and Rating Scale (OCAIRS)

- Gathers information on values, goals, personal causation, interests, habits, roles, skills, environmental, participation, long and short term goals, and adaptation
- Can be ordered through the MOHO Clearinghouse e-store *http://ascendant.cas.uic.edu/retail/*, or
  - Visit *www.moho.uic.edu*
  - Select menu item "MOHO Products"
  - Link to OCAIRS assessment for more information about the assessment and example assessment forms. To link to the MOHO Clearinghouse e-store, left-click on the "Buy Now" button.

Olaf: Using the OCAIRS to Guide Intervention and Discharge Planning

At age 23, Olaf was hospitalized for the first time in an acute psychiatric ward. His older sister, younger brother, and parents (who are professors) live in the same town in Sweden. Olaf moved to his own apartment 2 years earlier, when he began studying nursing at the local university. When he was younger, Olaf always had many friends. However, in the past 4 years he was very isolated, spending most of his time studying. For 6 months, Olaf had increasing difficulty keeping up with

FIGURE 17.1 Sample item (Interests) from the OCAIRS.

Interests

F	☐ Participates in many interests regularly outside of work ☐ High level of interest in primary occupation ☐ High level of satisfaction with level of participation in an interest(s)
A	☐ Participates in few, but clearly expressed, interests regularly outside of work ☐ Some interest in primary occupation ☐ Some satisfaction with level of participation in an interest(s)
I	☐ Few & vaguely defined interests outside of work, no regular participation ☐ Very little interest in primary occupation ☐ Very little satisfaction with level of participation in an interest(s)
R	☐ Does not participate in any identified interests outside of work ☐ No interest in primary occupation ☐ Dissatisfaction with level of participation

Key: **F** = Facilitates: Facilitates Participation in Occupation
A = Allows: Allows Participation in Occupation
I = Inhibits: Inhibits Participation in Occupation
R = Restricts: Restricts Participation in Occupation

his studies. Most recently, he complained of hearing a voice that told him to hurt himself because he was not good enough.

The occupational therapist used the OCAIRS to gather information about Olaf's occupational participation to help with planning during his anticipated 4-week hospitalization. Olaf was quite confused about what was happening to him. Several times during the interview he asked, "Do you think I'm schizophrenic?" Despite his confusion and fear, he was able to participate effectively in the interview. Olaf's scores on the OCAIRS are shown in *Figure 17.2*. The following qualitative information was also gathered during the interview.

When asked about his interests, Olaf noted that he used to like to listen to hard rock music, study, and read science literature, but he had not been able to do these

things for some time. He did have some goals. In particular, he wanted to begin his studies again. After finishing the nursing program, he wanted to enroll in management courses at the university and then start his own business. He said that it was very important to him to be smart and successful.

In contrast to his goal of beginning school again, Olaf's sense of personal causation was extremely low. He felt out of control. He feared that the voice he heard would control him. Although he felt compelled to return to his studies, he did not see how he could possibly succeed. Olaf indicated that he was no longer able to do anything well, and he could not point out any skills of which he was proud. He complained that he could not plan or organize his behavior to accomplish even everyday activities.

FIGURE 17.2 Olaf's Ratings on the OCAIRS.

	Facilitates	Allows	Inhibits	Restricts
Roles			✗	
Habits				✗
Personal causation				✗
Values			✗	
Interests		✗		
Skills			✗	
Short-term goals			✗	
Long-term goals		✗		
Interpretation of past experiences		✗		
Physical environment		✗		
Social environment			✗	
Readiness for change	✗			

Olaf previously was able to maintain a daily routine as follows. He attended the university in the morning and studied in the evening. He carried out his routine alone, remaining isolated during the weekend. He disliked cooking, so he mostly ate at the university canteen or a local restaurant. He noted that each day had been more or less the same for him for the past 4 years. He said, "I'm not a sociable person anymore." During the previous 6 months, Olaf had difficulty completing daily routines and concentrating on tasks. In the 3 weeks before being hospitalized, he remained in his flat alone, drinking tea and eating sandwiches, ignoring everything else, including his personal hygiene.

Olaf described actively avoiding other people, noting that he was very shy and felt uncomfortable initiating conversation. When asked about important people in his life, he hesitated and then finally mentioned his sister. He recalled that he had a girlfriend some years before. However, at the time, there was no person that he considered a significant support. While Olaf recalled a happy family life during childhood and adolescence, he felt that he no longer had anything to say to his parents. He admitted feeling very lonely and longed for more social contact.

Olaf liked his flat and very much wanted to return to it. He received a substantial amount of money from his grandmother when he bought his flat so he could furnish it the way he wanted. The flat was in the central part of the town, a location that he liked.

The interview helped the occupational therapist identify Olaf's strengths and weaknesses as shown in *Figure 17.2*. Although many aspects of his occupational life were quite eroded, his long-term goals and his physical environment were strong points. It was apparent in the interview that Olaf's greatest priorities were to:

- Engage in his studies again
- Take part in some social occupations
- Move back to his flat as soon as possible.

The OCAIRS also provided a structured way of helping the therapist start to plan Olaf's intervention. She planned to address his volitional status through structured graded occupations. Information about Olaf's occupational lifestyle gained from the OCAIRS was used to select the specific occupational forms/tasks used in intervention. These were things he indicated an interest in and that related to his long-term goals. She also chose occupational forms/tasks that were within his skill level so that he could experience success and thereby begin to rebuild personal causation. Given that Olaf felt he could not do anything, the therapist routinely provided Olaf with concrete feedback aimed at shaping his experience of doing things. Therefore, whenever he completed an occupational form/task, the therapist took time to review what he had accomplished and highlighted his strengths. She also carefully pointed out how his successes in therapy related to his long-term aims.

As Olaf gained some confidence, the therapist and he started to work together on his goal of returning to independent living in his own flat. He began by taking increased responsibility for self-care and care of his immediate environment. Since Olaf stated he was having difficulties maintaining a daily routine and completing his homemaker tasks, they developed a routine that included some of these tasks in the inpatient setting. Olaf followed this routine and reviewed it twice a week with the therapist. As he approached time for discharge, the therapist accompanied Olaf to his apartment several times to identify and practice homemaking tasks. Finally, Olaf was enrolled in several inpatient groups to increase his level of social interaction. While he remained quiet, his level of skill became adequate for social interaction once he regained some of his confidence for interacting with others.

The OCAIRS was also useful in planning for Olaf's discharge. His level of functioning was still not consistent with the demands of returning to university studies. However, given the importance to Olaf of being involved in studies, the therapist arranged for him to attend a supported educational facility for persons with psychosocial impairments. She worked with him to make choices for courses, focusing on those related to his long-term goals. She also helped Olaf plan a daily routine to accommodate attending the courses. Because of his poor sense of efficacy, she accompanied him to the school to sign up for the first day of classes. She also guided him to identify some groups at the school that he could join to have social contact. The therapist continued to make home visits with Olaf in his apartment after discharge to monitor the routine they had planned together so that he could manage his self-care and maintain the apartment.

In sum, the OCAIRS provided the therapist with information to gain an understanding of Olaf's occupational life, the challenges he faced, and his goals for the future. This information helped in identifying therapeutic goals and strategies and assured that therapy addressed what mattered to Olaf.

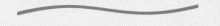

Occupational Performance History Interview—Second Version

As a historical interview, the Occupational Performance History Interview—Second Version (OPHI-II) (Kielhofner et al., 2004) gathers information about a client's past and present occupational adaptation. The OPHI-II is a three-part assessment that includes:

- A semi-structured interview that explores a client's occupational life history
- Rating scales that provide a measure of the client's occupational identity, occupational competence, and the impact of the client's occupational settings (environment)
- A life history narrative designed to capture salient qualitative features of the occupational life history

It is designed to give the interviewer a means of understanding the way a client perceives his or her life to be unfolding. The OPHI-II can be used with adolescents and adults who have a range of impairments.

As a semi-structured interview, the OPHI-II provides a framework and recommended questions for conducting the interview to assure that the necessary information is obtained. The interview is organized into the following thematic areas:

- Activity and occupational choices
- Critical life events
- Daily routine
- Occupational roles
- Occupational settings (environment).

Within each of these thematic areas, a possible sequence of interview questions is provided. The interview is designed to be very flexible so that therapists can cover the areas in any sequence or move back and forth between them.

The second part of the OPHI-II is composed of the three rating scales:

- Occupational identity scale
- Occupational competence scale
- Occupational settings (environment) scale.

The three scales provide a means of converting the information gathered in the interview into three measures. The occupational identity scale measures the degree to which persons have values, interests, and confidence; see themselves in various occupational roles;

and hold an image of the kind of life they want. The occupational competence scale measures the degree to which a person is able to sustain a pattern of occupational activity that is productive and satisfying. The occupational behavior settings scale measures the impact of the environment on the client's occupational life. A key form has been developed for these three scales that allows interval measures to be derived form the ordinal ratings made on the each of the scales (Kielhofner, Dobria, Forsyth, & Basu, 2005).

Administration

The OPHI-II is presented in a detailed manual designed to teach the therapist to administer the assessment. It includes detailed guidelines for conducting the interview and provides several resources for supporting the interview process. It also gives detailed instructions and examples for completing the rating scales and life history narrative.

The therapist begins by conducting the interview, which takes approximately 45 to 60 minutes. Although the OPHI-II is designed so that it can be completed as a single interview, therapists may conduct the interview in more than one part. Following the interview, the therapist scores the three rating scales consisting of a total of 29 items. The therapist rates each item with a four-point rating that indicates the client's level of occupational adaptation and environmental impact. The rating is completed by first noting criteria that describe the client for each item and then selecting the corresponding rating, as shown in *Figure 17.3*. Each of the three scales provides a profile of strengths and challenges related to identity, competence, and environmental impact, which is useful to planning therapy. Paper-and-pencil methods of generating client measures from each scale have been developed.

Finally, the therapist completes the life history narrative form that is used to report qualitative information from the interview. As part of this process, the therapist graphically plots the client's life story, thereby indicating the narrative slope, as discussed in Chapter 9. This allows the therapist to develop an appreciation of the plot of the occupational narrative underlying the client's identity and competence.

FIGURE 17.3 An example of scoring the OPHI-II scale: criteria are checked and the rating indicated by the criteria selected.

Item	Rating	Criteria
Has personal goals and projects	4	☐ Goals/personal projects challenge/extend/require effort. ☐ Feels energized/excited about future goals/personal projects.
	3	☐ Goals/personal projects fit strengths/limitations. ☐ Enough desire for future to overcome doubt/challenges. ☐ Motivated to work on goals/personal projects.
	②	☐ Goals/anticipated projects under/overestimate abilities. ☐ Not very motivated to work on goals/personal projects. ☒ Difficulty thinking about goals/personal projects/future. ☒ Limited commitment/excitement/motivation.
	1	☐ Cannot identify goals/personal projects. ☐ Personal goals/desired projects are unattainable given abilities. ☐ Goals bear little/no relationship to strengths/limitations. ☐ Lacks commitment or motivation to the future. ☐ Unmotivated due to conflicting/excessive goals/personal projects.

Key:
4 = Exceptionally competent occupational functioning
3 = Appropriate satisfactory occupational functioning
2 = Some occupational functioning problems
1 = Extreme occupational functioning problems

Occupational Performance History Interview—Second Version (OPHI-II)

. . . .

- Gathers information on client's life history with a focus on identity, competence, and environment.
- Can be ordered through the MOHO Clearinghouse e-store *http://ascendant.cas.uic.edu/retail/*, or
  - Visit *www.moho.uic.edu*
  - Select menu item "MOHO Products"
  - Link to OPHI-II assessment for more information about the assessment and example assessment forms. To link to the MOHO Clearinghouse e-store, left-click on the "Buy Now" button.

Christine: The OPHI-II As the Beginning of a Way Out

. . . .

Christine is an African-American woman in her mid-30s. Over the past several years, she has had a series of surgeries for recurrent nonmalignant brain tumors. In addition to repeated surgical removal of the tumors over several years, she has also received a shunt to alleviate elevated intraventricular pressure. As a consequence of her tumors and surgery, Christine has both mild cognitive impairments (mostly difficulty with short-term memory) and low vision impairment.

Following her most recent surgery, Christine was hospitalized in a short-term rehabilitation unit. During her stay, the occupational therapist focused on supporting Christine to use adaptive strategies to perform activities of daily living more effectively. As Christine neared discharge, she indicated to her therapist a desire to make some major changes in her life, specifically to return to work and live on her own.

The therapist referred Christine to an outpatient occupational therapy program, Work Readiness, designed to support clients who wished to achieve greater independence and move toward employment. As part of the

entrance to this program, Christine participated in the OPHI-II interview. Because the program was designed to assist clients in making major life changes, this historical interview was especially appropriate. It was routinely used both to help clients and therapists together decide whether the program was appropriate for the client and to help determine long-term goals and approaches.

The results of Christine's interview on the three rating scales are shown in *Figure 17.4*. Christine related a life story in which her strong occupational identity was partly eroded by her prolonged illness, impairments, and consequent loss of major occupational roles. Christine grew up on the south side of Chicago in a working-class family. She described her parents as warm and proud individuals with strong values. They instilled in their children a sense that they should make something of their lives, be leaders, and give something back to their community. As Christine put it, her parents not only expected their children not only to have a vision of their goals in life but also "to have a concrete plan for getting there."

Christine's father died when she was 12, which left the family in financial jeopardy. Christine recalls her father's death as both a tragic and defining moment in her life. According to her, "I walked to my father's coffin and looked down at him, pledging that I would never let my mother and sister go hungry or have to live on the streets." Christine was true to her vow. After earning a college degree in teaching, she still had part-time jobs in addition to being a full-time teacher in an inner city Head Start program. This she did to provide extra income for her mother and younger sister.

Despite the family challenges, Christine still remembers her adolescence fondly. She recalls that she, her sister, and her mother "found ways to be happy." For Christine, one of the key factors was her involvement in amateur acting. She joined a group that put on regular performances in a local community theater.

Whether in pursuing education, supporting her mother or sister, or finding ways to be happy, resourcefulness and self-reliance were key elements of Christine's experience during that early period. Then, one day in the classroom, everything changed. A peer teacher saw Christine do something strange. She attempted to pick up an object pictured on the page of a book she was reading to the children. Christine remem-

FIGURE 17.4 Summary of Christine's Scores on the OPHI-II

Occupational Identity Scale	1	2	3	4
Has personal goals and projects		X		
Identifies a desired occupational lifestyle				X
Expects success	X			
Accepts responsibility			X	
Appraises abilities and limitations		X		
Has commitments and values				X
Recognizes identity and obligations				X
Has interests				X
Felt effective (past)				X
Found meaning and satisfaction in lifestyle (past)				X
Made occupational choices (past)				X
Occupational Competence Scale	1	2	3	4
Maintains satisfying lifestyle	X			
Fulfills role expectations	X			
Works toward goals	X			
Meets personal performance standards	X			
Organizes time for responsibilities	X			
Participates in interests	X			
Fulfilled roles (past)				X
Maintained habits (past)				X
Achieved satisfaction (past)				X
Occupational Settings (Environment) Scale	1	2	3	4
Home-life occupational forms		X		
Major productive role occupational forms	Not Applicable			
Leisure occupational forms		X		
Home-life social group			X	
Major productive social group	Not Applicable			
Leisure social group		X		
Home-life physical spaces, objects, and resources			X	
Major productive role physical spaces, objects, and resources	Not Applicable			
Leisure physical spaces, objects, and resources		X		

Key: **1** = Extreme occupational functioning problems
2 = Some occupational functioning problems
3 = Appropriate, satisfactory occupational functioning
4 = Exceptionally competent occupational functioning

bers that she saw it as three-dimensional and real. This perceptual error, which led Christine to seek medical attention, and increasing headaches were the first signs of something awry in her brain. Christine still remembers the classroom incident both as her last day of teaching and as the turning point where the life she had crafted began to disintegrate.

Surgery to remove a tumor swiftly followed and left Christine with short-term memory loss and visual restrictions. Her job was gone, and she moved from her apartment back to her mother's house. The mother and sister, to whom Christine had offered financial support, now helped Christine through even her most basic daily routines. During several ensuing years, recurring surgeries and their cumulative sequelae left Christine increasingly impaired and more and more distanced from the life she once lived.

Christine was afraid to have others "see what I had become." She describes how, when people came to the house, she ran to the basement to "hide myself away." While Christine realized her incarceration was self-imposed, she saw "no way out." The person she once was and the life she once lived were gone forever. She described herself as "boxed in" by the fear of what others might see in her. She described the deep and painful frustration of being unable to pull out of herself what she used to be able to do. She had no other way to sum her life than the feeling of being "locked away."

Christine's daily routine reflected both her difficulties with short-term memory and her complete demoralization. She noted that the first big chore of the day was getting out of bed. This did not ordinarily occur without repeated entreaties from her mother. When she did finally manage to emerge from bed, the routines of daily life unfolded with excruciating slowness. Christine explained that the reason for her pace of performing was that she could not remember what she has just done. Things as simple as bathing became long, confusing trials in which she tried to tally each completed step and inevitably repeated herself several times to allay the anxiety that she has forgotten something. Christine was able to do little beyond self-care and helping out with chores around the house. She left the house only for medical appointments. Her former roles and routines were things of the past.

Christine still had a vivid image of the kind of life she wanted, even if she did not dare to hope for it. Christine longed to return to teaching children. She wanted to go back to a time when she was supporting her mother and sister instead of them guiding her through her day. She was explicit and articulate in expressing her continued desire to make a difference. At the same time, Christine could not reconcile the image of who she wanted to be with the impairments she experienced. So she was stuck, unable to get, in her words, "out of the box" in which she found herself. She longed for but could not see a "way out." Thus, while her goals were clear, they were not attainable.

As reflected in the OPHI-II ratings from *Figure 17.4*, Christine's identity had many strengths, along with the challenges of her compromised personal causation and her difficulty in formulating a realistic goal. The therapist recognized and built on these strengths and weaknesses in the course of Christine's involvement in the Work Readiness program. As discussed below, therapy focused on rebuilding her sense of capacity and efficacy and her selecting realistic goals for the future. Her competence was more severely affected in all aspects. Being "locked away," she did not pursue goals, enact roles and routines, or take on responsibilities as in the past. Finally, as Christine noted, she existed a long way from the high standards of performance that she inherited from her family. The course of therapy was designed to enable Christine to gradually rebuild these aspects of her competence.

Christine's removal from the world of work and her narrowed world of everyday life and recreation are reflected in the ratings on the occupational behavior settings scale. Her mother and sister were sources of guidance and comfort for her. As she notes, they kept her going and helped her "remember where I came from."

Christine's narrative slope, as depicted in *Figure 17.5*, has all the features of a tragedy. This woman, who drew strength from and rose out of the challenges of her early life to earn a college degree and take on a professional role, found herself sliding steadily downward. Christine's narrative also reveals a strong metaphor of entrapment (see discussion of metaphors in Chapter 9). Her feelings of being locked away found expression in her being house-bound and in hiding from others.

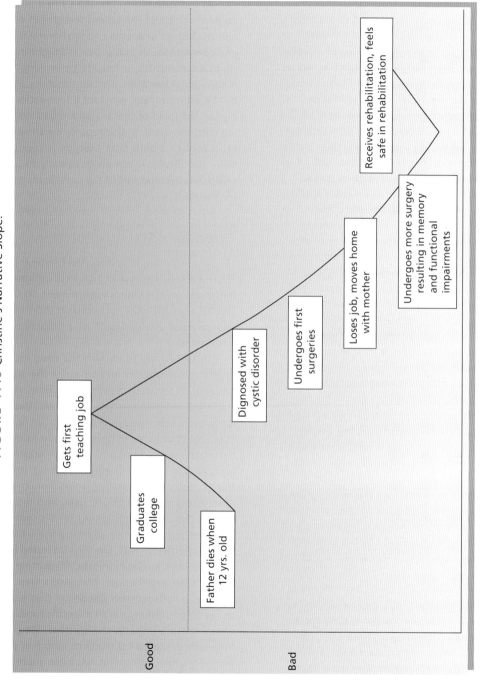

FIGURE 17.5 Christine's Narrative Slope.

Good

Bad

Father dies when
12 yrs. old

Graduates
college

Gets first
teaching job

Dignosed with
cystic disorder

Undergoes first
surgeries

Loses job, moves home
with mother

Undergoes more surgery
resulting in memory
and functional
impairments

Receives rehabilitation, feels
safe in rehabilitation

271

When the therapist shared these interpretations of Christine's life with her, she agreed that they were accurate. The metaphor of being locked away and its implied solution of needing to find a way out served as both an incentive for Christine to join the Work Readiness program and a recurrent theme in Christine's therapy. Through the course of therapy, Christine slowly rebuilt a routine by attending the program with increasing frequency. She learned with ongoing support how to monitor her performance and check for mistakes without repeating herself endlessly. After a couple of months, Christine attended the program daily and was able to join and perform in the presence of others. As she noted, she had found a "way out" through therapy.

When Christine had progressed to the point of considering a return to work, she had to find out for herself whether teaching was still a possibility. The therapist arranged a placement for Christine as a classroom volunteer. It was quickly apparent to Christine that her residual impairments made teaching unrealistic. Instead, in making her first foray into the world of work, Christine reached back to her old experiences of theatrical performance and secured a job in a casino, where her responsibilities included entertaining customers with a little "soft shoe." Christine had traversed the wide gulf from hiding away to presenting herself in a most public way. For her, this was an important journey.

Nevertheless, after a period of working in the casino, Christine longed for work that would more nearly match her value system. Taking advantage of the program's long-term follow-up services, she received support for a job search and eventually became an intake counselor in a program serving people with visual impairments. Having a visual disability herself, Christine found that she was able to put new clients at ease and to serve as a role model for what could be achieved despite impairments.

Christine also found her way back into the role of teaching as a lecturer in occupational therapy, speaking to students about the experience of disability and the client's perspective in undergoing therapy. She has gone on to create, in poetry, visual imagery, and film, teaching tools aimed at a variety of audiences to encourage the understanding of disability and how to cope with it. Her most recent accomplishment is becoming one of the authors of this chapter.

As this case illustrates, the OPHI-II provides a detailed chronicle of the salient features of a client's life and the impact of events and environment on identity and competence. It also provides insight into how the client interprets his or her life by evoking the client's occupational narrative. This information, as illustrated by the previous case, provides a foundation for determining the focus of therapy and negotiating its meaning with the client. In this regard, the OPHI-II is a powerful tool to assure that therapy is client centered. More specifically, it can allow therapy to address and effectively become part of the lives clients want to craft for themselves.

The School Setting Interview

The School Setting Interview (SSI) (Hemmingsson et al., 2005) is a semi-structured interview designed to assess the impact of the school environment on the student. The SSI uses MOHO's conceptualization of the social and physical environment as a framework for the assessment.

The SSI is used to identify the need for school setting accommodations and to assess the student-environment fit for students with disabilities. It is a client-centered interview that examines the student's interaction with the physical and social environments at school. It includes 16 items that make up a student's participation in school and together address the content areas of writing; reading; speaking; remembering things; doing mathematics; doing homework; taking examinations; going to art, gym, and music; getting around the classrooms; taking breaks; going on field trips; getting assistance; accessing the school; and interacting with the staff. The SSI is intended for students who are able to communicate adequately enough to discuss their experiences. This assessment is administered as a collaborative discussion that examines the student's performance with a specific focus on how the school setting impacts the student. Whereas it was originally designed for students who had physical impairments, the instrument has been successfully used with students who have emotional, developmental, and behavioral difficulties.

The SSI considers the student's occupational performance in all aspects of the school environment, such as the classroom, playground, toilets, lockers, gymnasium, corridors, and field trips. In addition to determining whether accommodations are necessary, the therapist gains a qualitative understanding of the student's experiences. Furthermore, the SSI guides the therapist to discuss with the students how they want to manage in school. The SSI empowers students to collaborate with the therapist in determining the types of accommodations they may need. It reflects the assumption that determining the student's preferences, values, needs, and interests is crucial to successful physical and social accommodations in the school setting.

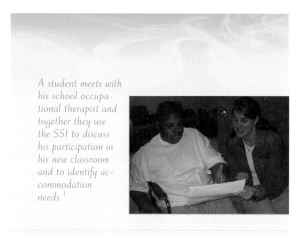

A student meets with his school occupational therapist and together they use the SSI to discuss his participation in his new classroom and to identify accommodation needs.[1]

[1]*Photo provided by Bridget Caruso, Occupational Therapist, University of Illlinois Medical Center at Chicago.*

Administration

Before beginning the interview, the therapist stresses to the student that the SSI is not designed to identify the student's weaknesses. The therapist explains that instead, the purpose of this assessment is to make sure the school is doing its best to assist the student to do well. In conducting the interview, the therapist explores each of the 16 items, asking the student:

- How he or she has functioned and currently functions in the area
- Whether the student perceives a need for accommodation to perform in the area
- Whether the student has an accommodation in this area

The SSI interview takes about 40 minutes, and the therapist records necessary information during the in-

terview. A form allows identification of whether there are accommodation needs in each area and whether they are met. Another form allows recording of recommendations for accommodation. This form indicates recommended changes to be made in objects, spaces, occupational forms/tasks, and social groups. It also records who will be responsible for each accommodation and how it will be implemented.

To give the therapist and other professionals a quick overview of student-environment fit and to track change, a summary form is provided. After the interview, the therapist indicates the extent of the student's accommodations, needs, and unmet needs on each item using a four-point rating scale.

School Setting Interview (SSI)

. . . .

- Gathers information on school environment impact and student–environment fit and identifies need for accommodations
- English-speaking therapists in the United States and Canada can order the SSI through the MOHO Clearinghouse e-store *http://ascendant.cas.uic.edu/retail/,* or
  - Visit *www.moho.uic.edu*
  - Select menu item "MOHO Products"
  - Link to SSI assessment for more information about the assessment and example assessment forms. To link to the MOHO Clearinghouse e-store, left-click on the "Buy Now" button.

Therapists outside of the United States and Canada can order the SSI from the Swedish Association of Occupational Therapists (FSA) by contacting Tina Poulsen at *TiPo.fsa@akademikerhuset.se.*

Thomas: Use of the SSI to Give Voice to a Student's Experiences and Needs

The principal of a high school in a Stockholm suburb invited the school occupational therapist to a routine planning meeting concerning Thomas, a first-year high school student. Thomas's parents, the school nurse, a special education teacher, and his language, physical education, and math teachers were also invited to attend. The therapist had known Thomas and his family for nearly 10 years.

At age 4, Thomas was diagnosed with muscular dystrophy. He always attended a regular school, and most things went well. Throughout primary school, he had a couple of good friends in his class. He also had a teacher who was empathic, flexible, and adept at including Thomas in class activities with the other children. The therapist had previously worked with Thomas and occasionally consulted with Thomas's mother by telephone.

Thomas's mother called the therapist, indicating that Thomas had asked her to make the call. The mother said that as far as she knew, everything was going fine with Thomas in his new school. Thomas then took the telephone and explained that he had heard of the upcoming meeting from his mother. As far as Thomas knew, he was not invited, and none of the teachers had spoken to him about it. He wanted to know what the meeting was about. The therapist explained that she understood the meeting to be a routine review meeting to assure Thomas was doing fine. When the therapist asked Thomas how he liked the new school, he responded, "It's okay, I suppose." Thomas's tone suggested otherwise, so the therapist made an appointment to meet Thomas after school that week.

The therapist then called the principal back to ask if there was some special preparation that he wanted her to do before the meeting. He explained again that it was a routine meeting. The principal was not aware of any problems. Thomas appeared to be doing fine and had not complained of anything. He expected the meeting to affirm that Thomas was performing well and adjusting to the new school.

Thomas's school was big and rather traditional, having been built in the beginning of the 20th century. When the therapist arrived for the appointment, Thomas was waiting at the entrance and appeared to be the only student present. He explained that it was the day of a sports outing. Thomas was not capable of going along, so he was there alone.

The therapist explained that since she was invited to the planning meeting next week, she wanted to interview Thomas to get his opinion about the school situation and how it affected his participation in school activities. As the interview progressed, it was obvious that Thomas found being in the new school a negative experience. Things that he readily did in his former school were now difficult or impossible for him. He had tried hard to adapt to the new circumstances and he had not wanted to complain, as he was afraid of drawing too much attention to himself. During the SSI interview, Thomas identified unmet needs and problems with student–environment fit in several areas, as reflected in the summary form shown in *Figure 17.6*.

In his previous school, Thomas's homeroom teacher taught the students in nearly all subjects. Therefore, she came to know his special needs and was able to integrate the accommodations he needed into her plans for the class. For example, in the area of writing, she always made a paper copy of any visual aids she used in class. She gave a copy of these to Thomas, since he wrote slowly and needed additional time to take notes. Now, in secondary school, Thomas had different teachers in nearly all subjects. He had informed some of his teachers about his need for paper copies of slides and overheads. However, the information had not reached some teachers or they had forgotten. Consequently, he rarely got paper copies of class audiovisuals. Thomas also needed more time for writing in examinations, but no such arrangements had been made in the new school.

Thomas was used to being able to participate in activities like field trips and outdoor activities, as his teacher always tried to include his needs in her planning. He had a powered wheelchair he could use on outings, since his walking was too labored for such events. There had already been several occasions in the new school when plans for special events were made without consideration of his needs. This meant that he

FIGURE 17.6 Thomas's identified needs and student–environment fit on the SSI Summary Form.

Student: Thomas				
Rating steps	**4**	**3**	**2**	**1**
Write				✗
Read		✗		
Speak	✗			
Remember things	✗			
Do mathematics		✗		
Do homework	✗			
Take exams				✗
Doing sport activities				✗
Doing practical subjects			✗	
Participating in the classroom			✗	
Participating in social activities during breaks				✗
Participating in practical activities during breaks			✗	
Going on field trips				✗
Getting assistance		✗		
Accessing the school			✗	
Interacting with staff				✗

Key: **1** = Unfit   **2** = Partial fit   **3** = Good fit   **4** = Perfect fit

was excluded. On the other hand, Thomas was very happy that he did not have to participate in gym, as he found it embarrassing that he could not dress himself.

Another big difference was that in his former school all of Thomas's classes were held in his home classroom. Now, in secondary school, he had to travel between classrooms. During the short breaks between classes, Thomas often had to go to a different floor or a different building. Ambulating made it difficult for him to carry books and other things that he needed in the next classroom. Neither his balance nor his strength was good enough to walk carrying a heavy bag. Of his own accord, Thomas had decided to start using his wheel-chair at school, which made it possible for him to carry his things between classrooms. Using a wheelchair in school had also made lunchtime easier, as he had difficulty standing in line in the lunchroom.

Using the wheelchair, however, created new problems. The organization of the school day required rather quick transfer between classrooms. To use the elevator was time consuming, and he had difficulty opening the manual elevator door. Moreover, there was only one wheelchair-accessible toilet, on the second floor of one building. Finally, there were only steps to the entrance of school, which forced him to take an otherwise unused side entrance that also increased the distance he had to travel when entering and leaving the building. Another problem related to frequent classroom changes was that Thomas and his personal equipment (e.g., assistive devices, special chair, special desk, and personal computer) were unfortunately seldom in the same classroom.

Finally, as part of the SSI interview, the therapist and Thomas collaboratively discussed ways that the school might address his unmet needs in each content area. The therapist suggested that Thomas be given an assistant who would carry his bag and take notes when needed or that he request a home classroom. However, Thomas did not want a personal assistant. He preferred to ask some classmates who were friends to assist him. He noted that they already helped him voluntarily sometimes without being asked. He also did not want to ask for a home classroom, as he thought it would adversely affect his relationships with classmates who would find it childish. He was most satisfied with the idea that the school be asked to schedule as many of his courses on the ground floor as possible to minimize his need to use the elevator.

The therapist then brought up to Thomas the risk of immobilization. She explained that if he constantly used the wheelchair, he increased the risk of contractures in his hip flexors. She pointed out that with his diagnosis immobilization even for short periods might cause permanent inability to walk. She pointed out that his use of the wheelchair in school, in combination with avoiding gym, was a serious risk. It was obvious that Thomas did not want to think about this. However, the therapist got his permission to talk with the physical therapist and with the gym teacher about arranging an individual gym program for Thomas.

Finally, they discussed ways that the school could become more aware of and attentive to Thomas's special needs. Thomas and the therapist decided together that the therapist should share the information from the SSI with the other team members at the planning meeting. She would be responsible to report to Thomas what happened.

Recommendations for Accommodation

At the staff meeting, the therapist presented the SSI results and discussed necessary accommodations for Thomas. The therapist recorded the results of this meeting on the SSI Environmental Accommodations and

Interventions Form, shown in *Figure 17.7*, and discussed later. The therapist began with presenting Thomas's need for classroom scheduling to keep him mostly on one floor. Second, she emphasized that all of Thomas's teachers needed better information about his special needs. She recommended that there be a written document about Thomas's needs (i.e., copies of slides, a desk suitable for a wheelchair, extra time in examinations, and consideration of his physical limitations when planning outdoor activities and field trips). The therapist recommended that the principal give this document to any new teacher. In addition, Thomas would receive copies that he could give to teachers as a reminder.

The therapist also requested on Thomas's behalf:

- Adapting one of the toilets on the ground floor

- A ramp at the entrance

- An automatic door opener to the elevator.

Finally, she brought up the serious risk of immobilization from constant use of the wheelchair in combination with not attending gym lessons.

Thomas's parents, teachers, and principal were surprised when the therapist described the results from the SSI. They had assumed that everything was fine, as Thomas had never complained. However, they appreciated the information and supported doing everything reasonable to adapt his learning environment. After discussion, the following decisions were made:

- The principal would investigate the logistics of reducing the number of classrooms and the number of teachers who taught in Thomas's classes. He was to consult with Thomas before he made any final decisions.

- The team agreed that a written document about Thomas's special needs was a good idea. The therapist agreed to write the document in cooperation with Thomas.

- The principal agreed to install a ramp at the entrance. As a ramp was needed immediately, the therapist offered to borrow for the school a ramp from a rehabilitation center until the school installed something more permanent at the entrance. The principal believed that the elevator alterations were prohibitively expensive.

FIGURE 17.7 Thomas's Intervention Planning Form.

Content Area	Environmental Adjustments				Team Members	Steps for Implementation: whom, when, where, and how
	Space	Objects	Forms	Groups		
1. Writing			Thomas is given photocopies of visual aides.		• OT • Teacher • Thomas • Principal	• OT and Thomas write his special needs report. • Principal informs Thomas' teacher about helpful strategies decided in the planning meeting.
7. Taking exams			Thomas is given more time to take exams.		• OT • Teacher • Thomas • Principal	• Same as above • PT consults with P.E. instructor and parents.
8. Doing sport activities			Alternative P.E. activities at school and home.		• PT • Teacher • Thomas • Principal	• PT, parents, and P.E. instructor regularly remind Thomas of contracture risks. • Regular assessment of Thomas' mobility by P.T.
9. Doing practical subjects			More time needed to complete art projects.		• Art teacher	• Art teacher will prepare activities that students can complete at their own pace.
10. Participating in the classrooms		Desk adjusted to fit wheelchair in more than one classroom.	Minimize the use of different classrooms.		• OT • Teacher • Thomas • Principal	• Principal, Thomas, and teachers discuss how to minimize the use of different classrooms. • OT orders appropriate desks.
11. Participating in social activities during breaks				Provide assistance to and from social activities so more time is spent having fun and not getting around.		• Thomas will identify some friends that can provide assistance to lunchroom, between classrooms, etc.
12. Participating in practical activities at breaks		Raised toilet seat, in bathroom at ground floor.			• OT • Thomas	• Decide on type of toilet seat and OT to order.
13. Going on field trips			Select field trip sites that are accessible to powered wheelchair.	Thomas will be included in class field trips.	• OT • Thomas • Teacher • Parents	• OT consults on selections of field trip sites. • Prior information from school to Thomas and parents to provide powered wheelchair.
15. Accessing the school	Ramp to the main door entrance. Automatic door opener to elevator.		Reduce transfer between different classrooms.		• OT • Thomas • Principal	• OT to provide temporary ramp. • Principal arranges for permanent ramp.
16. Interacting with staff				The school nurse provides mentorship to Thomas.	• Thomas • School nurse • OT	• School nurse to advocate on behalf of Thomas when needed. • The school nurse to cooperate with OT when needed.

277

- The gym teacher indicated that since he had limited experience with students who had physical impairments, he would need support to meet Thomas's needs. The physiotherapist was identified as the best person to consult with him.

- The physiotherapist agreed to assess Thomas's locomotion regularly and to consult with the school, Thomas, and his parents on how to avoid contractures.

- The school nurse was assigned the responsibility to serve as an advocate and coordinator to ensure that Thomas's needs were being met.

Finally, they decided to invite Thomas to the next planning meeting.

As this case illustrates, the SSI can be particularly helpful in identifying unmet needs for accommodation in the school setting. The framework of the interview, which gives students an opportunity to talk about their experiences, preferences, and needs, is well suited to this end.

Worker Role Interview

The Worker Role Interview (WRI) (Braveman et al., 2005) was first developed as part of a study designed to determine psychosocial variables influencing work success. Its usefulness as a client assessment quickly became apparent, and the instrument was further adapted for such use. The WRI is a semi-structured interview with an accompanying rating scale. The 16-item scale is rated according to the implications of each item for the client's likelihood of work success (either returning to a specific job or employment in general). The WRI is designed to collect data on six content areas:

- Personal causation
- Values
- Interests
- Roles
- Habits
- Perception of the environment.

The WRI was originally designed to gather data from an injured worker (Velozo et al., 1998). The most

current version was designed to be relevant to any person with a disability. The interview provides a solid foundation for planning intervention with a worker whose impairments are interfering with work (Fisher, 1999).

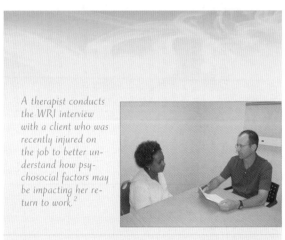

A therapist conducts the WRI interview with a client who was recently injured on the job to better understand how psychosocial factors may be impacting her return to work.[2]

[2]*Photo provided by Supriya Sen, Occupational Therapist, University of Illinois Medical Center at Chicago.*

Administration

The WRI is presented in a manual (Braveman et al., 2005) that provides background information as well as detailed instructions and guidelines for administration. An accompanying videotape provides an opportunity to see the WRI administered and to practice scoring the scale.

Therapists first administer a semi-structured interview that takes approximately 30 to 60 minutes. Interviews are provided specific to injured workers, as well as workers with longstanding illness or disability. In addition, the interview allows the therapist to simultaneously conduct the OCAIRS interview. Therapists then complete the rating scale, entering comments as appropriate. This instrument is designed for concurrent use with other assessments that provide information on work-related capacity. Because the WRI identifies psychosocial factors related to work that are not considered by most work assessments, it often reveals unique strengths and weaknesses that should be considered in therapy services aimed at enabling the client to achieve employment.

Worker Role Interview (WRI)

- Gathers information on values, interests, personal causation, habits, roles, and environmental perceptions as they affect returning to work or finding and keeping work.
- Can be ordered through the MOHO Clearinghouse e-store *http://ascendant.cas.uic.edu/retail/*, or
  - Visit *www.moho.uic.edu*
  - Select menu item "MOHO Products"
  - Link to WRI assessment for more information about the assessment, example assessment forms, or to link to the MOHO Clearinghouse e-store left click on the "Buy Now" button.

Peter: An Illustration of Use of the Worker Role Interview

Peter was a middle-aged man who lived in Gothenburg, Sweden. He was married and had a teenage son. Peter worked in a large company that made technological products. He had been employed in the company his entire working career. Previously, he worked with engineers in the product development department, work that Peter found very stimulating.

When the product development part of the company moved to another town, Peter's work responsibilities changed. He began working as an assembly line worker, doing piecework together with others. Peter did not find this type of work challenging or satisfying. After working for 5 years in this job, he developed low back pain due to degeneration in his lumbar discs. Nearly 3 years ago the pain increased to the point that he was absent from work for 6 months. Following this he was able to work part time for 1.5 years, but 7 months ago he had a recurrence of back pain and has been absent from work since then.

The Worker Role Interview was administered to Peter to assess his potential for return to work. Results of the interview are shown in *Figure 17.8*. The following qualitative information was gathered in the interview.

Peter felt as though he could not manage to do anything anymore, either at work or at home. When asked, he could not identify any tasks that he felt able to do at work. He had completely lost belief in his capabilities. Peter also could not see any solution to his problems as long as the doctors could not help his back pain. He did not see that there was anything he could do for himself. He felt that he would not be able to work again. Because Peter felt so out of control, he did not assume any responsibility for his situation. His only hope, as he saw it, was that some medical intervention would alleviate his pain.

It had always been important for Peter to do his share. By working, he had been able to achieve this and provide for his family, which was extremely important to Peter. That he had not worked made him feel ashamed. He stated, "I can't look other people in the eyes anymore." For Peter, it was also important to have a job that he could be proud of, where his skills as a craftsman were of use. When Peter worked at the product development department, he had many work-oriented goals. However, when he changed work responsibilities, much of his enthusiasm for the future of his career was lost. The only thing that was important for Peter at his present job was being able to do his fair share of work.

Working with the product development team had been interesting and involved exciting work tasks. He appreciated the freedom he had in his work and enjoyed working with the engineers. He had been expected to contribute creative ideas, which he really enjoyed doing, and he felt strongly supported by his supervisors. He found his present job responsibilities boring and described it as "a job that anyone could do." One of Peter's major leisure interests was sailing, an interest he shared with his family. Before the back pain started, he spent much time at the boat club. Peter was still often at the boat club. His boat was old and made of wood, which demanded upkeep that he found hard to manage because of his back. "At least I have the boat in the sea every year," he said. Nevertheless, he and his family did not sail much anymore.

FIGURE 17.8 Results of Peter's Worker Role Interview.

	Rating					Brief comments that support rating
Personal Causation						
1. Assesses abilities and limitations	SS	S	I	**SI**	N/A	Can identify any tasks he can perform Is not aware of his strengths
2. Expectation of job success	SS	S	**I**	SI	N/A	Doesn't think he can work at his present job anymore
3. Takes responsibility	SS	S	I	**SI**	N/A	The problem is beyond his control The doctors have to make him well and he can't do anything before that
Values						
4. Commitment to work	**SS**	S	I	SI	N/A	To work and provide for the family has been and is important for Peter
5. Work-related goals	SS	S	**I**	SI	N/A	Previously, Peter had work related goals, but not any longer
Interests						
6. Enjoys work	SS	S	I	**SI**	N/A	The present work isn't challenging at all Peter doesn't get any opportunities to use his skills
7. Pursues interests	SS	S	**I**	SI	N/A	Can't perform his interest on a satisfactory level
Roles						
8. Appraises work expectations	SS	**S**	I	SI	N/A	Peter can identify and knows what is expected of him at work
9. Influence of other roles	SS	S	I	**SI**	N/A	Strong sick role

FIGURE 17.8 Results of Peter's Worker Role Interview. (*continued*)

	Rating					Brief comments that support rating
Habits						
10. Work habits	SS	**S**	I	SI	N/A	Peter's work habits went along well when he was working
11. Daily routines	SS	S	I	**SI**	N/A	Has lost his structure Daily routines are not functional
12. Adapts routine to minimize diffculties	SS	S	I	**SI**	N/A	Only solution when he has pain is to go and lay down; it's his only strategy and he has not tried anything else
Environment						
13. Perception of work setting	SS	S	**I**	SI	N/A	Peter thinks that work environment is impossible to adjust for his needs Can't change working position enough in his work tasks
13. Perception of family and peers	SS	S	I	SI	**N/A**	Not enough information
14. Perception of boss	SS	S	**I**	SI	N/A	Peter thinks the boss needs an employee who can work at full capacity
13. Perception of coworkers	SS	S	**I**	SI	N/A	Doesn't want to make trouble for his co-workers and "destroy" their piecework

Key: **SS** = Strongly supports client returning to job
    S = Supports client returning to job
    I = Interferes with returning to job
    SI = Strongly interferes with returning to job
    N/A = Not applicable or not enough information to rate

Peter knew what was expected of him at work but did not like his current job. Despite being out of work, he still identified himself as being a worker. He noted, "I'd rather work than watch TV all day." He also saw himself in the role of the family provider, despite no longer being able to work. Peter also lost several other past roles. Before, he and his wife shared the responsibilities of taking care of the household (e.g., cooking, cleaning, and laundry). The only thing that Peter still did in the household was take care of the car. Peter also had taken on the sick role in that he spent a great deal of time seeking medical care, focusing on his symptoms, and looking to medical providers to find a solution to his pain.

Before Peter's back pain began, he had well-organized habits. His days were well ordered, and his work, family, household, and sailing constituted a full and satisfying routine. Peter's routine changed dramatically when he began to be absent from work. Watching TV was his main current daily activity. The only strategy Peter had for managing his pain was to lie down. He felt that the need to lie down regularly had restricted him socially. Previously, Peter and his wife often had friends over for dinner, but they seldom saw their friends anymore because he might have to lie down.

Peter described the physical work environment as "impossible to adjust to my needs." He needed to vary his body position more than was possible at work. Peter's boss was supportive. However, Peter said that he knew that the boss must have someone, unlike himself, who could do the job completely. Peter had always gotten along well with his coworkers. However, with the onset of his back pain, he could not "pull his weight," which adversely affected his coworkers' ability to get bonuses for team productivity. Consequently, he felt that while they did not say so, his coworkers would have preferred someone else in his position.

The interview revealed that Peter had both strengths and weaknesses related to work. His greatest liability was that he had lost control of his situation and confidence in himself and his capabilities. Work was important to Peter; therefore, therapy must restore his conviction that he could work. It also became apparent from the interview that the lack of enjoyment of his work was likely abetting the interference of his pain with

working. The rote work of his assembly line task encouraged him to concentrate on his pain. The therapist thought, therefore, that he should try a new form of work that required more problem solving. His lowered personal causation combined with taking on the sick role had also made Peter so passive that he was not applying his own natural ability and enjoyment of problem solving to figure out how to manage his pain. Therefore, the therapist planned to engage Peter more actively in coming up with solutions for being able to work and to manage his pain. Since Peter had lost his old routine and habits, the therapist also wanted to intervene in such a way that he could begin to reinstate a routine.

With the results from the WRI as the starting point, the therapist and Peter discussed how to go further with his situation. The therapist shared with Peter her understanding of his situation and what she thought he needed to do. She further recommended that Peter test out his work capability in a realistic environment that would also better match his interests. With support, Peter agreed to begin work practice at a company that contracted to maintain apartment buildings. The span of work included a wide variety of repair, grounds maintenance, and oversight of the general conditions and needs of the properties. Peter and the therapist together chose this particular workplace because the work there matched Peter's interest in planning and problem solving.

At first, he worked 2 hours per day. At the end of each week, Peter, his therapist, and the foreman met briefly to find out how the work was going for Peter and to make any necessary adjustments in how Peter did his job. By the end of 12 weeks, Peter had increased to working 4 hours per day.

This work practice period also helped Peter to redevelop his habits and structure his daily routines. Peter also developed a more realistic view of his work abilities and limitations. In the beginning of the work practice period, the occupational therapist educated Peter and his colleagues in lifting techniques and ergonomics. Although Peter still had pain in his back and had difficulty managing some work tasks (e.g., heavy lifting), he displayed an increasing confidence in his work capabilities.

He also learned new strategies for handling his pain. When he was at work, there were hardly any opportunities to lie down. Instead, Peter found out that by varying his work tasks, he could reduce his pain. Working as He also learned new strategies for handling his pain. When he was at work, there were hardly any opportunities to lie down. Instead, Peter found out that by varying his work tasks, he could reduce his pain. Working as a building caretaker suited Peter well, since he was able to use his technical and practical skills. He felt responsible to exercise judgment and able to intervene when problems arose in the buildings—a role that he liked. Consequently, his belief in his capabilities grew stronger. That he had found new strategies to handle the pain at work and home increased his sense of efficacy in both managing the pain and being able to be productive. At a final meeting of Peter and his rehabilitation team, it was concluded that he had a 50% work capacity and that he would receive a disability benefit for the other 50%.

As this case illustrates, the WRI provides information on volition, habituation, and perceptions of environment that influence work success and satisfaction. Thus, it is a useful complement to the performance capacity–oriented assessments that are often used in a work rehabilitation context. It identifies unique factors that influence a person's work success.

Work Environment Impact Scale

The Work Environment Impact Scale (WEIS) (Moore-Corner, Kielhofner, & Olson, 1998) is a semi-structured interview and rating scale designed to gather information on how individuals with physical or psychosocial disabilities experience their work environments. The WEIS is recommended for use with individuals who are currently employed and for indiviuals who are not curently working, but are anticipating return to a specific job or type of work. Typical candidates for this assessment are persons who are experiencing difficulty on the job and those whose work is interrupted by an injury or episode of illness.

The interview questions were not developed to be used with individuals who have been chronically unem-

ployed, because they ask respondents to reflect on how a given work environment affects them. Nonetheless, the WEIS may sometimes be useful to identify how past work environments impacted work productivity and satisfaction. In the end, the therapist must decide whether the WEIS is appropriate for a given client.

The WEIS is designed to provide a comprehensive assessment of how the qualities and characteristics of the work environment affect a worker. An important concept underlying this scale is that workers are most productive and satisfied when there is a fit or match between the worker's environment and the needs and skills of the worker. Hence, the same work environment may have a different impact on different workers. The WEIS does not assess the environment. Rather, it assesses how the work environment affects a given worker.

The WEIS is organized around 17 environmental factors, such as the physical space, social contacts and supports, temporal demands, objects utilized, and daily job functions. Consequently, it seeks to gain a comprehensive picture of how a wide range of features of the work environment affect a worker. These 17 factors are reflected in 17 items on the rating scale. Each of the items is scored with a four-point rating that indicates how the environmental factor affects the worker's performance, satisfaction, and physical, social, and emotional well-being. The scale provides a profile of which aspects of the environment negatively or positively affect the worker.

Administration

The WEIS is described in a detailed manual that provides background and detailed guidelines for completing the interview and rating scale. The manual also discusses how the WEIS can be used to identify the need for workplace modification to accommodate a disabled worker.

The therapist begins by administering a semi-structured interview. The interview must be done so as to capture the unique characteristics of the client's workplace and how they affect the client. After the interview, the therapist completes the rating scale and enters appropriate qualitative data. There is an optional summary sheet to identify environmental characteristics that facilitate or inhibit worker performance and satisfaction and may require accommodation. The summary sheet is a useful way to communicate the results and implications of the WEIS to other disciplines, the client, and the workplace. Conducting the interview and completing the assessment can take between 30 and 60 minutes.

The WEIS may be used as an independent tool when the work environment is a concern. However, the WEIS is often used in conjunction with the WRI. The two interviews can be combined, saving time in administration.

Work Environment Impact Scale (WEIS)

- Gathers information on work environment impact and identifies need for accommodations
- Can be ordered through the MOHO Clearinghouse e-store *http://ascendant.cas.uic.edu/retail/*, or
  - Visit *www.moho.uic.edu*
  - Select menu item "MOHO Products"
  - Link to WEIS assessment for more information about the assessment and example assessment forms. To link to the MOHO Clearinghouse e-store, left click on the "Buy Now" button.

Samantha: Using the WEIS to Identify Needed Workplace Accommodations

Samantha was a 36-year-old woman who was admitted to an acute-care inpatient unit with a diagnosis of major depression. She was admitted for noncompliance with medication, which resulted in increased isolation, decreased ability to care for herself, and increased flashbacks from earlier sexual abuse. This was her second admission to this unit in less than a year.

In the course of responding to the OCAIRS interview, Samantha indicated that she was working and that stress on the job had resulted in her current decompensation and need for hospitalization. She was unable to pinpoint the cause of her stress on the job to either the occupational therapist or the treatment team. Consequently, the

therapist decided that the WEIS would be useful to gain further information about Samantha's perception of her workplace. The therapist anticipated that the WEIS could be used to work with Samantha to identify specific areas on the job that were stressful and to determine whether changes or accommodations could be made to decrease the stress and increase her success in the worker role.

The WEIS was conducted approximately 1 week after her admission to the unit. Samantha was willing to engage in the interview and spoke openly. The WEIS rating scale as shown in *Figure 17.9* indicated that most factors in the work environment either supported or strongly supported Samantha's work performance and well-being. The primary negative factors of her work environment were her supervisor, the unclear expectations and rewards for performance, and her work schedule. The interview elicited the following qualitative information about Samantha's workplace.

Samantha worked in a corporate distribution center. Her three primary responsibilities were gathering and packing ordered items, replenishing inventory, and confirming orders. Overall, she reported that she enjoyed the work tasks, that she was able to complete tasks in a timely manner, and that she consistently exceeded productivity quotas. She reported some dissatisfaction in learning new jobs and equipment.

Samantha indicated that she was required to learn new tasks and equipment on her own because her supervisor and coworkers were not helpful in this area. Samantha had no need for regular contact with her coworkers to do her job. This was something she found supportive for herself, as she valued her independence and autonomy.

Samantha reported difficulty with her immediate supervisor. She perceived that his expectations and requests were unclear and that he did not communicate with her effectively. She also felt that he did not appropriately support her in the performance of her work tasks. Samantha indicated that the day before being admitted, she had to work late at her supervisor's request. When she went to ask her supervisor a question, he had gone home without indicating to her that he was leaving. She became tearful during the interview and kept saying, "I can't believe he went home." Samantha

FIGURE 17.9 Results of Samantha's Work Environment Impact Scale

	1	2	3	4	N/A	Comments
Time Demands: Time allotted for available/expected amount of work			✗			Able to complete things on time
Task Demands: The physical, cognitive, and/or emotional demands/opportunities of work tasks			✗			Limited support from others to learn work tasks
Appeal of Work Tasks: The appeal/enjoyableness or status/value of work tasks			✗			She enjoys the work
Work Schdedule: The influence of work hours upon other valued roles, activities, transportation, and basic self-care needs		✗				Ambivalent about work schedule
Coworker Interaction: Interaction/collaboration with coworkers required for job responsibilities					✗	Not required to interact with others
Work Group Membership: Social involvement with coworkers at work/outside of work					✗	Chooses not to interact
Supervisor Interaction: Feedback, guidance, and/or other communication/interaction with supervisor(s)		✗				Strained relationship with boss whom she does not see as supportive
Work Role Standards: Overall climate of work setting expressed in expectations for quality, excellence, commitment, achievement, and/or efficiency		✗				She routinely exceeds production goals, but receives no recognition or rewards. Expectations not clear
Work Role Style: Opportunity/expectations for autonomy/compliance when organizing, making requests, negotiating, and choosing how and what work tasks will be done daily			✗			Enjoys the autonomy
Interaction with Others: Interaction/communication with subordinates, customers, clients, audiences, students or others, excluding supervisor or coworkers					✗	
Rewards: Opportunities for job security, recognition/advancement in position, and/or compensation in salary or benefits		✗				Feels she has poor job security because of disability
Sensory Qualities: Properties of the work place such as noise, smell, visual, or tactile properties, temperature/climate, or air quality and ventilation			✗			Environment is noisy but it doesn't affect her
Architecture/Arrangement: Architecture or physical arrangements of and between work spaces and environments			✗			Has decreased negative effects

continued

FIGURE 17.9 Results of Samantha's Work Environment Impact Scale *(continued)*

	1	2	3	4	N/A	*Comments*
Ambience/Mood: The feeling/mood associated with the degree of privacy, friendliness, morale, excitement, anxiety, frustration in the work place			✗			*Generally positive atmosphere of cooperation*
Properties of Objects: The physical, cognitive, or emotional demands/opportunities of tools, equipment, materials, and supplies			✗			
Physical Amenities: Non-work-specific facilities necessary to meet personal needs at work such as restrooms, lunchrooms, or break room			✗			*Adequate, although she doesn't frequently use*
Meaning of Objects: What objects signify to a person			✗			

Key: **4** = Strongly supports return to job; **3** = Supports return to job; **2** = Interferes with return to job; **1** = Strongly interferes with return to job; **N/A** = Not applicable

saw this event as typical of his increasing lack of support.

She also expressed dissatisfaction with her work hours. The company was willing to decrease her work to 4 to 6 hours a day but indicated she could not work less. Samantha felt that her work schedule negatively affected other aspects of her life. She was able to accomplish little outside of work.

Following the interview, the therapist shared her perceptions of the impact of Samantha's work environment with her. Together, they agreed that these were the two main problems that needed attention:

● Decreasing her work hours

● Clarifying her relationship with her supervisor.

The therapist shared with Samantha that shorter work hours could be considered a reasonable accommodation and that it was within her rights under the Americans with Disabilities Act to request it. The therapist also recommended that she work with Samantha to identify what changes she wanted to occur in her supervision and how she would present these requests for changes to her supervisor. The therapist gave her an opportunity to role-play making the request.

The therapist also engaged Samantha in time management exercises. These were designed to assist her in prioritizing activities outside of work to increase her sense of efficacy and decrease feelings of being overwhelmed. Samantha also attended a stress management group at the therapist's recommendation.

The therapist shared the information that came from the WEIS with Samantha's outside case manager. The therapist recommended that if Samantha was unable to communicate her needs to her supervisor, the case manager should assist in this dialogue with the supervisor or with the employee assistance program at Samantha's workplace.

Samantha was able to act on these recommendations. She requested and was granted a shorter workday. This change helped her to manage her other responsibilities. Samantha had less success in obtaining more direct support and clarity from her supervisor. This was an issue that she continued to work on with her case manager. Nonetheless, Samantha demonstrated an increased ability to adapt to her job demands and has not required another inpatient hospitalization in the past 18 months.

Conclusion: Interviews in Perspective

This chapter presents and illustrates five interviews developed for different clients and different contexts. The variety of interviews allows the therapist to select the one or ones that will be most appropriate in a given setting or for a given client. These interviews are also designed to be flexible in use so that they can be adapted to each client.

Although interviews are not feasible for use with all clients, they do present opportunities to gather important information to achieve a client-centered focus. Hence, their use whenever possible is strongly encouraged. Interviews also actively engage clients in discussing and giving perspectives on their own situation, which helps them begin a collaborative role in their own therapy. Finally, they serve as important opportunities to build rapport. Although interviews take time, the time is well spent, given the kinds of information they yield and the opportunities they represent for beginning true collaboration with the client.

References

Braveman, B., Robson, M., Velozo, C., Kielhofner, G., Fisher, G., Forsyth, K., & Kerschbaum, J. (2005). *Worker Role Interview (WRI) (version 10.0)*. Chicago: Model of Human Occupation Clearinghouse, Department of Occupational Therapy, College of Applied Health Sciences, University of Illinois.

Fisher, G. S. (1999). Administration and application of the Worker Role Interview: Looking beyond functional capacity. *Work: A Journal of Prevention, Assessment & Rehabilitation, 12* (1), 25–36.

Forsyth, K., Deshpande, S., Kielhofner, G., Henriksson, C., Haglund, L., Olson, L., Skinner, S., & Kulkarni, S. (2005).

The *Occupational Circumstances Assessment Interview and Rating Scale (OCAIRS) (version 4.0)*. Chicago: Model of Human Occupation Clearinghouse, Department of Occupational Therapy, College of Applied Health Sciences, University of Illinois.

Hemmingsson, H., Egilson, S., Hoffman, O., Kielhofner, G. (2005). *School Setting Interview (SSI) (version 3.0)*. Swedish Association of Occupational Therapists. Nacka, Sweden.

Kaplan, K. (1984). Short-term assessment: The need and a response. *Occupational Therapy in Mental Health, 4* (3), 29–45.

Kaplan, K., & Kielhofner, G. (1989). *The Occupational Case Analysis Interview and Rating Scale*. Thorofare, NJ: Slack.

Kielhofner, G., Dobria, L., Forsyth, K., & Basu, S. (2005). The construction of keyforms for obtaining instantaneous measures from the occupational performance history interview rating scales. *Occupational Therapy Journal of Research, 25,* 23–32.

Kielhofner, G, Mallinson, T., Crawford, C., Nowak, M., Rigby, M., Henry, A., & Walens, D. (2004). *Occupational Performance History Interview-II (OPHI-II) (version 2.1)*. Chicago: Model of Human Occupation Clearinghouse, Department of Occupational Therapy, College of Applied Health Sciences, University of Illinois.

Moore-Corner, R., Kielhofner, G., & Olson, L. (1998). *Work Environment Impact Scale (WEIS) (Version 2.0)*. Chicago: Model of Human Occupation Clearinghouse, Department of Occupational Therapy, College of Applied Health Sciences, University of Illinois.

Velozo, C., Kielhofner, G., & Fisher, G. (1998). *Worker Role Interview (WRI) (version 9.0)*. Chicago: Model of Human Occupation Clearinghouse, Department of Occupational Therapy, College of Applied Health Sciences, University of Illinois.

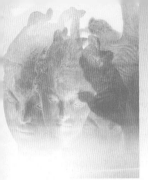

18

Assessments Combining Methods of Information Gathering

- Kirsty Forsyth
- Gary Kielhofner
- Patricia Bowyer
- Kathleen Kramer
- Annie Ploszaj
- Melinda Blondis
- Renee Hinson-Smith
- Sue Parkinson

This chapter discusses three assessments that combine different methods of gathering information:

- The Assessment of Occupational Functioning—Collaborative Version (AOF-CV)
- The Model of Human Occupation Screening Tool (MOHOST)
- The Short Child Occupational Profile (SCOPE)
- The Occupational Therapy Psychosocial Assessment of Learning (OT PAL)

Each of these assessments has a distinct format and purpose. The Assessment of Occupational Functioning—Collaborative Version (AOF-CV) was originally designed as an interview; it has been revised so that it can be administered as a self-report or an interview. The Model of Human Occupation Screening Tool (MOHOST) was initiated by a group of practitioners as a flexible means of gathering information on clients in a relatively short-term setting. The Short Child Occupational Profile (SCOPE) similarly provides flexible means of gathering information on children. The Occupational Therapy Psychosocial Assessment of Learning (OT PAL) incorporates observation along with brief teacher, student, and parent interviews to gather information on students.

The Assessment of Occupational Functioning—Collaborative Version

The original Assessment of Occupational Functioning was developed for use in long-term institutional settings (Watts, Kielhofner, Bauer, Gregory, & Valentine, 1986). Later revision of the assessment resulted in a more general version suitable for a variety of contexts (Watts, Brollier, Bauer, & Schmidt, 1989). The Assessment of Occupational Functioning—Collaborative Version (AOF-CV) is a semi-structured assessment that gives clients an opportunity to report about their occupational participation (Watts, Hinson, Madigan, McGuigan, & Newman, 1999). It is unique in that it may be administered as either an interview or as a self-report with follow-up from the therapist.

The AOF-CV is designed to yield a general overview of a person's occupational participation. It provides both qualitative information and a rating profile that reflect clients' views of their own strengths and limitations in personal causation, values, roles, habits, and skills. The assessment aims to efficiently generate a picture of numerous complex and interrelated factors that influence engaging in those things persons need and want to do. The AOF-CV can also identify areas that require more in-depth assessment.

Whereas the AOF-CV has been predominantly researched with psychiatric clients, the authors also recommend it for use in physical disability settings. As a screening instrument, it identifies those areas of a client's occupational functioning that require more in-depth evaluation. Therapists have reported that the AOF-CV is useful for assisting treatment and discharge planning within a range of settings. The AOF-CV is particularly useful for occupational therapists in acute care settings when there is pressure to develop specific, focused assessment protocols for each client.

view, the therapist treats the questions as a semi-structured interview, probing and asking additional questions as necessary. The questions, whether used as an interview or self-report, are designed to elicit the client's perception of his or her occupational functioning. The AOF-CV requires about 20 to 30 minutes when administered as an interview and about 12 minutes as a self-report with follow-up.

After the interview or self-report with follow-up is finished, the therapist completes a rating scale. The rating scale is in the form of questions about the client's functioning (e.g., "Does this person demonstrate personal values through the selection of well-defined, meaningful activities?") that are scored on a five-point scale. The rating scale provides a profile of strengths and weaknesses that is useful to guide treatment and/or discharge planning.

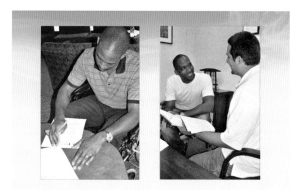

A client completes the written section of the AOF-CV before his next therapy session, and he discusses his responses with the therapist to identify current difficulties with his occupational participation.[1]

[1]*(Photos provided by Dianne F. Simons, PhD, OTR, Department of Occupational Therapy, Virginia Commonwealth University.)*

Administration

As noted previously, the AOF-CV may be administered either as an interview or as a self-administered questionnaire with follow-up from the therapist. It consists of 22 questions. When it is administered as a self-report, the client responds to the questions in writing. After reviewing the client's responses, the therapist briefly discusses them with the client to clarify and gather additional information necessary for completing the rating scale. When it is conducted as an inter-

*A*ssessment of Occupational Functioning—
Collaborative Version (AOF-CV)

. . . .

- Provides information on the client's view of his or her own strengths and limitations in personal causation, values, roles, habits, and skills. Yields qualitative information and a quantitative profile of factors affecting occupational participation.
- Can be downloaded from Virginia Commonwealth University (VCU) Occupational Therapy Department Web site at *http://www.sahp.vcu.edu/occu/aofcv.htm*, or
  - *Visit www.moho.uic.edu*
  - Select menu item "MOHO Related Resources"
  - Link to "Other Instruments Based on MOHO" to access link to VCU.

*P*hil: Using the AOF-CV to Gain Insight

. . . .

Phil was 36 years old. He was diagnosed with multiple sclerosis (MS) 4 years previously. Since then, he had been progressively debilitated with no remission. He was hospitalized during an exacerbation of MS and sub-sequently transferred to an intensive rehabilitation unit. Although he received outpatient occupational therapy and physical therapy in the past, this was his first inpa-tient rehabilitation admission. At the time he transferred to the rehabilitation unit, his physical limitations re-quired that he use a powered wheelchair for mobility. During hospitalization, he had attempted walking and stand/pivot transfers with very limited success, even with maximal assistance.

The therapist at the rehabilitation center adminis-tered the AOF-CV as an interview with Phil. She used the AOF-CV as a means of gaining insight into clients' views of their own situations and as a guide to make therapy more responsive to clients' needs. What the in-terview revealed is discussed later and Phil's ratings on the AOF-CV rating scale are shown in *Figure 18.1*.

Phil was divorced 2 years after his diagnosis was made. He was estranged from his youngest child, a daughter who lived in another state with her mother. Phil lived in a house with his two sons, aged 14 and 10. This house was not wheelchair accessible. Phil was previously employed full time as a roofer but could no longer work.

Phil reported that his two most important sources of meaning are his family and his work. However, both have been disrupted in the past 4 years. Phil's goals were to walk again and to participate in the things he did before the onset of MS. He avoided any suggestion that his ill-ness would likely progress and require accommodations. Consequently, he had no plans to adapt his home and had not considered the possible impact on his children.

Phil deeply wanted to be in control of his life. He re-luctantly admitted that he is greatly reliant on other people. He noted, "Other people make suggestions of what I should do in every aspect of my life, but I reserve the right to say yes or no, even though they are proba-bly right." Phil refused to discuss what was likely to be the course of his illness. He had almost no knowledge of MS and rejected the idea of learning about the dis-ease and its prognosis. Ironically, his lack of information greatly decreased his sense of control. He admitted that family members and friends often had to make medical and physical decisions on his behalf, since he would not become involved in anything pertaining to his illness and disability. Phil also reported feeling that his sons

were getting out of hand, since he could no longer watch or discipline them. His authority had been greatly eroded by the fact that he had to rely on them to per-form all of the household tasks as well as help him with aspects of his self-care.

Phil's previous interests all involved physical activity. He enjoyed playing golf and basketball, playing sports with his sons, helping neighbors with odd jobs, and working as a roofer. Participating in these interests was no longer possible or was radically altered. He contin-ued to watch sports on television and to attend sporting events. He tried to spend time with his sons but could-n't do things with them as before. Phil indicated that he had not attempted to find new things to do and in-sisted that he didn't want to explore things he might do from a wheelchair. Nonetheless, he reported feeling quite depressed at not having enjoyable things to do.

Prior to the onset of his illness, Phil had many roles, including parent, husband, worker, friend, sports partic-ipant, church member, and club member. His remaining role was parent, and it had been radically altered as he had become so dependent on his sons and had no con-tact with his daughter. He indicated being very de-pressed over the loss of these roles. Up until 4 months before his hospitalization, he independently performed his morning self-care, completed simple home manage-ment tasks such as cleaning and meal preparation, and cared for his children. During the most recent exacerba-tion, Phil remained in bed when his children were not home because he needed assistance to move around the house. For the past 3 years, he had a housebound routine except for occasional trips to sporting events and movies. He wanted to expand his routine to include more community activities when he felt better.

Phil's view of skills was fraught with conflict. His mounting impairments and swift decline in performance conflicted with his need to believe his condition would markedly improve. Consequently, he tended to deny his limitations, which further restricted his performance. He was able to communicate on a superficial level. However, he admitted having difficulty discussing per-sonal issues. He reported trouble discussing his illness with his sons. Phil admitted that his anger and poor communication had made his sons somewhat fearful and distant from him.

chapter 18

FIGURE 18.1 Phil's Ratings on the AOF-CV.

Volition					
Values	**5**	**4**	**3**	**2**	**1**
Does this person demonstrate his/her values throughout the selection of well-defined, meaningful roles?				X	
Does this person demonstrate his/her values through the selection of personal goals?				X	
Does this person demonstrate socially appropriate values through the selection of personal standards for the conduct of daily activities?		X			
Does this person demonstrate temporal orientation through expressed awareness of past, present, and future events and beliefs about how time should be used?	X				
Personal Causation	**5**	**4**	**3**	**2**	**1**
Does this person demonstrate personal causation through an expressed belief in internal control?				X	
Does this person demonstrate personal causation by expressing confidence that he/she has a range of skills?		X			
Does this person demonstrate personal causation by expressing confidence in his/her skill competence at personally relevant tasks?					X
Does this person demonstrate personal causation by expressing hopeful anticipation for success in the future endeavors?			X		
Interests	**5**	**4**	**3**	**2**	**1**
Does this person clearly discriminate between degrees of interests?		X			
Does this person clearly identify a range of interests?			X		
Does this person routinely pursue his/her interests?					X

Habituation					
Roles	**5**	**4**	**3**	**2**	**1**
Does this person demonstrate an adequate array of life roles (family member, student, worker, hobbyist, friend, etc)?					X
Does this person have a realistic concept of the demands and social obligations of his/her life roles?			X		
Does this person express comfort or security in his/her major life roles?					X
Habits	**5**	**4**	**3**	**2**	**1**
Does this person demonstrate habit patterns through well organized use of time?			X		
Does this person report that his/her habits are socially acceptable?				X	
Does this person demonstrate adequate flexibility in his/her habits?			X		

Occupational Performance Skills	**5**	**4**	**3**	**2**	**1**
Does this person have adequate motor skills necessary to move himself/herself or manipulate objects?					X
Does this person have adequate skills for managing events, processes, and situations of various types?				X	
Does this person have communication and interpersonal skills necessary for interfacing with people?				X	

Key: **1** = Very little **2** = Little **3** = Moderately **4** = Highly **5** = Very highly

Therapy Implications

The AOF-CV results made it clear that any successful re-habilitation had to begin with addressing Phil's view of his situation. Phil's unwillingness to address his physical limitations, combined with his poor prognosis, was his greatest liability. Before he could benefit from rehabilitation addressed at functional skills, his perspective on his disability and his future had to be addressed. Once Phil was able cognitively and emotionally to perform an accurate self-evaluation, he would be better able to plan for the future, communicate his needs, and participate in rehabilitation. From the evaluation, it was apparent that Phil's difficulty in facing his limitations and prognosis was exacerbated by his loss of participation in positive, meaningful activities. Therefore, the most likely point of intervention was to acknowledge these losses and to work with him to identify how he could reclaim some of his occupational participation without the necessity of regaining all of his physical abilities. Since Phil had lost meaning and self-confidence and felt most out of control in his parent role, this role was a possible beginning point. This was also a place to begin because his sons had expressed a willingness to help their father with his physical limitations, and they were at critical ages when his parenting was important to them. Once Phil began to feel a greater sense of control and possibility for his future, interventions such as environmental adaptation, energy conservation, and alternative activity exploration were undertaken. *Figure 18.2* illustrates the specific strategies for intervention derived from the AOF-CV that correspond to the areas assessed.

During the rehabilitation stay, the therapist had a degree of success in implementing her plans with Phil. The team was very supportive of the therapist's aims to address Phil's personal causation. The team as a whole worked to provide realistic information to Phil about his condition and prognosis. Additionally, because Phil was very much involved in a local church, his pastor worked with the team to provide Phil emotional support and spiritual guidance in coming to grips with his situation and its meaning for him. Phil was able to make some progress in facing the implications of MS and in collaborating to make changes to improve his function. Phil accepted and learned to use a number of adaptive aids to support toileting and bathing. Phil was given a narrow manual wheelchair to use in his narrow hallways and bedroom. He was reluctant to accept further adaptations at the time.

Phil returned to rehabilitation about a year later, severely impaired. The therapist revisited some key questions from the AOF-CV with Phil. At this point, he had come to grips with the reality of his MS and expressed fears about what it would mean. Phil noted that at home his older son was taking care of him. Since he had become too weak to transfer into or use his manual chair, until his sons came home Phil would lie in bed all day. Then the sons would cook meals, assist Phil with his activities of daily living, and help him do some activities out of bed. Phil acknowledged that this was not a satisfying way to live, and he was willing to try a variety of strategies to improve it.

Phil still very much wanted to attempt walking, and the team decided to validate his values by letting him try. He was fitted with braces but was unable to walk with them because his arm strength was limited. On the other hand, he did make some modest physical gains in rehabilitation that improved his performance capacity. However, the most important changes were based on adapting his environment to enhance his occupational participation.

The local Rotary Club adapted Phil's home, providing ramps, a new walk-in shower, a better bed, and widened hallways. They arranged to adapt the family vehicle so that it could accommodate Phil and his powered wheelchair. Phil also made plans in therapy for the kinds of things he wanted to do and problem-solved with his therapist to remove any obstacles. This whole process of environmental adaptation, planning for greater control, and focusing on how Phil could realize some of his values and interests in his everyday life gave him new hope. Phil returned home, and the next period was very good for him. His acceptance and increased knowledge of MS, newfound freedom in mobility within and outside his home, and increased ability to manage his own self-care gave him a measure of control over his life and allowed him less dependence on and greater involvement with his children. Phil's improved quality of life also affected his sons' lives after Phil died some months later.

After Phil's death, his older son lived independently and his younger son went to live with his mother and

FIGURE 18.2 Areas and strategies for intervention with Phil

Area	Strategies for Intervention
Values	• Identify with Phil his highest priorities for occupational participation • Assist Phil to develop realistic goals for occupational performance within areas of highest priorities • Begin process of long-term goal-setting strategies to accommodate for his prognosis of declining functional status, as he is able to cope with the prognosis and its implications
Personal causation	• Identify an area of great importance (e.g., parenting) and work with Phil to participate in this occupational area despite his impairments • As he can accept the information, increase Phil's knowledge of MS and functional implications • Work with Phil to plan for and adapt the home environment to enhance his performance and control
Interests	• Introduce modifications to past interests and explore their satisfaction with Phil • Provide opportunities for Phil to explore new areas of interest based on factors that provided him satisfaction in the past • Work with Phil to plan current and future increased participation in interests to reduce feelings of loss and depression

Area	Strategies for Intervention
Skills	• Identify in collaboration with Phil physical impairments and abilities with an aim to adapt the environment to minimize the impact of his limitations and to enhance his performance • Provide support and training to enhance Phil's interpersonal communication skills and ability to emotionally cope with his disability through better planning and communication
Roles	• Explore modifications of roles to allow Phil to retain as many roles as possible • Work with Phil to identify and plan for the self-care management role (see discussion in Chapter 5) and its implications for his ability to participate in other roles
Habits	• Educate Phil on energy conservation and adaptations to increase activity level • Work with Phil to plan and implement present routines and plan future routines

sister. The sons were grateful for the improved final months with their father. The therapist's use of the AOF-CV with Phil and others like him served as the basis for the occupational therapy department in this rehabilitation setting to garner team support for and to develop new programs addressing the psychosocial aspects of physical disability, which previously had not been systematically addressed. Clients on the rehabilitation unit have received the new programs positively.

As this case illustrates, the AOF-CV provides an efficient means of identifying the client's status and making apparent issues that should be addressed in therapy. It also points to areas that may necessitate further evaluation. This case in particular illustrates how issues that often go unattended and unresolved in physical rehabilitation can be approached. The AOF-CV is equally useful in identifying salient psychosocial issues in clients with a wide range of impairments in a variety of service contexts. The AOF-CV itself begins a collaborative dialogue with clients that can help the therapist design therapy that addresses the clients' greatest concerns and fears.

The Model of Human Occupation Screening Tool and the Short Child Occupational Profile

The MOHOST (Parkinson, Forsyth, & Kielhofner, 2006) and the SCOPE (Bowyer, Ross, Schwartz, Kielhofner, & Kramer, 2005) both gather information relevant to most MOHO concepts, allowing the therapist to gain an overview of the clients' occupational functioning.

Both instruments aim to capture the clients' relative strengths, highlighting the impact of volition, habituation, skills, and the environment on occupational performance. These instruments flexibly and efficiently gather information for screening referrals, identifying needs for further assessment and for treatment planning. They are also easy to administer again and can be used as outcomes measures. They can be used with a wide range of clients with psychosocial and/or physical impairments. The MOHOST is designed for adults, and the SCOPE is designed for pediatric populations. Depending on their needs and circumstances, adolescents may be appropriate for either assessment.

The MOHOST consists of a 24-item rating scale with items representing volition, habituation, skills, and environment; the SCOPE is similar but has an additional item for the environment scale that addresses the family routine. On both the MOHOST and SCOPE scales, each item is rated on a four-point scale. *Figure 18.3* illustrates the rating scale and some items from both instruments. As the items show, criteria for making the ratings are built into each item, thereby making the rating process more straightforward for therapists. Most of the information for completing the ratings can ordinarily be gained from informal observation of the client, but the MOHOST is designed so that the therapist can gather data through whatever means are most practical. There is a short form for recording the information gathered in the MOHOST, and this is illustrated in the case that follows.

Administration

The data collection methods for the MOHOST and SCOPE are designed to be flexible to meet multiple needs in practice. Therapists may use any dependable source of information. This information is often gained through observation; however, it may be supplemented or achieved through talking to the client, ward or residential staff, and/or relatives. Additionally, therapists may gather information from records, team meetings, or other sources. If necessary, therapists can build up an understanding of their clients' occupational participation over time to complete the assessments. When therapists have enough information, they complete the rating forms. Ratings can be recorded on the simple summary forms available for both assessments. These summary forms also have a place for a brief qualitative report. Because they are easy to administer and score, the MOHOST and SCOPE can be used at regular intervals to document the client's progress.

*M*odel of Human Occupation Screening Tool (MOHOST)

- Captures clients' relative strengths, highlighting the impact of volition, habituation, skills, and the environment on occupational participation.
- Can be ordered through the MOHO Clearinghouse e-store *http://ascendant.cas.uic.edu/retail/*,[1] or
  - Visit *www.moho.uic.edu.*
  - Select menu item "MOHO Products."
  - Link to MOHOST assessment for more information about the assessment and example assessment forms. To link to the MOHO Clearinghouse e-store, left-click on the "Buy Now" button.

[1]*When looking to purchase MOHO assessments, therapists can also inquire with their national association for purchasing information. For example, the British Association/College of Occupational Therapists has the MOHOST, along with several other MOHO assessments, available for purchase.*

*S*hort Child Occupational Profile (SCOPE)

- Captures clients' relative strengths, highlighting the impact of volition, habituation, skills, and the environment on occupational participation. Items are targeted to children, and the SCOPE includes an item regarding the child's family routine.
- To obtain a copy of the SCOPE, therapists should visit *www.moho.uic.edu* for the most recent information on the publication of the SCOPE, or e-mail moho_c@yahoo.com.

FIGURE 18.3 **A.** Sample items from the MOHOST.

Appraisal of Ability

Understanding of current strengths & limitations Accurate belief in skill, accurate view of competence Awareness of capacity	**F** **A** **I** **R**	Accurately assesses own capacity, recognizes strengths, aware of limitations Reasonable tendency to over/under estimate own abilities, recognizes some limitations Difficulty understanding strengths and limitations without support Does not reflect on skills, fails to realistically estimate own abilities *Comments:*

Routine

Balance Organization of habits Structure Productivity	**F** **A** **I** **R**	Able to arrange a balanced, organized and productive routine of daily activities Generally able to maintain or follow an organized and productive daily schedule Difficulty organizing balanced, productive routines of daily activities without support Chaotic or empty routine, unable to support responsibilities and goals, erratic routine *Comments:*

Problem-Solving

Judgement Adaptation Decision-making Responsiveness	**F** **A** **I** **R**	Shows good judgement, anticipates difficulties and generates workable solutions (rational) Generally able to make decisions based on difficulties that arise Difficulty anticipating and adapting to difficulties that arise, seeks reassurance Unable to anticipate and adapt to difficulties that arise and makes inappropriate decisions *Comments:*

Relationships

Co-operation Collaboration Rapport Respect	**F** **A** **I** **R**	Sociable, supportive, aware of others, sustains engagement, friendly, relates well to others Generally able to relate to others and mostly demonstrates awareness of others' needs Difficulty with co-operation or makes few positive relationships Unable to co-operate with others or make positive relationships *Comments:*

(continued)

FIGURE 18.3 **B.** Sample items from the SCOPE (*continued*)

Response to Challenge
The child engages in new activities and/or accepts the opportunity to achieve more, or perform under condition of greater demand.

		Comments:
F	The child spontaneously seeks and persists in new or more challenging activities.	
A	The child spontaneously attempts new or more challenging activities, but is easily frustrated and/or needs some support in order to persist.	
I	The child usually requires significant support to engage in new and more demanding activities and to overcome frustration and persist during such activities.	
R	The child avoids new or more challenging activities because they elicit a high level of frustration.	

Routine
The child has an awareness of routines and is able to participate effectively in structured daily routines.

		Comments:
F	The child demonstrates an awareness of the sequence and structure of regular routines, and can anticipate, initiate, and/or cooperate with activities related to these routines.	
A	The child requires occasional cueing and redirection in order to cooperate with the regular sequence and structure of routines in his/her life.	
I	The child is often unable to participate in the sequence and structure of regular routines.	
R	The child does not demonstrate an awareness of the sequence and structure of regular routines; does not anticipate, cooperate, and/or initiate routine activities.	

Problem Solving
The child demonstrates an appropriate ability to identify and respond to challenges.

		Comments:
F	The child consistently anticipates problems, generates workable solutions, and evaluates these solutions to determine the best course of action.	
A	The child can identify difficulties but needs step-by-step cues to generate an effective response.	
I	The child rarely anticipates and adapts to difficulties; needs on-going reassurance when problems are encountered.	
R	The child is unable to anticipate and adapt to difficulties; makes inappropriate decisions.	

Physical Space
Home, community, hospital/school areas.

		Comments:
F	Arrangement of the physical environment is accessible and provides opportunities to engage in various activities; stimulates and supports occupational participation in child's valued roles.	
A	Arrangement of the physical environment does not adequately support occupational engagement or is somewhat accessible; poses some limitations to the child's participation in valued roles.	
I	Arrangement of the physical environment affords a limited range of opportunities with limited accessibility and support for occupational engagement and participation.	
R	Arrangement of the physical environment is not accessible and restricts opportunities and prevents participation in the child's valued roles.	

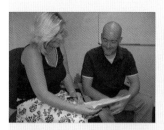

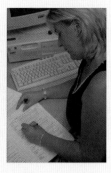

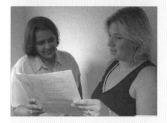

Katina, an occupational therapist and part of the mental health rehabilitation team, gathers information to complete a MOHOST. First she talks to her nursing colleague, John. Next, after reviewing the client's history in his records, she rates each item. Finally, she reviews the results with her manager, Lena, during a case meeting.

Andrew: Using the MOHOST to Gain a New Perspective

Andrew was in his late 30s and was diagnosed with schizophrenia 10 years ago. He completed an art degree but has never had a job or formed any major relationships. It was likely that he had impairments related to his mental illness for some considerable time before he came to the attention of psychiatric services. He was able to remain living in the community because he received substantial help from his parents.

Andrew had multiple psychiatric hospitalizations in his history. He was generally admitted to the hospital in an extremely distressed and agitated state, voicing paranoid delusions of a religious nature. He had never responded very well to medical treatment, and once, when the occupational therapist attempted to interview him during a previous hospitalization, Andrew answered most of the questions with "I don't know" or "I've never thought about it." Over the years, his symptoms became more florid, and he attempted suicide on several

occasions. He also assaulted staff when they questioned him regarding his symptoms or when they simply got in his way. Given that Andrew heard voices telling him to kill himself and that he had identified himself as living inside other people, he was thought to present a considerable risk both to himself and to the general public.

For much of his last inpatient admission he was uncommunicative and hostile. He neglected both his hygiene and his diet but would spend long periods writing furiously (and for the most part illegibly). Eventually, he made some improvement and started to attend the open art session on the ward for up to 10 minutes at a time. The artwork that he produced began to include some recognizable images in addition to apparently random scribbles. He expressed an interest in attending further occupational therapy, and after much deliberation, the team agreed that he could be accompanied to groups in the main day therapy area. His initial program was based on simple occupational forms that Andrew valued, where social interaction would not be the primary focus. These included art, yoga stretches, gardening, and table tennis.

The occupational therapist decided to use the MOHOST at this point to evaluate his progress and gain insight as to how to continue with him. The therapist completed the MOHOST based on her knowledge of Andrew from observing him in the groups and on the ward. Using the MOHOST as a structure, the therapist created the following account of Andrew's occupational performance. The MOHOST report she completed is shown in *Figure 18.4*.

Andrew appeared to be unaware of his limitations. He did not voice any difficulties in performance despite his overt impairments. He made no spontaneous reference to his future. He was able to make choices within structured situations (e.g., choosing art materials or getting a drink when thirsty). However, he still needed prompting to manage personal activities of daily living. Moreover, he occasionally engaged in activities that appeared to be the product of delusional impulse (e.g., shaving off all his body hair).

Andrew's long-held interest in art had recently resurfaced. He could be readily engaged in selected activities related to art and express satisfaction in these activities. He also enjoyed physical exercise and pursued activities independently, but he continued to express no

FIGURE 18.4 Andrew's ratings and analysis of strengths and limitations on the MOHOST.

ANALYSIS OF STRENGTHS & LIMITATIONS

Andrew does not express his feelings but has clear interests. He has also proved able to tolerate new situations and to demonstrate a degree of responsibility. His interactions remain limited but improve when there is a practical focus, and he is able to plan and organize activities with support. He continues to be restless and distractible, and has difficulty coping with a marked hand tremor.

Summary of Ratings

Motivation for Occupation				Pattern of Occupation				Communication & Interaction skills				Process skills				Motor skills				Environment: Inpatient Hospital			
Appraisal of ability	Expectation of success	Interest	Choices	Routine	Adaptability	Roles	Responsibility	Non-verbal skills	Conversation	Vocal expression	Relationships	Knowledge	Timing	Organization	Problem-solving	Posture & Mobility	Coordination	Strength & Effort	Energy	Physical space	Physical resources	Social groups	Occupational demands
F	F	F	F	F	F	F	F	F	F	F	F	F	F	F	F	F	F	**(F)**	F	**(F)**	**(F)**	**(F)**	**(F)**
A	A	**(A)**	A	A	**(A)**	A	A	A	A	A	A	**(A)**	A	A	A	**(A)**	A	A	A	A	A	A	A
I	I	I	**(I)**	**(I)**	I	I	**(I)**	I	**(I)**	**(I)**	**(I)**	I	**(I)**	**(I)**	I	I	**(I)**	I	I	I	I	I	I
(R)	**(R)**	R	R	R	R	**(R)**	R	**(R)**	R	R	R	R	R	R	**(R)**	R	R	R	**(R)**	R	R	R	R

Key:
F = Facilitates occupational participation
A = Allows occupational participation
I = Inhibits occupational participation
R = Restricts occupational participation

clear interest in his general surroundings. Likewise, he clearly valued the intervention of the occupational therapist, but the value that he placed on wider relationships was unclear. He still regularly asked his parents to leave when they came to visit him.

Andrew's sleep pattern had recently improved, and his ability to follow a routine was much better. He was aware of times and appointments and could cope with a certain amount of imposed structure. His responses had become much less unpredictable, and he had proved able to tolerate new situations. However, his interactions with the staff and his parents continued to

center on his immediate needs rather than any long-term social or productive focus.

There were several indications that Andrew's sense of responsibility had recently improved. He had accepted feedback and had made appropriate requests (e.g., for permission to take some art materials to the ward). He also regularly thanked the occupational therapy staff for their support.

Whereas Andrew had not previously made eye contact, he began to do so readily, but his gaze still tended to be fixed and his facial expressions and use of gestures continued to be limited. His progress was more evident in his improved ability to initiate and sustain conversation, to respond to greetings and disclose information appropriately, and to demonstrate basic listening skills. His speech was also much clearer and of a more normal rate and flow, although his intonation was flat and he interacted only when approached, continuing to isolate himself on the ward.

Andrew remained dependent on others to anticipate difficulties and make appropriate decisions. He continued to be antisocial at times. Therefore, his occupational therapy program was designed to reduce risk by minimizing any pressure to make complex decisions.

Andrew retained information given to him and showed some evidence of previous experience using art materials and practicing yoga. He initiated tasks but was unable to sustain concentration for any length of time when undirected. With encouragement, he would return to tasks to complete them, and he had been able to cope with a 30-minute yoga session. He was able to follow verbal instructions adequately, but his work was disorganized. He required prompts to tidy up.

Andrew's balance was reasonable and he was capable of running at speed, but there was a certain rigidity in his gait and posture. His movements lacked fluidity and appeared awkward and clumsy at times. Most noticeably, his hands shook uncontrollably when he was not engaged in activities requiring hand-eye coordination. He had no evident problems with strength and effort, however, and was able to calibrate force sufficiently well to play table tennis. Overall, Andrew remained restless, and he still had periods of overactivity when he would dance or perform press-ups. He also continued to write or draw at a furious pace before losing focus and ending activities abruptly.

Impact of Using the MOHOST

Completing the MOHOST helped not only the occupational therapist but also the multidisciplinary team to look at Andrew's skills afresh. If the tool had been used just a few weeks previously, it would have reflected primarily major problems with occupational participation. Now the MOHOST highlighted some strengths, providing a clear indication of Andrew's improvement.

The MOHOST also highlighted the importance of employing the following strategies in occupational therapy:

- Encouraging Andrew's interests and values

- Discussing Andrew's progress with him at regular reviews to help him to build on his success

- Supporting Andrew to rebuild a satisfying routine

- Introducing consideration of some occupational goals.

As the therapist implemented these strategies, Andrew responded as follows. He said that he wanted to use the gym and computing facilities. Later, he also wanted to join a baking group. The therapist recognized that these would provide opportunities to develop his motor, process, and communication/interaction skills and thus encouraged and supported his involvement.

His motivation to participate in these occupations was strong enough to allow the therapist and other staff to begin to negotiate with Andrew to make a number of positive changes. First, while Andrew had previously refused medication that could help to reduce his tremor, he agreed to take it when it was pointed out that it would probably enhance his performance. Moreover, the ward staff was also able to broach the sensitive issue of hygiene with Andrew and to work with him toward improving this. Andrew's hands were always heavily nicotine stained, and he took up his parents' suggestion to try nicotine gum, which helped him to smoke less. The occupational therapist shared with Andrew that she had observed him having difficulty seeing objects up close when engaged in therapy. Andrew consequently agreed to wear his glasses more, which undoubtedly helped him to be more aware of his surroundings and may have contributed to his handwriting becoming more legible.

Occupational therapy had led the way in achieving a rapport with Andrew that began to extend to other staff members. The MOHOST also gave a tangible way of measuring Andrew's progress and helped to boost everyone's hopes that Andrew was making some improvement. In particular, it provided growing evidence that Andrew was capable of responsibility, cooperation, and flexibility, which was crucial to the difficult decisions that the team had to make regarding risk assessment.

At the time that this case study was written, Andrew's recovery was far from assured. The therapist planned to continue using the MOHOST to document his progress and ensure a systematic, ongoing assessment of his occupational needs. In Andrew's case the MOHOST proved to be an effective assessment for guiding intervention and documenting his progress.

Ivan: Using The SCOPE as a Guide to Intervention

Ivan is a 4-year-old boy who was admitted to the hospital for a fever. Ivan was diagnosed with gastroscesis at birth. He was born at 32 weeks gestation. Due to surgeries and rehabilitation related to his condition, Ivan has spent most of his first 2 years in the hospital. He has a long history of hospital stays, with his most recent stay lasting 2 weeks. He had a small-bowel transplant at age 1, but his original transplant went into rejection, and he required a second small-bowel transplant at age 2 as well as a liver transplant. When not hospitalized, he lives at home with his mother, father, and younger sister. There he receives 16-hour nursing care every day of the week.

Since his last hospitalization 2 months ago, Ivan appeared to have acquired many new skills. Therefore, the occupational therapist working with Ivan chose to administer the SCOPE to evaluate his progress and to gain insight into new areas for intervention. The therapist specifically wanted to focus on interventions applicable to Ivan during his frequent hospitalizations and to identify possible environmental modifications for his hospital room.

The SCOPE was completed while observing Ivan in his hospital room and during play in the therapy room. Information was also gathered through informal discussions with the hospital staff who were familiar with Ivan from his current and previous hospitalizations. The profile of Ivan's strengths and challenges with participation are shown in *Figure 18.5*. A summary of the qualitative information gained from administering the SCOPE follows.

Volition

During the evaluation therapy session Ivan engaged in exploration of a toy when it was placed immediately in front of him for 5 to 10 minutes, and he freely explored familiar objects versus those that were unfamiliar. He showed clear enjoyment through facial expressions during activities. However, he did not associate any enjoyment with the outcomes of activities. Given his history of frequent and long-term hospitalizations, Ivan has not been afforded the opportunity to make choices and display preferences. He did not clearly request one object over another, and he responded similarly to any object given to him. While he showed no frustration at challenging tasks, he did not seek out challenging tasks after mastering other tasks. If given several objects (since he is usually only given one object at a time), it was unclear as to whether he would move on to a more or less challenging object.

Habituation

Ivan demonstrated understanding of and participated in all daily activities, including dressing, diaper changes, meals, and therapy sessions. He did not show distress during transitions between one activity and another, but he did require cues to end an activity. Ivan understood the hospital routine and participated in activities that made up his routine, such as dressing and eating. He sometimes required visual or verbal cues to follow through with sequences with routines (e.g., he did not indicate when he wanted his diaper changed). Ivan performed expected behaviors associated with his role as a patient. He complied with and understood the hospital routine. However, he did not display expected behaviors for any other roles, such as his role as a child (e.g., he did not understand how to play with traditional toys).

Communication and Interaction Skills

Ivan demonstrated some spontaneous nonverbal skills, but they were not always appropriate (e.g., he lifted his arms to be picked up, but also did this when he wanted something else, which made this behavior less effective). He needed many cues to show appropriate actions (e.g., when he wanted to play a game, he picked up the object, then looked at the therapist as if asking for the therapist to participate with him). When he was playing, he showed anticipation through his facial

FIGURE 18.5 Profile of Ivan's strengths and limitations on the SCOPE rating form.

Summary of Ratings

Volition				Habituation				Communication & Interaction skills				Process skills				Motor skills				Environment				
Exploration	Enjoyment	Preferences	Response to challenge	Daily activities	Response to transitions	Routine	Roles	Non-verbal communication	Verbal/Vocal expression	Conversation	Relationships	Understands & uses objects	Orientation to environment	Makes decisions	Problem solving	Posture & mobility	Coordination	Strength	Energy/endurance	Physical space	Physical resources	Social groups	Occupational demands	Family routine
F	F	F	F	F	F	F	F	F	F	F	F	F	F	F	F	F	F	F	F	F	F	F	F	F
A	A	A	A	A	A	A	A	A	A	A	A	A	A	A	A	A	A	A	A	A	A	A	A	A
I	I	I	I	I	I	I	I	I	I	I	I	I	I	I	I	I	I	I	I	I	I	I	I	I
R	R	R	R	R	R	R	R	R	R	R	R	R	R	R	R	R	R	R	R	R	R	R	R	R

Key:
F = Facilitates occupational participation
A = Allows occupational participation
I = Inhibits occupational participation
R = Restricts occupational participation

expressions. While many of his nonverbal expressions were inappropriate, he still used many effective behaviors, especially when cued by others. Ivan had an extremely limited vocabulary, and most of his vocalizations were echolalic. Ivan did engage in some meaningful interactions with adults, but did not always stay interested and was easily distracted. His expressions, both verbal and nonverbal, were not always appropriate or accurate, which affected his ability to have meaningful communication with others. The hospital environment did not provide any opportunity for age level–appropriate conversation. He showed no recognition of adults that he saw on a regular basis, which indicated his difficulty establishing and reciprocating relationships. It is important to keep in mind that each time Ivan is hospitalized there are many individuals in and out of his life during his stay, which contributed to his limited attachment to others. He did appear to recognize his family members as reported by hospital staff.

Process Skills

Ivan understood how to interact and orient himself with his environment as long as he received minimal cues from others. However, he did not seek or initiate opportunity to engage in the environment independently. When given an object that he had not seen before, Ivan would occasionally investigate it on his own. When asked to draw a picture with a marker, Ivan was confronted with a marker cap that was difficult to remove. He persisted at trying to get the cap off without getting frustrated and never looked to the therapist for help.

This indicated his limited ability to identify a challenge, since at a certain point it would have been appropriate for him to ask for help, which he did not.

Motor Skills

Ivan demonstrated trunk stability when seated; however, he lacked mobility and stability when standing and walking, which is necessary to fully participate in various play activities. These limitations are probably due to lack of opportunity to develop and practice his motor skills. Ivan's fine motor coordination appeared to be functional during play as evidenced by his successful manipulation of small objects. He recently began walking, and his gait appeared to be uneven, as he was observed to lean toward his left side. His uncoordinated gross motor skills make him unsafe in many gross motor activities during play. After passing through an obstacle course three times, Ivan was visibly winded. He seemed to lack the energy to persist at any task involving gross motor movements.

Environment

In the hospital environment Ivan was found to spend most of his time in his room, either in a crib or in a highchair into which he is strapped. Because of precautions taken to prevent further infection or to prevent the transmission of contagions to others, he is kept in his hospital room, restricting his opportunities for satisfying play. Hospital security and safety issues limit Ivan's opportunities to engage in play (e.g., he plays for extended periods with a single object, such as a medical syringe) or move around his environment. Because he had limited opportunities to interact with other children, Ivan was unable to develop any long-term relationships with peers or siblings. His parents did not visit often, which further complicated his ability to establish social relationships. In addition, Ivan did not seem to recognize the different roles that the various hospital staff play in his life, even though he may see the same person several times a day. His social context seemed to revolve only around the immediate needs that various individuals fulfill. The activities in which Ivan participated in the hospital did not afford him the opportunity to increase his performance skills and sense of competence. The environment was extremely under demanding, as most of his activities of daily living (ADLs) were performed by a caregiver

(nurse, other hospital staff). He had limited involvement in dressing and was not given the chance to practice toileting or participate fully in meals. Assistance with his ADLs was driven more by the workload of staff than by a routine that was compatible with Ivan. Although he participated when he could, such as putting on his socks, the occupational demands seemed to require passive participation from him. Because Ivan had spent a large portion of his childhood in the hospital, he had not had the opportunity to become part of a family routine. In addition, because his parents did not visit him much, when he was hospitalized, he had limited opportunity to develop his role as son and family member.

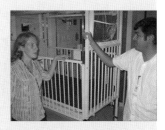

The occupational therapist working with Ivan discusses environmental modifications to his hospital room with the child life staff. The therapist identified the need to adapt Ivan's physical space after completing the SCOPE.[2]

[2]Photo provided by Meghan Suman, MS, OTR/L, University of Illinois Medical Center at Chicago.

Overall Findings from the SCOPE: Strengths and Limitations

The results of the SCOPE indicated that Ivan's strengths were in the areas of volition (exploration, enjoyment, and response to challenge), habituation (daily activities, response to transitions, and routines), and process skills (understands and uses objects, orientation to the environment, and ability to make decisions). Ivan's limitations were found to be in communication and interactions skills (verbal or vocal expression, conversation, and relationships), motor skills (posture and mobility, coordination, strength, energy, and endurance), and environment (physical space, physical resources, social groups, occupational demands, and family routines).

Impact of the SCOPE on Intervention

The SCOPE highlighted several of Ivan's strengths. These were his motivation to participate in play, his comfort level with daily activities and routines, and his ability to understand his environment. The SCOPE helped Ivan's therapist to develop intervention strategies that used his strengths to address his communication/interaction and motor skill limitations. The SCOPE also helped Ivan's therapist to identify that many of Ivan's behaviors were due to the limited amount of control that he had in the hospital environment. Therefore, intervention strategies included modifying and adapting his physical and social environment in collaboration with the hospital staff to allow more active participation and opportunity to engage in play. These are the specific interventions the therapist formulated:

The first goal was to increase Ivan's effectiveness with non-verbal communication and his use of verbal language. Ivan's therapist collaborated with the hospital staff to create the following change in his social environment. During meals, dressing, and bathing, staff would verbalize with Ivan, describing what they were doing and pointing to and naming objects. This change in how staff did their routine tasks would tap into Ivan's eagerness to interact with other people and his interest in communicating. Staff also agreed to look for and use opportunities to give Ivan more choices in daily care routines. Finally, staff agreed to respond to Ivan only when he used correct non-verbal communication and to correct him gently when he used inappropriate signs and gestures. Finally, to increase Ivan's social relationships and work on verbal skills, Ivan would be encouraged to learn the names of the health care providers who worked with him routinely in the hospital. To this end, the regular nurses and therapists were to tell Ivan their name and ask him to repeat it each time they worked with him.

The second goal was to improve Ivan's muscle strength and gross motor coordination through environmental modification. Because of the seriousness of his illness during the first 2 years of his life, Ivan was not afforded normal opportunities for free motor play. Because of safety concerns, Ivan was still not allowed to walk freely around his room without supervision. This meant that he usually sat passive for most of the day, which contributed to his lack of coordination and strength. However, the SCOPE revealed that Ivan enjoyed playing and would adapt well to more play time. To allow him to move about more freely, the occupational therapist arranged for an area of his room be gated off so Ivan could play in this space freely. Toys, in-

cluding a small tricycle, were kept in this area, encouraging Ivan to move about. The therapist set up a scheduled play time during which Ivan would have opportunities to play with another child to encourage social interaction. Finally, the therapist worked to involve Ivan's family by setting up scheduled family play times and teaching family members how to provide more stimulation in his hospital room.

Usefulness of the SCOPE

This case example demonstrates the effectiveness of the SCOPE in identifying a child's strengths and difficulties. The SCOPE was also a useful communication tool between the occupational therapist and other staff, caregivers, and family. The SCOPE gives a complete picture of the child and highlights both strengths and areas in which a therapist can intervene.

Summary: MOHOST and SCOPE

As these cases illustrate, both the MOHOST and SCOPE can provide a systematic framework for pulling together and documenting a client's occupational status. For clients with complex occupational problems who demonstrate difficulty functioning, it can highlight strengths on which therapy can build. Also, when progress is slow and uncertain, it can provide a concrete means of documenting change for the therapist, the client, and the team. Finally, when a new client's baseline level of functioning is unknown, the MOHOST or SCOPE can provide a valuable tool for gaining an overview of a client's occupational participation.

Occupational Therapy Psychosocial Assessment of Learning

The OT PAL (Townsend et al., 2001) is designed for use in a school-based setting with children aged 6 to 12 years. It is designed to assess students who are experiencing difficulty fulfilling expectations and roles in the classroom. The OT PAL is designed to capture information on psychosocial factors (beyond performance capacity) that influence a child's learning.

The OT PAL includes a quantitative rating scale consisting of 21 items that reflect a student's volition (ability to make choices) and habituation (roles and habits). This scale provides a profile of the student's volitional and habituation strengths and difficulties. Because the OT PAL does not gather information on performance capacity or skills, other assessments must be selected to provide this information.

The therapist collects information for completing the scale through observation supplemented with semi-structured interviews with the teacher, student, and parents. The interviews are designed to have the respondents offer different perspectives about the student's performance, behaviors, beliefs, and interests related to school. In addition to the rating scale, the OT PAL also provides the structure to gather and report qualitative information on these factors:

- The classroom
- The behavioral expectations in the classroom
- The teacher's style of teaching and managing the classroom
- The student's ability to meet these expectations
- The student's beliefs about his or her abilities as a learner within the school environment.

This information allows the occupational therapist to determine the quality of fit between the student and the classroom environment and how the latter affects the student's performance.

Administration

The OT PAL is designed so that it can be adapted to each child and school setting. The OT PAL includes the following forms:

- A preliminary (before observation) and environmental description worksheet that gathers information about basic characteristics of the student and the classroom
- The rating scale
- Brief teacher, student, and parent narratives that summarize the three interviews
- A summary form that summarizes student-environment fit, lists students' strengths and weaknesses, and describes any intervention plan.

Ordinarily, the therapist begins by preparing for the administration of the OT PAL (e.g., scheduling ob-

servation and interviews) and completing the pre-observation and environmental description forms. Next, the therapist observes the student in the classroom and other school settings as indicated and feasible. An observation of at least 40 minutes is generally necessary to gather sufficient information for completion of the rating scale. The teacher, student, and parent interviews are administered after the observation because part of their purpose is to gather information that supplements and confirms or corrects the observation. Each interview takes approximately 15 minutes. The parent interview may be conducted as a written questionnaire or via telephone. After the therapist finishes gathering information, he or she completes the rating scale and forms. This process leads naturally to development of intervention plans and recommendations to others in the school setting. Because of the comprehensive nature of the OT PAL, it is a useful assessment for giving input to the school team for planning how to best meet a child's educational needs.

O**ccupational Therapy Psychosocial Assessment of Learning (OT PAL)**

- Assesses students by capturing information on psychosocial and environmental factors that affect a child's learning. Focuses on volition (ability to make choices) and habituation (roles and habits).
- Can be ordered through the MOHO Clearinghouse e-store http://ascendant.cas.uic.edu/retail/, or
  - Visit www.moho.uic.edu
  - Select menu item "MOHO Products"
  - Link to OT PAL assessment for more information about the assessment, example assessment forms. To link to the MOHO Clearinghouse e-store left-click on the "Buy Now" button.

Gerald: The Use the OT PAL to Evaluate Adjustment to First Grade

Gerald was 7 years 11 months old and was in first grade. He was diagnosed at age 5 with acute lymphocytic leukemia and received chemotherapy for 2 years. Gerald was no longer receiving leukemia treatment but still had fatigue and weakness. He had also been identified as having sensory integrative dysfunction, which affected his attention span, arousal levels, spatial orientation, postural control, visual motor skills, visual perceptual skills, and bilateral integration. Gerald had several adaptations in his classroom environment to improve his organization and attention span. He also had a classroom aide during half of the school day to provide extra needed assistance.

Because Gerald faced numerous challenges in the classroom, the therapist decided to administer the OT PAL as a means of gathering information on his overall adjustment to first grade in anticipation of a school team review. The assessment illuminated both strengths and concerns for Gerald in the areas of making choices, habits and routines, and roles. A discussion of the information that was discovered through the OT PAL and its implications follows.

Volition

Gerald displayed a positive sense of personal causation with reference to his academic ability in certain aspects of classroom performance. His behaviors in the classroom clearly showed that he was highly motivated to demonstrate his competence. For instance, he actively participated in classroom discussion by consistently raising his hand in response to the teacher's questions. When observed, he volunteered to go up in front of the room during a classroom activity to write his answer to one of the questions on the board. The teacher reported that he took pride in his work and routinely drew attention to himself whenever he did well on a classroom task.

Although Gerald appropriately seized opportunities to display his competence in certain areas of academic performance, other actions indicated a challenge or

threat to his personal causation. For example, because he had difficulties focusing, organizing his school materials, and maintaining the pace of his individual work, he tended to rely heavily on his aide to scaffold his performance. Moreover, he had trouble when he needed to make self-directed choices and relied on his aide for guidance. In these situations, the more self-assured attitude he displayed when answering or performing publicly was replaced with a sense of insecurity.

He also did things that indicated that he either overestimated what he could do or attempted to hide his limitations. For example, Gerald offered to help another student carry the basket of lunches to the lunchroom (a job that the students do in each classroom), but he was unable to do his part because of limited strength and endurance. In addition, Gerald's teacher reported that students often rejected him during recess because of his limited motor capacities. For example, he wanted to play kickball, but the students did not want him on their team because he was not very good. Overall, Gerald appeared to be working very hard to maintain a public image of competency.

Sometimes he managed competent performance. On other occasions he failed publicly or lapsed into an insecure, dependent mode. While variation in belief in skill is typical of his age, Gerald fluctuated to extremes. This, combined with the negative social feedback he received because of his motor limitations, indicated that his personal causation was at risk.

Gerald strongly valued being able to perform in the classroom. For example, it was clear that he cared about receiving the symbolic star or smiley face on his assignments. It was also very important for Gerald to be looked upon and treated as "normal." He went out of his way to be involved in classroom activities and discussions just like other children. However, he had substantial difficulty maintaining involvement in some classroom activities and during recess. He got upset and frustrated when he could not do what other children did or was not invited to join in. Gerald also placed a high premium on his teacher's and parents' opinions of him as a student. The teacher and his parents saw him as working extra hard to earn their positive image of him as a student. For example, he was especially careful to follow classroom rules and to be seen as a good student.

Gerald named his favorite subjects without hesitation during the student interview. His reason for liking these subjects was that they were easy for him and he performed them well. While interests often coincide with what one does well, his stated reasons for interests in school highlight how the need to feel and be recognized as competent dominated Gerald's volition.

Habits and Routines

Figure 18.6 illustrates the habituation portion of the OT PAL rating scale as it was completed for Gerald. He readily described the routine of the school day. He showed a good understanding of what to do throughout the day, such as hanging up his coat and book bag when he arrived in the morning, going to his desk, and listening to the teacher's directions. He even explained that the daily schedule varies depending on the day (i.e., music lessons on Tuesdays and Thursdays).

However, according to Gerald's teacher, most of the time he struggled to keep up with his classmates in relation to school routines even with help from the part-time aide. Both his level of energy and difficulties with focusing, attending, and organizing hampered keeping up with routines. For example, he was generally slower than peers in writing and had difficulty arranging classroom materials to complete assignments. He was provided with a number of classroom adaptations to improve his organization and to help him find materials more efficiently, which only partly compensated for his difficulties. Gerald's teacher reported that he was not able to organize his assignments in keeping with classroom routines without the help of his part-time aide. The teacher reported that he also needed assistance making sure he was bringing home the necessary books or worksheets to do his homework. Another factor that contributed to Gerald's difficulty completing classroom activities within the allotted time was his periodic removal from the classroom for occupational therapy, physical therapy, and social work. As a consequence of these things, Gerald was often catching up on assignments during free time. This tended to mark Gerald as different from the other students, thus undermining his attempts to appear competent

Roles

Gerald strongly identified with and attempted to meet expectations of the student role in the classroom. He

accepted the teacher's authority, asked for help appropriately, tried hard as a student, and participated in activities and class discussions. Gerald had difficulty switching between group roles, particularly from leader to follower. He wanted to be in a leader role, apparently because it gave him a feeling of competence.

Gerald's teacher noted that his opportunities for interaction with peers, which are also part of the student role, were more challenging for him. His classmates generally accepted and interacted with him as a member of the classroom. However, he was sometimes teased, and others did not defend him when this happened. Moreover, only a couple of classmates would actually do things regularly with him outside of structured classroom activities. He was not invited to interact with others, and as noted earlier, was not welcomed as a participant in sport activities.

His teacher reported that aside from rare occasions of aggressive behaviors, Gerald managed to work adequately with his classmates. However, at the beginning of the year, he had much more difficulty. He used to touch students inappropriately and display aggressiveness. His touching inappropriately had stopped and his aggressiveness had decreased. His interactions with classmates gradually improved as Gerald became familiar with his classmates and they with him. Because of his trouble working with students in the beginning of the year, his teacher had some concerns about Gerald meeting and interacting with new students in second grade. She reported that if there was a problem between Gerald and another student, it was usually with a student who was not in Gerald's classroom.

Student–Environment Fit

Overall, Gerald's school environment supported his participation in school and learning. Gerald sat in the back of the room and at times had difficulty attending to the tasks at hand. However, this problem appeared more related to Gerald's need to move around at times and his short attention span rather than particular features of the classroom. Gerald was provided with and used a move-and-sit cushion (a pad he sits on to meet his need for movement and help increase his attention span). The pad improved his distractibility. In addition, Gerald used a desk that opened and closed, a basket, and a

FIGURE 18.6 Gerald's ratings and comments on the Habits/Routines section of the OT-PAL Rating scale.

II. Habits and Routines – The Student	N/O	4	3	2	1
A. Demonstrates school routines comparable to peers. Comments: *Gerald occasionally demonstrates the ability to keep up with his classmates in relation to the school routines, but often he struggles and needs assistance.*				X	
B. Adheres to routines within the school day. Comments: *Gerald is aware of routines within a school day. He periodically needs verbal cues to assist him with his routine.*			X		
C. Completes activities within time guidelines (e.g., finishes assignments/tasks in a timely manner). Comments: *Does not always complete task within time guidelines because he is often slower than his peers in writing tasks.*				X	
D. Maintains desk in a manner in keeping with classroom routines. Comments: *Even with adaptations, he still has trouble finding certain materials. It took him a longer time to find a book as compared to peers.*				X	
E. Maintains personal belongings in keeping with classroom routines. Comments: *Knows where his belongings should be kept, but his book bag and jacket were on the floor (not the appropriate place) during the observation.*				X	
F. Organizes assignments and projects in keeping with classroom routines. Comments: *tends to fall behind*	X				
G. Completes smooth transitions between routine activities (i.e., efficiently ends and begins another). Comments: *Gerald is often the last one in the class to complete a transition and often needs verbal cues regarding the new activity in which he just transitioned.*				X	
III. Roles – The Student	**N/O**	**4**	**3**	**2**	**1**
A. Demonstrates a well-established student role (i.e., accepts teacher's authority, asks for help appropriately). Comments: *Demonstrates many behaviors attached to the student role; however, he needs to be more self directed.*			X		
B. Demonstrates smooth transition between roles (i.e., switches smoothly from leader to follower). Comments:	X				
C. Responds acceptably to diverse roles adopted by others. Comments:	X				
D. Assumes roles consistent with classroom/school expectations. Comments:	X				

Key:
4 = Competent performance
3 = Questionable performance
2 = Ineffective performance
1 = Deficient performance
N/O = Not observed

part-time aide. The desk and basket enabled him to find supplies more easily and to be more organized. Gerald's part-time aide greatly supported his performance in the classroom. The classroom milieu was also highly structured, which helped Gerald to stay focused. Finally, the classroom provided some avenues for Gerald to feel a positive sense of personal causation related to his academic ability.

The desks in the classroom were arranged in groups of four (with assigned seating), facilitating Gerald's positive interactions with other students. Generally, Gerald could work with other students, although they tended to marginalize and sometimes tease him during open activities and recess.

Gerald was able to interact well with his teacher, readily asking for help and offering answers during group discussions. Gerald's teacher was a good match for him, as she has high expectations for all of the students but considers each student's circumstances. She considered each student individually, identifying their academic and emotional needs, and worked hard to meet those needs.

Implications of the OT PAL Assessment

The OT PAL identified Gerald's strengths and difficulties in the areas of volition and habituation. *Figure 18.7* summarizes Gerald's rating scale scores. Equally important to the profile of strengths and weaknesses is the qualitative information gathered about Gerald. His greatest strength was his desire to be a good student and the sense of efficacy he had concerning some aspects of his classroom performance. Gerald's volitional strengths were particularly important given his substantial habituation and performance capacity. However, aspects of Gerald's volition were at risk and needed to be supported and developed.

Supporting Gerald's volition meant paying attention to the strong values he held about being a student and bolstering his sense of personal causation. It was important to Gerald to be seen as a good and competent student, and this should be supported as much as possible. His limited motor performance barred him from a number of classroom and other activities, frustrating his attempts to be competent and to fit in. Additionally, a

number of factors in the classroom tended to make Gerald stand out, and these should be considered and minimized.

First, consideration was given to minimizing how Gerald's limited strength and endurance affected his performance and what could be done about it. Fatigue in particular is a common problem following chemotherapy, and its extent and duration vary greatly. Since the pace at which Gerald would regain these capacities was unknown, it was important to adapt circumstances in the interim to allow Gerald to participate more inside and outside the classroom. For example, carrying the lunch to the cafeteria was modified to involve pushing a cart.

Gerald at times relied heavily on his aide. Although this support was useful for him, it increasingly made him stand out from the other students. Moreover, growing independent of his aide in the future would further enhance his feelings of efficacy. The main function that Gerald's aide served was to help him organize his materials and focus on his schoolwork. Even though Gerald was provided with desk and basket adaptations to help him organize and find needed materials efficiently, he had not learned to use these resources optimally. The therapist and the aide worked together to develop an organization process that worked best for Gerald. Importantly, Gerald was involved in helping to plan this process. The therapist consulted with the aide concerning the importance of Gerald's growing more independent of her help and assisted her in planning how to gradually allow Gerald more responsibility and autonomy as he could handle it. This strategy enabled Gerald to develop habits to support his own competence in school.

Another area of concern was that Gerald needed to catch up on missed assignments during free time. It was important for Gerald to get free time to let off steam, which helped him focus throughout the rest of the school day. Moreover, having to work on schoolwork when other students were engaged in free activities set Gerald apart from the other students. Thus, an alternative schedule for Gerald to receive therapies that minimized interference with classroom work was developed.

FIGURE 18.7. Summary of Gerald's ratings on the OT PAL scale.

Volition — Student chooses to:										Habits and Routines — The student:							Roles — The student:			
Begin activity with direction	Begin self-directed activity	Stay engaged	Continue/transition with direction	Discontinue activity with direction	Discontinue self-directed activity	Engage with peers given direction	Engage with peers self-directed	Follow social rules	Show preferences	Demonstrates routines	Adheres to routines	Completes activities	Maintains desk	Maintains belongings	Organizes projects and assignments	Completes transitions	Demonstrates student role	Transitions smoothly between roles	Responds to diverse roles	Assumes school-related roles
N/O	N/O	N/O	N/O	N/O	N/O	N/O	N/O	N/O	N/O	N/O	N/O	N/O	N/O	N/O	N/O	N/O	N/O	**N/O**	**N/O**	**N/O**
(4)	4	4	(4)	(4)	4	4	(4)	(4)	(4)	4	4	4	4	4	4	4	4	4	4	4
3	3	(3)	3	3	3	(3)	3	3	3	3	(3)	3	3	3	3	3	(3)	3	3	3
2	2	2	2	2	(2)	2	2	2	2	(2)	2	(2)	(2)	(2)	2	(2)	2	2	2	2
1	(1)	1	1	1	1	1	1	1	1	1	1	1	1	1	(1)	1	1	1	1	1

Key: **4** = Competent   **3** = Questionable   **2** = Ineffective   **1** = Deficient   **N/O** = Not observed

As this case illustrated, the OT PAL can be very useful in the school context for identifying the status of volition and habituation and their contribution to how a child is adapting to school. The assessment also highlights factors in the school environment that support or constrain the student. Because of its focus, this instrument is well suited to complement capacity or performance-oriented assessments used in the school context.

Conclusion

This chapter presented three diverse assessments that have in common the combination of flexibility in the use of more than a single method of data collection. Each method of data collection has its strengths and weaknesses, and assessments that use a single method (interview, self-report, or observation) are designed to make the most use of the methodology they employ. These assessments, by combining or allowing alternative approaches to collecting information, are designed to maximize the use of mixed methods.

References

Bowyer, P., Ross, M., Schwartz, O., Kielhofner, G., & Kramer, J. (2005). *The Short Child Occupational Profile (SCOPE)* (version 2.1). Model of Human Occupation Clearinghouse, Department of Occupational Therapy, College of Applied Health Sciences, University of Illinois at Chicago, Chicago, Illinois.

Parkinson, S., Forsyth, K., & Kielhofner, G. (2006). *The Model of Human Occupation Screening Tool* (version 2.0). Authors.

Townsend, S. C., Carey, P. D., Hollins, N. L., Helfrich, C., Blondis, M., Hoffman, A., Collins, L., Knudson, J., & Blackwell, A. (2001). *The Occupational Therapy Psychosocial Assessment of Learning (OT PAL). (Version 1.0)* Chicago: Model of Human Occupation Clearinghouse. Department of Occupational Therapy. University of Illinois, Chicago.

Watts, J. H., Brollier, C., Bauer, D., & Schmidt, W. (1989). The Assessment of Occupational Functioning: The second revision. *Occupational Therapy in Mental Health, 8* (4), 61–87.

Watts, J. H., Hinson, R., Madigan, M. J., McGuigan, P. M., & Newman, S. M. (1999). The Assessment of Occupational

Functioning—Collaborative version. In B. J. Hempill-Pearson (Ed.), *Assessments in occupational therapy in mental health.* Thorofare, NJ: Slack.

Watts, J. H., Kielhofner, G., Bauer, D., Gregory, M., & Valentine, D. (1986). The Assessment of Occupational Functioning: A screening tool for use in long-term care. *American Journal of Occupational Therapy, 40,* 231–240.

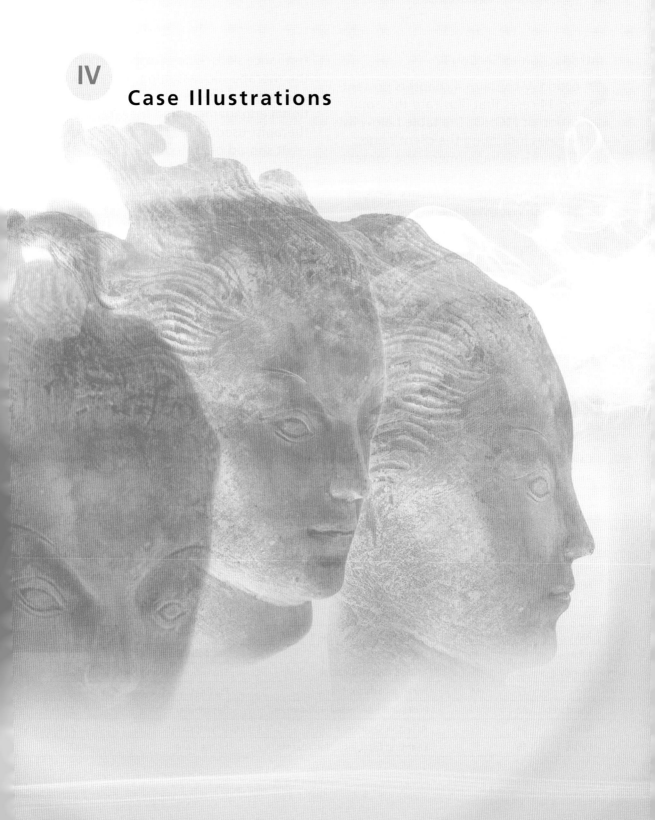

IV Case Illustrations

Introduction to Section IV

Section IV contains 4 chapters presenting 14 cases that illustrate the application of MOHO. The table below lists all the cases indicating the client's age, sex, diagnosis or impairment, the context in which therapy took place, and the chapter in which the case occurs. No single case employs every MOHO concept. Indeed, good use of MOHO involves recognizing those concepts that are most useful for a particular client and for deciding a course of intervention. Therefore, the cases should be viewed collectively as illustrations of a range of approaches to applying the model. Each case highlights an aspect of the process of therapy and change that occurs in therapy. For example, one case may have a stronger emphasis on volition, while another stresses performance skills. One case may emphasize the therapeutic reasoning process, while another emphasizes the client's occupational engagement and the strategies the therapist used.

It should be noted that some cases in this section have been partly fictionalized. We have changed some things about each client to preserve the person's confidentiality. Some of the cases are from the previous edition of this book. We still have included them because they are excellent examples. These cases were updated to reflect current concepts, terminology, and assessments. While not all details of each case are literal, each case faithfully presents the nature of the therapist's reasoning, the actual course of intervention, and the client's outcomes.

Case	Age	Sex	Diagnosis/Impairment	Context	Chapter
Alvaro	33	M	Schizophrenia	Community Agency	19
Barbara	33	F	Multiple Sclerosis	Rehabilitation Setting	19
David	8	M	Sensory Processing Difficulties Developmental Delay	Private Practice	21
Fredrick	23	M	Depression	Rehabilitation Unit	22
Haydée	50	F	Cerebro-Vascular Accident	Residential Setting	19
Jacob	85	M	Dementia, Hemiplegia, Aphasia Sensory Loss	Nursing Home	20
Jessy	22	F	Head Injury	Rehabilitation Setting	22
Joan	79	F	Congestive Heart Failure	Home Care	21
Julia	60	F	Cerebral Palsy	Residential Setting	22
Mandy	35	F	AIDS, Substance Abuse	Transitional Living Facility	21
Marc	27	M	Paranoid Schizophrenia	Psychiatric Setting	20
Margaret	22	F	Profound Intellectual Impairment	Residential Setting	20
Mary	84	F	Affective Disorder	Day Hospital	21
Paula	45	F	Learning Disability, Hemiparesis	Home Care	20

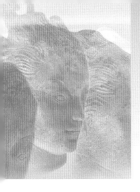

19

Recrafting Occupational Narratives

- Ana Laura Auzmendia
- Carmen Gloria de las Heras
- Gary Kielhofner
- Claudia Miranda

This chapter contains three cases. They each illustrate the process of rebuilding occupational adaptation in the face of significant life challenges. In each case, the client's occupational identity has been significantly eroded. Consequently, the course of therapy involved helping clients recraft occupational narratives for themselves and finding ways to put these narratives into action. The cases provide insight into the process of rebuilding occupational narratives as well as the complexities and challenges involved.

Haydée: Recrafting a Narrative

Haydée was the widowed mother of three grown children and grandmother of seven. She led an active and independent life in Mar del Plata, Argentina, working as a school principal. Five days after her 50th birthday she had a cerebral vascular accident resulting in left hemiplegia. She received acute services at a local hospital and was transferred to a rehabilitation institute, where she made limited progress. The physician in charge of Haydée's rehabilitation wrote in her chart that she would need to use a wheelchair for the rest of her life.

Haydée was transferred to a nearby public geriatric residence. She was unable to get out of bed. Her impairments were significant. For example, she had lateral rotation and deviation of her neck due to contractures and she drooled uncontrollably. In addition, Haydée was severely depressed and withdrawn.

Initial Information Collection and Therapeutic Reasoning

Considering Haydée's physical impairments and her emotional status, the therapist decided to first establish a relationship with her through a series of brief unstructured interviews in which she could learn about, validate, and encourage her. In these conversations, Haydée sometimes talked of suicide. At other times she wanted to overcome her despair but did not know where to begin. Haydée's thoughts and feelings reflected her severely compromised volition. She felt totally robbed of control over her life. She had no interest in anything around her. She felt all her life plans as well as the lifestyle she valued had been destroyed.

Engaging Haydée

Because of her compromised volition, the only goal Haydée could see as possibly improving her life was to walk again. Therefore, her therapist decided not to negotiate a goal more in line with her current physical status. Rather, she met Haydée where she was and validated her one desire at the time, agreeing to see what could be done. Gait training services were not available in the nursing home. Consequently, the therapist attempted to refer Haydée to physical therapy, which was available through the rehabilitation facility. However, Haydée did not meet criteria for outpatient services because of the prognosis she had been given. Moreover, Haydée did not have the resources to purchase private physical therapy in the residence.

Therefore, the therapist found an occupational therapy colleague who had the background to work with Haydée on walking and who agreed to see Haydée for a reduced fee that she could afford.

Because the therapist demonstrated to Haydée a willingness to attend to her desires, she gained Haydée's trust. She was able to use this as a foundation for advising Haydée to engage in other aspects of occupational therapy. The therapist worked with Haydée to enhance her occupational performance, through engaging her in doing things she enjoyed that also improved her scapular and neck mobility and sitting posture. The therapist also felt it was important to address the fact that Haydée had isolated herself from others because of her depression. Thus, she advised Haydée of the importance of involving herself with others and persuaded her to join a creative activity group.

Haydée rapidly improved over the next few months. As she began to experience the return of her motor function, her volition improved as well. She felt more in control, enjoyed things she did, and saw herself as achieving things that mattered to her. Haydée showed such gains that she was admitted to rehabilitation services on an outpatient basis while still living in the geriatric home.

Through concentrated rehabilitation efforts, Haydée continued to improve her upper extremity motor skills and occupational performance. In everyday activities such as eating she was beginning to use her left arm as an assist. She also began to walk with a tripod cane and the assistance of another person. Haydée became more socially active and regularly attended occupational therapy groups at the geriatric residence.

Dealing with a Devastating Setback

During radiography to monitor her osteoarthritis and osteoporosis (conditions she had before her stroke), the technician fell with Haydée while assisting her to transfer from her wheelchair to a gurney. In the fall, Haydée fractured her affected left wrist. Six weeks later, when the cast was removed, Haydée had lost many of the fine motor abilities she had previously gained in her hand. Realizing her loss in function, Haydée became depressed and withdrawn again. Haydée's still vulnerable volition was clearly affected by this turn of events over which she had no control

and which had such negative consequences for the functional gains she had worked so hard to achieve. At this point, Haydée was not able to identify any goal for herself because she did not see how working toward something would really help her.

The therapist decided that Haydée needed an exploratory intervention (as discussed in Chapters 10 and 13) that would allow her to regenerate some sense of control, regenerate some feelings of satisfaction in doing things, and experience something of value. Because Haydée had such disrupted volition, it was clear that she would need a highly supportive environment that could support her volition by providing external sources of confidence, interest, expectation, and value. The therapist also reasoned that this environmental support could best be achieved in a group context. Therefore, she began to encourage and persuade Haydée to join a group project.

Turning the Corner Through Engagement in a Group Project

At first Haydée was reluctant. However, with constant encouragement and statements of expectations that Haydée could and should do this for herself from the therapist, she agreed to join a project called "the Puppet Workshop." A number of residents of the facility had planned, with the leadership of an occupational therapist, to implement a musical puppet show. For this project, they would make the puppets and stage, adapt the script of the musical for puppets, rehearse, and perform the show.

Becoming involved in this project provided the necessary momentum for Haydée. Moreover, she became an essential part of the group, so that the group members began to provide the expectation for Haydée to participate that the therapist previously provided. Over time she improved her sense of efficacy and gained a feeling of satisfaction in doing things. Since she had more education than most residents, Haydée was recruited to write the adaptation of the play's script. At first she hesitated, but with some coaching and encouragement from the therapist, Haydée soon found that she was quite good at writing. Bolstered by her success in this task, she also showed interest in performing with puppets. When she first tried, it was difficult because of the functional restrictions of her left arm. However, with environmental adaptations and coaching, she was able to manipulate a puppet. Thus, she became a puppeteer.

The first puppet show was held at the geriatric residence for other residents and for family members. It was a great success. The puppet group was subsequently invited to perform seven more shows hosted by different community settings. One of the settings was the school where Haydée formerly was the principal. Haydée had suggested this setting. Performing there meant that she had to face the emotionally difficult challenge of re-encountering her former colleagues and students. Going to the school and seeing the children and teachers enjoy the puppet show was a great boost for Haydée. Once again, she began to feel that she could do something worthwhile.

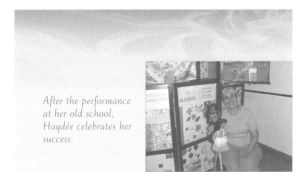

After the performance at her old school, Haydée celebrates her success.

Going back to her old school was only one of many social and physical challenges Haydée faced because of the puppet performances. For example, she also had to cope with a variety of architectural barriers that made it difficult to get onto the stages. With all of these challenges and successes, the puppet project was an important achievement for Haydée. Working on the script and doing the performance stimulated Haydée's feeling of efficacy and enjoyment in writing. She began writing poetry and essays in occupational therapy. Moreover, her excursions into the community provided her with the opportunity to know that many barriers, physical and social, could be faced and overcome.

During this period, as Haydée began to show regeneration of her volition, the therapist also worked with her to establish a routine and to enhance her performance of self-care. Haydée was able to make steady progress. After some time, she indicated a desire to be-

gin thinking about her future and what she would do with the rest of her life.

Administering the Occupational Performance History Interview— II (OPHI-II)

Because of Haydée's progress, the therapist felt it was an ideal time to administer the OPHI-II. Haydée had shown enough progress to be able to reflect on her life history and look to the future. The therapist did not complete the occupational settings (environment) part of the OPHI-II since Haydée already had indicated a desire to move to a new living environment. As the OPHI-II scores on *Figure 19.1* show, Haydée had begun to rebuild her occupational identity, but her competence was still limited.

The process of engaging in the interview was important for Haydée. It allowed her to put into perspective the experiences of her life and to be reminded of her own strengths. Furthermore, through the process of telling her life story, Haydée was able to identify goals she wanted to strive toward in the future. The following is the occupational narrative that Haydée told in the interview.

Haydée began her story with her family, expressing that she had a wonderful childhood. Her parents were poor and worked hard to support 10 children. Haydée was the only one of her siblings to finish high school. She went on to obtain a diploma in teaching through her own fierce determination. Soon thereafter, Haydée married and had her first child. She went to work in a car dealership, since it allowed more flexibility than teaching. In the years that followed, she had a warm and loving relationship with her husband and together they had two more children.

However, with the birth of Haydée's youngest child, things began to change dramatically. Her son was born prematurely, became dehydrated, and had convulsions. Then, when her son was 13 months old, her husband was killed in a car accident. Simultaneously, after 10 years of working for the dealership, she was suddenly laid off along with seven other persons.

Haydée even had to fight to receive a pension to which she was entitled. As she notes, "I never had time to grieve as I should have. Two days after my husband's death, I took my bike and went to apply for my pen-

FIGURE 19.1 Haydée's strengths and challenges on the OPHI-II Occupational Identity and Competence Scales.

Occupational Identity Scale	1	2	3	4
Has personal goals and projects			X	
Identifies a desired occupational lifestyle			X	
Expects success				X
Accepts responsibility				X
Appraises abilities and limitations				X
Has commitments and values			X	
Recognizes identity and obligations			X	
Has interests				X
Felt effective (past)				X
Found meaning and satisfaction in lifestyle (past)				X
Made occupational choices (past)				X
Occupational Competence Scale	1	2	3	4
Maintains satisfying lifestyle			X	
Fulfills role expectations		X		
Works toward goals		X		
Meets personal performance standards			X	
Organizes time for responsibilities			X	
Participates in interests			X	
Fulfilled roles (past)				X
Maintained habits (past)				X
Achieved satisfaction (past)			X	

Key :
4 = Exceptionally competent occupational functioning;
3 = Appropriate, satisfactory occupational functioning;
2 = Some occupational functioning problems;
1 = Extreme occupational functioning problems

sion. I didn't have time to cry." This incident typifies Haydée's view of herself as both a fighter and positive person. She refers to herself as both optimistic and obstinate.

Mustering her strength, Haydée immediately found a job teaching. It was difficult to be both a full-time worker and a single mother of three small children. As she saw it, she had no time for herself and in-

sufficient time for her children. Nonetheless, Haydée excelled as a teacher, advancing to a substitute principal position. Her successes during this period in managing her household and raising children, while doing well as a teacher, greatly increased her sense of efficacy. She was very proud of her ability to set and achieve goals. As her children grew up and left home, she set two important goals for herself. First, she wanted to become a school principal. Second, she wanted to begin taking courses at a local university.

Shortly after Haydée reached the first of these goals, she had the stroke. The life she had worked so hard to build collapsed, leading her to despair and forcing her to live in a geriatric residence at age 50. Haydée saw the past months in the residence, and especially her experiences in the puppet workshop, as allowing her to begin rebuilding her life again. Her success was reflected in her current routine, which was organized and balanced with various leisure, self-care, and rehabilitation activities. She engaged in a variety of interests and had goals to:

- Improve her walking
- Manage herself in a house
- Obtain a disability pension
- Work part-time as a writer.

She acknowledged that she had difficulty staying focused on and sustaining energy for achieving her goals, so talking about them helped her commit to them.

As illustrated in Haydée's narrative slope (*Fig. 19.2*) she made significant progress in reversing the tragic consequences of her stroke. Once again, she was finding a way to rise above adversity in reconstructing a vision of a life she wanted. Also, in beginning to think about her future narrative, Haydée was able to reflect on her past, identifying what she would like to do differently. For example, she noted how she had been so focused on her career, explaining, "I often would get only 4 hours of sleep. I was obsessed with work." Now she wanted to live her life in a less extreme way. She saw her stroke as an opportunity to reflect on her life and think about how she would live in the future. The therapist advised Haydée of the picture of her occupational narrative that came from the interview, and Haydée heartily agreed with it. She also came to the conclusion with

FIGURE 19.2 Haydée's narrative slope.

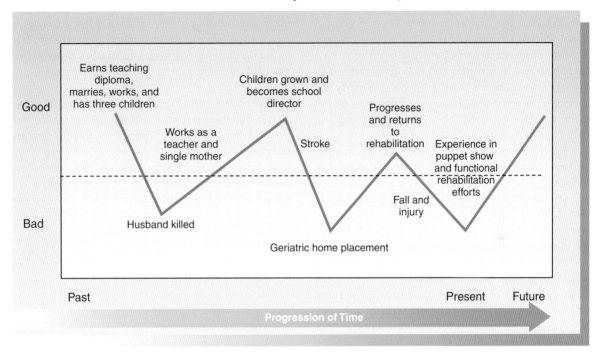

the therapist's advice and encouragement that she would focus in the coming months on realizing the future she envisioned for herself.

Building a New Occupational Narrative

In the following months, Haydée worked hard to achieve the competence she envisioned in her narrative. She improved performance of her self-care activities, achieving independence in everything except bathing. She used her wheelchair to get around in the facility and walked around in her room with a tripod cane. Haydée undertook a 500-km trip on her own to complete the legal procedures to receive her pension.

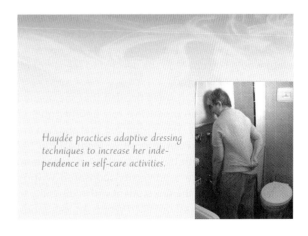

Haydée practices adaptive dressing techniques to increase her independence in self-care activities.

During this time, Haydée continued to write. She completed a private book of essays and prose. To write effectively on the computer, she worked in occupational therapy to improve her motor skills for typing. Haydée continued to participate and often took on a leadership role in activities and outings organized by the geriatric residence. At the New Year's party she danced for the first time. Haydée also began to go out alone to shop regularly, using a taxi that accommodated her wheelchair.

Finally, Haydée achieved one of her most important dreams. She traveled by bus with her three children back to her hometown. There she encountered relatives and old friends that she had not seen for years. She also visited the cemetery where her parents and husband were buried. Haydée returned very enthusiastic with the plan to move to her native city in a short time.

The occupational therapist was concerned that it was not clear how the move would fit into the identity Haydée was constructing for herself. It seemed that Haydée was caught up in the emotion of the visit. Nonetheless, the therapist realized the importance of allowing Haydée to make her own decision and the need to support her to make a good decision. Consequently, she advised Haydée that she should make this decision very carefully, since a move to a new environment could have many unanticipated effects on her. She negotiated with Haydée that she should take time with this decision. They agreed that Haydée would travel back one more time to gather more information about what her life could be like there before making this important occupational choice. Haydée made the trip with her daughter, traveling by bus. During this visit, she was able to reinterpret the situation, realizing that her initial plan was not realistic. As she put it, "Everyone has his or her life set up; what place would I occupy?" So she decided to search for alternatives for her future.

After reflection, Haydée decided that she needed to focus on her main productive role and her goal of living independently. She recognized that she had enjoyed writing and received positive feedback on her writing abilities. With her therapist's encouragement, she decided to take a university-sponsored writing course. She became the first student with a disability to attend a literary workshop called Words Amidst Hands.

During this time she also continued in occupational therapy, practicing her skills in using the computer and focusing on her self-care. After a couple of months she became totally independent in self-care, including bathing. She began to practice other activities of daily living such as sewing, washing, and ironing.

All of these efforts not only moved Haydée closer to her objective but also allowed her to realize her longstanding values of independence, vitality, and accomplishment in what she did. Haydée still had some highs and lows. Nonetheless, despite occasional fears and uncertainties, Haydée continued to strive to live her occupational narrative. In the words of one of her poems:

Sometimes . . . .

I feel like:
Laughing or crying.
And I laugh or cry.
Sometimes . . .
I feel like:
Walking, running or dancing.
And I walk, run or dance.
Sometimes . . .
I feel like:
Going back to the classroom,
And seeing the eager gaze,
Of the children, waiting for their work.
And I go back to the classroom.
To enjoy those gazes.
Sometimes . . .
I feel like:
Going back to my city.
And going through its streets.
And I return and go through its streets.
Sometimes . . .
I feel like:
Being with my parents,
In our home.
And I am with my parents.
Sometimes . . .
I feel like:
Going to the beach, with my grandchildren.
And I go to the beach,
With my grandchildren.

Sometimes . . .
I feel like:
Dreaming . . .
And . . . I dream awake.

Haydée in Perspective

The case of Haydée illustrates how the most effective occupational therapy must be timed according to the client's needs and readiness for change. Haydée's therapist correctly reasoned that initial assessment was best done through informal means and only later chose to do the OPHI-II, at a point when she felt Haydée could emotionally face and benefit from reviewing her life. Haydée also illustrates that the course of therapy is not always linear. There are often times when a client will regress or have difficulty moving forward as a result of complex combinations of personal and environmental factors. In particular, the process of rebuilding one's occupational narrative is extremely difficult when the onset of a disability has completely altered it.

Barbara: Transformation from Victim to Heroine

Barbara was a 33-year-old single mother, diagnosed with multiple sclerosis 3 years earlier. For 5 years before her diagnosis she had intermittent symptoms, such as weakness and pain in her back and lower extremities, blurred vision, and some slurring of her speech. Barbara was recently admitted to a rehabilitation center after several months of exacerbation. During the exacerbation she experienced dramatically decreased endurance and ascending muscle weakness that sometimes made it hard for her to breathe and swallow. During the worst of this period, she was unable either to walk on her own or to propel a wheelchair.

When the therapist first met Barbara, Barbara was depressed and anxious but able to express her thoughts and feelings. She felt out of control, had lost her involvement in her everyday activities, and was terrified of what the future had in store for her. Consequently, the occupational therapist was quite concerned not only about Barbara's physical condition but also about her severely impacted volition.

Despite her depression and anxiety and even though she had no idea how to go about it, Barbara expressed a willingness to do all she could to get her life back in order. In large measure this was fueled by the fact that she was responsible for two children. The therapist reasoned that it would be useful to examine Barbara's occupational narrative along with her to help figure out where her life had been and might go in light of her disability. She first interviewed Barbara using the OPHI-II and then collaborated with Barbara to complete the Interest Checklist and the Role Checklist. Because the impact of Barbara's environments could not be determined until her future performance capacity was better known, the therapist did not complete the occupational settings (environment) portion of the OPHI-II. Her plan was first to get an overall picture of Barbara's life and how the multiple sclerosis had affected it, then to go on to assess Barbara's physical capacity and performance, gathering other information as needed.

Barbara's Occupational Narrative

During her interview, Barbara related the following narrative. During her senior year in high school she became pregnant. After graduation she married the father; her daughter was born soon thereafter. Barbara had only worked briefly as a waitress on weekends during school. Barbara did not enjoy this job. She disliked working with customers on a daily basis, since she was a private person. For the next 2 years, Barbara's time was taken up with being a homemaker and mother. She had a second daughter 2 years after her first.

In the meantime, Barbara's relationship with her husband deteriorated badly. He was an alcoholic and physically abused Barbara. He also had not been able to hold a steady job because of multiple absences and a temper that got him into trouble with supervisors. Financial stress, combined with her husband's self-destructive drinking and his abuse of her, made life practically unbearable for Barbara. It became increasingly clear that her husband was not going to do anything about his drinking and abuse. Moreover, he had no prospects for work. Therefore, Barbara decided she would be better off alone with the children. Shortly after the birth of her second daughter, she divorced him.

Forced by the financial realities of being a single mother without the benefit of child support, Barbara returned to work. She found employment as a secretary in a construction firm, filing papers, typing, bookkeeping, and acting as a receptionist. With a great deal of effort, she managed to balance the demands of being a single mother of two children, working full-time, and maintaining a household. She did this for nearly a decade. During this time Barbara viewed herself as a fighter and a survivor who overcame a number of hurdles to be a good mother and provider.

Barbara was forced to resign her job 3 years earlier. Her multiple sclerosis had progressed to the point that she was unable, despite extreme effort and a supportive work environment, to fulfill her job responsibilities. In the 2 years before her resignation, Barbara frequently missed work because of fatigue and weakness.

In retrospect, Barbara realized she had enjoyed her job. She liked the moderate contact with other people that her job demanded and thought she did it well. She felt a sense of accomplishment in being able to hold the dual role of single parent and family breadwinner. Although it was hard, it was a source of great satisfaction to her that she had pulled her life together. However, Barbara had also felt guilty about not being with her children during the day. Barbara's values were organized around her view of her responsibility as a mother and her hard-won independence. Her children and the family which she and they constituted were of central importance. Fiercely independent, she wanted to be financially secure, and therefore not reliant on anyone else.

The advent of multiple sclerosis threatened all of Barbara's most basic values. She was plagued by the idea that she could be neither a good mother nor a source of income for her family. The entire life story she had constructed and lived had come crumbling down. Her financial picture had worsened as she lost her income and had to rely on social security income. She had grown dependent on her children and her parents. The independence and self-reliance she had worked so hard to achieve after leaving her husband had disappeared.

Just before her hospitalization, Barbara spent three-quarters of her waking day in bed watching television or talking to family members on the telephone.

The other major portion of her day was spent talking with her children or directing them to get household chores completed. Barbara had no set schedule for meals or self-care activities. Household chores were completed sporadically by her children or her parents. When Barbara had enough energy, she would get up and spend an hour or two folding clothes or straightening the house. As a consequence, she would be exhausted for the next 2 or 3 days.

Overall, her low energy level and tendency to tire easily meant that Barbara was unable to sustain even a resemblance of the active lifestyle she previously had when working as a single mother. Moreover, she no longer had access to the occupational forms/tasks that she enjoyed and valued and which gave her a sense of competence. Finally, the highly organized habits that had supported her earlier function had disintegrated to a haphazard and passive daily routine.

The impact of multiple sclerosis on Barbara's occupational identity and competence are illustrated in *Figure 19.3*, which shows the ratings the therapist gave her on the OPHI scales along with comments written by the therapist. At this point, Barbara felt her life was in a shambles. She was unable even to take care of herself. The future loomed ahead as a great blank. Despite the great strength Barbara had shown in the past, when confronted with the life change wrought by multiple sclerosis, she had no idea of where to begin in imagining a future for herself. This is illustrated in Barbara's narrative slope, which is shown in *Figure 19.4*.

Information From Other Assessments

On the Role Checklist (*Fig. 19.5*) Barbara identified family member as her only continuous role for the past, present, and future. At this time, her daughters were 14 and 12 years old. She had been completely out of touch with her husband for 12 years and had depended only on the occasional support of her parents to assist in child rearing. Nonetheless, she did not indicate on the form that she was a caregiver to her children. When her therapist questioned why she did not consider herself in the role of caregiver to her children, she responded, "No, I'm inadequate. I can't handle those responsibilities. My parents are their caregivers."

FIGURE 19.3 Therapist ratings and comments regarding Barbara's strengths and challenges on the OPHI-II.

Occupational Identity Scale	1	2	3	4	Comments
Has personal goals and projects	X				Before MS had ongoing goals and projects, now has none since future is unclear
Identifies a desired occupational lifestyle		X			Desires previous lifestyle, but has no idea of what is possible now
Expects success	X				Feels hopeless about the future
Accepts responsibility			X		Has done her best in the face of disease process, does not know what to do now to be in control of life
Appraises abilities and limitations	X				Has no idea what they will be in future
Has commitments and values				X	Taking care of children, working
Recognizes identity and obligations				X	Strong sense of responsibility as a mother
Has interests			X		Mostly revolves around work and children
Felt effective (past)				X	Felt very effective in managing her substantial responsibilities
Found meaning and satisfaction in lifestyle (past)				X	Managed a challenging but satisfying and meaningful life as a working single mother
Made occupational choices (past)				X	Took control of her life with major choices
Occupational Competence Scale	**1**	**2**	**3**	**4**	
Maintains satisfying lifestyle	X				All areas affected by current limitations
Fulfills role expectations	X				"
Works toward goals	X				"
Meets personal performance standards	X				"
Organizes time for responsibilities	X				"
Participates in interests			X		"
Fulfilled roles (past)				X	Worker and single mother roles
Maintained habits (past)				X	Well-organized life despite multiple demands
Achieved satisfaction (past)				X	Satisfied with meeting challenges of her life

Key : **4** = Exceptionally competent occupational functioning; **3** = Appropriate, satisfactory occupational functioning; **2** = Some occupational functioning problems; **1** = Extreme occupational functioning problems

Barbara identified the following roles as disrupted: worker, caregiver, home maintainer, and friend. She had lost her friends, who became uncomfortable as her disease progressed. Barbara very much missed social contact with others outside her family.

Barbara rated the roles of caregiver, home maintainer, and family member as very valuable. When the therapist pointed this out, Barbara agreed that if she could choose her future, these would be the roles she wanted to fulfill. Discussing the Role Checklist, the therapist pointed out that Barbara's biggest concern

was being a burden to her children. They were just coming to an age when they needed more independence. Her concern about being a burden was even more acute, since she very much wanted for her daughters to have a better start in life than she had.

Together, the OPHI-II and the Role Checklist gave a detailed picture of how Barbara's life had been transformed by the steady progress of her multiple sclerosis. A previously self-reliant and determined woman, she had been transformed into someone who felt victimized and helpless. This transformation was also re-

FIGURE 19.4 Barbara's narrative slope.

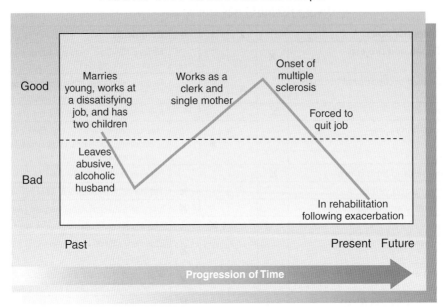

flected in her change from a life filled with valued roles to one filled with losses.

Barbara identified 8 strong interests on the 80-item Modified Interest Checklist (*Fig. 19.6*). These interests mostly centered on family life, socialization, and sports. Despite Barbara's regular involvement in these interests in the past, she had recently participated in only one interest, watching television. She agreed with her occupational therapist's advice that she needed to identify, develop, and pursue new interests. As suggested in her Interest Checklist responses, Barbara had seen a significant decline in the quality of her everyday occupational participation.

Barbara's Functional Decrements

Multiple sclerosis imposed functional limitations that severely affected Barbara's occupational performance. At admission, Barbara could not completely dress herself or bathe; she reported that she had not been in a shower for well over a year and instead took sponge baths. She was unable to transfer from her wheelchair without assistance and could only propel it about 200

feet on a level surface, requiring two or three rest stops to catch her breath.

Since Barbara's major life role at the time was homemaker, the occupational therapist continued an ongoing informal evaluation of Barbara's homemaking performance. Barbara reported that for the past 5 months she had managed to make only two or three meals for her family and had relied on her children or parents to do most homemaking tasks. She confessed that she was unsure how to approach these tasks from a wheelchair. During an informal observation of her performance in the kitchen, Barbara was unable to maneuver her wheelchair effectively to transport items from the cabinets, stove, or refrigerator. It took her about 15 minutes to transport a single item from the refrigerator to a counter across the room.

Course of Therapy

Barbara came to occupational therapy twice a day. She came in a wheelchair or on a stretcher if she was too fatigued to sit. Her occupational therapist concluded that the overall focus of her therapy would be to help

FIGURE 19.5 Barbara's responses on the Role Checklist.

Role	Role Identity			Value Designation		
	Past	Present	Future	Not at all Valuable	Somewhat Valuable	Very Valuable
Student	X					
Worker	X		X			
Volunteer				X		
Caregiver	X		X			X
Home Maintainer	X		X			X
Friend	X		X		X	
Family Member	X	X	X			X
Religious Participant				X		
Hobbyist/Amateur				X		
Participant in Organizations					X	
Other						

her find a way out of her story of victimization and helplessness and to reinstate life roles. She realized that this would mean enabling Barbara to maximize her performance and participation despite her motor impairments. This would require adjustments in her environment.

Barbara's occupational therapy was developed to coordinate with physical therapy and nursing care. It was modified weekly according to Barbara's endurance level and strength. Her various therapies and self-care activities were scheduled hourly, with half-hour rest periods between them. Barbara was unable to envision what was possible for herself or how her therapy should unfold. Consequently, the therapist collaborated with her by giving her routine feedback on her progress and its implications, advising her about new goals and approaches, and then negotiating with Barbara to modify or refine them in ways that increasingly gave Barbara control over the course of her own therapy.

The occupational therapist began by advising Barbara about multiple sclerosis: the symptoms, possible precursors to exacerbations, and how she would need to have a flexible habit pattern in the future to accommodate fluctuations in her motor skills. In relating this information to Barbara, her therapist also began to portray ways in which she could retake control over her life and reinstate important parts of her former life. She began to encourage Barbara to reframe her occupational narrative by considering future scenarios. Throughout the hospitalization, Barbara's children and parents were also informed about multiple sclerosis and encouraged to support Barbara to envision her life in a more positive way.

Before Barbara relearned any self-care or homemaking skills, the therapist coached her in how to integrate work simplification principles into what she did. Once she had the basic information, Barbara practiced work simplification in the hospital routine and occupational therapy sessions. Barbara also explored objects that would compensate for her limited motor skills (e.g., a reacher, a dressing stick, and a long-handled bath sponge).

During self-care and homemaking tasks, Barbara practiced planning her actions ahead of time so that she could complete an occupational form/task with efficiency and minimal energy expenditure. With her therapist's advice, Barbara also identified when it was acceptable to ask for help from her children or parents to complete tasks. Before each weekend at home, Barbara developed a schedule with the advice of the occupational therapist. In doing this, Barbara learned

FIGURE 19.6 Barbara's responses to items on the Modified Interest Checklist in which she showed a past or present interest.

Activity	What has been your level of interest?						Do you currently participate in this activity?		Would you like to pursue this in the future?	
	In the past ten years			In the past year						
	Strong	Some	No	Strong	Some	No	Yes	No	Yes	No
Listening to popular music	X			X			X		X	
Holiday activities	X			X				X	X	
Swimming	X					X		X	X	
Bowling	X				X			X	X	
Visiting	X			X			X		X	
Cycling	X					X		X	X	
Child care	X				X			X	X	
Cooking/baking	X				X			X	X	

the value of both planning and of being flexible with her time according to her strength and endurance.

The occupational therapist worked to help Barbara gradually identify a future for herself. Together they explored what roles and activities were most important to her, using these as a basis to set goals. Barbara decided to set daily, weekly, and monthly goals and to identify which of these were of highest priority for her. In selecting occupational forms/tasks to use in the course of therapy, her therapist had two interrelated goals:

- Giving Barbara an opportunity to explore things that might become new interests
- Improving her strength, coordination, and endurance

Barbara chose to learn macramé. She learned the basic knots while sitting at a table and then was able to macramé with her arms up in the air, with the macramé secured to an overhead stationary object. As her strength and endurance improved, time spent doing macramé was increased and the wheelchair seat belt and armrests were removed. Later, she sat on the edge of a plinth while doing macramé to increase her stability.

As Barbara's motor skills improved, her occupational therapist began to advise her on ways that her environment could be modified to accommodate her limitations. Her therapist helped her to choose bathroom

equipment that would enable her to be independent in self-care. The therapist fitted Barbara for an appropriate wheelchair and cushion, and she coached Barbara while she practiced wheelchair control and maintenance.

In preparation for her return home, Barbara also planned environmental adjustments to her house to improve accessibility. Finally, she began to participate in community excursions, during which she was able to put together all she had learned about energy conservation, work simplification, and use of adapted equipment. For example, she shopped in a local grocery store using a wheelchair grocery cart. In the final stage of her therapy, Barbara identified that she wanted to be independent in getting around in her community and needed to be able to drive a car. She received driving instruction and learned to drive with hand controls.

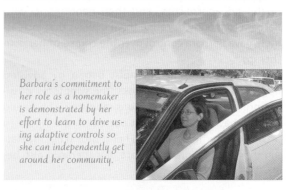

Barbara's commitment to her role as a homemaker is demonstrated by her effort to learn to drive using adaptive controls so she can independently get around her community.

Barbara had to face the fact that the occupational narrative she had crafted and would have preferred to continue living was not going to be possible. The therapist validated Barbara's pain in coming to grips with this. At the same time, the therapist advised and encouraged Barbara to envision a new life story, which included probable further decrements in capacity and periods of exacerbation. Barbara commented that she had successfully faced adversity before when she became a single mother and that by doing it again she would continue to enact for her daughters a powerful example. Over time, Barbara was able to reframe her experiences in this way and increasingly saw herself as a heroine struggling against a mighty adversary. The transformation from victim to heroine in her occupational narrative enabled Barbara to go on with her life.

Preparing for the Return Home

Approximately 2 weeks before her discharge, Barbara's occupational therapist accompanied her on a home visit. Barbara's parents met Barbara and the therapist to participate in the review of possible home modifications. Barbara lived in a one-floor ranch house. Neither of the two entrances to the home was wheelchair accessible, but a ramp and sidewalk could be constructed at the front entrance. The house was small and crowded with furniture. By rearranging the furniture all the rooms were made wheelchair accessible except the utility room and the bathroom. Since neither of these rooms could be modified for improved accessibility, Barbara and the occupational therapist identified and practiced a system of transfers onto a chair and the commode. They were able to determine that the transfers were feasible so that Barbara could use the bathroom independently.

Barbara's father and mother were impressed with the improvement in Barbara's ability to transfer and her mobility throughout the house. They made suggestions for further possible home modifications. Both of Barbara's parents were extremely supportive. Her father planned to make the necessary home modifications with the help of Barbara's two brothers who lived nearby. Both of Barbara's daughters were accepting of their mother's illness and did extra household chores with few complaints. Her family admitted that in the past their willingness to help Barbara might at times

have made her overly dependent and agreed to cooperate with her in the future to maintain the level of independence that she wanted to have in her life.

Constructing an Acceptable Life

As therapy proceeded, Barbara continued to recognize and accept her reduced capacities and other consequences of her disease. Importantly, she had begun to develop an image of how she could have a satisfying life that operationalized her value of independence. In part, this meant that she had a new definition of independence which allowed her to rely to some extent on her family while being on her own in every way that she reasonably could. Her occupational narrative and long-term goals were organized around being an independent homemaker and a caregiver to her children. She solidified the image of herself as an example of how to rise above adversity. She was able to enact this new narrative and to achieve her homemaker and mother roles, albeit in altered ways.

At discharge, Barbara was independent in self-care, homemaking, and wheelchair management. She could propel her wheelchair up and down ramps, on flat level surfaces, and over rough terrain. She was able to maneuver the chair around objects and through small hallways. She had completed adapted driving training, was able to drive using hand controls, and was able to put her own wheelchair in and out of her car. She identified this accomplishment as her "ticket to freedom." After discharge, Barbara was referred to a vocational counselor at the department of rehabilitation services. Her goal of independent homemaking was recognized as a vocation. Therefore, the department financed the recommended home modifications and the hand controls for the car.

Barbara no longer required her parents' assistance on weekends, and she managed the cooking and cleaning and self-care independently, with minimal help from her children. She began socializing again with some of her old friends and neighbors and joined a bimonthly bridge club. Barbara continued her newfound interest in macramé and gave away many of her projects as gifts.

Barbara in Perspective

Barbara recrafted her occupational narrative by identifying an acceptable lifestyle for herself and reinstating her most important roles. This required her to reframe what had happened to her. It also required that she redefine her roles and find new ways to enact values. In the end, her struggle with multiple sclerosis became another episode in which her fierce determination allowed her to prevail and create the kind of life she wanted.

The therapist enabled Barbara to envision a future life and to work toward achieving it. Improving motor skills, making environmental modifications, and learning energy conservation all became ways for Barbara to achieve occupational competence. However, without a narrative to enact, these practical approaches would have lacked the cogency they had for Barbara. As noted in Chapter 9, occupational identity is a prerequisite for occupational competence.

Alvaro: Realizing Values and Interests

Alvaro was a 33-year-old Chilean man when he began occupational therapy. He was the youngest of three children and lived with his mother, a homemaker, and his father, a pilot. As a child and adolescent, Alvaro was an outstanding student who showed musical talent from a young age. He was gregarious and had many friends.

When Alvaro was 18 years old, he had a first psychotic episode and was diagnosed with schizophrenia. He became paranoid and withdrawn. He experienced unpleasant side effects from prescribed medication and consequently resisted taking it. His family did not understand Alvaro's illness, and his relationship with his father, who could not comprehend or accept his illness, became particularly strained. Alvaro's mother was very supportive and stood by him through four suicide attempts.

For 15 years Alvaro's psychosis continued unabated. He developed obsessive and delusional ideas that he interpreted as blasphemous. These symptoms where particularly unsettling to him because he had deep religious values. At this time he "preferred death to having such thoughts and feelings." He felt overwhelming desperation, anxiety, and guilt.

When clozapine became available in Chile, Alvaro began to take it, and for the first time his symptoms abated. Around this time Alvaro met an occupational therapist at a conference about the importance of active participation in treatment and rehabilitation of people with mental illness and their families. Following the conference, Alvaro and a number of other young persons with mental illness asked the therapist to assist them in organizing a self-help group. Subsequently, the group began to meet regularly with the guidance of the occupational therapist, who also provided services to the clients. Alvaro was an active member who took on the role of encouraging other members. Nonetheless, he still had difficulty concentrating and focusing himself.

Initial Assessment

Because Alvaro was not actively psychotic, had a long history of illness, and had been referred to a long-term community setting, his occupational therapist chose to begin his assessment with the OPHI-II. *Figure 19.7* shows his ratings on the OPHI scales.

SUMMARY OF THE RESULTS OF THE OPHI-II

After the onset of Alvaro's mental illness, he attempted studies at University of Chile, School of Music. He began his studies over four times. Each time the demands of study, examinations, and relating to professors and classmates led to an exacerbation of his psychosis and subsequent dropping out of the program. During this time and when he was able, Alvaro also sang in the Chamber Chorus of Chile and volunteered in a nursing home, where he performed religious songs. Through all this period Alvaro had a variety of psychotic symptoms, including paranoid delusions (e.g., that he was being followed). Despite his symptoms, Alvaro's faith, values, and intense passion for music carried him forward.

Occupational Identity

Alvaro's sense of efficacy was eroded by his repeated failures. Thus Alvaro's volition was characterized by a gap between his strong values ("living life and using talents God gave me") and interests (a passion for music) and his personal causation, which was dominated by negative expectations for the future. He was particularly fearful that his schizophrenic symptoms would come back and ruin anything he attempted.

Alvaro showed a high sense of obligation in what he perceived as his ongoing role responsibilities. These

FIGURE 19.7 Alvaro's strengths and challenges on the OPHI-II occupational identity, competence, and settings (environmental) scales.

Occupational Identity Scale	1	2	3	4
Has personal goals and projects				✗
Identifies a desired occupational lifestyle			✗	
Expects success	✗			
Accepts responsibility				✗
Appraises abilities and limitations		✗		
Has commitments and values				✗
Recognizes identity and obligations				✗
Has interests				✗
Felt effective (past)		✗		
Found meaning and satisfaction in lifestyle (past)			✗	
Made occupational choices (past)				✗
Occupational Competence Scale	**1**	**2**	**3**	**4**
Maintains satisfying lifestyle		✗		
Fulfills role expectations			✗	
Works toward goals				✗
Meets personal performance standards	✗			
Organizes time for responsibilities		✗		
Participates in interests		✗		
Fulfilled roles (past)		✗		
Maintained habits (past)		✗		
Achieved satisfaction (past)		✗		
Occupational Settings (Environment) Scale	**1**	**2**	**3**	**4**
Home life occupational forms			✗	
Major productive role occupational forms			✗	
Leisure occupational forms			✗	
Home life social group			✗	
Major productive role social group			✗	
Leisure social group			✗	
Home life spaces, objects, and resources				✗
Major productive role spaces, objects, and resources			✗	
Leisure spaces, objects, and resources				✗

Key: **1** = Extreme occupational functioning problems
 2 = Some occupational functioning problems
 3 = Appropriate satisfactory occupational functioning
 4 = Exceptionally competent occupational functioning

included taking care of his mother as a good son and being an uncle to his nephews, volunteering, and being responsible for his own treatment and recovery. He was too fearful of the future to have goals or a vision of life that he really thought he could live. During the interview, Alvaro stated that he still wanted to return to his studies at the University of Chile. However, he was extremely fearful that he would only fail again. His years of living with schizophrenia had led him to a compromised sense of his life story—one in which he simply struggled to enact his values as best he could.

Occupational Competence

He often felt that he could not meet these role obligations as he should. Moreover, his father continued to devalue him, and Alvaro felt that he would never live up to his father's expectations for a son. While maintaining a routine of self-care and family and volunteer involvement, these occupations did not afford him a satisfactory quality of life, since they didn't fit with his occupational identity. Overall, Alvaro was not living the life he would have liked were it not for his impairment. Instead he was doing the best he could to live the best kind of life he could.

Occupational Settings (Environment)

Alvaro's social environment consisted mainly of his mother, the singers of Chamber Chorus of Chile, and the group of old people he helped in his volunteer role. He identified them as being very supportive and giving. The major negative aspect of his social environment was his father's devaluing attitude toward him. The tasks he performed in each of these environments provided a level of satisfaction, but they did not meet Alvaro's hopes for what he wanted to do. He was also aware that his strained relationship with his father made his mother very sad. Alvaro did have financial resources from his family that allowed him to have the things he needed and valued. He owned a classical guitar and had money to attend concerts.

Occupational Narrative

Alvaro's occupational narrative is dominated by a constant quest for realizing his values. His narrative slope (*Fig. 19.8*) illustrates a downward trend followed by a period of struggles in which he fights against his symptoms, repeatedly fails at school, and yet maintains a level of participation. Given the significant impact of his impairment on his life course and all the failures Alvaro has accumulated since adolescence, his narrative is also dominated by a sense of fear about what the future will bring, even as he struggles on.

Additional Evaluation

Because informal observation indicated that Alvaro was having difficulty with motor, process, and communication interaction skills, the occupational therapist decided to observe Alvaro using the Assessment of Motor and Process Skills (AMPS) and the Assessment of Communication and Interaction Skills (ACIS). She also decided to use the Volitional Questionnaire (VQ) to gather more details about his volition.

INFORMATION GATHERED FROM THE AMPS

The occupational therapist chose to modify the administration of the AMPS. This allowed her to observe Alvaro outside the standard AMPS task doing things he was highly motivated to do. She chose to approach the assessment in this way because she had noted that his performance was highly variable depending on his level of motivation for the task. In addition to observing him making a sandwich (a standard AMPS task) she also observed him serving tea for his mother and during a music rehearsal involving his peers.

During these observations, Alvaro was competent in seeking and using knowledge and organizing time. He had difficulty attending to the task at hand and could not effectively pace himself. He was generally competent at arranging his environment to support tasks, but he was ineffective at adapting and often failed to notice circumstances in the environment that required him to modify his actions. He also had difficulty with motor skills (i.e., regulating the speed and force of actions so that he bumped furniture, accidentally banged his guitar, and dropped dishes). He did not appear to learn from his mistakes during the task.

INFORMATION GATHERED FROM THE ACIS

Figure 19.9 shows the results of Alvaro's ACIS observations. He was observed with his mother and father during a group activity and at a mental health conference. He was a charming person, very expressive and sensitive

FIGURE 19.8 Alvaro's narrative slope.

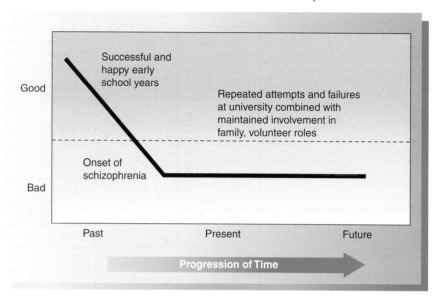

to others. He collaborated and related well. He demonstrated competence in the domains of physicality and relations. Alvaro's main problems were in the area of information exchange. He had difficulty being assertive, articulating, modulating, and speaking. Alvaro had problems voicing his opinions because he feared rejection and worried about offending others. He often had to repeat himself and still ended up confusing others. He vacillated between being too loud or almost silent when talking. His problems with articulating (due to side effects of medications) meant that others often had to ask him to repeat what he said. Despite his areas of difficulty, he got on well with others because of his strengths.

The one exception to these observations was when Alvaro interacted with his father. In this circumstance, his communication and interaction skills deteriorated, and he became totally passive. Alvaro was unable to finish a conversation with his father and retreated to his bedroom. The occupational therapist administered the ACIS to Alvaro twice more to track changes in his communication and interaction skills (*Figs. 19.10* and *19.11*).

INFORMATION GATHERED FROM THE VOLITIONAL QUESTIONNAIRE

The occupational therapist observed Alvaro using the VQ while he was volunteering at a mental health confer-

ence, during a group activity, and doing activities with his mother and father. *Figure 19.12* shows his VQ ratings.

When participating in known and supportive environments, Alvaro demonstrated spontaneous volition, except for items most clearly related to personal causation (i.e., showing pride, trying to solve problems, and trying to correct his own mistakes). He received higher scores in some items that ordinarily reflect high volition (e.g., staying involved and seeking additional responsibility) because the activities were so closely tied to his values. In this instance he persisted despite worries about being ineffective. In contrast to other situations, his volition was very low when doing social activities with his father. The VQ observation confirmed the therapist's suspicions that Alvaro's motivation was largely bolstered by his strong values despite his strong sense of inefficacy. The occupational therapist administered the VQ twice more to track changes in his volition across contexts (*Figs. 19.13* and *19.14*). As the repeated administrations of the VQ reveal, after intervention, Alvaro's volition still decreased when faced with situations that were unstructured and ambiguous, such as interacting with his father and waiting for a response from his school. However, in his major roles, such as student and worker, he began to demonstrate his volition spontaneously.

FIGURE 19.9 Alvaro's ratings from the first administration of the ACIS in four observational settings. Summary of all observations in each situation.

	With his father				With his mother				With the group				At a conference			
Physicality	1	2	3	4	1	2	3	4	1	2	3	4	1	2	3	4
1. Contacts				X				X			X					X
2. Gazes				X				X			X					X
3. Gestures				X				X			X					X
4. Maneuvers				X				X			X					X
5. Orients				X				X			X					X
6. Positions				X				X			X					X
Information exchange	1	2	3	4	1	2	3	4	1	2	3	4	1	2	3	4
7. Articulates		X				X					X			X		
8. Asserts	X				X					X						X
9. Asks	X							X			X					X
10. Engages	X							X			X					X
11. Expresses	X							X			X					X
12. Modulates		X				X				X				X		
13. Shares			X					X				X	N/A			
14. Speaks		X				X				X					X	
15. Sustains	X							X			X				X	
Relations	1	2	3	4	1	2	3	4	1	2	3	4	1	2	3	4
16. Collaborates				X				X			X					X
17. Conforms				X				X			X					X
18. Focuses				X				X			X					X
19. Relates				X				X			X					X
20. Respects				X				X			X					X

Key: **1** = Deficit   **2** = Ineffective   **3** = Questionable   **4** = Competent

The Therapist's Conceptualization of Alvaro's Situation and Identification of Treatment Goals

The occupational therapist concluded that despite Alvaro's significant impairment, he had managed a level of occupational participation because of his volitional strength, in particular his values. As a consequence he had been able to participate in his meaningful roles, such as group member and coordinator, volunteer, family member, and amateur musician. Alvaro's problems and challenges included his weak personal causation and difficulties with process and communication/interaction skills. When the therapist shared this conceptualization with Alvaro and identified what she considered were his strengths and weaknesses, Alvaro agreed. Together they negotiated the following goals for Alvaro:

- Achieving a career as a musician at University of Chile
- Gaining the respect of his father
- Continuing with his volunteer role
- Contributing to the development of a self-help center.

FIGURE 19.10 Alvaro's ratings from the second administration of the ACIS in four observational settings. Summary of all observations in each situation.

	With father				Forming center				Musical group				Applying to school			
Physicality	1	2	3	4	1	2	3	4	1	2	3	4	1	2	3	4
1. Contacts				X				X				X				X
2. Gazes				X				X				X				X
3. Gestures				X				X				X			X	
4. Maneuvers				X				X				X				X
5. Orients				X				X				X				X
6. Positions				X				X				X				X
Information exchange	1	2	3	4	1	2	3	4	1	2	3	4	1	2	3	4
7. Articulates		X					X			X					X	
8. Asserts	X					X				X						X
9. Asks	X							X				X				X
10. Engages	X							X				X				X
11. Expresses	X							X				X				X
12. Modulates		X				X				X					X	
13. Shares				X				X				X				X
14. Speaks		X					X				X				X	
15. Sustains	X							X			X				X	
Relations	1	2	3	4	1	2	3	4	1	2	3	4	1	2	3	4
16. Collaborates				X				X				X				X
17. Conforms				X				X				X				X
18. Focuses				X				X				X				X
19. Relates				X				X				X				X
20. Respects				X				X				X				X

Key: **1** = Deficit **2** = Ineffective **3** = Questionable **4** = Competent

Working with Alvaro

Alvaro agreed with the therapist that he needed to develop his sense of efficacy to achieve his goals. His course of therapy followed the remotivation process (de las Heras, Llerena, & Kielhofner, 2003). This meant that Alvaro needed to begin with goals that were close to his volitional and skill levels, in familiar environments, and doing tasks in which he felt satisfaction and efficacy. Additionally, it was important that his occupational therapist validate his fears and encourage him, demonstrating her belief that he could succeed. Alvaro was very motivated by the idea of helping to develop the community-based self-help center, Reencuentros. The occupational therapist was working with a small group of people, including Alvaro, to develop this center; she asked each member to take on different roles according to their unique skills. Alvaro, who knew musicians and locations where music was performed, agreed to work on developing a strategy for doing concerts and other musical events to raise money. He even began to play his classical guitar during these events in front of many people. At the time he did these activities, Alvaro was anxious but always satisfied with what he could accomplish. He told the therapist,

FIGURE 19.11 Alvaro's ratings from the third administration of the ACIS in four observational settings. Summary of all observations in each situation.

	With father				Educational program				With professors				At work			
Physicality	1	2	3	4	1	2	3	4	1	2	3	4	1	2	3	4
1. Contacts				X				X				X				X
2. Gazes				X				X				X				X
3. Gestures				X				X				X			X	
4. Maneuvers				X				X				X				X
5. Orients				X				X				X				X
6. Positions				X				X				X				X
Information exchange	1	2	3	4	1	2	3	4	1	2	3	4	1	2	3	4
7. Articulates			X				X				X				X	
8. Asserts	X						X				X					X
9. Asks	X							X				X				X
10. Engages	X							X				X				X
11. Expresses	X							X				X				X
12. Modulates			X			X					X				X	
13. Shares				X				X				X				X
14. Speaks		X					X				X				X	
15. Sustains		X						X				X				X
Relations	1	2	3	4	1	2	3	4	1	2	3	4	1	2	3	4
16. Collaborates				X				X				X				X
17. Conforms				X				X				X				X
18. Focuses				X				X				X				X
19. Relates				X				X				X				X
20. Respects				X				X				X				X

Key: **1** = Deficit   **2** = Ineffective   **3** = Questionable   **4** = Competent

"I have never done so many things in my entire life." In response, the therapist gave Alvaro feedback that in her opinion Alvaro had done much in the past to continue functioning despite his illness. This helped Alvaro reexamine his narrative of failure.

Over time through participating in real-life occupations that resonated with his values and interests, Alvaro showed an increased sense of efficacy. He was more spontaneous in trying new things and trying to solve problems. He was able to stick with increasingly challenging tasks until they were completed. His therapist coached him and provided him feedback throughout the process to help him make choices to

take on appropriate challenges and to recognize when he succeeded.

The therapist also provided feedback to help Alvaro better understand the challenges he faced in communication/interaction, motor, and process skills. She identified ways he could perform more effectively. At first the therapist had to coach Alvaro consistently and provide him feedback about environmental cues he had missed. Eventually he was able to perform, monitoring himself and the environment. Together they identified that if he wrote down the steps and environmental demands of any new task, Alvaro was able to be more aware and thus monitor himself and the en-

FIGURE 19.12 Alvaro's ratings from the first administration of the Volitional Questionnaire.

Indicators	Conference					Self help group					Activities with mother					Activities with father				
1. Shows curiosity	P	H	I	**S**	N/O	P	H	I	**S**	N/O	P	H	I	**S**	N/O	**P**	H	I	S	N/O
2. Initiates actions/tasks	P	H	I	**S**	N/O	P	H	I	**S**	N/O	P	H	I	**S**	N/O	**P**	H	I	S	N/O
3. Tries new things	P	H	I	**S**	N/O	P	H	**I**	S	N/O	P	H	I	**S**	N/O	**P**	H	I	S	N/O
4. Shows pride	P	**H**	I	S	N/O	P	**H**	I	S	N/O	P	**H**	I	S	N/O	**P**	H	I	S	N/O
5. Seeks challenges	P	H	I	**S**	N/O	P	**H**	I	S	N/O	P	H	I	S	**N/O**	**P**	H	I	S	N/O
6. Seeks additional responsibilities	P	H	I	**S**	N/O	P	H	I	**S**	N/O	P	H	I	**S**	N/O	**P**	H	I	S	N/O
7. Tries to correct mistakes/failures	P	H	**I**	S	N/O	P	H	**I**	S	N/O	P	H	I	S	**N/O**	**P**	H	I	S	N/O
8. Tries to solve problems	P	H	I	S	**N/O**	P	H	**I**	S	N/O	P	H	I	**S**	N/O	**P**	H	I	S	N/O
9. Shows preferences	P	H	I	**S**	N/O	P	H	I	**S**	N/O	P	H	I	**S**	N/O	**P**	H	I	S	N/O
10. Pursues an activity to completion/accomplishment	P	H	I	**S**	N/O	P	H	I	**S**	N/O	P	H	I	**S**	N/O	**P**	H	I	S	N/O
11. Stays engaged	P	H	I	**S**	N/O	P	H	I	**S**	N/O	P	H	I	**S**	N/O	**P**	H	I	S	N/O
12. Invests additional energy/emotion/attention	P	H	I	**S**	N/O	P	H	I	**S**	N/O	P	H	I	**S**	N/O	**P**	H	I	S	N/O
13. Indicates goals	P	H	I	**S**	N/O	P	H	I	**S**	N/O	P	H	I	S	**N/O**	**P**	H	I	S	N/O
14. Shows that an activity is special/significant	P	H	I	**S**	N/O	P	H	I	**S**	N/O	P	H	I	**S**	N/O	P	H	I	**S**	N/O

Key: **P** = Passive   **H** = Hesitant   **I** = Involved   **S** = Spontaneous   **N/O** = No opportunity to observe

vironment during his performance. Over time Alvaro's personal causation increased and he once again felt ready to tackle his goal of once again studying music at the University of Chile. Attending the university meant that he must prepare himself for a very demanding environment in which he would have to do such things as take examinations in front of classmates and professors, learn classical guitar techniques that demand sophisticated motor and process skills, and interact and communicate in a new environment. Alvaro's improvements in communication and interaction skills, particularly in the area of communication exchange, are illustrated in *Figures 19.10* and *19.11*.

Alvaro, conscious of all of these challenges, decided he wanted to continue at Reencuentros part-time while attending university part-time. Together Alvaro and his therapist inquired as to whether the school of music at the university would allow part-time study. This was a very difficult process, since the program was very selective and rigid. Over 2 months, Alvaro went to the school weekly and called daily to remind administrative staff about his request. The thera-

pist encouraged and sometimes accompanied him, especially at the beginning. During this time Alvaro continued helping Reencuentros to raise money and took on the role of coordinator of the music group that performed in pediatric hospitals and nursing homes. This new role demanded higher level performance and personal causation.

Alvaro showed an increasing sense of efficacy in different environments; he needed less support and encouragement from his therapist to face challenges in new and much more demanding environments. He began taking initiative to apply strategies he had learned to improve his skills.

Despite this, the occupational therapist still observed that Alvaro's symptoms interfered with his process skills. She met with and advised Alvaro, his family, and doctor that he was still having some difficulty with psychotic symptoms and suggested consideration of a change in medication. Alvaro and his mother agreed with this, and the physician altered his prescription. The change in medication helped Alvaro to better organize his thoughts and communication.

FIGURE 19.13 Alvaro's ratings from the second administration of the Volitional Questionnaire in more challenging situations.

Indicators	Talking on radio	Participation in fundraising	Playing guitar at events	Learning skills
1. Shows curiosity	P H I **(S)** N/O	P H I **(S)** N/O	P H I **(S)** N/O	P H I **(S)** N/O
2. Initiates actions/tasks	P H **(I)** S N/O	P H I **(S)** N/O	P H **(I)** S N/O	P H **(I)** S N/O
3. Tries new things	P H I **(S)** N/O	P H **(I)** S N/O	P H I **(S)** N/O	P H **(I)** S N/O
4. Shows pride	P H **(I)** S N/O	P H **(I)** S N/O	P H **(I)** S N/O	P **(H)** I S N/O
5. Seeks challenges	P H I **(S)** N/O	P H **(I)** S N/O	P **(H)** I S N/O	P H **(I)** S N/O
6. Seeks additional responsibilities	P H I **(S)** N/O	P H I **(S)** N/O	P H I **(S)** N/O	P **(H)** I S N/O
7. Tries to correct mistakes/failures	P H **(I)** S N/O	P H **(I)** S N/O	P H I **(S)** N/O	P H **(I)** S N/O
8. Tries to solve problems	P H I **(S)** N/O	P H **(I)** S N/O	P H I **(S)** N/O	P H **(I)** S N/O
9. Shows preferences	P H I **(S)** N/O	P H I **(S)** N/O	P H I **(S)** N/O	P H I **(S)** N/O
10. Pursues an activity to completion/accomplishment	P H I **(S)** N/O	P H I **(S)** N/O	P H I **(S)** N/O	P H I **(S)** N/O
11. Stays engaged	P H I **(S)** N/O	P H I **(S)** N/O	P H I **(S)** N/O	P H I **(S)** N/O
12. Invests additional energy/emotion/attention	P H I **(S)** N/O	P H I **(S)** N/O	P H I **(S)** N/O	P H **(I)** S N/O
13. Indicates goals	P H I **(S)** N/O	P H I **(S)** N/O	P H I **(S)** N/O	P H **(I)** S N/O
14. Shows that an activity is special/significant	P H I **(S)** N/O	P H I **(S)** N/O	P H I **(S)** N/O	P H I **(S)** N/O

Key: **P** = Passive   **H** = Hesitant   **I** = Involved   **S** = Spontaneous   **N/O** = No opportunity to observe

With this, Alvaro's sense of efficacy increased, even in demanding social situations such as interacting with his father.

At Reencuentros, Alvaro began to use the services of the Integration Educational Program, which helped members to examine their volition, skills, habits, and environmental options and demands in relation to their desires. As he participated in this program, he continued appealing to the university for part-time admission. He shared the process with his peers, who encouraged him to continue.

Finally, the university gave a positive response. Alvaro celebrated with his parents, who were both happy and a bit frightened at the news. Consequently, at one of the regular meetings with his parents, the therapist shared her assessment of how much Alvaro's volition and skills had improved and the effect of these improvements on his occupational participation. She also explained that Alvaro would continue receiving the support to help him succeed at school.

Alvaro's Occupational Life at School

Alvaro began to attend school on a regular basis, taking three courses each semester. As expected, the courses were difficult for him. However, Alvaro spoke with his professor, who allowed the occupational therapist to observe some classes. The therapist informed the instructor of Alvaro's challenges in learning to play. The instructor agreed to modify his teaching style and to provide individual classes with Alvaro. Together the instructor and Alvaro negotiated the pace and sequence of learning that accommodated his challenges.

This kind of flexibility was totally new to the music program at the university. However, when the director and professors met and got to know Alvaro's strengths and courage, they agreed to the necessary accommodations. Alvaro persisted at his studies and finally graduated 7 years later. During this time he continued to receive support at Reencuentros, where he also volunteered as coordinator of the musical group.

FIGURE 19.14 Alvaro's ratings from the third administration of the Volitional Questionnaire.

Indicators	Negotiating with school					Coordinating musical group					Role of student and worker					Activities with father				
1. Shows curiosity	P	H	I	**S**	N/O	P	H	I	**S**	N/O	P	H	I	**S**	N/O	**P**	H	I	S	N/O
2. Initiates actions/tasks	P	**H**	I	S	N/O	P	H	I	**S**	N/O	P	H	I	**S**	N/O	P	**H**	I	S	N/O
3. Tries new things	P	H	I	S	**N/O**	P	H	I	**S**	N/O	P	H	I	**S**	N/O	**P**	H	I	S	N/O
4. Shows pride	P	H	**I**	S	N/O	P	H	I	**S**	N/O	P	H	**I**	S	N/O	**P**	H	I	S	N/O
5. Seeks challenges	P	**H**	I	S	N/O	P	H	I	**S**	N/O	P	H	I	S	**N/O**	**P**	H	I	S	N/O
6. Seeks additional responsibilities	P	H	**I**	S	N/O	P	H	I	**S**	N/O	P	H	I	**S**	N/O	**P**	H	I	S	N/O
7. Tries to correct mistakes/failures	P	H	**I**	S	N/O	P	H	I	**S**	N/O	P	H	I	**S**	N/O	**P**	H	I	S	N/O
8. Tries to solve problems	P	H	**I**	S	N/O	P	H	I	**S**	N/O	P	H	I	**S**	N/O	**P**	H	I	S	N/O
9. Shows preferences	P	H	I	**S**	N/O	P	H	I	**S**	N/O	P	H	I	**S**	N/O	**P**	H	I	S	N/O
10. Pursues an activity to completion/accomplishment	P	H	I	**S**	N/O	P	H	I	**S**	N/O	P	H	I	**S**	N/O	P	H	**I**	S	N/O
11. Stays engaged	P	H	I	**S**	N/O	P	H	I	**S**	N/O	P	H	I	**S**	N/O	P	**H**	I	S	N/O
12. Invests additional energy/emotion/attention	P	H	I	**S**	N/O	P	H	**I**	S	N/O	P	H	I	**S**	N/O	**P**	H	I	S	N/O
13. Indicates goals	P	H	I	**S**	N/O	P	H	I	**S**	N/O	P	H	I	**S**	N/O	P	H	I	**S**	N/O
14. Shows that an activity is special/significant	P	H	I	**S**	N/O	P	H	I	**S**	N/O	P	H	I	**S**	N/O	P	H	I	**S**	N/O

Key: **P** = Passive **H** = Hesitant **I** = Involved **S** = Spontaneous **N/O** = No opportunity to observe

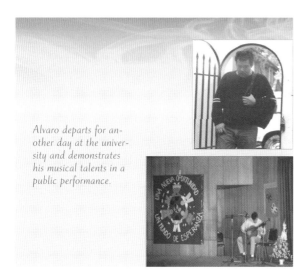

Alvaro departs for another day at the university and demonstrates his musical talents in a public performance.

His psychiatrist, people he met at Reencuentros, his therapist, and his mother went to Alvaro's final examination, which consisted of giving a concert to a large audience at the University of Chile. He made a great effort, playing four long pieces. While playing the last piece, the one he knew best, he began to make mistakes on pacing because of fatigue and anxiety. However, he continued playing the piece until it was done and received a warm and enthusiastic round of applause.

Alvaro's father died 2 years before he finished school. While his father did not see his final achievement, Alvaro felt he would know anyway. Alvaro took his father's death with pain but also with strength. His memories of his father were realistic, emphasizing the best of him as a person.

Integrating Work and Education

Following graduation, Alvaro committed himself to finding a job. He was confident despite the lack of opportunities in Santiago. He applied for a job as music director of a youth center at Santiago. The occupational therapist helped Alvaro to prepare a résumé and practice for the job interview. She helped him arrange for references and supported him by phone the day of the interview.

Alvaro got the job and began working part time. He was responsible for arranging the sound for all musical plays and concerts given at the center. One night when working there, he did not notice a piece of furniture and fell, breaking his right leg. Although he had to be out of work for the month, the center waited for him to return. The staff and youth all valued Alvaro's personality and social attitudes. When the center closed because of financial problems, Alvaro went on to work as coordinator of music at different centers over the years.

Alvaro in Perspective

Alvaro is now 45 years old. Since beginning helping to found Reencuentros more than 12 years ago, he has remained involved. Any time he was needed for an event to raise money or to put on a concert, Alvaro was happy to volunteer. Recently his former therapist and director of Reencuentros told Alvaro that the center would have to close because it had insufficient funding. As one of Reencuentros' founders, Alvaro tried desperately to find some means to prevent the closure. Finally Alvaro helped with the closing of the center. He prepared for and ran the closing ceremony. It was a bittersweet ending for Alvaro, who had gained and given

so much. Nonetheless, the story had come full circle and Alvaro was able to go on with confidence to do the things he valued, despite the acknowledged uncertainty of the future.

Conclusion

Each of the cases in this chapter illustrated the human potential that exists even in the face of extreme adversity and personal failure. Life stories can be retold and rebuilt. However, the extent of the devastation of life faced by each of the clients in this chapter required substantial and long-term efforts on the part of their occupational therapists.

Reference

de las Heras, C. G., Llerena, V., & Kielhofner, G. (2003). *Remotivation process: Progressive intervention for individuals with severe volitional challenges (Version 1.0).* Chicago: Model of Human Occupation Clearinghouse, Department of Occupational Therapy, College of Applied Health Sciences, University of Illinois.

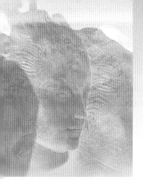

20

Applying MOHO to Clients Who Are Cognitively Impaired

- Gary Kielhofner
- Susan Andersen
- Dalleen Last
- Deborah Roitman
- Jutta Brettschneider
- Luc Vercruysse
- Noga Ziv

Clients who have cognitive impairments are not always recognized and treated as individuals with desires and preferences who need something meaningful to do. Since persons with cognitive limitations can lack the personal resources to advocate for their own perspectives and desires, therapists must advocate on their behalf and seek to empower them. This means putting in the time and effort to learn about their volition, habituation, performance capacity, and environmental context.

As the cases in this chapter will illustrate, there are a number of formal and informal ways of gathering information on such clients that can help reveal their identities, desires, fears, and so on. These cases will also illustrate how gathering this information can lead to an understanding of clients that informs effective intervention.

Jacob: Rediscovering Volition

Jacob is 85 years old. He was born in Rumania in 1920 and went to Israel with his wife and two children in 1958. He had a little textile shop in Rumania and contin-

ued to work in textiles and fashion in Israel. In his free time he loved to dance (including the Hungarian czardas, for which he won a prize), listen to music, take care of the family garden, spend time with his family and friends, go on trips, and according to Jacob's daughter, enjoy good food and "everything that was beautiful."

His son was killed in the Yom Kippur war (1973). Shortly after that Jacob had a stroke, which left him with hemiplegia on the right side (including lack of sensory perception). Since the stroke, he has also been aphasic. He was subsequently diagnosed with dementia. Jacob lived at home until his wife, who was his caretaker, died in 2002. Since then Jacob has lived in the total care ward of a nursing home. His daughter visits him daily, and he has a private caregiver for 2 hours every day.

Jacob has severe dementia and has also developed osteoporosis (leading to repeated spontaneous fractures and associated pain). He is almost completely blind and deaf (i.e., with minimal residual hearing in his right ear). These conditions, combined with his hemiplegia and aphasia, mean that Jacob functions at a very low level. When the occupational therapist first saw Jacob, he had no functional language or gestures. He was almost completely unresponsive and managed only passive compliance with nursing staff to complete his activities of daily living, including feeding.

Volition and the Choice of Treatment Environments

MOHO stresses that volition is particularly important in lower-functioning clients, who cannot advocate for their own wishes and desires. Since Jacob was so passive and unresponsive, the therapist decided it would be useful to explore the possibility of using a special intervention context, *Snoezelen* (Chung, Lai, Chung, & French, 2002; van Diepen et al., 2002). *Snoezelen* refers to a controlled multisensory environment, defined by Shapiro and Bacher (2002) as a room in which the nature, quantity, arrangement, and intensity of stimulation are controlled by the therapist.

Treatment in this kind of environment is referred to as "controlled multisensory intervention." The therapist who works in the room is a *responsive therapist*, specially trained in the art of working with individuals who have severe difficulties in communication. The *Snoezelen* therapist projects empathy, exhibits skilled observation, and does not dominate the treatment process. Rather the therapist is an active partner in the process, demonstrating patience and an underlying commitment to understand the client's behavior (Shapiro & Bacher 2002).

The concept of volition is particularly useful in understanding why the *Snoezelen* intervention is often so useful with clients like Jacob. When sensory, motor, and cognitive deficits limit a person's sensory access to and control over the environment, volition can diminish. A client loses the sense of capacity and efficacy. Even when a client's dementia means that he or she cannot process thoughts about personal competence and control as before, individuals are still capable of feelings of helplessness. Moreover, the sense of satisfaction and pleasure associated with enacting values and interests wither, as the individual is not able make choices for action based on his or her inner volitional propensities. In a sense, then, volition shuts down and the individual is cut off from making choices about engaging the external world.

In many instances the environment becomes a subtle conspirator in this process. Caretaking environments such as nursing homes are staffed with individuals who must complete daily routines (e.g., feeding, cleaning, and toileting) with clients who have limited capacity for these activities of daily living. Staff tend to do these things on behalf of clients, since this is the most efficient strategy and avoids mistakes or problems that emanate from limited capacity (Kielhofner, 2005).

Baseline Assessment

To get a baseline of Jacob's volition, his therapist chose to administer the Volitional Questionnaire (VQ) while observing Jacob in an environment in which he spent substantial time, the dining room of the unit, which also doubles as an activity room. The room was brightly lit and noisy. The objects were familiar (food, drinks, eating utensils, tray tables, and objects used for various simple activities). The room was populated with Jacob's peer residents and caregivers, most of whom are familiar to Jacob. Because Jacob is so impaired, staff have found it easier to feed him than to try to assist Jacob to feed himself. During activities he sits passively by. As illustrated in *Figure 20.1*, Jacob's volitional behavior is either passive or hesitant in this context. Informal observation in other parts of the unit confirmed that Jacob was similarly passive throughout the day.

In collaboration with Jacob's daughter the occupational therapist set the goal of providing Jacob with one environmental context in which he could express volitional behavior (i.e., exercise some control and feel a sense of pleasure and meaning within the limits of his cognitive and other impairments).

The Intervention Context and Process

The *Snoezelen* room is an indoor room. Both light and sound can be controlled by the therapist. Objects in the room are designed to provide simple, soothing sensory stimulation. Intervention is done one-on-one. Jacob was introduced to the room, and his therapist was guided by his responses. The aim of the intervention was to discover and facilitate Jacob's volition. The following is a description of a typical intervention session after Jacob became familiar with the room.

Therapy in the Snoezelen Room

Jacob enters the *Snoezelen* room together with his assistant, who pushes the reclining wheelchair. His left hand holds the right hemiplegic arm tightly to his

FIGURE 20.1 Jacob's ratings on the Volitional Questionnaire in the dining room.

Environmental Context: Dining Room				
1. Shows curiosity	P	**H**	I	S
2. Initiates actions/tasks	**P**	H	I	S
3. Tries new things	**P**	H	I	S
4. Shows pride	**P**	H	I	S
5. Seeks challenges	P	**H**	I	S
6. Seeks additional responsibilities	**P**	H	I	S
7. Tries to correct mistakes	**P**	H	I	S
8. Tries to solve problems	**P**	H	I	S
9. Shows preferences	P	**H**	I	S
10. Pursues activity to completion/accomplishment	**P**	H	I	S
11. Stays engaged	P	**H**	I	S
12. Invests additional energy/emotion/attention	**P**	H	I	S
13. Indicates goals	**P**	H	I	S
14. Shows that an activity is special or significant	P	**H**	I	S

Key: **P** = Passive **H** = Hesitant **I** = Involved **S** = Spontaneous

body. The expression on his face changes within seconds from indifference to interest and curiosity. Jacob seems to know what is coming and is ready for his weekly adventure.

The occupational therapist takes his left hand with a firm touch and speaks in his right ear: "Shalom, Jacob." Jacob usually responds with "shalom" or "toda raba" [thank you] or "heifa" [a nonsense term]. These are his three available verbal expressions, but he manages to communicate a fair amount with them. The therapist asks him how he is doing, and the tone of his "toda raba" tells her he is well. Jacob is often in severe pain, and his verbalizations provide cues about his level of pain. Today's friendly "toda raba" suggests there is not so much pain and so the therapist increases the volume of the music. With the help of his assistant she leads him to a water bubble pillar in the corner of the room. His responses in the past suggest that he is able to discern the changing colors in the pillar.

The occupational therapist sits on his non-hemiplegic side and reaches out for his hand. His face starts to relax, and Jacob begins to lead the movement with the rhythm of the music. He starts to move in a dance that involves more and more of his body. The therapist gently guides his left arm to touch his hemiplegic arm and both legs. Jacob quickly takes over this sequence of movements. He first smiles and then breaks into a laugh as he continues with this new sequence.

After a while, the therapist goes over to his hemiplegic side. With a gentle nudge from the therapist, Jacob takes hold of his hemiplegic hand with his left hand. He moves both hands, along with the therapist's hand, in rhythm with the music. Jacob, who usually appears marginally conscious, is completely awake at this point, and he demonstrates adequate trunk control. His occupational therapist releases his wheelchair belt.

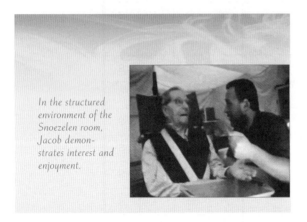

In the structured environment of the Snoezelen room, Jacob demonstrates interest and enjoyment.

The occupational therapist asks Jacob if he is ready to get up and get closer to the water pillar. Jacob raises his eyebrows and then winks. The therapist interprets this as a yes. With his assistant, the therapist helps Jacob out of the wheelchair, transferring him to sit next to the water pillar so that he can touch, listen, and see the colors and water bubbles more closely.

Jacob puts his right ear on the pillar and listens. After a while they transfer him to the other side of the pillar and he hugs the pillar and starts moving his hand up and down the pillar. On his face is an expression of intense listening and a deep smile. The transfer back to the wheelchair is easy.

Jacob's daughter arrives toward the end of the session, and she and the occupational therapist agree on another treatment 2 days later. In that session, Jacob and his daughter play with glass marbles and laugh together. Then his daughter, with tears in her eyes, kisses her father on the cheek. He takes her hand and showers it with gentle kisses.

Jacob in Perspective

To illustrate the change in Jacob's behavior when he is in the *Snoezelen* environment, the therapist completed the VQ a second time. The results shown in *Figure 20.2* indicate that Jacob's volitional behavior is now mostly spontaneous or involved. For Jacob and others who have severe sensory, perceptual, motor, and cognitive impairments, the highly controlled environment of the *Snoezelen* provides a unique volitional opportunity. The participation of some clients can also be enhanced in other contexts if they are modified to be supportive and more accessible, mimicking the features of the *Snoezelen* environment that facilitate interaction.

Marc: Recapturing Freedom

Marc, a 27-year-old Belgian man, was diagnosed with paranoid schizophrenia. According to the institutional records, Marc was the younger of two children. As a child, he had difficulty making friends. He felt inferior and was often teased, in response to which he became physically aggressive. As a teenager Marc had problems at school, took drugs, and got into trouble with authorities.

Marc had a very difficult relationship with his father, who had schizophrenia and who was hospitalized multiple times. His father died suddenly when Marc was 19 years old. His mother, a teacher, found it very hard to manage the family after the death of her husband. At age 22, Marc was first hospitalized, complaining of constantly hearing voices that dominated his life. While hospitalized he began a relationship with another patient, and following discharge he lived mostly in her apartment in Brussels. During this time he began training in carpentry but stopped because he developed paranoid suspicions toward fellow trainees.

Shortly thereafter, Marc had to be readmitted to the hospital because he could not handle growing tensions between himself and his girlfriend. After a period of hospitalization he was discharged to a psychosocial center that provided partial residential care. While living there he began regularly using marijuana with two fellow residents and stopped taking his medication. His symptoms soon became so severe he was admitted to long-term psychiatric care. Marc spent the next 3 years in a psychiatric ward. During that period, he was socially isolated, sometimes even refusing to see his mother and girlfriend when they visited the hospital. Marc only rarely left the hospital, and his ability to do anything beyond minimal self-care was extremely restricted. Even the slightest demands for

FIGURE 20.2 Jacob's ratings on the Volitional Questionnaire in *Snoezelen* environment.

Environmental Context: *Snoezelen* Treatment				
1. Shows curiosity	P	H	(I)	S
2. Initiates actions/tasks	P	H	I	(S)
3. Tries new things	P	H	(I)	S
4. Shows pride	P	H	I	(S)
5. Seeks challenges	P	H	(I)	S
6. Seeks additional responsibilities	(P)	H	I	S
7. Tries to correct mistakes	(P)	H	I	S
8. Tries to solve problems	P	(H)	I	S
9. Shows preferences	P	H	(I)	S
10. Pursues activity to completion/accomplishment	P	H	(I)	S
11. Stays engaged	P	H	(I)	S
12. Invests additional energy/emotion/attention	P	H	(I)	S
13. Indicates goals	P	(H)	I	S
14. Shows that an activity is special or significant	P	H	I	(S)

Key: **P** = Passive   **H** = Hesitant   **I** = Involved   **S** = Spontaneous

performance exacerbated his symptoms. Over time his symptoms, especially the auditory hallucinations, worsened.

Just before being transferred to a ward designed for the most therapy-resistant clients, he deteriorated even further. The overall focus of this new ward and its therapy services was to help clients find some comfort in life despite severe intractable psychiatric disability. When he came to the ward, Marc had more or less constant auditory hallucinations. The voices he heard accused and gave orders to him. Marc also had ongoing paranoid delusions. Despite taking medications, Marc remained very psychotic and frightened.

Marc lost all interest in doing things. His only activity was pacing or wandering about agitated. He rarely allowed any social contact with others. Most of the

time he isolated himself, fretting over the voices he heard. After a few weeks, a medication change had a modest improvement on Marc's psychosis so that he became somewhat more approachable. At this point the therapist began to invite Marc into the therapy workshop, but Marc always declined.

The therapist consistently greeted Marc and had short conversations with him in an attempt to validate him and develop some rapport and trust. As Marc became more comfortable having short talks with the therapist, the therapist decided to administer the Occupational Performance History Interview—II (OPHI-II) to Marc in the hope of finding a way to reach him. Although Marc had some difficulty attending and giving a detailed life history, some very useful information was revealed in the interview.

Marc told the therapist that there was a period between when his father died and his first hospitalization when he was able to function. This was the best period of his adult life. During that time he worked for a while as a truck driver. He found his job stressful, but it gave him a feeling of freedom that he very much appreciated. After the trucking job, he also worked for a while on a farm, which he liked because of the feeling of freedom he got from working outdoors. He also spoke about feeling free during a short period when he lived on his own in a room he could decorate himself.

However, this freedom period did not last long. His psychiatric symptoms became worse, and he began to isolate himself in the room, listening to records. When he was not doing that, he wandered around in the city and frequented pubs. The people he met in the pubs reintroduced him to drugs, which contributed to his getting worse and ending up hospitalized.

One of the highlights of the interview was Marc's revelation that he had a strong interest in photography. Marc had taken a class in photography. He had even arranged a darkroom at home. He recalled that he had greatly enjoyed developing black-and-white pictures that he made himself. His hobby was interrupted by an exacerbation of his illness.

As shown in *Figure 20.3*, Marc's ratings on the occupational identity and competence scales reflect his severe impairment. The only area in which he did not have a major problem was interests, and this was due to his identified interest in photography. Collaborating together, Marc and his therapist created his narrative slope (*Fig. 20.4*), which showed that Marc's one clearly positive life period was his freedom period when he lived in a room of his own, worked, and took up photography.

Based on Marc's history, the therapist reasoned that photography might be a way to engage Marc in doing something. The therapist explained to Marc that taking pictures would allow him to walk about freely and capture some impressions that he could later develop in the darkroom. The idea, the therapist explained, was to see if he could recapture some of his old feeling of freedom from the good period of his life. When presented with this idea, Marc agreed to explore photography. This was the first time in years he had chosen to undertake something.

FIGURE 20.3 Marc's ratings on the OPHI-II.

Occupational Identity Scale	1	2	3	4
Has personal goals and projects	✗			
Identifies a desired occupational lifestyle	✗			
Expects success	✗			
Accepts responsibility	✗			
Appraises abilities and limitations	✗			
Has commitments and values	✗			
Recognizes identity and obligations	✗			
Has interests		✗		
Felt effective (past)		✗		
Found meaning and satisfaction in lifestyle (past)		✗		
Made occupational choices (past)		✗		
Occupational Competence Scale	1	2	3	4
Maintains satisfying lifestyle	✗			
Fulfills role expectations	✗			
Works toward goals	✗			
Meets personal performance standards	✗			
Organizes time for responsibilities	✗			
Participates in interests	✗			
Fulfilled roles (past)	✗			
Maintained habits (past)	✗			
Achieved satisfaction (past)		✗		

Key :
1 = Extreme occupational functioning problems
2 = Some occupational functioning problems
3 = Appropriate, satisfactory occupational functioning
4 = Exceptionally competent occupational functioning

With coaching from his therapist, Marc went to the library in the nearby village and found some books on photography. He checked out these books and began coming to therapy, during which time he read the books. Next, his therapist and he planned for Marc to go home for a weekend to find his old photography equipment. They located a small room in the occupational therapy building that they outfitted as a darkroom.

The therapist and Marc together decided to begin with developing some pictures from old negatives he still had from his schooldays. This turned out to be dif-

FIGURE 20.4 Marc's narrative slope.

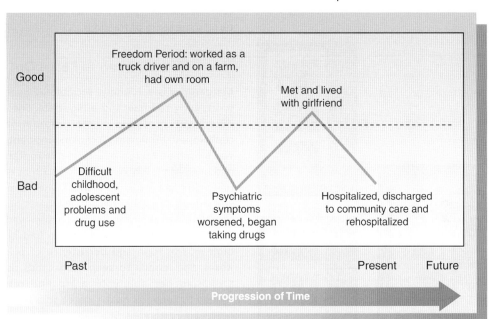

ficult for Marc because it brought back painful memories. After validating Marc's reaction, the therapist negotiated that he would find another source of negatives for Marc to develop. Consequently, some of the occupational therapy staff members brought negatives in with the request that Marc develop them and enlarge them. Marc did this for a couple days, but then indicated that he was not thrilled with the routine of developing old negatives.

He indicated that he would much rather develop pictures he took himself. The therapist then negotiated with Marc that he could go outside the hospital to take pictures, provided he was willing to join the organized excursions with other patients. Marc agreed. He began going on outings with other patients, taking pictures and even engaging in some social interaction with the others.

Up to this point the therapist had accompanied Marc into the darkroom, but since Marc had improved, the therapist suggested that Marc could begin developing the pictures on his own. Marc began to do this but soon found that his auditory hallucinations became very upsetting to him when he was alone in the darkroom. The therapist supported and coached Marc to think about possible solutions to this problem. Marc

identified the idea of taking a small portable radio with him into the darkroom. He tried this and found that it made him much more comfortable.

Soon the therapist asked Marc if he would be willing to take pictures of other patients on these excursions. These pictures would be used in a newsletter that was regularly published by the patients in the hospital. Marc chose to do this and felt a sense of pride that he was asked to take on this role. During this time Marc began to improve in other areas. He became more social and more attentive to self-care. He began to take regular walks in the nearby village to shoot pictures.

Over time, Marc showed that he had a unique talent for photography. He made wonderfully expressive pictures and received praise for them from staff and patients alike. Bolstered by all this feedback, Marc decided, with encouragement from the occupational therapist, to organize an exhibition of his pictures. He put together a beautifully designed exhibition in the hospital, which also served as his farewell. Shortly thereafter he was discharged to a psychosocial center in the village of Elsene. As a going-away present, Marc gave his occupational therapist some framed pictures he had taken and developed.

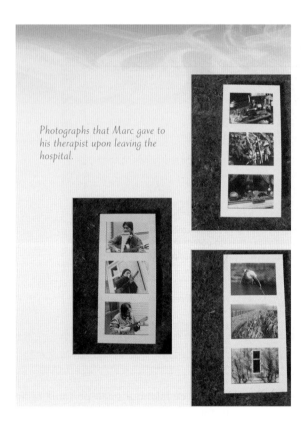

Photographs that Marc gave to his therapist upon leaving the hospital.

Epilogue

Five years after this case was written, Marc is living in a sheltered house in Brussels. He is attending a day activity center a few days a week to structure his day.

Marc in Perspective

Marc's case was particularly challenging, since his occupational identity and competence were so completely impaired. At the time he began therapy, Marc had no volitional desire to do anything. The value of learning about a client's past is underscored, since it was a past interest from the one good period in Marc's life and the idea of recapturing some of the feeling of freedom from that period that engendered his desire for action. When clients cannot narrate for themselves a vision of a future, the therapist can sometimes find such a vision from the client's past, as Marc's therapist was able to do. While the severity of Marc's psychiatric disability is such that he will likely always need a supportive envi-

ronment, at this writing he has functioned well for 4 years in the community center. There he has recaptured some sense of freedom.

Margaret: Learning to Reach Out

Margaret was a friendly, sociable 22-year-old with short, curly red hair and a big smile. She was diagnosed with profound mental retardation and encephalopathy following a choking incident when she was a toddler. Margaret was unable to stand or walk and needed maximum assistance for mat or bed mobility. She had a custom manual wheelchair that she was unable to propel herself. Margaret had very little active movement in her legs and moved her arms with great difficulty because she had abnormally high muscle tone and persistence of primitive reflexes. She tended to keep both hands fisted, compromising her ability to grasp and release. She tended to keep her head rotated to the left with her neck hyperextended. She had difficulty bringing her head to midline during grooming or looking down during tabletop activities. Although Margaret had very little expressive speech, she could understand some of what was being said to her, and she did produce vocalizations to communicate.

Margaret lived in a facility for individuals with profound physical and mental disabilities and attended a developmental training program. In this setting the occupational therapist mainly evaluated clients and consulted to direct care staff. Margaret also received services from an occupational therapy assistant in a small-group setting every 2 weeks. This case discusses the therapist's use of MOHO in an annual evaluation and consultation process.

Although Margaret's physical and cognitive limitations were very evident, these were not the only problems that had to be addressed to allow her to participate more actively. She also demonstrated low volition, as evidenced by her initial score on the VQ (*Fig. 20.5*). When the therapist observed Margaret during grooming and other activities, it was clear she did not have confidence in her ability to do them, even with assistance. Nor did she appear to have any desire to take an active role in doing these things.

Instead, her satisfaction came from interactions with and reactions of the direct care staff. For instance,

FIGURE 20.5 Margaret's VQ ratings initially and 1 year later.

Client: Margaret
Diagnosis: Profound mental retardation, Encephalopathy

Environmental Context	Initial Observation				Observation 1 year later			
1. Shows curiosity	P	H	I	**S**	P	H	I	**S**
2. Initiates actions/tasks	P	**H**	I	S	P	H	**I**	S
3. Tries new things	P	**H**	I	S	P	**H**	I	S
4. Shows pride	P	**H**	I	S	P	H	**I**	S
5. Seeks challenges	**P**	H	I	S	P	**H**	I	S
6. Seeks additional responsibilities	**P**	H	I	S	**P**	H	I	S
7. Tries to correct mistakes	**P**	H	I	S	**P**	H	I	S
8. Tries to solve problems	P	**H**	I	S	**P**	H	I	S
9. Shows preferences	P	H	**I**	S	P	H	**I**	S
10. Pursues activity to completion/accomplishment	**P**	H	I	S	**P**	H	I	S
11. Stays engaged	P	**H**	I	S	P	**H**	I	S
12. Invests additional energy/emotion/attention	P	**H**	I	S	P	**H**	I	S
13. Indicates goals	**P**	H	I	S	P	H	**I**	S
14. Shows that an activity is special or significant	P	**H**	I	S	P	H	I	**S**

Rating Key: **P** = Passive; **H** = Hesitant; **I** = Involved; **S** = Spontaneous

she would laugh when a staff member encouraged her to try to move her arms to press a switch or to perform hand-over-hand assisted fine motor activities. She did not even attempt to look at what she was doing. Instead, she watched the reaction on her caregiver's face.

Margaret would indicate pride in her accomplishments (by smiling or laughing) only with much staff encouragement and rarely expressed a desire to try something again. She would rarely initiate any action except with a great deal of staff encouragement. She rarely indicated goals such as how she wanted to do something or what she wanted to do. Despite her low personal causation, it was clear that Margaret had some interests and values. The most obvious was her interest in her personal appearance and her value of social interaction.

Because of her extreme physical limitations, the staff members tended not to expect or require much participation on her part. Also, because it was hard to know which activities were really enjoyable to Margaret, they did not readily try to elicit choices from her.

Recommending Goals and Intervention

The therapist recognized that Margaret needed an approach that would tap into her volitional strengths while providing physical support to facilitate her movement. Thus, the therapist devised goals and strategies for the staff to implement, based on using her strong interest in personal appearance and value of social interaction to encourage. The focus of these goals was to allow Margaret to participate in self-care more actively. For example, the therapist recommended the goal that Margaret would keep her hands open during the application of nail polish. The combination of physical facilitation techniques (e.g., hand massage) and Margaret's interest in getting a manicure proved successful. She not only reached this goal but also began to demonstrate increased ability to grasp and release, particularly in her dominant right side.

The therapist also recommended the goal that Margaret brush her hair with a long-handled hairbrush with assistance while looking in a mirror. Again, the combination of physical facilitation to relax her muscle tone with Margaret's pride in her beautiful curly red hair enabled Margaret to achieve success with this goal. She also demonstrated improved ability to bring her head to midline to look in the mirror during this activity.

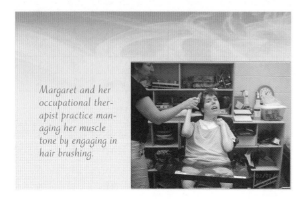

Margaret and her occupational therapist practice managing her muscle tone by engaging in hair brushing.

Because of Margaret's value of social contact, the therapist also recommended the goal that Margaret would reach at least to midline with her right hand to shake hands with staff who approached her. To facilitate this goal, Margaret received physical facilitation, such as stretching on a therapy ball and passive range of motion in diagonal patterns. Margaret enjoyed this interaction with staff immensely and eventually attempted to shake hands as staff approached, without any verbal cueing. With practice she increased her skill in timing the opening of her hand with reaching for a staff member's hand.

Margaret was clearly pleased with her success and began to demonstrate active attempts to reach, grasp, and release in other activities. She was also beginning to make choices and to assert her need for physical assistance to do things she wanted to do. This in turn made staff more inclined to ask her to try new things.

A year later, Margaret had shown enough volitional desire and progress in occupational performance that she was moved from her developmental training classroom to a more vocationally oriented day program for higher-functioning clients. This new environment placed more emphasis on productive activities and put Margaret in contact with higher-functioning peers. A number of these clients had augmentative communication devices and/or power wheelchairs. Some were

even able to talk. Instead of being in a classroom of 12 clients, Margaret joined nearly 30 clients in this new environment. This required her to further develop the skill of asserting herself to get her needs met.

Margaret began to thrive in this new environment. Her vocalizations increased, and she used them to gain staff attention. She also showed an increase in visual motor attention. Her ability to use her hands continued to improve with practice. With coaching, she could pick up an object, bring her arm across her body, and drop it in the appropriate container. This allowed her to do new occupational forms/tasks, such as sorting clips or filling potpourri sachets. Margaret showed her new volitional strength by becoming very vocal if she was not given an opportunity to participate when other clients were doing these kinds of things.

Finally, Margaret showed her increased volition by deciding on her own goal. She was able to communicate that she wanted to learn to do assisted tooth brushing. This occupational form/task was especially difficult for Margaret because she could not easily relax her right arm to flex her elbow to get the toothbrush to her mouth. Nevertheless, Margaret insisted that this be one of her new goals and was eventually able to achieve it.

During her last annual evaluation, Margaret's volition was again assessed using the VQ. As shown in *Figure 20.5*, her volitional ratings were significantly higher. She required less assistance to initiate actions and spontaneously showed that activities were significant to her. She showed pride and indicated goals with less cueing. She even sought challenges on occasion, when given encouragement. Margaret also indicated her preferences more consistently.

Direct care staff members noted the changes in Margaret. They saw that she was much more insistent on getting her needs met or in voicing her opinion by giving a yes or no response in a group setting. She insisted on being allowed to participate and derived pleasure from her accomplishments. Margaret also became popular with other clients, particularly one of her male classmates. She began independently reaching out to hold hands with him.

Margaret in Perspective

Margaret illustrates the extent to which volition can be an asset in achieving basic gains in motor capacity. She also illustrates how clients in long-term settings can settle into patterns of unnecessary passivity. Such patterns are often locked into place by the clients' lack of a sense of efficacy and by staff members' low expectations of clients.

Paula: Getting Control of Life

Paula was a 45-year-old woman who lived with her mother in the Cotswolds area of England. She had a mild learning disability, epilepsy, and right-sided hemiparesis. Paula was referred to the occupational therapist because her mother was aging and Paula's sisters wanted her to become more independent in homemaking.

The therapist first made an informal home visit to discuss the referral with Paula and her mother. She also planned to begin collecting information informally and to identify the most appropriate formal assessment tools. It quickly became clear that her family determined Paula's routines. Her two sisters who lived nearby had set days for shopping, gardening, and visiting Paula and her mother. Paula had organized her schedule to fit in with the family's routines. She volunteered 2 days a week but otherwise spent many hours alone in her room listening to music or watching videos.

Paula reported that she had mild right-sided weakness and had minor problems handling and gripping things with her dominant right hand. Her speech was unclear at times, especially when she was anxious. Paula reported that her difficulty pronouncing words sometimes prevented her from communicating as freely as she would have liked. During this visit, the therapist asked Paula if she could observe her doing some household tasks, and Paula agreed. From the observation, Paula's process skills appeared adequate, although she complained that the medication (anticonvulsants) she took made her feel groggy and confused sometimes.

Although Paula showed no significant problems in performing, her mother intruded regularly, directing and correcting Paula throughout the task. The therapist could see that this was very frustrating for Paula. Moreover, it increased her anxiety, which made it harder for her to focus on her performance. Later, Paula complained, "This always happens." Despite her

clear annoyance at her mother's intervention, Paula did not express to her mother her wish to continue alone in the task.

As a result of this visit, the therapist determined that Paula had the ability to self-report accurately and effectively and needed an opportunity to express her own views of her life. Consequently, the therapist decided to administer three assessments:

- The Occupational Self-Assessment (OSA)
- The OPHI-II
- The Role Checklist.

The therapist explained to Paula that she wanted to meet with her alone the next time to ask some questions and give Paula an opportunity to tell about her life. Paula liked this idea and agreed to an appointment time.

Occupational History

Paula responded to the OPHI-II interview with short but passionate responses. The life story she reported was as follows. Paula reported having motor and learning problems from an early age. Her first seizure occurred when she was 6 years old. She painfully recalled how at school her classmates ridiculed her because of her seizures and speech impediment. Things got somewhat better when she went to the senior school, because she found and confided in a supportive school counselor. This person helped Paula develop coping strategies and bolstered her self-confidence.

Paula left school at the age of 16. Some years later, she found a job in a warehouse. More than anything, working improved her life. She earned an income and felt capable and useful. Paula also made a number of friends at work with whom she shared hobbies and spent time.

Paula had always lived with her mother. Although Paula and her mother enjoyed a generally positive relationship, Paula felt that her mother dominated her decision making. Moreover, her mother did most household tasks, since she lacked confidence in Paula's abilities and worried about her having a seizure while doing something. Of late, Paula's seizures had become more frequent. Consequently, her mother pressured Paula to further diminish engagement in any household and leisure activities. For example, Paula had always used a bicycle as her major form of transportation, but she gave it up at her mother's urging to avoid the possibility of having a seizure while riding.

The most critical event in Paula's life was the loss of her job a few months before. Paula had worked for 22 years in a warehouse where she operated light machinery. She had performed well at work. Despite occasional seizures, she had never had any injuries or problems. Paula's supervisors were very supportive. Unfortunately, two events converged that led to her job loss. The first was a change in management structure that occurred when a larger corporation bought the company. The second was that Paula had a number of severe seizures at work. The new manager directed Paula's immediate supervisors to dismiss her on the grounds that her seizures made her an injury risk.

Paula was devastated by the loss of her job. She began to do volunteer work 2 days a week but deeply wanted to return to employment. Paula felt that she had lost the main area of her life in which she felt valued and effective. Moreover, her other occupational roles had been affected by her job loss. She lost friendships and leisure opportunities, since most of her friendships and leisure pursuits had been shared with work colleagues. Her role within the family had reverted to being the disabled member rather than a financial contributor. Her only interests at this point

were listening to music and watching television. She spent long periods alone in her room, which contributed to her increasing feeling of isolation.

Paula's entire sense of efficacy was organized around her work in the past. Now that she was confined mostly at home, where she had little access to the persons and things she had liked to do, Paula's life took a dramatic downward plunge, as illustrated in her narrative slope (*Fig. 20.6*). She also internalized many of the fears that her mother expressed about her becoming injured if she had a seizure. Although Paula had always managed life with some seizures, the convergence of her job loss, the increased frequency of seizures, and the growing concern expressed by her family led Paula herself to feel that everything was threatened by her seizures.

Paula had little control over her home environment. She felt hemmed in by expectations of her family members. For example, although Paula absolutely hated gardening, she was expected by her mother and sisters to maintain a large garden. Rather than create conflict or disappoint her family, Paula did the work without complaining.

Paula acknowledged that her mother and sisters were the most significant people in her life. However, she felt very ambivalent about her relationship with

FIGURE 20.6 Paula's narrative slope.

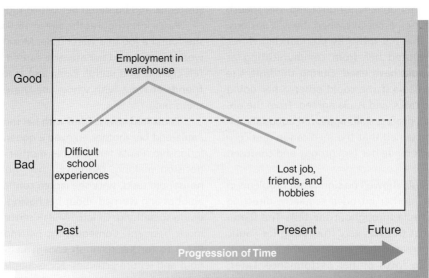

them. On one hand, she valued being part of the family group, but she also resented the restrictions and obligations put on her by her mother and sisters. She was also disturbed because her mother and sisters did not seem to recognize her abilities or place any value on her role within the family.

Paula's ratings on the OPHI-II are shown in *Figure 20.7*. Her occupational identity was impaired by her

FIGURE 20.7 Paula's ratings on the OPHI-II.

Occupational Identity Scale	1	2	3	4
Has personal goals and projects			✗	
Identifies a desired occupational lifestyle				✗
Expects success		✗		
Accepts responsibility			✗	
Appraises abilities and limitations			✗	
Has commitments and values				✗
Recognizes identity and obligations		✗		
Has interests			✗	
Felt effective (past)				✗
Found meaning and satisfaction in lifestyle (past)				✗
Made occupational choices (past)				✗
Occupational Competence Scale	**1**	**2**	**3**	**4**
Maintains satisfying lifestyle	✗			
Fulfills role expectations		✗		
Works toward goals	✗			
Meets personal performance standards	✗			
Organizes time for responsibilities	✗			
Participates in interests	✗			
Fulfilled roles (past)				✗
Maintained habits (past)				✗
Achieved satisfaction (past)				✗
Occupational Settings (Environment) Scale	**1**	**2**	**3**	**4**
Home-life occupational forms	✗			
Major productive role occupational forms		Not Applicable		
Leisure occupational forms	✗			
Home-life social group		✗		
Major productive social group		Not Applicable		
Leisure social group	✗			
Home-life physical spaces, objects, and resources		✗		
Major productive role physical spaces, objects, and resources		Not Applicable		
Leisure physical spaces, objects, and resources		✗		

Key :
1 = Extreme occupational functioning problems
2 = Some occupational functioning problems
3 = Appropriate, satisfactory occupational functioning
4 = Exceptionally competent occupational functioning

loss of work, and her competence was dramatically affected, as shown in the difference between the items reflecting the past and those reflecting the present. Finally, the negative impact of her environment is apparent in the ratings. She no longer had her work environment, and the opportunities for her occupational participation were quite constrained at home.

Paula filled out the Role Checklist and discussed it with the therapist. As shown in *Figure 20.8*, Paula's past roles were student, worker, friend, and hobbyist, to which she gave a value rating of very important. Her present roles were volunteer, home maintainer, and family member. Notably, she rated the volunteer role and family member role as only somewhat important. She explained that since the work she did was unpaid, she was not contributing to the family budget as she always had.

In further discussing her responses, Paula noted that she desperately wanted to return to paid work. She also indicated somewhat guiltily that she wanted to move out of her mother's home and become a home maintainer in her own right. Paula also indicated that she wanted to get back to being involved in her roles as a friend and hobbyist. It was notable that she did not foresee a very significant involvement in the family member role. Paula explained that her mother was elderly and ill. Paula did not think she would have an ongoing close relationship with her sisters following her mother's death.

OCCUPATIONAL SELF-ASSESSMENT

From the OPHI-II, it was clear that Paula felt she had lost control over her life. The therapist felt that it was important to begin giving control back to Paula. Therefore, when she presented the OSA to Paula, the therapist advised Paula that the OSA was her own assessment, since only Paula knew all the answers to the questions. The therapist also explained that doing this assessment would give Paula a say in what she wanted her life to be and in the kind of services she received from the occupational therapist.

This was very empowering to Paula, as she realized that she could influence the outcome of the assessment and the focus of her therapy. She worked through the forms eagerly with coaching from the therapist (*Fig. 20.9*). In the discussion that followed, Paula wanted to talk about her total health needs and services. She was deeply concerned that her seizures were getting out of control. She felt isolated and increasingly self-conscious about her speech problems, since she no longer had access to the coworkers who were accustomed to and comfortable with her speech. She felt bored and useless. Finally, she felt very lonely, as she did not really see her mother and sisters as friends or companions with whom she could do leisure things. Together, the therapist and Paula set the following immediate goals:

FIGURE 20.8 Paula's responses on the Role Checklist.

Role	Role Identity			Value Designation		
	Past	Present	Future	Not at all valuable	Somewhat valuable	Very valuable
Student	X					X
Worker	X		X			X
Volunteer		X			X	
Caregiver						
Home Maintainer		X	X			X
Friend	X		X			X
Family Member	X	X	X		X	
Religious Participant						
Hobbyist/Amateur	X		X			X
Participant in Organizations						

FIGURE 20.9 Paula's responses on the OSA.

Myself	Competence				Values			
	Lots of problems	Some difficulty	Well	Extremely well	Not so Important	Important	More Important	Most Important
Concentrating on my tasks			✗		✗			
Physically doing what I need to do		✗			✗			
Taking care of the place where I live		✗					✗	
Taking care of myself		✗						✗
Taking care of others for whom I am responsible			✗			✗		
Getting where I need to go		✗					✗	
Managing my finances			✗		✗			
Managing my basic needs (food, medicine)	✗							✗
Expressing myself to others	✗							✗
Getting along with others			✗			✗		
Identifying and solving problems		✗			✗			
Relaxing and enjoying myself			✗				✗	
Getting done what I need to do			✗			✗		
Having a satisfying routine		✗				✗		
Handling my responsibilities		✗					✗	
Being involved as a student, worker, volunteer, and/or family member			✗					✗
Doing activities I like			✗				✗	
Working towards my goals		✗			✗			
Making decisions based on what I think is important			✗		✗			
Accomplishing what I set out to do			✗				✗	
Effectively using my abilities	✗				✗			

My Environment	Environmental Impact				Value of Environment			
	Lots of problems	Some problems	Good	Extremely good	Not so Important	Important	More Important	Most Important
A place to live and take care of myself	✗							✗
A place where I can be productive (work, study, volunteer)			✗			✗		
The basic things I need to live and take care of myself				✗				✗
The things I need to be productive		✗				✗		
People who support me and encourage me			✗					✗
People who do things with me		✗					✗	
Opportunities to do things I value and like		✗					✗	
Places where I can go and enjoy myself		✗					✗	

- Get Paula's seizures under better control
- Get help to reduce her speech difficulties
- Increase her leisure activities, especially outside the home
- Identify companions with whom to spend time and make more friends.

Completing the OSA and setting goals empowered Paula to take more control over her health services. She attended a meeting of the interdisciplinary community team during which she asserted herself, expressing her own preferences and values.

The Therapist's Conceptualization of Paula's Situation

From the information gathered, the therapist constructed the following conceptualization of Paula's situation. Despite a previous pattern of positive occupational participation, Paula had recently undergone a contraction in all areas of participation. Paula had entered a negative spiral that began with the loss of her job and finding herself isolated back home, where she had little control over her life.

Paula clearly knew what she valued, but because of her family's dominance of her decision making and her own fears of being hurt during a seizure, she had increasingly restricted participation in the things she most enjoyed and valued. The most significant limiting factor in her performance was her fear of doing things. Her family reinforced and maintained her anxiety and sense of inefficacy. As Paula herself had identified on the OSA, her main priority was to undertake things that would increase her feeling of being capable of managing her life once again. When the therapist shared her conceptualization with Paula, she agreed and noted that she needed to "strengthen herself as a person" by undertaking things that she valued.

Intervention

Following the plan they had outlined when completing the OSA, the therapist and Paula began by addressing the medication issue. The therapist, working in conjunction with the community nurse, supported Paula in getting her medication adjusted. It was known from her previous medical history that Paula became stressed when a change in her drug therapy regimen

was indicated. The therapist sought to put Paula in control as much as possible. The community nurse had advised Paula on how to chart her seizure activity. This identified that there was a definite pattern of seizure frequency during the month. Consequently, Paula and her therapist developed a schedule so that doing things that were new or potentially stressful was kept to the times of the month that were most likely to be seizure free.

Paula had told the therapist that her primary concern was that she might be injured if she had a seizure when using electrical equipment. Consequently, she had quit doing most household tasks that required use of such equipment. The therapist advised Paula that they would be able to find special appliances that would reduce this risk. However, as they explored purchasing such equipment, Paula decided that she wanted to use ordinary appliances, focusing instead on precautions that enhanced her safety. With support of the therapist, Paula planned a visit to a business that sold equipment with automatic electricity cutoff.

The therapist next helped Paula refer herself to speech therapy. Since Paula had identified this as a problem she wanted to address, the therapist felt she would have a greater sense of control if she did a self-referral rather than having a speech therapist found for her. Paula found a therapist and began speech therapy. The speech therapist identified that Paula showed dysarthric and dyspraxic features in her speech. She developed a set of recommendations to help Paula with her speech problems. She also gave Paula a set of exercises to improve her speech control.

Next, the occupational therapist addressed Paula's last two goals of finding friends and increasing her leisure participation. The therapist accompanied Paula to a Disability Resource Center where they accessed a database. Paula had never used a computer before and was very proud of this achievement. In the database they found information about local social clubs. Paula chose one to attend but expressed anxiety about going alone. The therapist accompanied her for the first three visits. Paula enjoyed this club and subsequently made arrangements to be picked up at her home by special transportation. In the next few months, she began to attend the group regularly and went on several trips with the group.

Coping with Life Changes

Paula's mother's health deteriorated to the point that she had to go into a nursing home. With the help of the therapist, Paula found a situation where she could live with a family as a paying guest. Paula hoped this would be temporary and that she could someday manage a household herself. Because she had not been given opportunities when living with her mother, Paula had not learned many of the necessary skills to live alone. Consequently, at the advice of the therapist, Paula began to attend a day center once a week where she had the opportunity to shop with others, plan, and cook lunch. The therapist also began working with Paula on other aspects of the homemaker role. Paula had identified ironing, sewing, and budgeting as areas she wanted to develop.

As her personal causation improved, Paula also identified that she would like to explore the possibility of working again. She expressed a desire to work in a library. The therapist helped Paula refer herself to an employment service for persons with learning disabilities. Paula soon began working two part-time jobs at a local university library and at the city library.

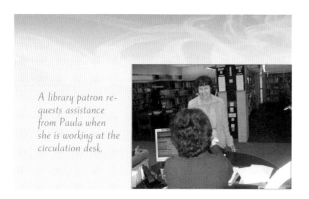

A library patron requests assistance from Paula when she is working at the circulation desk.

Shortly after she began working, the family with whom Paula was living moved to a nearby town and Paula moved with them. The distance required Paula to travel by bus to work and day care, which she found stressful. Also, another paying guest joined the family, and Paula felt this person intruded on her privacy. Finally, the teenage son in the household began to make fun of Paula, bringing back angry memories of her earlier victimization at school.

Paula's seizures began to increase, as they did whenever she was stressed. Paula was determined to find herself other accommodations and enlisted the help of the therapist. However, even before the therapist could assist her, Paula found a flat to rent. Although apprehensive about living alone, she decided that with some continued assistance from her therapist, she could manage.

Epilogue

Five years after this case was written, Paula is living independently in a subsidized apartment. The apartment has been adapted to suit physical needs and safety aspects regarding epilepsy. She now has a part-time paid job in a library and is active in her hobbies. Her work is going very well, although occasionally a seizure prevents her from attending or necessitates going home early. Paula continues regular visits with her family and meets up with them for holiday and family celebrations. She receives some support from a care agency, which she pays for herself. Her life has changed so much from days when Paula felt totally controlled from the outside. Now, she decides what outside support she needs. While her epilepsy still gives her cause for concern, she is involved with its management.

Paula in Perspective

Paula's therapy exemplifies client-centered practice in which a therapist can empower a client to take control of life. It also illustrates how important it is for therapists to serve as advocates for clients when they are faced with social barriers. However well intentioned others' concerns about Paula were, she needed to be able to decide what reasonable risks she would take. The therapist's most important role was to support Paula in making the decisions that put her in control of her life.

Conclusion

When their clients have cognitive limitations, occupational therapists have a mandate to work toward comprehending and advocating for the client's volition. In some instances, cues may be found in a person's past.

Volition may be revealed in the subtle ways a client responds to circumstances in the environment. It is, however, always discoverable. No matter how impaired persons are, their volition exists. In their own ways, they experience and express it.

Some cases in this chapter illustrated that therapists can find ways to understand and reach the client. With effort, therapists can discover things about their lower-functioning clients that not only make their volitional thoughts and feelings evident but also provide essential information for designing effective therapy. Other cases illustrated the importance of advocating for client's volition when it is not being fully addressed in the environment. Together the cases illustrated how, by respecting clients' volition, therapists can open up possibilities for truly client-centered practices that empower clients to more fully participate in occupational life.

References

Chung, J. C., Lai, C. K., Chung, P. M., & French, H. P. (2002). Snoezelen for dementia. *The Cochrane Database of Systematic Reviews. 4.*

Kielhofner, G. (2005, July). The remotivation process. Seminar presented at the Conference of the Israeli Occupational Therapy Association, Jerusalem.

Shapiro, M. and Bacher, S. (2002). *Snoezeling: Controlled multi-sensory stimulation –A handbook for practitioners.* Israel: Beit Issie Shapiro.

van Diepen, E., Baillon, S. F., Redman, J., Rooke, N., Spencer, D. A., & Prettyman, R. (2002). A pilot study of the physiological and behavioural effects of Snoezelen in dementia. *The British Journal of Occupational Therapy, 65(2),* 61–66.

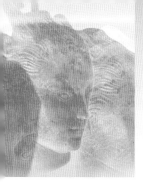

21

Facilitating Participation Through Community-Based Interventions

- Gary Kielhofner
- Mara Levin
- Brad Egan
- Alice Moody
- Camille Skubik-Peplaski
- Laurie Rockwell-Dylla

This chapter presents four cases in which therapists provided services to clients in community contexts. What most links the cases together is the extent to which therapy capitalizes on and enables the clients to participate more fully in settings of home, family, neighborhood, and workplace. The cases span childhood to old age and present a range of cognitive, emotional, and physical problems and challenges.

The course of therapy for each of these clients takes place over several weeks or months. It naturally proceeds within the unfolding lives of the clients. Each of the cases illustrates in a different way how therapy can facilitate clients' occupational participation in a community context.

David: Increasing Motivation for Participation

David was a 9-year-old boy with a diagnosis of developmental delay. Whereas David achieved early developmental milestones on schedule, he always tired easily, talked constantly, and was impulsive. His parents noted that David still was very clumsy and had a poor attention span. He was very uncomfortable with any changes in his routines and had difficulty learning new tasks. Finally, David's parents described him as fearful

of being hurt in everyday situations that were not actually physically threatening. David attended a regular third grade class and received speech therapy services in school. There had been discussion of holding him back in school because of his fine motor deficits.

David was seen privately by his occupational therapist. His parents sought out occupational therapy services to address problems stemming from David's sensory processing difficulties. The therapist initially assessed David with a battery of motor and perceptual instruments and an observational guide for use with the sensory integration model. When evaluated from the perspective of sensory integration (Ayres, 1979; Bundy, Lane, & Murray, 2002), David displayed auditory, gustatory, and tactile defensiveness. This meant he had difficulty integrating sound, taste, and touch and perceived these sensory stimuli as uncomfortable and threatening. He was hypersensitive to many forms of sensory stimulation, such as loud noises. His diet was limited to a small range of foods he could tolerate (pasta, hamburgers, creamy peanut butter, white bread, and ketchup). He was unable to eat almost anything that was firm or crunchy.

David also displayed gravitational insecurity and vestibular deficits. He was very uncomfortable doing anything that involved moving away from the ground, such as climbing or swinging. Merely watching a merry-go-round would make him dizzy. He avoided most playground equipment. As a consequence of these limitations of performance capacity, David's performance was quite restricted. For example, he could not manipulate buttons or tie his shoes. Moreover, David's handwriting was very poor.

The following discussion illustrates how the occupational therapist employed MOHO concepts as a component of her therapy. Sensory processing difficulties are typically interwoven with volitional problems (Kielhofner and Fisher, 1991). Moreover, as discussed in Chapter 6, there is a lived body experience of having these difficulties. Finally, the long-term impact of therapy on a child like David must involve enabling him to choose to do things that facilitate sensory processing challenges with performance.

Therefore, while his therapist used sensory integrative principles and strategies as the major focus of David's therapy, MOHO concepts were also used. Since our aim is to show how MOHO supported and complemented the sensory integrative approach, we will discuss only those details of the sensory integrative approach that were most intertwined with the therapist's use of MOHO.

Evaluating David's Volition

The therapist began to evaluate David's volition through informal observation. Since therapy involved engaging David in various sensorimotor activities, the therapist had constant opportunity to observe David's volition in action. Additionally, discussions with David's parents provided information about David's volition, especially his sensorimotor likes and dislikes.

In the area of personal causation, David was keenly aware that he lacked skills that other children possessed. He had an especially difficult time in gym class, where his poor coordination made him stand out. David had little that was positive to say about his capacities. As his parents indicated, David was extremely fearful of occupational forms/tasks that required motor actions.

David had few interests. His main pastimes were playing Nintendo and watching television. Because David had difficulty performing in a wide range of contexts, he attempted to dismiss as unimportant many of the things that other children his age found meaning-

ful and valuable. For example, he disavowed any interest in going to the playground in the park. However, he was also very aware of being different from other children in other ways. For example, he was unable to tolerate or manipulate ordinary clothes, so he wore sweat clothes and sneakers with Velcro closures. David was clearly disturbed by these differences, as he very much valued being like other children.

David made very restricted decisions for engaging in ordinary childhood occupations. In particular, he avoided participating in games with other children that involved gross movement. He did not participate in any of the childhood sports that his peers enjoyed. Clearly, David's volitional problems included these:

- Feelings of lack of control, especially in motor performance
- Lack of enjoyment in performance and failure to develop a range of age-appropriate interests
- Attempts to avoid the pain of not being able to do things valued by others by disavowing their importance
- Feeling threatened by sensory stimulation from his environment.

These problems were critical to address because they affected David's quality of life.

Any changes he might achieve in his performance capacity would depend on David choosing to perform in ways that would enable him to develop his capacity and skills.

Intervention

David attended occupational therapy once a week. His therapist engaged him in doing things that were indicated from a sensory integrative perspective. At the same time, the therapist also focused on goals. David would do the following:

- Demonstrate that he felt in control and expected to succeed while engaging in ordinary childhood occupations that involved motor challenges
- Show greater enjoyment and a greater desire to do things involving motor challenges
- Be able to do more things that he valued and found meaningful.

Because David's volition was so limited, the therapist began all intervention at the exploration level and progressed toward competence and achievement—the continuum of change discussed in Chapter 10.

David's therapy began with simple movement patterns on objects that were close to the ground and had small radiuses of movement (i.e., therapy ball, platform swing, scooter boards). To address David's volition, these movement activities were integrated into games that the therapist created and played with him. These games were designed to allow David to physically explore the environment in a safe context with minimal performance demands. To maximize his feeling of control, David was allowed to make up the rules of the games. Over time, David showed increasing enjoyment in his therapy sessions and was able to make up new games.

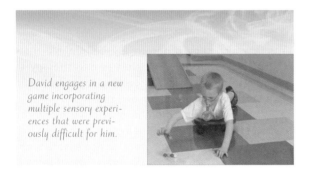

David engages in a new game incorporating multiple sensory experiences that were previously difficult for him.

After a period of therapy, David cautiously expressed an interest in sports. In response the therapist began to incorporate basketball and baseball themes into the same kind of safe therapy games. As he became more comfortable with gross motor games, David played with increasing ease and intensity, willingly choosing to do such things as swinging, rolling in barrels, and jumping off a loft into foam pillows. During this phase, the therapist coached David's parents to replicate some of the same safe opportunities for exploration at home and the playground. She also began to explore new foods with him and helped David's mother figure out ways to allow him to try different foods at home. His diet became more diverse, and he was increasingly willing to try new foods.

Given David's progress in the gross motor area coupled with his increased sense of efficacy, the therapist decided to address some of the fine motor challenges that he faced. Concurrent with this change, the therapist recognized that David's performance capacity and volition had improved to the point that he

could handle competency-level demands. During the competency stage of change, she expected David to begin to handle greater performance demands by improving his performance. As noted in Chapter 10, striving for competence leads to skill development and the organization of these skills into habits. Competency affords an individual a growing sense of personal control. As persons strive to organize their performances into routines of competent behavior that are relevant to their environment, they immerse themselves in a process of becoming, growing, and arriving at a greater sense of personal mastery.

David's therapist began by adding performance demands requiring fine motor capacity. For example, she suggested that they play Star Wars and dress up in costumes. This allowed her to introduce buttoning and unbuttoning. David started with oversize buttons and then progressed to smaller ones. During this phase, she also negotiated with David's parents to work with him to practice things he was learning in therapy.

The therapist initiated a program aimed at enhancing David's handwriting. This program used principles consistent with the lived body concept discussed in Chapter 6. In the program (Benbow, 1999), the therapist gave David visual and verbal feedback so that he could feel each letter as he wrote it. The therapist developed and taught David to do a warmup exercise program before writing in school that prepared his hands for handwriting. Over time, he was able to copy sentences from a paper, and then from the chalkboard, with improving accuracy. Eventually, David's handwriting improved significantly, and he found that it took much less effort to write. David was especially excited when he realized that the improvement in his handwriting had contributed to the decision not to hold him back in school.

The therapist also initiated a program to help David learn to monitor, maintain, and change his level of alertness in different situations. The program helped David become more aware of his inner experiences and to control them. This allowed him to better attend and learn in the classroom and to interact more effectively with other children. David actively worked to learn to do this, as it gave him a greater sense of control. With time and practice, the handwriting warmup exercise and the self-monitoring of his alertness became habits.

Next, David began to show signs of moving to the achievement level (i.e., being able to face greater challenges and risks). For example, David found ways to vary his performance and challenge himself to do more than what he was already able to do. He increasingly attempted new things he had never done before. As he saw peers in therapy do something he had not yet done, he would want to do it.

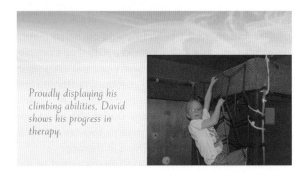

Proudly displaying his climbing abilities, David shows his progress in therapy.

Achievement also means having greater control and integrating new skills and habits for managing everyday life. David was showing signs of this as well. For example, he increasingly sought out his therapist's advice and coaching to help him improve his performance in areas of daily life.

Recognizing David's readiness for the achievement level, the therapist decided to offer David even more control over the aims of therapy. She invited David to complete the Child Occupational Self-Assessment (COSA). In addition to giving him a voice in stating how he saw himself and what he most wanted to address in therapy, the COSA would also allow David to see the progress he had made in therapy.

The therapist administered the COSA orally. David was initially shy when asked the COSA questions, but as the assessment progressed, he was able to identify how he felt about his performance and what was important to him (*Fig. 21.1*). The assessment provided an important opening to set goals that David found important. On the COSA David identified many areas wherein he had some problems. However, the COSA did provide him an opportunity to note some areas that were okay and others in which he had strengths.

When David and his therapist discussed his responses to the COSA, David identified that he felt his relationships with his peers would be improved if he could do more of the things they did and was able to dress like them. As a result they developed three new goals for therapy:

- To manage a button and zipper independently so he could wear jeans like his peers
- To tie his shoes independently so he could have the kind of sneakers that many of his peers wore
- To learn and use strategies that would help him calm down to learn at school.

The therapist's acknowledgment of these goals as being important to David and her assurance that they would work toward them in therapy were highly motivating for David.

The therapist worked out a plan with David's parents in which they progressively bought him new clothes. David brought the clothes into therapy to work on necessary skills for getting them on. David learned to manage his button and zipper and to tie his shoes over the next 2 months. In another month he learned to tie double knots. His mother then purchased him a pair of the fancy sneakers his peers were wearing. Throughout this stage of therapy, David increasingly felt effective in accomplishing goals.

As his personal causation was enhanced, David continued to identify new occupational forms/tasks that he wanted to learn in therapy. When he did so, the therapist allowed him to work on these self-initiated goals. In this way, David began to direct his own therapy. For example, he wanted to be able to make his own snack. Thus, in therapy he practiced making a peanut butter sandwich until he mastered it.

Near the end of therapy, David told the therapist he wanted to have his birthday party at a local indoor play area, since his peers were having their parties there also. He shared his concern over whether he would be able to handle himself okay on the playground. In response, the therapist secured approval from the insurance company to do a therapy session at this play area. With his therapist's encouragement and coaching, David tried each play apparatus (e.g., climbing tube, rope ladders, ball pits, drawbridge, and swings). With practice David managed to master each piece of equipment during the session. Importantly, this gave him confidence to go ahead with the birthday

FIGURE 21.1 David's initial responses on the COSA.

CHILD OCCUPATIONAL SELF ASSESSMENT (COSA)
Summary Rating Form

Name: **David**   Gender: ☒ M ☐ F   Age: 9

Myself	I have a big problem doing this	I have a little problem doing this	I do this ok	I am really good at doing this	Not really important to me	Important to me	Really important to me	Most important of all to me
Keep my body clean	✗				✗			
Dress myself	✗							✗
Eat my meals without any help	✗				✗			
Buy something myself	✗				✗			
Get my chores done	✗				✗			
Get enough sleep			✗		✗			
Have enough time to do things I like	✗					✗		
Take care of my things	✗					✗		
Get around from one place to another	✗				✗			
Choose things that I want to do	✗					✗		
Keep my mind on what I am doing	✗						✗	
Do things with my family	✗							✗
Do things with my friends		✗				✗		
Do things with my classmates		✗				✗		
Follow classroom rules	✗						✗	
Finish my work in class on time	✗					✗		
Get my homework done	✗					✗		
Ask my teacher questions when I need to	✗							✗
Make others understand my ideas	✗					✗		
Think of ways to do things when I have a problem	✗				✗			
Keep working on something even when it gets hard		✗				✗		
Calm myself down when I am upset	✗							✗
Make my body do what I want it to do		✗						✗
Use my hands to work with things	✗							✗
Finish what I am doing without getting tired too soon	✗							✗

party. During his birthday party, he was able to enjoy himself and use the equipment along with the other children.

Also near the end of therapy, the therapist administered the COSA again to review progress with David and to identify goals David would continue to work on himself. As shown in *Figure 21.2*, most areas were now adequate, and he was able to identify a number of strengths. He noted only two areas in which he still had some problems: doing what his parents told him and playing with friends.

In the follow-up discussion with the therapist, he identified two goals for his future. He noted that he wanted to improve his ability to "shift his engine to just right" so he could meet these goals:

- Finish school work in allotted time
- Adjust his behavior to play with other kids.

David was able to plan how to address both of these goals. This included, for instance, using sour candy to "shift his engine."

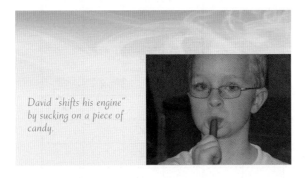

David "shifts his engine" by sucking on a piece of candy.

By the time therapy came to an end, David had successfully played baseball on a school team. He preferred basketball because he was the best player on the court for his age. When terminating therapy, David's final comment on how things had gone in therapy was he could "do lots of stuff." David also announced that he had decided to become an artist when he grew up. As noted in Chapter 10, one of the important developmental steps for latency-aged children is occupational choice. It requires that the child have both interests and some sense of efficacy. Before he began therapy David rarely picked up a pencil or crayon.

David's Therapy in Perspective

David's therapy illustrates the concept of occupation-based practice using MOHO. Sensory integrative theory is readily integrated into therapy by identifying David's performance capacity challenges and blending them with his occupational needs and preferences. This case emphasized volition, since for David it was so critical. Habituation, lived body, and environmental concepts were also used to guide the therapy process. The concept of volition was critical both because it illuminated an area in which David needed to achieve changes and because the volitional process was important for the success of the sensory integrative aspects of the therapy. A child can benefit from sensory integrative strategies only when he or she is volitionally engaged (Kielhofner & Fisher, 1991).

David's therapy also illustrated how client-centered therapy takes on different forms over time. Early in therapy, David was unable to choose goals because he did not believe in his ability to achieve goals. Consequently, the therapist needed to understand David's volition and his limitations of performance capacity to set goals on his behalf. Only later, when David's volition had improved, could he actively participate in deciding on goals for therapy.

Joan: Recreating the Meaning of Home

Joan was a 79-year-old woman with myxedema (an extreme and disabling edema due to a thyroid abnormality) and a history of congestive heart failure. A couple of weeks earlier, Joan's condition worsened to the point that she was hospitalized and treated with medications aimed at eliminating some of the edema. She was given the choice to receive rehabilitation in the hospital or at home. Joan opted to return home to receive physical and occupational therapy services. This discussion describes the course of Joan's home-based intervention. It interweaves the themes of occupational identity and the meaning of home. Moreover, it demonstrates how therapy can enable persons to reclaim their lives and their environments.

The therapist arrived at Joan's home in a middle-class suburb of Chicago. There she first encountered Joan's two adult daughters, Anne and Debbie, and Joan's 87-year-old husband, Art. Debbie led the therapist into

FIGURE 21.2 David's final responses on the COSA.

CHILD OCCUPATIONAL SELF ASSESSMENT (COSA)
Summary Rating Form

Name: David　　Gender: ☒ M ☐ F　Age: 9

Myself	I have a big problem doing this	I have a little problem doing this	I do this ok	I am really good at doing this	Not really important to me	Important to me	Really important to me	Most important of all to me
Keep my body clean			✗		✗			
Dress myself			✗		✗			
Eat my meals without any help			✗			✗		
Buy something myself				✗	✗			
Get my chores done			✗			✗		
Get enough sleep			✗		✗			
Have enough time to do things I like		✗				✗		
Take care of my things		✗				✗		
Get around from one place to another		✗				✗		
Choose things that I want to do			✗			✗		
Keep my mind on what I am doing				✗	✗			
Do things with my family			✗					✗
Do things with my friends	✗					✗		
Do things with my classmates		✗				✗		
Follow classroom rules			✗		✗			
Finish my work in class on time		✗			✗			
Get my homework done				✗		✗		
Ask my teacher questions when I need to				✗	✗			
Make others understand my ideas		✗				✗		
Think of ways to do things when I have a problem		✗				✗		
Keep working on something even when it gets hard		✗				✗		
Calm myself down when I am upset				✗	✗			
Make my body do what I want it to do		✗			✗			
Use my hands to work with things				✗				✗
Finish what I am doing without getting tired too soon				✗				✗

the living room, where the shades were down and curtains closed. Joan was sitting in a recliner in a nightgown and robe. She sat with her shoulders hunched, clearly having trouble breathing. A fan in the corner of the room was blowing. Debbie explained that the fan helped reduce the moisture in the air, easing her mother's breathing.

The centerpiece of the former living room was a queen-size bed with a comforter and embroidered pillows. While attractive, the bed evidenced that the living room had been transformed into a sickroom. Other objects completing the transformation were a bedside commode next to the television and a table that held pills, a cup of water, and a bell for summoning help.

Joan's History and Current Performance

The therapist decided to conduct the Occupational Performance History Interview—II (OPHI-II) as a group interview. She began the interview during the first visit and continued it over time as she continued to talk with Joan and her daughters. Since home health services extended over several visits, the ongoing interview allowed the therapist to build rapport and increasingly learn about Joan.

The following narrative emerged out of the interview. Many years ago, Joan developed a thyroid condition that Joan's physician thought had been cured with a newly approved medication. For several years, she had no symptoms and engaged in her normal routine of taking care of her family and her house, which had always been the focus of Joan's life. She had a satisfying life filled with cooking, cleaning, pursuing her hobby of crochet, and socializing with her family and friends.

Joan's illness recurred a year ago. The swift decline that followed led to the transformation of the living room into a sickroom and to a dramatic alteration of all their lives. Debbie recalled how her mother's eyes began to look buggy and how she began to retain so much fluid that her legs had become four times their previous size. As the edema progressed, Joan had increasing difficulty breathing and became increasingly fatigued with each passing day. Her symptoms progressed to the point that she was unable to cook or do heavy housework. From then on, she relied on help from her daughters.

Debbie and Anne both decided to restructure their lives, moving back home to become full-time caretakers. Debbie was single, had her own condominium, and worked as a freelance artist. She was spending increasing amounts of time at her family home rather than her own residence, so she decided it was best just to move back home. Anne was divorced and did not have children. She relinquished her apartment to return home and help her sister take care of their increasingly frail parents. They shared responsibility for meeting the medical, physical, and emotional needs of their mother and father as well as the responsibilities of maintaining the household.

As the year unfolded, Joan came to need help not only with homemaking, but also with her own personal care. She found it increasingly difficult to climb up and down the 14 steps to her bedroom and bathroom, so the family decided to move the bed down to the living room.

Joan's world slowly shrank to her former living room. She ate her meals there. She was sponge-bathed in the adjacent partial bathroom. She watched television from her recliner chair most of the day. She spent restless nights in her queen-size bed. Nearly immobilized, she had not been to other parts of the house for some time. Joan's occupational narrative was one of loss and retreat. As Joan and her family saw it, she had lost both life and her home as she retreated into her sickroom.

After hearing this story of Joan's decline and observing Joan's fragile physical condition, the therapist explained her role and asked the family what they hoped to gain from therapy. The daughters told the therapist that it would help if their mother could become less reliant on them for her personal daily tasks. They all agreed together that this would be the primary goal of therapy.

The therapist next evaluated Joan's performance by asking her to demonstrate how she did her daily tasks. The observation revealed that Joan's edema, combined with her severely limited strength and endurance, made performing even her basic self-care routines nearly impossible. The therapist knew that achieving the overall goal of more self-reliance would require engaging Joan in occupational forms/tasks she valued, but Joan had such limited performance capacity that she could not effectively do them.

Course of Therapy

The therapist explained to Joan that to become able to do more things for herself, she would need to increase her strength and endurance. However, Joan was not convinced that she could do so and benefit from an exercise program on her own between therapy sessions. At the second visit, Joan admitted she was unable to follow through on the recommended exercises. She seemed very defeated when talking about her physical condition. In contrast, as they talked about Joan's lifestyle in her younger and healthier days, Joan enthusiastically reminisced about how she loved to cook and conjure up new recipes.

Since Joan did not have the physical capacity to get to the kitchen, much less participate in cooking, the therapist decided on the following strategy. She led Joan to participate in simple exercises for building strength and endurance while simultaneously enlisting Joan to share her store of expert knowledge about cooking. These conversations during exercise began Joan's return to the occupational form/task of cooking. The therapist did this by asking Joan for advice and suggestions about recipes and referring to Joan as her "cooking mentor." This process highlighted Joan's remaining capacity, her store of expert cooking knowledge. Consequently, Joan could experience culinary competence even though she did not have the motor capacity necessary to do the cooking itself. It also took her mind off the exercises and allowed her to put forth more effort.

As soon as Joan had enough capacity, the therapist encouraged Joan to try some cooking together with her. Joan agreed and referred to the process as getting her "kitchen coordination" back. Initially, Joan needed substantial assistance to do the cooking. Nonetheless, her position as the "cooking mentor" who supervised the therapist allowed Joan to feel satisfied with her performance.

Soon, Joan was regularly watching cooking shows and would share the latest recipes with the therapist when she came. One day, the therapist arrived to find Joan in the kitchen in the process of making chop suey. Joan had not independently made a sandwich—much less a whole meal—in well over a year! Joan enjoyed preparing the meal but found that it was overtaxing. Thereafter, she was content to assist her daughters with preparation of dinner, which was more in line with her physical abilities.

After the initial success with cooking, the therapist decided to find another occupational form/task from Joan's past for which she might have the physical ability. Joan had also shared with the therapist how she had loved to crochet and give her projects away as gifts. Her daughters showed the therapist beautiful and intricately designed afghans, curtains, towels, doilies, and pot holders that Joan had crocheted. Joan said that she had lost interest in crocheting because her diminished eyesight made it difficult.

Nonetheless, the therapist encouraged her to try crocheting again and advised Joan that if she started doing it, she might discover that she still enjoyed it and could do it. At the therapist's suggestion, Joan's daughters bought crochet yarn and set it on her table, just in case she wanted to try it. The presence of the crocheting objects in the environment gave Joan the opportunity and resources she needed. Eventually, she tried it. Joan found that she could still crochet by relying on her sense of touch to compensate for her failing vision.

The therapist had learned over the sessions how important Joan's home had always been to her and the care with which she had decorated and maintained it. She advised Joan that it was possible for her now to reclaim her home. Joan enthusiastically responded to this idea as the next goal for therapy. As Joan's endurance and strength improved, the occupational therapist began to encourage and physically support Joan during each therapeutic session to walk to a different room of her home using her walker.

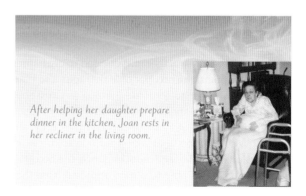

After helping her daughter prepare dinner in the kitchen, Joan rests in her recliner in the living room.

During these walks, Joan's husband offered encouraging comments, predicting, "Soon you'll be running around here." The walks also provided occasions for Joan to talk about the rooms and things that transpired in them, incorporating them once again as part of her life space. Next, the therapist persuaded Joan that since she was able to maneuver around her house, she should get back into the routine of having dinner in the dining room with her family. By incorporating the use of this space in her daily routine, Joan took a first step forward to restoring some of her previous lifestyle.

Soon, her walking had progressed to the point that her physical therapist thought she was ready to tackle the biggest physical barrier that faced her—the 14 steps leading to the upper level of her home. Joan not only had to overcome fatigue, but she had also experienced panic attacks with the physical therapist during sessions aimed at stair climbing. She clearly faced a personal causation hurdle related to walking up the stairs. She was afraid she would not make it up the stairs and would have to be carried down. She also had fears that she would not be able to make it back down the stairs and would be stuck upstairs. This prospect upset her, since she had not been up the stairs in over a year and it had become foreign territory.

Given the fears that dominated Joan's personal causation with reference to climbing the stairs, she needed a great deal of encouragement from both the physical therapist and the occupational therapist. Joan mastered three, then four, then five steps over the course of a few weeks. She gained not only strength but also an increased sense of efficacy related to stair climbing. The occupational therapist and a physical therapist were both present when Joan finally made it all the way to the top.

When Joan demonstrated the ability to climb all the steps, the physical therapy goals were accomplished, and the physical therapist decided to discharge Joan. At this point, the occupational therapist also had to consider whether to continue therapy services. She consulted with Joan and the family and it became clear that Joan was not yet as self-sufficient as they all wished. With the goal that Joan continue to increase her functional mobility and independence, the occupational therapist was able to obtain approval from the insurance company to continue with therapy.

During the next phase of therapy, the therapist's goal was to help Joan be more independent once she was upstairs. To emphasize that Joan was moving from the sick role into her former homemaker role, the ther-

apist framed the next phase of therapy as shopping. Together, they shopped for appropriate adapted bathroom equipment, looking through pamphlets and catalogs. The therapist also arranged a demonstration of adapted equipment in her home. Together, the therapist and Joan collaborated to choose equipment that served Joan's physical needs and preserved her safety and that met her concerns that the equipment should complement the aesthetics of her home and not be institutional looking. With the addition of the equipment, Joan needed much less assistance from her daughters.

The therapist and Joan collaborated to identify her next goal, which Joan phrased as "going outside to get a breath of fresh air and feel the sunshine." Joan was able to climb down the front steps with coaching from the therapist. She then transferred into her wheelchair, which she used to visit the neighborhood. The therapist instructed the daughters on how to use the same procedure to assist Joan to get outside on a more regular basis. In some of her final sessions, Joan progressed to walking with her walker in the garden to look at flowers her husband had planted and in front of the house to reestablish friendships with neighbors she had not seen in months.

Conclusion of Services

Occupational therapy services were concluded when the therapist, in collaboration with Joan and her daughters, concluded that their initial goal had been achieved. Joan's progress was evidenced by increased independence in self-care; assisting and supervising meal preparation; once again engaging in previous leisure pursuits; and getting around her home, yard, and neighborhood. Finally, Joan started taking a more active role in household decisions.

Joan in Perspective

This case example has several features worth commentary. First of all, community contexts often provide opportunity for and call on the therapist to address as clients not just the disabled person, but also family members and others. The therapist effectively incorporated Joan's daughters and husband into assessment, goal setting, and intervention.

Second, the therapist was initially faced with a common dilemma. Joan did not have sufficient capacity to engage in the occupational forms/tasks that had meaning for her. The approach the therapist used (i.e., having Joan begin to reengage in cooking by sharing her expertise orally during exercises that prepared her occupational engagement) was a creative and effective way to resolve the problem. Moreover, while the therapist had to consider biomechanical factors throughout therapy, it was important that she framed the experience of therapy in response to Joan's occupational narrative as reclaiming Joan's life and her home. This kept the process motivating for Joan, as it allowed her to construct the competence to enact her identity.

Finally, the therapist had to decide on and justify continuation of therapy after the physical therapist discontinued her intervention when Joan reached the functional goal of climbing stairs. The occupational therapist's decision to continue therapy was based on an understanding that for Joan and her family, function meant reclaiming the competence to enact her identity. From this perspective, the therapist was able to justify and continue services to the point of achieving a better outcome for Joan and her family.

Mandy: A Journey Toward Work

Mandy is a 35-year-old resident in a 2-year transitional living facility for adults with HIV/AIDS who are homeless or at risk for homelessness. The facility offers on-site case management, recovery, spiritual care, and occupational therapy. In addition to offering several weekly groups, occupational therapy services consist of the Resident Trainee Employment Program (RTEP). The RTEP provides 12 weeks of part-time paid employment for residents of the facility. Because many of the residents have little or no work experience, the trainee program assists in establishing a work history, reviewing employment interests, addressing transferable work skills and habits for future employment, and identifying potential barriers associated with returning to work.

After seeing a job posting for a kitchen trainee, Mandy scheduled an appointment with the occupational therapist. After describing the job duties in detail, the occupational therapist administered the OPHI-II and the Worker Role Interview (WRI) to gain a better understanding of Mandy's life history, future expectations, values, and priorities for change. The therapist conducted a single interview that included the content of both these assessments. For the environmental sections of these instruments, the therapist focused on Mandy's current environment (including the RTEP program), since Mandy would be moving, if all went well, to a type of environment that was new to her. The following is the occupational narrative that resulted.

Mandy's Occupational History

Mandy was raised in Chicago with an older sister, two older brothers, and five younger siblings. She describes her father as being a "philanderer," and her parents divorced when she was young. During this time she was molested by her family's landlord. She never told her mother or father about the abuse but was able to confide in one of her sisters. Despite these difficulties, Mandy feels she has remained close with her family.

After her parents' divorce, Mandy's grandmother came to live with them. These times were better for Mandy "because there was always a roof over my head and my grandma took care of me." One of the occupations she shared with her grandmother was cooking. With limited knowledge of meal preparation, Mandy began preparing chicken, lasagna, greens, and casseroles. Mandy explained, that her grandmother "didn't use anything to measure. We just had to keep tasting and adding things until it was right. We had so much fun in the kitchen . . . I guess I became somewhat of a good cook, too."

Though Mandy was always a "smart kid," in the 9th grade, at age 14, she became pregnant and stopped attending school. The following year, Mandy met a pimp. She had already bonded with local prostitutes and had become intrigued with their flashy outfits and access to drugs, particularly marijuana, which she was now smoking on a regular basis. She left her baby with her mother and grandmother and became a child prostitute. She began using harder drugs and eventually sold street drugs in addition to her prostitution. During this time, she shared an apartment with other prostitutes or stayed in hotels. She reports she never really lived on her own, since she always had someone with her and never paid her own bills.

Over the next 18 years, Mandy had 5 children, 3 of whom were "trick babies" (i.e., pregnancies that resulted from her prostitution). Her illegal activities led Mandy to a felony conviction and several stays in prison, the longest being 9 months. While Mandy was in prison, she was able to earn her GED and take some college courses. During this time, her sister raised her children. Though she has contact with all five of her children, she believes that her absenteeism as a mother negatively impacted her children.

At age 33, Mandy was exhausted by her lifestyle, and she voluntarily entered a 3-month inpatient rehabilitation program. She began a 12-step program and maintained her sobriety for 7 months. When sober, Mandy noticed she would not prostitute herself as much, and she would give her mother money for her children. She found employment as a food server, and though she enjoyed her work and got along well with her coworkers, Mandy did not like her supervisor. She found that he gave her too much direction in her job. She states that she prefers a supervisor who is more hands-off and follows through on payment for her work. She was fired after 3 months for having a bad attitude.

Mandy then started using drugs and prostituting herself again. She soon developed a persistent cough and often felt feverish and achy. Eventually, Mandy was hospitalized with pneumonia. It was during this hospitalization, at age 34, that Mandy received her AIDS diagnosis. Mandy noted that finding out she had AIDS was the worst time in her life, and she described her mental state as being fragile during this time. She became so depressed that after she was stabilized medically, she was transferred to the hospital's inpatient psychiatric unit to ensure she would not harm herself. There, she worked with a psychiatrist to determine a psychiatric drug regimen that could help with her depression and also with a doctor to determine a drug regimen for her AIDS. She was also offered counseling services for her new diagnosis of AIDS, which she participated in minimally.

Mandy was discharged to a 6-month residential drug treatment program that specifically worked with people with HIV/AIDS. From this program, at age 35, she applied to her current housing situation, the transitional living facility for people living with HIV/AIDS. Mandy could not identify a time when things were at their best. She stated that she has never had a "good" period in her life and reckoned that her current situation was the best she had experienced.

Mandy reported that her current routine is not satisfying. She spends her time fulfilling program requirements, attending sobriety meetings, visiting with family, watching television, cooking, reading, and playing cards or Scrabble. She feels she does not have a lot of control over her life decisions at the transitional living facility but believes the structure can help her determine her next step. She has some close friends at the transitional living facility but does not mingle with others very much, as she likes to keep to herself. At the time of the interview, Mandy had celebrated 8 months of sobriety, consistently worked with a sponsor, and attended recovery support groups daily. In addition, she had minimal side effects from her current drug regimen, and her viral load remained undetectable. With a favorable health status and sobriety milestones under her belt, Mandy felt ready to ponder the idea of working on a part time or seasonal basis.

As shown in her OPHI-II scale scores (Fig. 21.3), Mandy's current occupational identity and competence were more intact than in the past when she was using drugs and prostituting. Her scores indicated that her occupational identity is not yet fully formed, though she has developed interests and recognizes the need to fulfill her current obligations. This conclusion was supported by her limited engagement in a variety of occupations and her uncertainty of what her next step in life should be. Mandy's competence scores also reflect her limited past achievements and her feelings that she has failed in certain life roles.

Mandy's WRI scores (Fig. 21.4) indicate that she has strengths in the areas of interests and taking responsibility. Her personal causation is weak because of her limited work history and job loss. Overall, the WRI scores reflect Mandy's inexperience in a traditional worker role, her uncertainty of success in this role, and her lack of routine.

Finally, Mandy's narrative slope (Fig. 21.5) illustrates the stagnation in the majority of her life with an attempt to move from her circumstances, followed by her AIDS diagnosis and recovery to a more positive place than she had occupied previously. She was beginning an upward slope and hoped it would continue with her new goal of participating in RTEP.

The therapist gave Mandy feedback on her OPHI and WRI scores and her narrative slope. Mandy agreed with the therapist's understanding of her occupational

FIGURE 21.3 Mandy's ratings on the OPHI-II.

Occupational Identity Scale	1	2	3	4
Has personal goals and projects		✗		
Identifies a desired occupational lifestyle		✗		
Expects success		✗		
Accepts responsibility		✗		
Appraises abilities and limitations		✗		
Has commitments and values		✗		
Recognizes identity and obligations			✗	
Has interests			✗	
Felt effective (past)	✗			
Found meaning and satisfaction in lifestyle (past)	✗			
Made occupational choices (past)	✗			
Occupational Competence Scale	**1**	**2**	**3**	**4**
Maintains satisfying lifestyle		✗		
Fulfills role expectations		✗		
Works toward goals		✗		
Meets personal performance standards		✗		
Organizes time for responsibilities		✗		
Participates in interests		✗		
Fulfilled roles (past)	✗			
Maintained habits (past)	✗			
Achieved satisfaction (past)	✗			
Occupational Settings (Environment) Scale	**1**	**2**	**3**	**4**
Home-life occupational forms		✗		
Major productive role occupational forms	Not Applicable			
Leisure occupational forms		✗		
Home-life social group		✗		
Major productive social group	Not Applicable			
Leisure social group			✗	
Home-life physical spaces, objects, and resources		✗		
Major productive role physical spaces, objects, and resources	Not Applicable			
Leisure physical spaces, objects, and resources		✗		

Key: **1** = Extreme occupational functioning problems
2 = Some occupational functioning problems
3 = Appropriate satisfactory occupational functioning
4 = Exceptionally competent occupational functioning

FIGURE 21.4 Mandy's ratings on the Worker Role Interview.

Worker Role Interview Summary Form	SS	S	I	SI	N/A
Personal Causation					
Assess abilities and limitations			X		
Expectation of job success			X		
Takes responsibility		X			
Values					
Commitment to Work			X		
Work-related goals			X		
Interests					
Enjoys work		X			
Pursues interests		X			
Roles					
Appraises work expectations			X		
Influence of other roles			X		
Habits					
Work habits				X	
Daily routines			X		
Adapts routine to minimize difficulties			X		
Environment					
Perception of work setting					X
Perception of family and peers			X		
Perception of boss					X
Perception of coworkers					X

Key:
SS = Strongly supports
S = Supports
I = Interferes
SI = Strongly interferes
N/A = Not applicable

narrative and circumstances. Together they discussed what might help or hurt Mandy's continuation on a positive trajectory. Mandy saw the following barriers to obtaining a paid position in the community:

- Lack of education
- Lack of work history
- Difficulty communicating effectively with others
- Criminal history
- Difficulty maintaining sobriety
- Social prejudice and discrimination toward her HIV status.

Mandy also believed that applying for the resident trainee kitchen position would support a continued upward trajectory to her narrative. She identified the following benefits of working at her place of residence:

- Transportation to and from work would not be an issue
- Her AIDS status is already known and accepted by staff
- She would have access to the occupational therapist, who could provide onsite job support

FIGURE 21.5 Mandy's narrative slope.

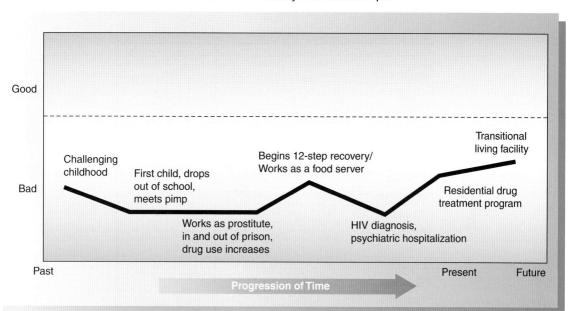

- Her criminal history is already known to staff
- She would have access to her medications and could adhere to her current medication schedule
- She would still be able to make all of her recovery meetings because the hours were flexible
- She could begin a traditional work history to use on a résumé and for references when applying to other jobs.

Mandy felt that this opportunity could be the doorway to finding paid external employment and help her achieve her goal of living independently in the community. After again describing the job duties in detail, the therapist recommended that Mandy review the potential benefits and barriers to returning to work. A followup appointment was scheduled for the following week.

A week later, Mandy was still eager to apply for the kitchen trainee position. Because she identified that she had difficulty communicating effectively with others, the occupational therapist completed the Assessment of Communication and Interaction Skills (ACIS). Also, to clarify Mandy's self-perceptions and priorities, Mandy completed the Occupational Self Assessment (OSA). Both of these assessments would aid Mandy and the therapist in setting long- and short-term goals.

Mandy's scores on the ACIS (*Fig. 21.6*) indicate that her skills in the three areas of physicality, information

exchange, and relations were generally ineffective, supporting Mandy's self-perception of having poor communication skills. The therapist noted, however, that when Mandy made an effort, she had the underlying ability to communicate effectively with others. Her problem was that she had difficulty sustaining an effective communication and interaction style.

On the first, Myself, part of the OSA (*Fig. 21.7*), Mandy identified four problem areas she would like to change:

- Managing my finances
- Expressing myself to others
- Having a satisfying routine
- Accomplishing what I set out to do.

Discussing her responses, Mandy stated that she had problems following through with her goals and often quit for fear of failure. She stated that she "self-sabotages" her efforts to improve herself, and she acknowledged that she needed to let go of some control to maintain sobriety and improve her life situation.

On the second, Environment, section of the OSA (*Fig. 21.8*), Mandy identified three areas she would like to change:

- A place to live and take care of myself
- The things I need to be productive
- Opportunities to do things I value and like.

FIGURE 21.6 Mandy's scores on the ACIS.

	4	3	2	1
Physicality				
Contacts			✗	
Gazes			✗	
Gestures			✗	
Maneuvers		✗		
Orients			✗	
Postures			✗	
Information Exchange				
Articulates			✗	
Asserts			✗	
Asks		✗		
Engages			✗	
Expresses			✗	
Modulates		✗		
Shares			✗	
Speaks			✗	
Sustains			✗	
Relations				
Collaborates			✗	
Conforms		✗		
Focuses		✗		
Relates			✗	
Respects			✗	

Key:
1 = Deficit   **2** = Ineffective   **3** = Questionable   **4** = Competent

In discussing this section, Mandy noted that she was satisfied with her living situation but knew she would have to leave the facility after her 2 years of residence. Therefore, she wanted to ensure she would be able to move into her own apartment and felt she should start addressing this need as soon as possible.

Using the results from the ACIS and OSA and considering the objectives of the RTEP, Mandy and her therapist identified the following long-term goals:

- Before entering the RTEP Mandy will identify recovery meetings that support her work schedule so she can to maintain sobriety
- Mandy will create a résumé to apply for the RTEP

- Mandy will obtain her kitchen sanitation certification to allow her to work in food services by the end of the 12-week program
- Within 2 months Mandy will access services from a local organization that helps formerly incarcerated individuals enter the workforce
- Mandy will practice appropriate and assertive communication through role-play to increase her ability to communicate effectively in the workplace
- Mandy will demonstrate understanding of her rights in employment and disclosure under the Americans with Disabilities Act (ADA) by the end of the 12-week program.

FIGURE 21.7 Mandy's ratings on the Myself section of the OSA.

Myself	Competence				Values				Priority
	Lot of problem	Some difficulty	Well	Extremely well	Not so important	Important	More important	Most important	
Concentrating on my tasks			✗			✗			
Physically doing what I need to do			✗				✗		
Taking care of the place where I live			✗				✗		
Taking care of myself			✗					✗	
Taking care of others for whom I am responsible									
Getting where I need to go				✗			✗		
Managing my finances	✗						✗		✓
Managing my basic needs (food, medicine)			✗					✗	
Expressing myself to others	✗							✗	✓
Getting along with others		✗					✗		
Identifying and solving problems		✗					✗		
Relaxing and enjoying myself		✗					✗		
Getting done what I need to do		✗					✗		
Having a satisfying routine	✗						✗		✓
Handling my responsibilities		✗						✗	
Being involved as a student, worker, volunteer, and/or family member		✗						✗	
Doing activities I like		✗					✗		
Working towards my goals		✗						✗	
Making decisions based on what I think is important		✗					✗		
Accomplishing what I set out to do	✗							✗	✓
Effectively using my abilities			✗				✗		

Phase I: Applying for the Resident Kitchen Trainee Position

Mandy's insubstantial work history made drafting a traditional résumé challenging. After explanation, Mandy decided to create a functional résumé that focused on transferable skills and strengths instead of chronological work history. Mandy thought this option best shifted attention away from the gaps in her limited employment history. Mandy also worked with the therapist to practice interviewing strategies and interview protocols. After reviewing all applicants, the staff offered Mandy the resident trainee kitchen position at 20 hours per week. Excitedly, Mandy accepted.

FIGURE 21.8 Mandy's ratings on the Environment section of the OSA

Step 1: Below are statements about things about your environment (where you live, work, go to school, etc.) For each statement, circle how this is for you. If an item does not apply to you, cross it out and move on to the next item.	There is a lot of problem	There is some problem	This is good	This is extremely good	Step 2: Next, for each statement, circle how important this aspect of your enviroment is to you. This is not so important to me	This is important to me	This is more important to me	This is most important to me	Step 3: Choose up to 2 things about your environment that you would like to change (You can also write comments in this space) I would like to change
A place to live and take care of myself	Lot of problem	Some problem	**Good** (circled)	Extremely good	Not so important	Important	More important	**Most important** (circled)	✓
A place where I can be productive (work, study, volunteer)	Lot of problem	**Some problem** (circled)	Good	Extremely good	Not so important	Important	**More important** (circled)	Most important	
The basic things I need to live and take care of myself	Lot of problem	Some problem	**Good** (circled)	Extremely good	Not so important	Important	More important	**Most important** (circled)	
The things I need to be productive	**Lot of problem** (circled)	Some problem	Good	**Extremely good** (circled)	Not so important	Important	More important	**Most important** (circled)	✓
People who support and encourage me	Lot of problem	Some problem	Good	**Extremely good** (circled)	Not so important	Important	More important	**Most important** (circled)	
People who do things with me	Lot of problem	Some problem	Good	**Extremely good** (circled)	Not so important	Important	**More important** (circled)	Most important	
Opportunities to do things I value and like	Lot of problem	**Some problem** (circled)	Good	Extremely good	Not so important	Important	More important	**Most important** (circled)	✓
Places where I can go and enjoy myself	Lot of problem	Some problem	**Good** (circled)	Extremely good	Not so important	Important	**More important** (circled)	Most important	

Phase II: Becoming the Kitchen Trainee

Being in the kitchen reminded Mandy of being with her grandmother. However, given the restrictive dietary needs for HIV drug efficacy and general health needs, Mandy wasn't able to cook many of her grandmother's favorite recipes. In the beginning of her employment, Mandy mostly assisted with the prep work, cleaning, and simple dessert recipes provided by the kitchen supervisor. The kitchen supervisor frequently praised Mandy's efficiency and ability to follow directions. The kitchen supervisor then decided to change Mandy's job duties to include bringing in new recipe ideas for the menu and preparing main courses.

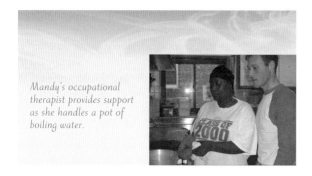

Mandy's occupational therapist provides support as she handles a pot of boiling water.

Mandy informed the staff during a check-in that she was enjoying her kitchen position and was still able to fulfill all of her other obligations. However, upon hearing the additional job duties, Mandy decided to schedule a meeting with the occupational therapist. She discussed her uneasiness with increased job responsibilities, noting, "Expectations scare me and make me feel like I don't know what I am doing." Moreover, she did not know where to find recipes and did not feel confident in her skills to prepare the main courses. Mandy worked with the therapist to identify resources for recipes, such as television cooking programs, Internet recipe sites, and free community cooking classes. Mandy and the therapist also discussed the possibility of gradually increasing her job duties with the kitchen supervisor.

To present this idea of gradually increasing work responsibilities, Mandy and the therapist used role playing to help Mandy plan how she could effectively communicate her needs to her supervisor. As a result, Mandy was initially only required to find two recipes a week that she thought she would be able to prepare

and make one entree with the assistance of the kitchen manager. Mandy and the therapist continued to discuss different strategies of communication and how communication skills can help to produce a successful work experience. As she became more conscious of her interaction style, Mandy noticed that her kitchen supervisor seemed more willing to accommodate her schedule requests and more receptive when Mandy needed help. Mandy was eventually able to request a schedule change of her supervisor, without assistance from the occupational therapist, to attend a doctor's appointment.

Mandy's added job responsibilities meant she would work paid extra hours. She described the extra money as "not even noticeable because it just means that my family asks for more." As money started to cause friction between Mandy and her family, she began to question the benefits of going back to work. Mandy was becoming resentful because she had initially thought of her family as a support to her returning to work and now concluded that they were taking advantage of her employment. As a result, the occupational therapist and Mandy discussed the need to establish appropriate boundaries with her family. They also worked together to develop an appropriate budget that would allow Mandy to keep up with her bills rather than fall deeper in to debt.

During the last 5 of her 12 weeks in the kitchen, Mandy enrolled in the Kitchen Sanitation Certification program at the community college. The occupational therapist assisted her in creating a daily schedule that included work, school, meetings, and time for studying. Upon completion of her traineeship, Mandy took the sanitation certification examination. Unfortunately, she did not achieve her certification.

As a consequence, Mandy canceled her occupational therapy sessions for the next 2 weeks and avoided all contact with the occupational therapist. During this time, the occupational therapist continued to leave reminders about their meetings and the weekly occupational therapy groups in Mandy's mailbox, but chose not to confront Mandy about her poor attendance. After 1 month of limited contact, Mandy attended an occupational therapy group. The occupational therapist asked Mandy if she would stay after the group to talk, and Mandy agreed. Mandy opened up to the therapist about the shame and humiliation she felt after having failed the certification examination. The occupational therapist validated Mandy's feelings and then worked with her to identify positive outcomes of her traineeship, such as completing the 12-week program, earning increased responsibilities, effectively communicating with her supervisor, and so on.

During this conversation, Mandy was able to reexamine her experiences in the trainee program and recognize her myriad achievements during the 12-week program. Mandy stated she did not want to retake the certification examination at this time but was willing to continue with her goal of finding employment in the community by following up with a local organization that helps formerly incarcerated individuals reenter the workforce .

Postscript

Three months after completing the RTEP, Mandy began looking for seasonal work and found a job with a florist delivering orders during Valentine's Day, Easter, Mother's Day, Thanksgiving, and Christmas. Her work assignments usually lasted 2 to 3 weeks and provided just enough money until the next holiday period. Mandy liked the short intervals associated with seasonal work. She said, "I feel like I work enough times out of the year to consider myself productive. Because the assignments only last 2 to 3 weeks, I don't find myself getting bored. Before I know it, the assignment is over and I can go back to my normal life with a little more cash in my pocket until the next holiday rolls around." Mandy also continued to work with the organization that helps formerly incarcerated individuals reenter the workforce to find continuous part-time employment. She has not retaken the sanitation certification test.

Mandy In Perspective

Like many people with occupational histories marked by significant deviant behavior and failure, Mandy faced a major challenge trying to find a new and satisfying pattern of occupational performance. At the time she began therapy, Mandy had an overwhelming sense of failure and limited work experience. In addition, she had a history of sabotaging efforts to improve her life situation and an aggressive and confrontational man-

ner when communicating. Finally, she had had a narrative in which she was able to follow through with something successfully and improve her life. She had to completely reorganize her values, interests, life roles, and habit patterns and occupational narrative.

Consequently, a seamless transition into a new occupational lifestyle was not to be expected. Rather, Mandy's occupational therapy service plan had to be flexible to accommodate her pace and direction of change and to recognize and support what she was able to accomplish. Although she never received her certificate in kitchen sanitation or job offers in a related field, Mandy was able to make her support meetings, complete the RTEP, request job modifications, follow through on sealing and expunging past charges on her criminal record, and independently seek out and maintain seasonal work. These were major accomplishments for her, and they contributed to a significant improvement over her past occupational life—an improvement in which Mandy rightfully takes pride.

Mary: Reinvesting in Valued Roles

Mary is 84 years old and lives in a beautifully maintained house in a small town in England with her husband. She has a 40-year history of depressive illness with agitation and mood swings. Despite this, she has led a fruitful and interesting life.

Three years ago Mary began a marked withdrawal from some of her interests. A year and a half ago, she was referred to a day hospital for older people with functional mental health problems. At this point she had prolonged low mood, apathy, and lack of energy during the day. She was frequently agitated and exhibited antisocial behavior such as shouting during the night.

By this time, she was doing very little for herself and her husband had assumed full responsibility for the running of their home. On questioning, Mary described herself as resting. Her husband reported that Mary's day generally consisted of eating and sleeping.

Mary's Background

During Mary's initial involvement in the day hospital, the occupational therapist used unstructured interviewing to slowly get to know Mary while building rapport. The following information emerged about Mary's past occupational life. She started her working life as a teacher after earning a university degree in history. However, she tired of teaching and wanted something more challenging for a career. She set her mind on a career in law and completed her qualification in law in a year's less time than was the norm. Mary enjoyed a prestigious career in the practice of law. As one of few women in her field at the time, Mary served as a role model and mentor to young women who aspired to enter the male-dominated profession. Her branch of law required that Mary spend a great deal of time in the public arena. She became a well-known and highly respected figure in the region.

In addition to her career, Mary pursued a number of interests. She enjoyed writing, and some of her work was published. She was an expert gardener who specialized in cacti. She also enjoyed reading literature, wrote her own recipes, and was an accomplished piano player.

On retirement, Mary continued to enjoy several of these interests and in addition took up baking and dressmaking, creating a whole new wardrobe for herself. She had managed to be active and involved until the point of her sudden decline 3 years earlier.

As Mary settled into the day hospital, she appeared to enjoy the social contact it afforded. While she was reluctant to engage in activities, she was quite social and took advantage of every opportunity to talk to others about her past occupations. Her husband reported an improvement in her agitation, possibly due to new medication and the change of environment during the day.

Despite this improvement, Mary refused to engage in activities in the day hospital and remained almost completely passive at home. The team asked the occupational therapist to focus on reengaging Mary in her previous interests. Mary's occupational therapist arranged a home visit to meet with Mary and her husband in their own environment. She wanted to gather more information and to establish what they saw as problem areas. During the home visit, the occupational therapist found out more about Mary's past and saw some of Mary's published works.

The therapist chatted separately with Mary and her husband about their life at home. According to Mary, there were no problems. She noted that after all, she was retired and this meant "resting". In contrast, her husband described a downhill struggle over the past 2 years, during which time Mary became increasingly unwilling to do things around the home and became increasingly agitated. The husband was quite willing to be caretaker for Mary, but found her agitated and combative behavior difficult to manage.

With the information that had been gathered at this point, the occupational therapist began to formulate a number of questions: Why did Mary begin to withdraw from the occupations she had valued and enjoyed? Was Mary's description of "resting" a sign that something had changed in her volition? The therapist further wondered if a subtle change in functional capacity might be underlying her choice to withdraw from her occupations.

Administration of the Model of Human Occupational Screening Tool

The therapist decided to assess Mary initially through informal observation. In the day hospital, the therapist gently encouraged Mary to participate in more active pursuits based on her previous interests. For example, she asked Mary to help with potting plants and to bake some simple scones for herself and her husband. During these and other activities, it became apparent that Mary had severe process skill deficits. Moreover, after initially trying these tasks, Mary became angry and hostile and refused to return to the day hospital.

The occupational therapist visited Mary at home. She avoided any discussion of her functional capacity, as it was clear that this topic gave her high levels of distress. After several sessions of gentle discussion, Mary was persuaded to return to the day hospital once a week. She clearly stated that she had no desire to participate in cooking, crafts, or gardening and only enjoyed group discussions. If asked to do anything she didn't want, she would telephone her husband and ask him to come get her immediately. Then she would refuse to attend for several days.

Her husband reported that her agitation increased whenever she was not attending day hospital. Staff at the day hospital felt that they had been put in a difficult position. The program was built around a philosophy of engaging clients in activities. However, when asked to engage in an activity, Mary would withdraw from the day hospital and her husband would suffer her increased agitation.

To try to understand Mary's behavior, strengths, and weaknesses and make sense of the situation, the occupational therapist used the information she had gleaned from the home visit, informal discussions with Mary and her husband, and observations to complete a Model of Human Occupational Screening Tool (MOHOST). The MOHOST assessment allowed her to gain an overview of Mary's occupational functioning (*Fig. 21.9*). The qualitative report her therapist wrote follows:

VOLITION

Mary's scores were low in this area and reflect a mismatch between her personal causation and her performance skills. Mary viewed herself very positively based on her previous high-achieving lifestyle. She presents her abilities as though they were all intact. Although able to talk about a variety of past interests, Mary makes it very clear that she does not wish to engage in any of these, preferring to sleep or chat. It appears that Mary either (1) is unable to face her limitations and avoids activities as a means of avoiding the pain of admitting her loss of capacity or (2) wants to avoid the public disgrace of being seen as incompetent by others. It is also possible that some combination of these two factors is involved. In either case, Mary cannot manage to reflect on her current skill levels and incorporate an accurate understanding of her limitations into making choices about her occupational life.

She actively defends her volitional status by arguing that she is "resting" upon retirement. In addition, Mary argues that she had previously been driven to participate in her chosen occupations by monetary gain and success. Thus, she notes that her previous interests are "not appropriate in retirement." She has managed a rather elaborate strategy to guard herself against the personal pain and public embarrassment of admitting her limited capacity. This strategy is consistent with a history of having achieved highly and publicly in a number of

---

areas despite a chronic illness. As a consequence of her decision to do nothing in order to preserve her previous volitional image of herself, she has become totally inactive and reliant on her husband in order to meet her daily goals.

HABITUATION

Mary stated that her daily routine consisting of "rest" suited her well and that she did not wish to change this. As previously discussed, she had withdrawn from her previous roles and became hostile when required to face any responsibility. She did not seem aware of the impact that this had on her husband.

COMMUNICATION AND INTERACTION SKILLS

Mary was generally able to exchange information adequately, though she was observed to experience word-finding difficulty which became worse when she was feeling frustrated. She was however, able to read aloud written information (e.g., a poem) perfectly. Mary's body language and tone were sometimes overly assertive or demanding, which negatively impacts on her ability to establish positive relationships within the day hospital.

MOTOR SKILLS

Mary's motor skills are generally as expected for her age. She walks slowly, and sometimes awkwardly with a stooped posture, using a walking stick for support. She has some difficulty coordinating her movements, and a slight tremor is evident in both arms on movement. Mary's energy level is very low and she remains inactive at home.

PROCESS SKILLS

Clear cognitive impairment is apparent during activity. She has difficulty selecting tools for a task (e.g., picking up a paintbrush to paint with), and required much verbal and visual prompting to plan and sequence. Mary was observed to try to dip the paintbrush into a pot of paint when the lid was still on. Following errors such as this, Mary has become unwilling to participate in any further activity-based sessions, which ruled out further more formal assessment of her process skills.

ENVIRONMENT

Mary's home environment offers a variety of opportunities for occupational participation including books, her piano, a garden and well-maintained comfortable surroundings and furniture. Despite a previously active social life, she remains isolated from the "outside world" other than the company of her husband and peers and staff within the day hospital. Her isolation from previous colleagues, acquaintances, and friends appears to emanate from her volitional situation as discussed above.

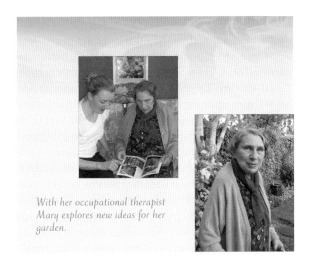

With her occupational therapist Mary explores new ideas for her garden.

FIGURE 21.9 Mary's ratings on the Model of Human Occupation Screening Tool.

Summary of Ratings																							
Motivation for Occupation				Pattern of Occupation				Communication & Interaction skills				Process skills				Motor skills				Environment: *Home & Day Hospital*			
Appraisal of ability	Expectation of success	Interest	Choices	Routine	Adaptability	Roles	Responsibility	Non-verbal skills	Conversation	Vocal expression	Relationships	Knowledge	Timing	Organization	Problem-solving	Posture & Mobility	Coordination	Strength & Effort	Energy	Physical space	Physical resources	Social groups	Occupational demands
F	F	F	F	F	F	F	F	F	F	F	F	F	F	F	F	F	F	F	F	**F**	**F**	F	F
A	A	A	A	A	A	A	A	**A**	**A**	**A**	A	A	A	A	A	A	A	A	A	A	A	A	A
I	I	I	I	I	I	I	I	I	I	I	**I**	**I**	I	I	I	**I**	**I**	**I**	I	I	I	**I**	I
R	**R**	**R**	**R**	**R**	**R**	**R**	**R**	R	R	R	R	R	**R**	**R**	**R**	R	R	R	**R**	**R**	R	R	**R**

Key:
F = Facilitates occupational participation
A = Allows occupational participation
I = Inhibits occupational participation
R = Restricts occupational participation

Development of an Intervention Plan

When Mary's therapist shared the results of the MO-HOST with the multidisciplinary team, they better understood Mary's choices and behaviors. Mary's occupational identity, particularly her sense of capacity and values, were strongly shaped by her previous roles and life achievements, which were earned in the face of an ongoing affective disorder. Her beliefs about her personal effectiveness and her ability to feel valuable and valued remained rooted in the past. Given Mary's age, the likelihood of further cognitive decline, and her husband's willingness to care for her so long as her agitation was managed, trying to challenge or change Mary's volition was not considered a useful strategy. Rather, the team felt that Mary's and her husband's quality of life would be enhanced by supporting her volition as it was constructed.

This reformulation of Mary's refusal to participate in the activity program of the day hospital allowed the team to view her day hospital attendance in a much more positive light. Because many of her past roles involved functioning in a very public arena, the following kind of interventions were implemented. Mary was given the opportunity to discuss her past achievements. She was asked to read out loud some of her written work. Mary enjoyed reading aloud some of her work within the day hospital and gaining positive feedback from others. Over time, she was even gently persuaded to participate in simple creative writing sessions in a group. She enjoyed listening to the contributions of others as well as reading out loud her own. Given the opportunity to reflect on her past and demonstrate her remaining competence, she became enthused and animated in the day hospital.

Mary continues to attend the day hospital and participate in these low-key activities with enthusiasm, and as a result, her agitation levels dramatically decreased. She returns home in a calm, content state of mind. Staff in the day hospital do not push Mary to participate in activities in which she would fail or struggle. Current intervention aims to preserve Mary's occupational identity.

Conclusion

This chapter presented four cases that represent applications of MOHO in a community-based context. In presenting the cases, we sought to emphasize how therapists achieved client-centered practice that respected the client's views and desires. We also tried to point out how community-based practice inevitably draws therapists into dealing with the contexts in which clients work, play, and do their activities of daily living: home, school, neighborhood, community, and workplace.

References

Ayres, AJ. (1979). *Sensory Integration and the Child*. Western Psychological Services, Los Angeles.

Benbow, M. (1999). *Loops and Other Groups: A Kinesthetic Writing System*. San Antonio, TX: Psychological Corp.

Bundy, A.C., Lane, S.J., & Murray, E. (Eds.) (2002). *Sensory Integration: Theory and Practice* (2nd ed.). Philadelphia: FA Davis.

Kielhofner, G., & Fisher, A. (1991). Mind-brain-body relationships. In A. Fisher, E. Murray, & A. Bundy (Eds.), *Sensory integration: Theory and practice* (pp. 27–45). Philadelphia: FA Davis.

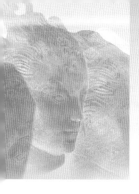

22

Enabling Clients to Reconstruct Their Occupational Lives in Long-Term Settings

- Gary Kielhofner
- Christiane Mentrup
- Claudia Miranda
- Daniela Schulte
- Jayne Shepherd

This chapter presents three cases from inpatient physical and psychiatric rehabilitation. A common theme throughout the cases is how therapy enabled these persons to envision and live their lives differently. While the nature of the clients' impairments varied, they shared a common challenge. Each had to reorganize volition, reconstruct habit patterns, revise or reengage in life roles, and find new ways to effectively perform and participate in occupational life.

The therapists often had to gently nudge clients toward new ways of experiencing and seeing things, toward recognition of painful realities, and toward making hard decisions and compromises. They were able to help their clients to change through careful understanding of their situation made possible through the concepts and tools provided by MOHO.

Fredrick: Finding a Way to Trust Therapy

Clients do not always see the value of therapy. For a variety of reasons, they may feel that therapy is unnecessary or unhelpful. Fredrick came to therapy with serious doubts. Consequently, his therapist had to take special care to build a sense of trust and motivate him to collaborate in therapy. This case illustrates how MOHO provides a useful set of concepts and tools for under-

standing and building trust with a client who is not positively motivated toward therapy.

At age 23, Fredrick was admitted to a psychiatric ward of a general hospital in a small northern German city. He was diagnosed with depression, which he had had since childhood. Before this admission he spent 3 weeks in a psychiatric ward of another local hospital but left against medical advice. The next day he attempted suicide.

Fredrick had an understandably negative attitude toward psychiatric institutions. When Fredrick was 9 years old, his mother committed suicide in a psychiatric ward. His mother's death and doubts about the meaning of his own life dominated Fredrick's thoughts and feelings as a young man. Because he had little faith in the worth of psychiatric care, Fredrick had always been ambivalent at best about receiving psychiatric services. He regularly dismissed the advice of those attempting to provide him psychiatric services. He rarely followed through on their recommendations.

Guiding Questions and Initial Assessment

Fredrick's history suggested that he had longstanding problems of occupational adaptation. Therefore, the therapist's main questions focused on understanding

Fredrick's occupational identity and competence. Furthermore, she realized that his cooperation with therapy would depend on her understanding of his volition and being able to engage him in terms of his own view of himself and his world.

Because of Fredrick's history and perspective on psychiatric care, the occupational therapist was particularly concerned with beginning assessment in a way that might build some trust and give him confidence in the therapist's genuine desire and ability to offer help. One advantage of MOHO-based assessments is that they focus on everyday occupational life rather than on illness or disability; they are aimed at revealing the client's unique perceptions, desires, and experiences. Using these assessments can often help to build trust and confidence.

The occupational therapist decided to begin assessment with the Occupational Performance History Interview—II (OPHI-II). She reasoned that it would give Fredrick a chance to tell his own story and enable her to begin to build rapport with him. Also, it provides a level of detailed information that is often important to thoroughly understanding the perspective of a client.

At the beginning of the interview, Fredrick was aloof and skeptical. As he began to tell his occupational narrative and saw the interest of the therapist in his viewpoint, he became more open.

The OPHI-II pointed toward difficulties Fredrick had in enjoying life and feeling connected to roles. Therefore, the therapist decided to ask Fredrick to complete the Interest Checklist and the Role Checklist next. She chose these assessments because they allowed Fredrick to actively report about himself. To underscore this point, the therapist gave these assessments to Fredrick to fill out on his own. She explained them as opportunities for him to reflect on and record how he viewed these two important aspects of his life. The therapist also informally observed and had conversations with Fredrick on the ward and in occupational therapy. The sections that follow describe the assessment process and the understanding of Fredrick's occupational circumstances that the therapist was able to construct along with him.

Fredrick's Occupational Identity and Competence

Fredrick began his occupational narrative when he dropped out of high school. He saw no purpose and had no interest in school. For a while after leaving school he did nothing. Then he was accepted as a carpentry apprentice. A 3-year apprenticeship with a master carpenter is the traditional way to learn this trade in Germany. However, after only 4 weeks, Fredrick quit because he had second thoughts about whether he really wanted to learn carpentry.

Following this, Fredrick was unemployed. After almost a year, he decided to undertake training as a car mechanic. After successfully completing general mechanics training, he went on to take specialized courses in truck mechanics. Not long after he began employment as a mechanic, he quit the job. He had chronic back pain that he attributed to spending much of the day bent over his work. He was also disillusioned with his lack of satisfaction on this job.

Fredrick was unemployed for the next 6 months. During this time he sought treatment for his back pain at a German spa. Fredrick's physician also advised that he not return to mechanics because of his back problem. Thus, Fredrick began working as a janitor's assistant in an administration building complex. The pay was good, but he soon found himself once again disillusioned with his work. He quit the janitorial job, which was his last form of employment.

Fredrick related his occupational narrative as a series of failed attempts to find meaningful work. He complained of being unable to find enjoyment and satisfaction in what he did, even when he tried hard. He had not developed a clear sense of what he might find satisfying and had no clear identification with a work role or career. He lacked confidence in his ability to find something meaningful and stick with it. Along with the pattern of repeated unsuccessful attempts at work, Fredrick saw the future as gloomy. He expected more of the same and accordingly did not see a reason for trying.

Fredrick was convinced that any effort he made would ultimately result in the same disappointment and disillusionment as before. He could not recall a time in his life when things were really good. Most of his everyday life patterns had been bland and unfulfilling to him. He could not imagine a life that he would find satisfying.

Along with his extreme difficulty in constructing an occupational identity, Fredrick had ongoing difficulty sustaining occupational competence (i.e., a pattern of everyday action that supported being productive and satisfied). His problems in occupational identity and competence are reflected in the first two scales of the OPHI-II as shown in *Figure 22.1*.

Fredrick's Volition

During the OPHI-II interview, Fredrick initially expressed skepticism about the merits of occupational therapy. The therapist offered to show him the areas where ther-apy took place and the things that were available there for him to do. He agreed to take a look. When he saw the therapy crafts room, he indicated that he had always had an interest in arts and crafts but never had an opportunity to follow up on this interest. With encour-

FIGURE 22.1 Fredrick's ratings on the OPHI-II scales.

Occupational Identity Scale	1	2	3	4
Has personal goals and projects	X			
Identifies a desired occupational lifestyle		X		
Expects success	X			
Accepts responsibility		X		
Appraises abilities and limitations			X	
Has commitments and values			X	
Recognizes identity and obligations		X		
Has interests		X		
Felt effective (past)	X			
Found meaning and satisfaction in lifestyle (past)	X			
Made occupational choices (past)	X			
Occupational Competence Scale	1	2	3	4
Maintains satisfying lifestyle		X		
Fulfills role expectations		X		
Works toward goals		X		
Meets personal performance standards		X		
Organizes time for responsibilities		X		
Participates in interests		X		
Fulfilled roles (past)	X			
Maintained habits (past)	X			
Achieved satisfaction (past)	X			
Occupational Settings (Environment) Scale	1	2	3	4
Home-life occupational forms		X		
Major productive role occupational forms	X			
Leisure occupational forms			X	
Home-life social group				X
Major productive social group		X		
Leisure social group		X		
Home-life physical spaces, objects, and resources				X
Major productive role physical spaces, objects, and resources		X		
Leisure physical spaces, objects, and resources				X

Key: **1** = Extreme occupational functioning problems
   2 = Some occupational functioning problems
   3 = Appropriate, satisfactory occupational functioning
   4 = Exceptionally competent occupational functioning

agement from the therapist, he decided to work on some clay projects during an open activity group.

His attraction to doing creative activities was also reflected in his responses to the Interest Checklist (*Fig. 22.2 A, B & C*). Similarly, during the OPHI-II interview he mentioned creative interests but again noted that he had never followed up on them. The Interest Checklist also indicated that Fredrick was inclined toward sports, arts, and culture.

During the OPHI-II interview, Fredrick indicated that his personal values included having freedom to make his own choices and making good use of his leisure time. Nevertheless, he noted that he lacked confidence in his own decision-making ability and had not used his leisure time well for a long time. It was also clear that he wanted to have a work career but felt defeated in reaching this goal after all his failures.

Fredrick showed very poor personal causation. He doubted his capacity and felt he had been very ineffective in the past. Fredrick felt no control over the events in his life. He was quite hopeless about the possibility of success in the future. His long history of difficulties and failures left him with little energy to try anything new or to work toward goals.

Fredrick's Habituation

Fredrick indicated on the Role Checklist (*Fig. 22.3*) that he moderately to strongly valued the roles he had occupied recently and that he planned to fulfill them in the future. These included his roles as a friend, as a sportsman in an athletic club, and occasionally as a caretaker (baby sitter) for his sister's children. For many years, Fredrick had been living with a group of four friends in a rented house. He was very satisfied with this living arrangement and was accepted by the friends. This positive environmental impact is noted in his OPHI-II ratings (*Fig. 22.1*). Fredrick's family member role involved some contact with his sister, who lived 20 km away. He saw his father infrequently. He reported no other friends or social contacts. He felt his friend role was limited and expressed a longing to be able to have more intense human contact and to build up an extended circle of friends. Fredrick wanted to reenter the worker role and hoped to find a job that would fulfill him more than the others had.

Fredrick was dissatisfied with his former habits, which he described as lacking structure. The only scheduled activities he indicated were attending karate class 3 times a week and meeting friends once a week. However, for some time before his admission, he was not doing either of these things.

Fredrick's Performance Capacity, Performance, and Skill

Fredrick did not report any major limitations of capacity. He complained about mild back pain, but it did not interfere with his performance. He also noted that attending the karate class had had a relaxing and pain-relieving effect. He wanted to reinitiate his involvement in karate.

Fredrick chose to begin doing ceramics in occupational therapy. His therapist observed his performance informally to note whether he had any identifiable performance problems. Initially, Fredrick worked slowly, but this appeared related mainly to his continued depression. Nonetheless, he worked on his clay projects independently. Despite his stated desire to be involved in creative activities, Fredrick approached the tasks rather mechanically and without any obvious creative expression. Moreover, when he encountered problems with a new activity, he was reluctant to ask for help or information from the therapist or others.

Goal Setting

The occupational therapist shared her understanding of Fredrick's situation with him, and to a large extent he agreed. Fredrick clearly recognized that the therapist had made an earnest and successful effort to understand his perspective and to make sense of his circumstances. Consequently, he agreed that he would be willing to work with the therapist to accomplish some goals. Fredrick and the therapist together identified the following long-term goals and shared them with the multidisciplinary team:

- Fredrick will develop new perspectives for restructuring his occupational identity
- Fredrick will undertake vocational retraining in a more creative and less physically demanding area
- Fredrick will have a greater degree of satisfaction in everyday life
- Fredrick will increase the number of his friends and increase his involvement with others.

FIGURE 22.2A Fredrick's responses on the Interest Checklist.

Activity:	What has been your level of interest?						Do you currently participate in this activity?		Would you like to pursue this in the future?	
	In the past ten years			In the past year						
	Strong	Some	No	Strong	Some	No	Yes	No	Yes	No
Gardening/yardwork			x			x		x		x
Sewing/needlework			x			x		x		x
Playing cards		x				x		x	x	
Foreign languages	x				x			x	x	
Church activities			x			x		x		x
Radio		x			x		x		x	
Walking		x			x		x		x	
Car repair		x			x			x		x
Writing			x			x		x		x
Dancing			x	x				x	x	
Golf			x			x		x		x
Football			x			x		x		x
Listening to popular music		x			x			x	x	
Puzzles			x			x		x		x
Holiday activities	x			x				x	x	
Pets/livestock			x			x		x		x
Movies			x			x		x		x
Listening to classical music		x			x			x	x	
Speeches/lectures			x			x		x		x
Swimming		x		x			x		x	
Bowling			x			x		x		x
Visiting		x			x			x	x	
Mending			x			x		x		x
Checkers/chess			x		x			x	x	
Barbecues			x			x		x		x
Reading			x		x			x	x	
Traveling			x			x		x		x
Parties		x			x			x	x	

continued

FIGURE 22.2B Fredrick's responses on the Interest Checklist (*continued*)

Activity:	What has been your level of interest?						Do you currently participate in this activity?		Would you like to pursue this in the future?	
	In the past ten years			In the past year						
	Strong	Some	No	Strong	Some	No	Yes	No	Yes	No
Wrestling			X	X				X	X	
House cleaning			X			X		X		X
Model building			X			X		X		X
Television			X			X		X		X
Concerts	X			X			X		X	
Pottery		X		X			X		X	
Camping	X					X		X		X
Laundry/ironing			X			X		X		X
Politics			X			X		X		X
Table games			X		X		X			X
Home decorating		X		X				X	X	
Clubs/lodge		X			X			X	X	
Singing		X			X			X		X
Scouting			X			X		X		X
Clothes			X			X		X		X
Handicrafts		X			X		X		X	
Hairstyling			X			X		X		X
Cycling		X		X				X	X	
Attending plays			X			X		X		X
Bird watching		X			X			X		X
Dating	X			X				X		X
Auto racing			X			X		X		X
Home repairs		X			X			X	X	
Exercise		X			X			X	X	
Hunting			X			X		X		X
Woodworking		X			X			X		X
Pool		X			X			X	X	
Driving		X			X			X	X	

FIGURE 22.2C Fredrick's responses on the Interest Checklist (*continued*)

Activity	What has been your level of interest						Do you currently participate in this activity?		Would you like to pursue this in the future?	
	In the past ten years			In the past year						
	Strong	Some	No	Strong	Some	No	Yes	No	Yes	No
Child care		✘			✘			✘	✘	✘
Tennis			✘			✘		✘		✘
Cooking/baking		✘		✘				✘	✘	
Basketball	✘				✘			✘	✘	
History		✘			✘			✘	✘	
Collecting			✘			✘		✘		✘
Fishing			✘			✘		✘		✘
Science			✘			✘		✘		✘
Leatherwork			✘			✘		✘		✘
Shopping			✘			✘		✘		✘
Photography			✘			✘		✘		✘
Painting/drawing		✘		✘			✘		✘	

FIGURE 22.3 Fredrick's responses on the Role Checklist.

Role	Role Identity			Value Designation		
	Past	Present	Future	Not at all valuable	Somewhat valuable	Very valuable
Student	X		X		X	
Worker	X		X		X	
Volunteer				X		
Care giver	X		X		X	
Home maintainer	X		X		X	
Friend	X	X	X			X
Family member	X	X	X		X	
Religious participant				X		
Hobbyist/Amateur	X		X		X	
Participant in organizations				X		
Other:	X	X		X		

To work toward these long-term goals, the therapist and Frederick developed short-term goals and a plan of therapy. These were refined as the course of therapy unfolded.

Course of Treatment and Outcome

Fredrick remained in psychiatric rehabilitation for 10 weeks. Consistent with his history, he periodically expressed his ambivalence about psychiatric care with sarcastic remarks and by challenging hospital staff. Fredrick did participate in occupational therapy throughout this period. Initially, however, he was wary, and his attitude toward therapy was inconsistent.

Four weeks after admission he attempted suicide again, by cutting a gash in his neck. Immediately after harming himself, he panicked and sought nursing assistance. Following this incident, Fredrick was transferred to a more structured rehabilitation unit. This event proved to be a turning point for Fredrick. He began to recognize that he needed to do something to change his life. With encouragement, he slowly began to open up to the possibility that with help he might be able to improve his life. Since the occupational therapy department provided services to clients in several units, Fredrick was able to continue with the same therapist and the same therapy plan. Over the next 6 weeks,

Fredrick became increasingly invested in occupational therapy.

Fredrick attended craft groups regularly, working with clay. He became more able to accept coaching and feedback from the therapist to improve his performance. On his own, he chose to start reading books about working with clay. With time, his technique improved and he became more relaxed and creative when he worked with the clay. He also learned to seek advice and suggestions and to ask for help when he encountered a new problem. As a result, he was able to produce pottery objects that he found pleasing. His sense of efficacy in doing something of value increased over time. He began to feel a sense of pleasure and satisfaction.

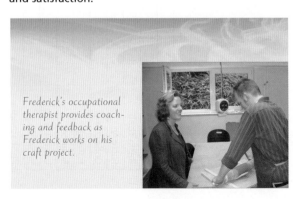

Frederick's occupational therapist provides coaching and feedback as Frederick works on his craft project.

During this time, Fredrick expressed concern to the therapist about his difficulties interacting with others. Based on his concerns and her own observation of his tendency to isolate himself, the therapist informally interviewed him about this aspect of his performance. Fredrick admitted that he was greatly distressed and felt very uncomfortable around people, with the exception of the long-term friends with whom he lived. He was also able to recognize that this discomfort was an obstacle to his goal of establishing new friends and intensifying his social contacts.

Fredrick identified that he felt very insecure about his skills for interacting with others. At this point, the therapist advised Fredrick that the Assessment of Communication and Interaction Skills (ACIS) could help identify his social strengths and weaknesses. Fredrick acknowledged that while he lacked confidence in his social skills, he had no idea what his strengths and weaknesses were. He agreed that such information would be useful.

They decided on the following approach. Since Fredrick had developed some good skills for working with clay, the therapist suggested that it would be a good learning experience for him to lead a small ceramics group. Fredrick was reluctant at first but then agreed to do it. The therapist and Fredrick decided to videotape the group so that they could review his performance afterward. Fredrick was able to lead the group, giving initial instructions and supporting the other clients when they needed it.

Afterward, Fredrick and the therapist together used the ACIS to rate his communication/interaction skills while watching the videotape. Because of Fredrick's history of distrust of therapy, the therapist administered the ACIS in this way to give Fredrick a greater sense of control and responsibility for recognizing his own strengths and weaknesses. She invited Fredrick to rate himself and then offered to compare his views with hers. To allow Fredrick to do the rating, the therapist explained the meaning of each item.

Figure 22.4 shows both the therapist's and Fredrick's ratings, illustrating that they were in close agreement. Using the ACIS in this way allowed Fredrick to concretely see his own limits in sustaining communication and in providing verbal support and information to others. He recognized some of his obstacles to being able to engage and respond to other persons' needs.

The occupational therapist also gave him feedback concerning strengths that he showed in this situation. Fredrick considered this exercise a success, since it reassured him of social abilities he did possess and gave him some concrete feedback on areas to improve. He was proud to have done it despite his initial reservations. Moreover, he found it a positive experience to see himself on videotape successfully leading the group.

The assessment exercise increased his confidence in his social skills. He came to recognize that even with some weaknesses, he could get along with people. At the same time, he became aware of the fact that he needed some time to retreat and that when he allowed this for himself, he was more motivated and better able to interact with others. He identified a necessary rhythm between doing solitary things and being socially involved.

Fredrick collaborated with the occupational therapist to examine his habit patterns and to plan for a more productive and satisfying use of his time. At first, Fredrick was unable to plan for himself, so he agreed to allow the occupational therapist to structure a weekly plan with him that reflected things that had been positive for him in the past. Then they worked together to see how this schedule could be modified to reflect his growing interests, role involvement, and occasional need for some private space. By the time the team was planning discharge with Fredrick, he had completely taken over responsibility for sustaining his daily structure. He was highly motivated to keep planning and sustaining his daily routine.

Over the course of therapy, Fredrick showed increased efficacy, enjoyment, and satisfaction with his performance. He was able to plan and expect success in projects. As he became more regularly involved in performance and had some success, he was able to identify an increasing range of interests and to explore new things. By the time of his discharge, he showed markedly improved personal causation. As Fredrick put it, he realized that he "had adequate skills but just didn't use them."

Fredrick also came to realize how much his preoccupation with anxiety about performance and his conviction that life had no meaning had interfered both with his performance and enjoyment of the things he did. He focused on approaching performance with a positive attitude and on relaxing and enjoying what he

FIGURE 22.4 Therapist ratings and Fredrick's self-ratings on the Assessment of Communication/Interaction Skills.

Physicality	4	3	2	1
Contacts	X			
Gazes	X			
Gestures		X		
Maneuvers		X		
Orients	X			
Postures		X		
Information Exchange	**4**	**3**	**2**	**1**
Articulates		X		
Asserts		X		
Asks			X	
Engages		X		
Expresses		X		
Modulates		X		
Shares			X	
Speaks		X		
Sustains		X		
Relations	**4**	**3**	**2**	**1**
Collaborates		X		
Conforms		X		
Focuses	X			
Relates	Not Applicable			
Respects	X			

Key: **4** = Competent; **3** = Questionable; **2** = Ineffective; **1** = Deficit

☐ Self-Assessment |X| Therapist Assessment

did. In collaboration with Fredrick, the therapist used his responses on the Interest Checklist as a guide for him to try out new things. Fredrick realized that many of the things he thought he might like to do he had never or only partly tried. Consequently, he explored a variety of interests during his hospitalization and was able to identify the things that were most enjoyable to him.

As his confidence increased and as he identified things he enjoyed, he was able to identify three major goals for himself to pursue after discharge. These were to improve his karate skills, to learn to play a musical instrument, and to learn a second language. Before discharge, Fredrick, in collaboration with the social worker and the occupational therapist, took the initia-tive to contact the local labor department for an appointment. There he began to plan for vocational training in an area that would allow him more creativity. He identified getting this training as another major goal to pursue after discharge.

Fredrick in Perspective

Fredrick began therapy with a very poor occupational identity. It included feelings of inability, lack of interest and enjoyment in life, difficulty identifying goals combined with limited role involvement, negative experiences in the worker role, and an unsatisfying daily routine. All of these elements of occupational identity were woven into a narrative in which the dominant theme was a series of failed attempts with no prospect for a positive future. This narrative also included a viewpoint that therapy would not help him.

The therapist earned Fredrick's trust and engaged him by giving him a voice and a degree of control. She initially did this by engaging him in assessments that allowed him to tell his story and write down his own view of things. Moreover, her interest in learning how he saw things and her efforts to understand his situation helped to win Fredrick's trust.

One notable strategy was the therapist's use of the ACIS. Engaging the client in completing the ratings with her was not only a good way to enable him to have a voice but also an effective means to involve him in developing a more realistic understanding of his strengths and weaknesses. In fact, it was not his lack of skills that primarily isolated him but rather his sense of incapacity and inefficacy in interacting with others. Once he was able to change his thoughts and feelings about his social effectiveness, the problem of social isolation was largely ameliorated. In addition, he was aware of areas of weakness that he would attempt to improve.

Clients should never be written off as uncooperative and noncompliant. They are always acting from their own narratives and with the rationale those narratives provide. Successful therapy means giving those narratives voice and working within them. This, of course, is almost always a difficult task that requires tact and patience on the part of the therapist. The potential payoff of such efforts is made apparent by this case. Once the therapist earned Fredrick's trust and respect, he was able to begin to recognize and to address each of his problems and challenges. He was able to begin to develop a positive occupational narrative for himself in which there was hope for the future. That is, he came to envision himself as enjoying life, finding satisfying work, and developing more friendships and social involvement. Finally he identified personal projects for himself (learning a language, taking karate, and learning to play a musical instrument). Constructing an occupational identity that envisioned a positive future was a major accomplishment for Fredrick. Although much of the challenge of enacting this identity (i.e., occupational competence) remained to be realized after discharge, he had a story to realize—something that was formerly absent.

Julia: Rediscovering Volition

Julia is a 60-year-old Argentine woman with cerebral palsy. She has moderate dysarthria resulting in difficulty making herself understood. Her motor impairment has prevented her from being independent in activities of daily living. Thus, she has always required substantial assistance. Nevertheless, Julia has maintained a remarkable history of occupational participation. She recently moved to a residence for older adults, a situation that has significantly altered her quality of life.

The residence is in the city of Mar del Plata. It houses 70 people whose average age is 85. The residents have a wide range of diagnoses, but a large percentage of them have cognitive impairments and dementia. Consequently, the institution's daily routine is highly structured. At home Julia used to wake up later in the morning and go to bed late, so that she could watch the television programs she enjoyed. However, the residential facility wakes residents early and puts them to bed early.

Julia was initially assigned to a room she shared with three other residents with whom she did not feel very comfortable. Soon after, she was transferred to a smaller room that she shared with a 90-year-old woman who talked to herself, had severe hearing loss, and advanced severe dementia. Moreover, the physical space of the room did not allow Julia to move around in her wheelchair, nor was the bathroom accessible to her. Upon being institutionalized, Julia also lost control over her finances.

Julia's wheelchair was too wide to pass easily through doorways. At home Julia was accustomed to maneuvering the wheelchair with her legs facing backward, but staff were afraid she would bump into and injure one of the elderly residents. Although she required only moderate assistance, she was required to eat in the small dining room with those who had severe motor and cognitive impairments and who required a great amount of assistance to eat. She was very upset that she was not allowed to join the others in the general dining room.

The staff of the facility had not worked with anyone with this diagnosis before, and they knew little about her impairment or her abilities. Julia's dysarthria and involuntary movements increased in severity as a result of the stress brought on by institutional life. Other residents, especially the older adults, began to think she had a mental impairment, and Julia quickly picked up on their comments, such as "Poor woman, what a shame." Julia frequently complained, "They don't understand me; they think I am stupid. Don't treat me like I'm stupid!"

Julia was understandably demoralized by her situation. The occupational therapist decided to begin her assessment of Julia by informally talking with her about her life history.

Julia's Story

Julia's mother was a principal at a school, and her father was a commissioner and inspector for the police. They were always very affectionate with their daughter, supporting her development by providing a stimulating environment, even though she required assistance to participate in activities of daily living.

Julia refers to her infancy and adolescence as being a period that was full of emotions, affection, and occupations. As a young girl she had many friends. When she played at their houses, they helped her with her needs without her having to be accompanied by an assistant. On her fifteenth birthday, her parents had a celebration, as was the tradition. Their friends and family came. She wore the traditional dress, and she danced the traditional waltz with her father.

She attended the local community primary school and was able to complete her homework with help from a personal assistant. Later, through a specialized program, she completed 2 years of high school. Julia enjoyed studying Castilian literature and botany and really stood out in these areas. She left school when she was about 20, which is also the time her father died. Her family then moved to the capital of Argentina.

Julia spent her free time pursuing many of her interests, such as going for walks in her wheelchair, window shopping, going to the movies or theater, or going out for a drink. She was able to do all of these activities with the help of a hired personal assistant.

She had a strong sense of personal causation and saw herself not as a disabled person who required an assistant but as a person capable of an autonomous life. She wanted to work, to marry, and to have children.

In time, Julia met a man who lived near her house and they began to date. A few months later, when Julia was 26, they decided to marry. After the wedding, they lived in a roomy apartment with her mother, brother, and the constant involvement of her personal assistant. Julia became pregnant and gave birth to a son whom she breast-fed and cared for with some assistance. However, her marriage did not go well. Her husband, an alcoholic, eventually became physically violent toward her. As a result, they separated after 2 years of marriage. In retrospect, Julia reflected, "I married on a whim, to demonstrate that I could get married like everyone else . . . to stop their gossip."

Julia began corresponding with another man over a long time, and when she was 31 years old, she met him in person. He lived in another city and had to keep his identity private for political reasons. They began to go out and 4 months later decided to live together.

Julia became pregnant. Her mother was skeptical of her having another child, since she had taken on a large role in the care of her first grandson. It was clear that they would all share in the care of this new child, since the couple lived in the house with Julia's mother. A girl was born. With the help of her husband and an assistant, Julia took on a more active role as a mother.

When her children were adolescents, Julia's husband died of pulmonary disease and her mother also died. A short time later Julia was diagnosed with a malignant tumor in her breast, which required an operation and followup treatment. This was a difficult stage in Julia's life, but she went on.

When Julia was about 55 years old, her daughter married, moved to another city, and had her first child. Julia continued living with her son, along with the help of a personal assistant. She began a small business selling goods from her home with the help of her neighbors. Julia felt that she had finally developed a worker role.

Julia deeply missed her daughter, and when asked, Julia moved to live with her daughter's family in a property Julia bought in Mar del Plata. Four years later, Julia's daughter, under the weight of caring for her own children and coping with marital problems, asked Julia to consider moving to an adult residential home. The idea was that Julia could spend some days living in the facility and the other days living in her daughter's house.

Julia agreed to move to the facility, which was the only option available to her. Her daughter's restricted finances and obligations for her own children meant that she could not travel to visit Julia as frequently as she had hoped.

The Impact of the Environment on Julia's Occupational Adaptation

Based on informal conversations with Julia and observations of her in the home, the occupational therapist concluded that the institutional environment had had major negative impacts on Julia's previously strong volition:

- A decrease in her personal causation characterized by feelings of loss of control over her life
- Lack of opportunities to enact her interests
- Inability to realize her values of autonomy, intellectual challenge, and close affectionate communication, along with feeling devalued by other residents, by staff, and by activities that she perceived as "silly games."

Establishing Goals

The occupational therapist decided to begin with a formal assessment that would most likely empower Julia. She proposed that Julia complete the Occupational Self-Assessment (OSA) to analyze her own occupational function. The environmental form of the OSA was also completed with Julia to gather additional information to inform therapeutic goal setting and intervention planning related to the influence of her new environment on her performance. After assisting Julia to complete it (*Figs. 22.5 A & B* and *22.6*) the therapist helped Julia identify her priorities for occupational therapy. This self-reflective evaluation served to validate Julia's feelings.

Together Julia and the occupational therapist discussed strategies for making changes, and Julia identified what she considered the most important to work on in therapy. With respect to herself, Julia had a long list of goals:

- To complete what I need to do
- To choose where to eat
- To take care of others
- To participate in a volunteer role

- To get around myself
- To manage my finances
- To express myself and fit in well with others
- To relax and enjoy myself
- To have a satisfying routine.

With respect to her environment Julia's goals were as follows:

- Have things I need to be productive
- Have people who help me and encourage me
- Have opportunities to do things that I value and that I like.

In discussing these goals, Julia emphasized performing in a volunteer and/or caregiver role. She identified that she had carried out the caregiver role for her children and grandchildren. She also recounted that in the past she had felt very satisfied doing charitable work for a large poverty-stricken family.

In fact, despite Julia's concerns about being "lumped together" with the elderly residents, she had taken to informally helping those with marked deterioration, keeping them company and advising the infirmary aides if a problem arose that required their presence. Similarly, she came up with voluntary tasks that she carried out. She spent a great amount of time in the entrance of the residential facility, functioning as a "lookout" where the professionals and other supporting staff could seek her out for information. For example, they could ask her if a certain professional had left. When they discussed this together, the occupational therapist suggested that Julia should formally develop a secretary–informant role.

The Course of Therapy

In collaboration with Julia, the occupational therapist decided on a course of therapy that would enhance the match between Julia and her new environment as well as give Julia resources to better manage this environment. First, the occupational therapist began to inform the facility personnel, visitors, and older residents who had most contact with Julia of her limits and abilities. In particular this meant informing them that her impairment was motor and not cognitive and that Julia was an intelligent and capable woman who had lived a full and productive life.

At the same time the therapist instructed Julia about aging and the limitations and potential of those

FIGURE 22.5 Julia's ratings on the Myself section of the OSA

Occupational Self Assessment
Myself

Name: ___Julia___   Date: _____

Step 1: Below are statements about things you do in everyday life. For each statement, circle how well you do it. If an item does not apply to you, cross it out and move on to the next item.				Step 2: Next, for each statement, circle how important this is to you.				Step 3: Choose up to 4 things about yourself that you would like to change (You can also write comments in this space)
	I have a lot of problem doing this	I have some difficulty doing this	I do this well	I do this extremely well	This is not so important to me	This is important to me	This is more important to me	This is most important to me	I would like to change
Concentrating on my tasks	lot of problem	some difficulty	**well**	extremely well	not so important	**important**	more important	most important	
Physically doing what I need to do	lot of problem	**some difficulty**	well	extremely well	not so important	**important**	more important	most important	
Taking care of the place where I live	lot of problem	some difficulty	**well**	extremely well	not so important	**important**	more important	most important	
Taking care of myself	lot of problem	some difficulty	**well**	extremely well	not so important	**important**	more important	most important	
Taking care of others for whom I am responsible	lot of problem	**some difficulty**	well	extremely well	not so important	**important**	more important	most important	*Grandchildren, older adults*
Getting where I need to go	**lot of problem**	some difficulty	well	extremely well	not so important	**important**	more important	most important	✓
Managing my finances	lot of problem	some difficulty	well	extremely well	not so important	important	**more important**	most important	*Right now this is a problem because they manage my finances; I want to regain control in this area*
Managing my basic needs (food, medicine)	lot of problem	**some difficulty**	well	extremely well	not so important	important	**more important**	most important	*Choosing where I eat*
Expressing myself to others	lot of problem	**some difficulty**	well	extremely well	not so important	important	**more important**	most important	*That they understand me better*
Getting along with others	lot of problem	**some difficulty**	well	extremely well	not so important	**important**	more important	most important	*I would feel better living here if they didn't think I was dumb*
Identifying and solving problems	lot of problem	some difficulty	**well**	extremely well	not so important	**important**	more important	most important	

FIGURE 22.5B Julia's ratings on the Myself section of the OSA (continued)

Myself

Name: _Julia_   Date: _____

	Step 1: Below are statements about things you do in everyday life. For each statement, circle how well you do it. If an item does not apply to you, cross it out and move on to the next item.				Step 2: Next, for each statement, circle how important this is to you.				Step 3: Choose up to 4 things about yourself that you would like to change (You can also write comments in this space)
	I have a lot of problem doing this	I have some difficulty doing this	I do this well	I do this extremely well	This is not so important to me	This is important to me	This is more important to me	This is most important to me	I would like to change
Relaxing and enjoying myself	lot of problem	**some difficulty**	well	extremely well	not so important	**important**	more important	most important	✓
Getting done what I need to do	lot of problem	**some difficulty**	well	extremely well	not so important	**important**	more important	most important	✓
Having a satisfying routine	**lot of problem**	some difficulty	well	extremely well	not so important	**important**	more important	most important	
Handling my responsibilities	lot of problem	some difficulty	**well**	extremely well	not so important	**important**	more important	most important	
Being involved as a student, worker, volunteer, and/or family member	lot of problem	some difficulty	well	extremely well	not so important	important	**more important**	most important	_I would like to become a volunteer in this environment_
Doing activities I like	lot of problem	some difficulty	**well**	extremely well	not so important	important	**more important**	most important	
Working towards my goals	lot of problem	some difficulty	**well**	extremely well	not so important	**important**	more important	most important	
Making decisions based on what I think is important	lot of problem	some difficulty	**well**	extremely well	**not so important**	important	more important	most important	
Accomplishing what I set out to do	lot of problem	some difficulty	**well**	extremely well	not so important	important	**more important**	most important	
Effectively using my abilities	lot of problem	**some difficulty**	well	extremely well	not so important	**important**	more important	most important	✓

393

FIGURE 22.6 Julia's ratings on the Environment section of the OSA.

My Environment

Name: _____ Julia _____   Date: _____

Step 1: Below are statements about things about your environment (where you live, work, go to school, etc.) For each statement, circle how this is for you. If an item does not apply to you, cross it out and move on to the next item.

Step 2: Next, for each statement, circle how important this aspect of your environment is to you.

Step 3: Choose up to 2 things about your environment that you would like to change (You can also write comments in this space)

	There is a lot of problem	There is some problem	This is good	This is extremely good	This is not so important to me	This is important to me	This is more important to me	This is most important to me	I would like to change
A place to live and take care of myself	lot of problem	**some problem**	good	extremely good	not so important	**important**	more important	most important	*My room and roommate*
A place where I can be productive (work, study, volunteer)	lot of problem	some problem	**good**	extremely good	**not so important**	important	more important	most important	
The basic things I need to live and take care of myself	lot of problem	some problem	**good**	extremely good	not so important	**important**	more important	most important	
The things I need to be productive	lot of problem	**some problem**	good	extremely good	not so important	important	**more important**	most important	✓
People who support and encourage me	lot of problem	**some problem**	good	extremely good	not so important	important	**more important**	most important	*I would like only one person to help me*
People who do things with me	lot of problem	**some problem**	good	extremely good	not so important	**important**	more important	most important	*Many people here are much older and have more disabling conditions than me*
Opportunities to do things I value and like	lot of problem	**some problem**	good	extremely good	not so important	**important**	more important	most important	*Watching TV late at night, chatting with my friends, eating with everyone else*
Places where I can go and enjoy myself	lot of problem	some problem	good	extremely good	not so important	important	more important	most important	*Not applicable*

who had slight or moderate dementia. The therapist then introduced the idea of developing a role of a secretary for Julia to the professional team, pointing out the importance of this role for Julia. Some responded positively, while others seemed resistant.

The therapist also successfully negotiated with the head administrator and personnel to modify Julia's daily routine so that Julia could wake up later and stay in the den watching television until 11:30 at night.

The occupational therapist also requested a smaller wheelchair that could be more easily maneuvered and a room that would allow her more mobility and social interaction. After a short time Julia was moved to a room that provided more space in which to move around, access to her bathroom, and the opportunity to communicate with her (higher functioning) roommates.

The therapist also recommended that Julia eat in the main dining room. However, administration did not agree to this change, since it would have required extra staff to be available in the main dining room to assist Julia.

Julia attended occupational therapy twice a week. Having learned that Julia would like to decorate her new living space, the therapist suggested that she make a collage, using pictures of her grandchildren. The therapist supported Julia physically while she chose the materials, forms, and colors. The therapist also coached Julia while she practiced how to maneuver her wheelchair in tight spaces without bumping other residents.

The occupational therapist worked together with the assistant activities coordinator to get Julia's children more involved. They conducted interviews with Julia's daughter and son, who visited her sporadically because he lived in another city. At first they negotiated more regular visits by Julia's daughter and then pursued the original plan that Julia would spend a few days in the house with her daughter's family. After a while, Julia began spending some time at her daughter's house.

Reexamining Her Approach

After 3 months, Julia's occupational therapy consisted of attending groups and individual counseling sessions. The occupational therapist observed that Julia had be-

come very demanding, possibly due to her renewed sense of control and her desire to meet her higher-level goals. Julia had increased the frequency and number of requests, some of which were not appropriate in the context of therapy and which required the occupational therapist's constant assistance. The occupational therapist gave feedback to Julia about her behavior while validating her feelings. She also helped Julia reexamine her most important priorities in light of the limitations of the institutional environment. Also, she helped Julia reflect on the difference between her past personal assistants and the staff in the facility, who could not be as personally attentive because of the needs of the other residents. The therapist pointed out to Julia that sometimes her constant need of assistance resulted in negative reactions from staff who were also trying to attend to other residents. With coaching from her occupational therapist, Julia learned to moderate her demands and to communicate her needs more effectively.

Julia's Progress

During the year that followed her individual intervention, Julia increased her occupational participation by learning a new sport, bocce ball; by exploring puppetry classes; and in "therapeutic breakfast," an activity the social worker created to stimulate verbal communication among the residents. Julia was actively involved in the preparation of the residence newsletter, contributing various articles.

Julia also attended a falls training and prevention workshop that stimulated her to work on improving her motor skills. Over time she developed better trunk control and was able to sit in a regular chair with moderate assistance. She began to participate in ball exercises using the arm she could better control to catch and to throw.

She also became involved in and enjoyed the sociocultural activities, such as outings, going out to eat, recreational walks in the fresh air, and birthday parties. She was able to develop more meaningful relationships with other residents with whom she socialized, taking part in card games and chatting with them.

Exploring New Roles

Upon returning from vacation, the occupational therapist learned that Julia had negotiated an agreement

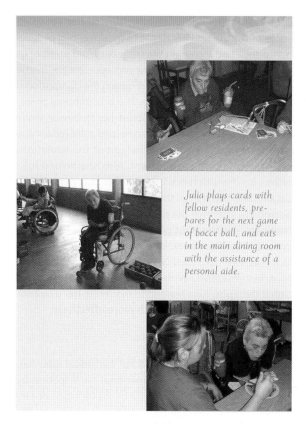

Julia plays cards with fellow residents, prepares for the next game of bocce ball, and eats in the main dining room with the assistance of a personal aide.

with the geriatric aides to assist her once they finished assisting those in the smaller dining room. This meant that she could sit and interact with the others in the main dining room while she waited for an aide to assist her with eating. It was clearly evident that her personal causation had dramatically improved and that Julia had to a large extent achieved her initial goals.

During their next session, the occupational therapist gave Julia feedback about her goal attainment and advised her that it might be a good idea to come up with new goals. So they decided to brainstorm together. Julia reflected that she had always liked studying and wished she had finished high school. She also mentioned that she had thought about writing a book about her life story to reach out to others with similar challenges. The occupational therapist acknowledged these goals and also suggested that Julia might want to expand her bocce playing into the role of being an amateur. She told Julia about a local sports academy for people with disabilities. One of the sports was bocce ball, and if one reached a certain skill level, one could

participate in regional events. The therapist also pointed out that it was possible to earn a scholarship to the academy based on financial need.

Julia agreed to visit the academy and to have an entrance evaluation. As it turned out, the academy had not only a sports program and physical therapy but also elementary and high school education programs. She was offered immediate admission into the sports program and was also given the option of attending the full-time educational program. The social worker from the residence initiated the process of applying for aid that would cover her tuition.

Julia also began to work on her book; she started telling her story to her roommate, who recorded it for her. After a while, Julia told the therapist that she wanted to devote more time to the book than her roommate could afford. The occupational therapist coached Julia in contacting a volunteer organization to provide someone to assist her writing efforts.

While Julia acknowledges that she has made important improvements in her life, she recently revealed that she really could not see herself living the rest of her life in the residence. The occupational therapist validated Julia's thoughts and feelings regarding her future and helped her to consider other possibilities. Obviously, Julia's occupational narrative is not yet finished. Whatever her challenges, Julia has redeveloped a strong volition that will help carry her through them.

Jessy: Reentering Life

Jessy was 22 years old when she sustained a closed head injury in an automobile accident. She was referred to occupational therapy 7 days after the accident while still in the intensive care unit (ICU). As sequelae to left intracerebral hemorrhage, Jessy had right hemiparalysis, aphasia, and multiple contractures. She remained comatose for 4 weeks and semicomatose and confused for 7 weeks while in acute care. Because of the nature of her problems, the therapist used the biomechanical, motor control, and cognitive-perceptual models (Katz, 2005; Kielhofner, 2002; Mathiowetz & Haugen, 1994; Trombly & Radomski, 2002) to guide much of therapy as it pertained to Jessy's performance capacity throughout her rehabilitation. The therapist used MOHO as an overall framework to guide efforts to help Jessy reclaim elements of her former occupational life and to fashion a new occupational identity and competence. This discussion illustrates how her therapist incorporated MOHO concepts and tools throughout Jessy's therapy.

Initial Information Gathering and Intervention During Acute Care

The therapist began by interviewing Jessy's family members and some visiting friends to get information on Jessy's interests and valued activities, roles, and routines. They described Jessy as an attractive, intelligent, and active young woman who enjoyed rock music and cared about animals and nature.

Since Jessy was still minimally responsive, her therapist's first goal for her volition and habituation was to provide an enriched environment that would begin to orient her to the external rhythm and structure of everyday life. Her therapist developed a program of environmental stimulation using rock music along with objects and pictures of animals and nature. The therapist taught the nursing staff and family members how to position Jessy and how to provide her this environmental stimulation.

Initially, Jessy was dependent on others for all aspects of her care including feeding, bathing, toileting, dressing, bed mobility, and transfers. She made no attempt to speak; her only expression was that she often cried. She was unable to sit up for more than 5 minutes without going into a pattern of total extension and sliding out of the chair. Jessy had to be restrained, as she often thrashed around and would fall out of bed. Initially, Jessy did not respond to any sensory stimuli except pain.

As she became semicomatose, Jessy remained in decorticate posturing with marked spasticity and contractures of all extremities. Hence, she was still severely limited in performing any voluntary, controlled movement. However, she did begin to show favorable responses to visual, auditory, and tactile stimulation. She was still very confused and could not follow one-step instructions. When possible during therapy, her restraints were removed or she was seated in a chair.

The therapist initiated a swallowing and feeding program, coaching Jessy on how to eat with adaptive equipment. The therapist also began to engage Jessy in completing simple self-care, which was soothing to her

since it evoked familiar habits. As she progressed, Jessy was able to express herself with the aid of a picture communication chart. Toward the end of her stay in acute care, Jessy could attend to a task for 2 to 3 minutes, following one-step verbal directions approximately 50% of the time. She also began to use facial expressions and other physical gestures to communicate. Finally, Jessy could perform some basic self-care with assistance and supervision.

Information Gathering and Intervention During Rehabilitation

When Jessy was medically stable she was transferred to a rehabilitation center in the same facility. In the rehabilitation phase, Jessy's therapist first gathered data through informal observations that revealed the following: Jessy often dropped items, was unable to write with her left hand, and could not button even large buttons. Her dominant right hand was severely limited by a frozen shoulder that hurt with any movement. She could roll side to side in bed using the bed rails but could not sit up on her own. She required assistance to transfer. The left side of Jessy's face was paralyzed and she drooled constantly.

Because her skills were initially so limited, Jessy's therapist informally observed her motor, process, and communication/interaction skills as she worked with her each day. Her reacquisition of skills was uneven, and her performance thus required constant surveillance, structuring, and coaching. For example, as she was relearning to eat, her therapist observed that with a scoop dish and a built-up spoon, Jessy was able to feed herself, but she needed coaching and encouragement to stay focused on the task and to properly grip the spoon and her cup. Otherwise, Jessy would be easily distracted or might drop the spoon or cup. Jessy was still having flexion contractures, spasticity, incoordination, and poor balance, which severely constrained her motor skills in other self-care activities, such as bathing and dressing. Her occupational therapist first focused on having Jessy cooperate with these occupational forms/tasks. As she observed any progress, she encouraged Jessy to begin doing small steps.

Jessy initially communicated by gesturing, shaking, or nodding or by pointing at objects, letters, words, or pictures. Her awareness of the environment increased daily. With time, Jessy could attend to simple activities for about 10 minutes. Beyond this, she easily became agitated and frustrated. Because of her limited tolerance for performance, the therapist saw Jessy for 10 to 15 minutes two to four times a day. Jessy still sometimes became confused and had difficulty heeding the goal of even simple two-step tasks. Approximately half the time she did not get to the second step. An illustration of her process skill difficulties at the time is that Jessy could gather the items needed to brush her teeth but could not correctly sequence the steps of this occupational form/task correctly.

At this point, Jessy's performance was also impaired because she was often agitated. For example, she was constantly moving around and would often be crying with her hand on her forehead. Clearly, her sense of capacity and efficacy was severely shaken. Consequently, she had a low frustration tolerance and would give up on tasks that were difficult for her. Furthermore, she seldom initiated anything because of her feelings of limited capacity. For example, because communication posed such a challenge for her, she would not initiate interaction with others.

Even as Jessy progressed, the effects of her altered sense of personal causation were apparent. Although Jessy's communication skills improved and she was able to speak, her interactions with others were very helpless and childlike. She became embarrassed easily and often giggled nervously. When she had difficulty expressing her feelings, she resorted to crying, pouting, or yelling. It was clear that these behaviors were not consistent with what she deeply desired. For example, despite often acting helpless, it was clear she resented being bossed around (as she called it) when others sought to assist or direct her. This was a tumultuous time marked by irregular progress. When she became very distressed, Jessy developed migraine headaches that kept her in bed for up to 2 days at a time.

Discovering the Original Jessy

Once Jessy had sufficient communication skills to tell her therapist about her life before the accident and could tolerate it emotionally and cognitively, the therapist interviewed her using the OPHI-II. This assessment helped identify both Jessy's previous occupational life and how her life had been altered since her injury. The therapist also asked Jessy to fill out the Role Checklist, and they

later discussed it. Together, these assessments provided the following picture of Jessy before her accident.

Jessy was a bright and high-achieving student who completed high school with honors. She was a senior at a prestigious New England university, majoring in chemistry at the time of her accident. During college, she had worked part-time for 3 years as a waitress in a restaurant. Jessy had previously worked as a baby sitter, a sales clerk, and a housekeeper to earn money. She had enjoyed all of her jobs, as she liked working with people. Jessy had planned to be a chemist, working in a university laboratory doing research. She saw her accident as delaying this goal but not obliterating it. Jessy's strong interests included crafts, nature, animals, cooking, and socializing.

Jessy was the oldest of three children. Before entering college, she often baby-sat her 9-year-old brother. She had lived with her brothers, mother, and stepfather until 2 years ago, when she moved out of the house. Before the accident, she lived on campus in an apartment with her boyfriend, and they shared financial costs and household chores. Her choice to live with her boyfriend in defiance of her parents' desires evidenced Jessy's strong-willed nature. In addition to working in a fast-food restaurant, Jessy volunteered at the local humane society, worked on the school newspaper, and maintained a high grade point average. All in all, her occupational history revealed a talented, willful, and energetic young woman with a strong past occupational identity.

As shown in *Figure 22.7*, Jessy still retained many elements of her past occupational identity, but it had been dramatically affected by her trauma and its sequelae. She had all but lost her sense of efficacy, feeling very out of control. While hoping to reconstitute the life she previously lived, her ability to envision how realistic it was or how she would go about reestablishing her life was extremely limited. Her personal causation was particularly affected, as she had no clear idea of what her future capacities would be and was unsure what success she would have in the future. Jessy's occupational competence, which had been strong, was severely compromised.

Figure 22.8 summarizes Jessy's responses on the Role Checklist. While the pattern of role change tells a story of its own, discussion of Jessy's responses gave her therapist useful insights into the transformation that

FIGURE 22.7 Jessy's ratings on the OPHI-II scales.

Occupational Identity Scale	1	2	3	4
Has personal goals and projects			✗	
Identifies a desired occupational lifestyle			✗	
Expects success		✗		
Accepts responsibility		✗		
Appraises abilities and limitations	✗			
Has commitments and values				✗
Recognizes identity and obligations			✗	
Has interests			✗	
Felt effective (past)				✗
Found meaning and satisfaction in lifestyle (past)				✗
Made occupational choices (past)				✗
Occupational Competence Scale	1	2	3	4
Maintains satisfying lifestyle	✗			
Fulfills role expectations	✗			
Works toward goals	✗			
Meets personal performance standards	✗			
Organizes time for responsibilities	✗			
Participates in interests	✗			
Fulfilled roles (past)				✗
Maintained habits (past)				✗
Achieved satisfaction (past)				✗

Key : **1** = Extreme occupational functioning problems
2 = Some occupational functioning problems
3 = Appropriate, satisfactory occupational functioning
4 = Exceptionally competent occupational functioning

took place after the accident. What follows is a summary of their discussion.

Whereas Jessy previously was actively involved in a number of roles, the accident removed her from those roles and placed her in a dependent patient role. Moreover, Jessy no longer had control over any of her previous role responsibilities. Her parents had been appointed by the court as her legal guardians during her comatose and semicomatose periods, and consequently, they controlled her finances. They also controlled other details of her life, such as who her visitors were and when they came and what mail and phone calls she received.

Before the accident, Jessy was extremely active. Her typical day included getting up at 6:00 A.M., studying, going to classes or work, volunteering, or working on the school paper. She had no set times for meals or household chores, and she saw her boyfriend erratically, as he also had a part-time job. Jessy's day was now dictated by the hospital routine. She was awakened at 6:00 A.M. and bathed, dressed, and given breakfast. For 8 hours, she attended therapies. She had only 30 minutes of free time during the day, but evenings were generally free except for 45 minutes of self-care activities before bedtime.

Jessy's view of her previous life is highlighted by the four things she valued most, in the following order of importance: independence, being with her boyfriend, having pets, and living away from home. In many ways she was a typical young adult making the transition to constructing her own life and moving toward family roles of her own. In addition, her priorities also showed what a high premium she placed on her independence and self-reliance. In this context, the im-

FIGURE 22.8 Jessy's responses on the Role Checklist.

Role	Role Identity			Value Designation		
	Past	Present	Future	Not at all valuable	Somewhat valuable	Very valuable
Student	X	X				X
Worker	X		X			X
Volunteer	X		X			X
Care giver	X		X		X	
Home maintainer	X		X			X
Friend	X	X	X			X
Family member	X	X	X		X	
Religious participant	X				X	
Hobbyist/Amateur	X		X		X	
Participant in organizations	X		X		X	
Other: NA						

pact of her current situation became more apparent. Jessy had been robbed of what she most valued. The life of independence and self-reliance she had been living had come to a halt. She was forced to depend on others for almost all aspects of her life. Overall, she felt severely constrained and confined. Most of all she felt, as she put it, "like a prisoner" in her own body. Her occupational narrative was clearly one of entrapment.

Jessy fiercely wanted to be released from her confinement. With coaching and encouragement from her therapist, Jessy was able to translate this desire into concrete goals. Jessy's long-term goal was to walk on her own in 6 months. Her immediate goals were to be able to wash and dress herself and to have a weekend pass to her apartment. Jessy recognized that her valued life of independence and self-reliance could be reestablished only after she could care for herself and walk on her own.

While Jessy recognized the importance of these goals, her immediate sense of efficacy was still a problem. Jessy repeatedly complained of her lack of control over her life. She felt as if she had lost the past 2 years of independence from her family and had been returned to childlike dependence. She was plagued with anxieties that she would be permanently limited, de-pendent on others, and incapable of taking control of the direction of her life.

Regaining Control

As her attention span and concentration level increased, Jessy came to occupational therapy twice a day for 90-minute sessions. Therapy initially took place in a room where distractions were eliminated as much as possible to enhance Jessy's ability to attend. Also, because of her limited ability to heed the purpose of a task, brief activities were used and a new task was introduced about every 20 minutes. This structuring of the environment also gave Jessy a greater feeling of control. Being able to complete a task successfully helped eliminate her frustration and agitation.

The occupational forms/tasks used to help Jessy increase her range of motion, coordination, and strength were based on Jessy's previous interests and her personal concerns. For example, early on Jessy engaged in rolling cookie dough and sanding a project to increase voluntary control, strength, and range of motion. These activities reflected her interest in crafts and cooking and therefore also had the effect of enhancing her enjoyment in therapy and giving her experiences that helped reinforce the idea that she was by degrees beginning to reenter the kind of life she previously had. Later, as more voluntary movement returned, she took up new activities, such as cross-stitch, preparing meals, and doing leather work, that still reflected her interests but provided more appropriate motor and process challenges. Slowly, Jessy could manage a wider range of occupational forms/tasks, including such things as cooking. She practiced tuning out distractions and attending to performance for longer periods.

The therapist and Jessy set and reviewed goals weekly according to Jessy's improvements and her personal desires. Throughout this process the therapist was careful to give Jessy opportunities to be in control and to have her desires validated. The following illustrates this. One day, a month into rehabilitation, the therapist asked Jessy what she wanted to cook. She indicated sugar cookies. When the therapist offered her a sugar cookie mix, Jessy became horrified. She had been a gourmet cook and would not think of using a mix! The therapist validated her desire to bake cookies from scratch. Although she struggled with process skills limitations that made following the recipe difficult, her volition counterbalanced these difficulties. When the cookies were done, Jessy was clearly bolstered by the fact she was able perform according to her own standards.

Jessy continued to become upset at times when she encountered her limitations and what felt to her like painfully slow progress. Her therapist worked to encourage her, to give feedback on her progress, to underscore the times that were enjoyable, and to celebrate the small triumphs that came when she mastered something that she could not previously do. These efforts helped to locate Jessy in a narrative in which she could see herself progressing toward a life she wanted. They also helped reduce her frustration about the distance she still needed to go. For example, when Jessy's ataxia decreased, she was once again able to write; however, it was initially inaccurate. To reduce her frustration over the discovery that her writing was impaired, it was important to give her feedback that reframed it as sign of progress from the time she could not write at all. The therapist also helped her to envision her impaired writing as a phase on the way to being able to write competently. By helping Jessy interpret her experience this way, her therapist enabled Jessy to feel a greater sense of efficacy even while her

capacities were still limited. Eventually, Jessy's right arm became sufficiently coordinated so she could write effectively.

Throughout this phase of therapy Jessy made simultaneous, although uneven, gains in a number of areas. Each week brought new surprises and new frustrations. With her therapist's assistance, she was able to place all these experiences in a larger story in which she was making her way back toward a way of life she enjoyed and valued.

As Jessy's process skills improved, her therapist modified occupational forms/tasks and environmental support to give her more challenge. Her therapist also provided necessary memory aids. As Jessy's motor skills increased, she was able to do such things as dress, bathe, style her hair, brush her teeth, and shave her legs. However, for quite some time she required standby assistance for all transfers, as she often lost her balance when standing.

Jessy progressed from living with a roommate to modified independent living and finally to staying in the hospital's apartment before discharge. Jessy was given increasing responsibility for her own care and worked with her therapist to develop and follow a routine that allowed her to establish new workable habits. This routine included making her bed, doing her laundry, keeping her room organized and clean, making and keeping her own appointments, taking her own medicine on schedule, and cooking one meal a day. Mnemonic aids were still necessary to assist Jessy in carrying out this routine. In the last 3 weeks of her hospitalization, Jessy planned her own schedule, setting up her own therapies, bedtime, self-care, and leisure time.

Jessy persisted in wanting to return to her previous lifestyle. In particular, it was important to her to be in control and self-sufficient. Therefore, the occupational therapist collaborated with Jessy to develop an inventory of all her previous responsibilities. Together Jessy and her therapist put them in order of priority, considering both the importance and the feasibility of each. Following the creation of this priority list, Jessy began to work toward recapturing her previous responsibilities.

For example, Jessy lost control of her own finances when her parents took over that responsibility. Consequently, regaining financial responsibility became a goal. Jessy and her therapist agreed to tackle this initially through simulating the kind of financial responsibilities she had when living on her own. To this end, her therapist and Jessy worked out a hypothetical budget and Jessy had to "pay weekly bills" to different people for rent, food, electricity, water and sewage, phone, therapies, entertainment, clothes, toiletries, transportation, and savings. Her therapist monitored and gave Jessy feedback on her ability to follow through on these financial management activities. At the time of discharge, Jessy was writing checks correctly and balancing her checkbook, although she continued to forget payments unless reminded or sent an overdue bill.

In similar fashion, Jessy and her therapist identified a host of objects and occupational forms/tasks, large and small, that she sought to master once again. For example, she practiced the use of a phone book, a newspaper, a dictionary, an encyclopedia, and a vending machine. She engaged in occupational forms/tasks such as filling out a job application, doing functional mathematics, filing paperwork, reading maps, giving directions, writing letters, and reading bus schedules. She also practiced performing in occupational settings such as the library and supermarket.

By the time she was discharged, Jessy's performance in a range of occupations was greatly improved. However, Jessy still had difficulty attending and noticing. Moreover, she sometimes became flustered, which further impaired her performance. While Jessy desperately wanted total control of her life, she had to accept that her memory loss and process skill deficits meant that she needed some supervision. Moreover, she required standby assistance when she walked because she was still unsteady and at risk for falling.

Jessy was still having difficulty communicating and interacting with others. Sometimes she was too passive to get her needs met or to receive necessary assistance. Other times she lost control and had outbursts with those around her. Jessy's therapist worked with her to identify and practice appropriate assertiveness and socially appropriate behavior. This was done in a variety of settings, with Jessy's therapist giving her instruction and feedback. Jessy relearned how to initiate conversations in different situations and how to participate in community outings to a variety of occupational behavior settings. Jessy was a naturally engaging person. Consequently, as she relearned expected behavior, she readily became friends with numerous patients and staff members. She often advocated for and encouraged other patients.

One of the biggest challenges for Jessy was to come to grips with what her discharge status would likely be. Her ongoing impairments limited how much independence and self-reliance was safe for her. To ease Jessy toward acknowledging and accepting this reality, she went on numerous weekend trips home before discharge. Jessy's therapist gave her family a list of things Jessy could do independently so they would both allow and expect her to do them. This helped ensure that Jessy's most important social group at the time, her family, would support and expect the level and kind of occupational performance of which Jessy was capable. Additionally, the therapist worked with Jessy and her family to develop a schedule for her at home. This schedule allowed Jessy to do what was most important to her and provided structure for both Jessy and her family so that she could be supervised without too much interference.

Reentering Occupational Life

Jessy returned to live at home with her parents and brothers. She was followed up as an outpatient in occupational therapy. As part of that followup, the therapist decided to administer the Role Checklist again to see whether Jessy was reentering roles as she had intended. The checklist and subsequent discussion indicated that Jessy had not followed through on her plans to reenter the student and volunteer roles (i.e., she had planned to enroll in a community college class and volunteer at the local humane society). Her therapist learned that Jessy was also having difficulty structuring her day.

On the positive side, Jessy had become reacquainted with some old friends and had gone to the movies and out to eat with them. She had pursued her leisure interest of cross-stitching and frequently played games with her younger brothers. Nonetheless, Jessy felt she could do more than her parents were allowing her to do and that her parents were limiting her occupational competence.

While Jessy clearly knew how she wanted her life to turn out, she was quite unsure of the immediate future. Therefore, therapy focused on helping Jessy develop a clearer idea of what she wanted her life at the time to be and on setting short-term goals. Jessy would make a list of what she wanted to achieve by her next scheduled therapy, then she would report her accomplishments or problems to the therapist. She developed lists incorporating her values and interests and became increasingly realistic about her capabilities.

As time went on, Jessy decided she wanted some kind of vocational training that would allow her to obtain a job. She also wanted to pursue opportunities to live somewhere other than at home. With help from her therapist she found and began attending a vocational training center where she could live in a dormitory. During this time she continued to return for periodic followup in occupational therapy. At the vocational training center, she received 6 months of training in computer skills. She continued to practice her habits and skills and worked toward her goal of personal independence. She was able to take over her personal finances at this point, including managing the investment of funds she had received from an insurance settlement related to her accident. During this time, in occupational therapy, she learned to drive again.

Reinventing Her Occupational Narrative

A year and a half after her head injury, Jessy had partially reclaimed her previous life. Importantly, she was also able to recraft her occupational narrative in necessary ways. Jessy had largely come to grips with the reality of her continuing limitations. Considering these, she felt she had rebuilt some significant portions of her previous life. Still, there were losses. Her old boyfriend was unable to handle all the changes in Jessy, and their relationship had ended. Jessy realized that she would never become the chemist she had aspired to be before the accident.

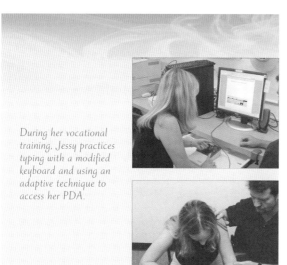

During her vocational training, Jessy practices typing with a modified keyboard and using an adaptive technique to access her PDA.

Jessy became increasingly reconciled to the fact that she was not exactly the same person she had been. Her right hand was still impaired. She could walk on her own but needed a cane. She was able to do all her self-care and basic homemaking and had developed new habits that supported her daily living tasks and work. However, she continued to have some trouble with process skills. This required her to accept minimal supervision for daily tasks.

Jessy moved to a group of supervised living apartments where she had her own room and shared household chores with other residents. She took the bus to her part-time job as a computer operator. She continued to make friends easily and had a new boyfriend. She lobbied those in charge of the supervised living apartments to secure permission for residents to have pets; this was a big accomplishment for her.

Jessy felt that her schedule allowed a level of activity that she could handle and that she had a good mix of work and leisure time. She talked with her family two times a month and had demonstrated to their satisfaction that she could be semi-independent. Although Jessy had to relinquish the image of herself as a chemist–researcher, she was inventive in sustaining involvement in chemistry as part of her life story. She volunteered as a technical aide in a junior high school chemistry club.

Jessy was content with the life she had managed to compose for the time being. Nonetheless, in her future story she would be living on her own. In that story she would get around in her own car with her cocker spaniel in the back seat!

Jessy in Perspective

Jessy's course of therapy involved a long and complex process of change. While much of the therapy consisted of restoration of her motor, process, and communication/interaction skills, it was equally important that her volition be supported throughout and that necessary changes in personal causation and values were also attended to in therapy. Finally, the redevelopment of her habits and roles was essential.

Like many persons who incur permanent and significant impairments, Jessy was not able to return to the life she had previously lived and desired. Therefore, successful therapy had to enable her to reconstruct her occupational identity and build a new occupational competence that took into account her remaining abilities and lingering limitations. By doing this, therapy enabled Jessy to be living an occupational narrative that she could accept and find satisfying. Happily, several years later, Jessy was working 30 hours per week as a computer operator doing data entry and basic analysis for a researcher at a research center. She had held the job for 5 years, needed only minimal job coaching, and was considered an extremely reliable worker. She was trying to piece together her experience of trauma and recovery and planned to write about it for others so they would know what the experience is like. And she had four pets.

Conclusion

As noted at the outset of this chapter, the cases described herein presented complex challenges. Because of the difficulty and painful issues faced by each client, success in therapy was far from guaranteed. The success of each case reflects the fact that the therapist took the time and used the tools necessary to fully understand clients and how best to approach them. Thus, the cases represent good examples of how to use MOHO to make sense of clients' circumstances and to devise a thoughtful approach to the therapy process.

References

Katz, N. (2005). *Cognition and Occupation Across The Life Span.* Rockville, MD: AOTA.

Kielhofner, G. (2002). *Conceptual foundations of occupational therapy* (3rd ed.). Philadelphia: FA Davis.

Mathiowetz, V., & Haugen, J. B. (1994) Motor behavior research: Implications for therapeutic approaches to central nervous system dysfunction. *American Journal of Occupational Therapy, 48,* 733–745.

Trombly, C., & Radomski, M. (2002). *Occupational therapy for physical dysfunction* (5th ed.). Philadelphia: FA Davis.

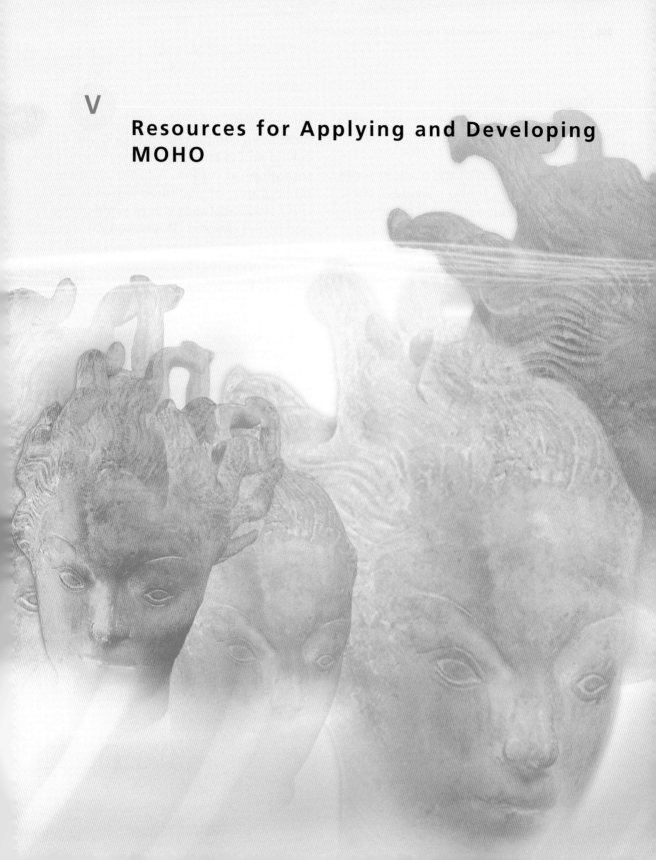

V

Resources for Applying and Developing MOHO

Introduction to Section V

This final section of the book includes five chapters. It also provides information about additional resources that can be accessed by persons interested in learning more or finding out the latest about MOHO theory, research, and application.

Chapter 23 discusses issues of communication and documentation of one's use of MOHO. Chapter 24 discusses how MOHO can guide the program development process. Three examples of programs developed in the United States and Canada are provided. The chapter is also a resource for understanding how a conceptual practice model is used in program development. The examples illustrate different ways that MOHO can be used to create programs in both institutional and community-based settings.

Chapter 25 discusses evidence based practice for therapists using MOHO. It contains materials that allow easy reference of evidence related to MOHO.

Chapter 26 discusses MOHO-based research. This chapter begins by providing an overview about why research is important to a conceptual practice model and what types of research are typically undertaken to examine and develop a model. Then, the types of research that have been completed on MOHO are discussed and exemplified through brief presentations of studies. A comprehensive bibliography of published research with brief study abstracts is contained at the end of the chapter. This chapter is a detailed resource for anyone who wishes to understand the research base of MOHO and anyone who is considering undertaking research related to MOHO.

Chapter 27 discusses the relationship of MOHO to the American Occupational Therapy Association Practice Framework and the World Health Organization ICF system. This chapter will help therapists understand the similarities and differences between MOHO and these two widely used frameworks.

The Appendix follows this section, and includes an introduction to the Model of Human Occupation Clearinghouse and website, as well as a comphrenesive bibliography. The MOHO Clearinghouse distributes MOHO information and resources to support practice and research, and the website is one of the primary ways this occurs. The MOHO bibliography contains contains English language articles, books, and chapters that discuss MOHO. The body of more than 220 citations is constantly growing. This bibliography is updated monthly, and a current bibliography can be found on the web site.

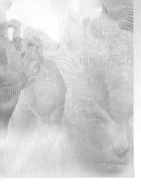

23

Communication and Documentation

- Kirsty Forsyth
- Gary Kielhofner

ommunication and documentation are essential to occupational therapy. The following are a few examples of typical requirements for communication and documentation:

- Explaining to a client why you want to administer a particular assessment
- Reporting the results of an assessment
- Writing down treatment goals and strategies in the medical record (or other intervention record)
- Explaining your recommendations for intervention to family members of your client
- Discussing a complex case with an occupational therapy colleague to "think though" the best approach to therapy
- Sharing your understanding of a client's situation with the client to receive feedback and validation
- Presenting your therapy plan at an interdisciplinary or multidisciplinary meeting
- Advising a client on how to use strategies that worked in therapy beyond discharge or termination of therapy
- Presenting one of your clients as a case at a professional meeting with the aim of demonstrating the impact of therapy.

In each of these and other instances, occupational therapists who use MOHO will need to put into words one or more of the stages in the therapeutic reasoning process discussed in Chapter 11:

- Generating theory-based questions about the client
- Collecting information about and from the client to answer the questions one has generated
- Using the information gathered to create a conceptualization of the client, including strengths and challenges

- Identifying goals and strategies for therapy
- Implementing and monitoring therapy
- Determining outcomes of therapy.

Thus, the essence of communication and documentation is to share with someone else the internal thought processes that make up one's reasoning about the client and the client's therapy. If one is actively using MOHO as a theory to guide this thought process, communication and documentation entail sharing theory-based ideas and rationales. It stands to reason, then, that one's communication and documentation can only be as good as one's underlying reasoning. Thus, in this chapter we will talk about these as interrelated topics.

The chapter is organized so that we first discuss the communication and documentation implications of each of the steps of therapeutic reasoning. After this, we discuss a number of additional issues related to communication and documentation, such as use of terminology and forms. Finally, in discussing documentation, we will not adhere to a single format. Many different documentation formats are used across settings and in different countries. In this chapter we seek to represent a range of those formats.

Communicating and Documenting the Process of Evaluation

Communicating MOHO Theory and Theory-Based Questions to Clients

Therapists should begin to communicate to clients the theory they are using from the beginning of therapy. Consider that from the first encounter most clients begin forming impressions about the kind of support and assistance they may receive from the therapist. It is important that the client have an understanding of and expectations for occupational therapy that are as accurate and realistic as possible.

How much one says and how to frame it depend on the client. Most of the time, however, therapists use everyday language to explain their theoretical approaches. The following are examples of how therapists might orient a client to the theory and questions they will be using.

Sara

Sara was a college-educated 44-year-old woman recently diagnosed with multiple sclerosis. Her therapist introduced MOHO as follows:

> As an occupational therapist, I work from a perspective that is concerned with how multiple sclerosis has affected your ability to participate in the things that are important to you—for example, your work, taking care of yourself, your leisure activities. I'll want to get to know what is important to you and how you feel your illness has affected your ability to do what you need to do and like to do. I will also want to know something about your major life responsibilities and your everyday routines.
>
> We'll work together to figure out ways we can minimize any problems in your everyday life and how you can best go on with life in a meaningful way. We can make changes in your environment or in how you go about doing things that allow you to be more effective in getting done what you need and want to do.

Melissa

Melissa was a 65-year-old woman who had limited cognitive capacities due to Alzheimer's disease. Her therapist used a much briefer explanation: "My job is to help

you manage things and be able to do what's most important and enjoyable to you."

Mike

For Mike, a 10-year-old with cerebral palsy, introduction to the school therapist's use of MOHO was as follows:

> I'm here to make sure you are managing okay in school and liking it. I want to find out how you are doing with such things as getting to your classes, doing homework, dressing for gym, eating lunch, getting along with your classmates and your teacher. I'd also like you to tell me what you do well and what is harder for you. And I want to know what's most important to you and what you like in school.

As the examples illustrate, it is possible to give clients, in terms suited to their ability to understand, an indication of the therapist's concepts and approach. Even though terms like volition and personal causation were not used in these explanations, the therapists nevertheless conveyed to the clients that they were concerned with volitional issues.

Explanations of MOHO concepts may be expanded or simplified depending on the response of the client. The point is to meet clients where they are, respecting their emotional states, cognitive abilities, background, and other characteristics. When clients are nonverbal, communication may occur primarily through the therapist's actions. This means, for example, conveying one's intention to know what the client values and enjoys by responding to any indication of these things by the client. Similarly, one conveys concern for personal causation by respecting a client's need to feel some sense of personal control.

Clients who are uncooperative present some of the largest challenges. One of the best tools a therapist has for dealing with uncooperative clients is the concept of volition. What appears to be lack of cooperation from the therapist's viewpoint is always a volitionally driven decision by the client. No single strategy will work, but respect for the client's viewpoint, however different from that of the therapist, is a constant principle. If therapists can understand the client's volitional perspective, they can often develop appropriate strategies.

The process of communicating with the client only begins with the first encounters in therapy. As time goes on, therapists should reveal more and more to their clients about their perspectives. Once again, how this is done should be based on what the client is able to grasp and integrate.

Communicating MOHO Theory and Questions to Other Professionals

It is useful and important to make known one's theory and approach to gathering information to others such as peer professionals. This can be done in a variety of ways. One might do so formally by giving a presentation at a team meeting or by providing in-service training. One can also do it informally by sharing anecdotal information about clients in which theoretical concepts are embedded. Discussing clients in team meetings or when consulting with another professional often provides an excellent opportunity to mention and explain the concepts one is using.

In the end, it is important that other service providers and professionals have some understanding of one's theoretical perspective and its implications for what one does in therapy. Others' interests or abilities to understand MOHO concepts will, of course, vary. Therefore, one must judge when and how to communicate the information to others.

Explaining Assessments to Clients

It is extremely important to explain planned assessments to the client if at all possible. Clients often perceive a large power differential between themselves and the therapist. Assessment can seem mysterious and frightening to a client. Clients may have no idea why the therapist is asking questions or gathering information. They may fear that the therapist will discover something negative about them. Clients may be concerned that the therapist will gain information that affects them (e.g., where they can live, how much freedom they have, how much help they receive).

Consequently, the therapist should explain these points to the client (and/or family member) in terms that can be understood:

- Why the assessment will be done
- What is entailed in doing the assessment
- What the assessment is likely to reveal
- How the information will be used.

Also, the therapist should assure the client (and/or family member) that the information learned in the assessment process will be shared with the client. Most MOHO assessments gather information on the client's viewpoint, concerns, and desires. Therefore, it is appropriate to inform the client that one of the main aims of assessment is to clarify the client's desires and needs and ensure that they will be addressed seriously in therapy.

The following are examples of how the therapist might explain the use of assessments to a client.

THE OCCUPATIONAL SELF-ASSESSMENT (OSA)

It would be very helpful for me if you would complete a short form called the Occupational Self-Assessment. It will take you about 10 to 15 minutes. The form asks you to look at a number of statements about how you do things in your everyday life. You will indicate on the form how well you do the things listed and how important they are to you. I'm asking you to fill out this form because I want to know what's important to you. I also want to know where you think things are going okay and where you feel you have some problems. When you have finished this part of the form, we will look at it together and then you and I will use it to decide what things you would most like to change about your life.

THE OCCUPATIONAL PERFORMANCE HISTORY INTERVIEW—SECOND VERSION (OPHI-II)

As we begin therapy, I'd like to get to know you better. I'm interested in how [name the injury or disability] has affected your life. I would also like to know how you see your future and what we can do in therapy to make things better for you. To do this, it would be very helpful for me to sit down with you for a while and talk about your life. After we have done so, I will fill out some forms and share them with you. This might not only help me understand you better but give you some new ways to think about your life.

THE ASSESSMENT OF COMMUNICATION AND INTERACTION SKILLS (ACIS)

You and I have agreed that sometimes it is not so easy for you to talk and get along with others. It would be really helpful for me to see you in different social situations to gain a better understanding of what actually happens. After I've spent some time with you in these situations, I will fill out some forms. We will look at these forms together to see what things you do well and what things you might want to work on in therapy so you can feel more confident about getting along with others.

These examples only illustrate how one may introduce an assessment. Therapists should develop their own styles of doing so and modify what they say according to each client's unique characteristics. A client who is anxious may need to be reassured. A client who is cognitively disabled or confused will need a simple explanation. Of course, it is not always possible to explain the intended assessment to the client. Some clients are too cognitively or emotionally constrained to understand or accept the information. Other clients are uncooperative. In these situations, therapists must make careful decisions about how to proceed with assessment. For example, a therapist may decide to discreetly observe a client with the aim of gaining information helpful to intervention or to achieving a more collaborative relationship with the client.

Explaining Assessments to Other Professionals

Explaining the use of assessments to other professionals should also be aimed at elucidating the purpose, process, and content of assessments. Some professionals will be interested to know whether the assessments can be used in a reliable way and whether valid interpretations can be made from the assessment findings. MOHO assessments have been or are in the process of careful development and study. This should be emphasized when explaining them to other professionals. Knowing the kinds of research that has been done to ensure the dependability of an assessment is useful for being able

to speak to its value. This does not mean that a therapist should be prepared to recount all the research, but it is a good idea to know something about how an assessment has been studied.

When a therapist decides to use an assessment regularly, it is a good idea to become familiar with the kinds of studies that have led to the development of the assessment. The information provided in Chapter 25 is a useful beginning. Also, most MOHO-based assessments have manuals that discuss the research behind the assessment in ways that therapists and other professionals can readily understand.

Documentation provides an excellent opportunity to explain assessments to other team members. In documentation, the value of the assessment in identifying client problems can be readily demonstrated. The following is a summary report of an ACIS evaluation with Rachel, who before a psychotic episode was actively involved in her community. She was having difficulty effectively engaging in social activities.

Rachel

Rachel wanted to be able to return to her community-based activities, which were largely social. Rachel was observed in social activities using the ACIS. It revealed the following strengths and challenges: Rachel's nonverbal interactions (i.e., eye contact, gesturing, touching others) were appropriate. She maintained interactions even when she felt disoriented. She was able to engage others and readily initiated conversation with others. She had trouble focusing during conversation (i.e., jumped from one topic to another). When distressed, she increased the pace and volume of her speaking to the effect that others became uncomfortable. She had difficulty picking up others' cues and respecting their needs or desires in social interaction. Her skill difficulties significantly affected her ability to engage in social activities.

As the example illustrates, sharing what an assessment reveals about a client demonstrates its utility.

Communicating One's Conceptualization of a Client's Situation to Professionals

As discussed in Chapter 11, conceptualizing the client's situation requires synthesis of information collected with MOHO concepts to create a unique explanation or understanding of each client. One important resource in creating a conceptualization of the client is the client's strengths and problems/challenges that are listed in the Therapeutic Reasoning Table following Section 2 of this text.

This step is best illustrated through a detailed example. The following is an account of how the first author conceptualized a client's occupational circumstances.

Ruth: Part I

. . . .

Ruth was 70 years old and had experienced a stroke that resulted in left-sided hemiplegia. When the occupational therapist joined the team and took over Ruth's therapy, Ruth was 4 weeks into a rehabilitation program. Nursing staff described Ruth as initially strongly motivated for therapy. However, she had become withdrawn, noncompliant, and depressed. The physician was considering antidepressive medication. Nursing staff also considered Ruth a safety risk, as she would try to do things for which she had questionable capacity. Consequently, nursing staff indicated that they "had to keep a constant eye on her." They also noted that Ruth had stated her intention to discharge herself from the hospital against medical advice.

Given Ruth's mood and apparent dis-interest in rehabilitation, the therapist decided to assess her using selected portions of the OPHI-II and informal observation. The therapist felt that asking Ruth to do anything more would not be successful, given her withdrawal and apparent intention to discharge herself.

During the interview, which was conducted as an informal conversation, the therapist emphasized to Ruth the importance of her being able to say how she really felt about her situation. This was reinforced through active listening and an attitude of empathy to Ruth's experience and viewpoints.

Ruth characterized her mood as being "fed up." When asked to explain what this meant, Ruth described herself as previously being a very independent person who now was "useless." She had lived alone without family and always made her own decisions and looked after herself. She also valued her privacy and felt that her most private self-care routines were now exposed to "strangers."

Moreover, she complained that staff kept telling her she could not do things for herself, which made her feel even worse. She stated she had been a "doer" all her life and was now reduced to a "watcher." Even at 70, she kept her own apartment, went out every day on public transportation, assisted two friends with domestic chores, was actively involved in her church, and had a busy social life.

She felt that being in the hospital was a waste of time, since all she was doing was sitting around feeling bored. She questioned the value of the rehabilitation hospital when she could feel more comfortable at home and could at least try to do things on her own there. Ruth stated that she had no interest in occupational therapy, since being in therapy would only reinforce what she could not do. She also admitted to fears that the therapist might discover something that would prevent her from being allowed to go home.

From informal observation, it was apparent that Ruth's motor skills were so limited that she could not perform even basic personal care. When attempting transfers and walking, she was clearly at risk for falling.

With this information, the therapist was able to construct the following conceptualization of Ruth's situation. Ruth's personal causation was extremely limited because she felt incapable and unable to effect outcomes she desired. Because this was so emotionally painful for her, she was unable to fully think about the extent of her limitations. She also experienced her environment on the ward as constraining her choices to do things. Her social environment (nurses) was reinforcing this on a regular basis. Moreover, her previous experience in occupational therapy had led to her focus on her limitations, reinforcing her lowered personal causation. Ruth's value system made the loss of capacity, privacy, and independence particularly painful for her.

Ruth's former active routine and roles such as a home maintainer, religious participant, caretaker, and friend had all been eliminated by her stroke and the routine in the rehabilitation hospital. Her loss of a familiar and stimulating routine and of occupational roles had left her feeling bored and alienated. Moreover, her current routine was passive and without meaning or satisfaction, so that it further eroded her already compromised volition.

Ruth's rehabilitation experience was extremely demoralizing for her, since it assaulted rather than supported her volition. She was forced into losing choices and being passive. She was confronted with her limitations. Ruth's lack of role-related responsibilities and routine contrasted with the high level of activity from which she previously achieved satisfaction. Being forced to sit and watch when her volition was organized around actively doing things was intolerable for her.

If she returned home, she would be extremely limited. Given that Ruth had only recently had the stroke and had started to regain movement, the best way forward was to have Ruth engage in a rigorous therapy program. Going home at this point would not only compromise possible gains in her performance capacity but would likely result in further deterioration of her volition and habituation. Ruth would therefore be very unlikely to be able to live independently, requiring institutional placement.

This conceptualization of Ruth's circumstances made it apparent that unless things were radically altered, she would discharge herself with the likelihood that she would be permanently reduced to a passive and dependent state. In this case, with only the limited information that could be gathered given Ruth's depressed mood and lack of interest in therapy, the therapist was able to construct a conceptualization of Ruth's circumstances. We will see later how the therapist used this information.

Communicating One's Conceptualization to the Client

Sharing one's conceptualization with the client is particularly important for any client who is able to understand and emotionally deal with the information. In addition to letting the client know how the therapist understands the client, sharing this information allows the therapist to validate with the client whether it is accurate.

Negotiating with the client at this stage to arrive at a common understanding of the situation is often critical to support the next steps in therapy. Of course it is not always possible to share all details of the therapist's conceptualization. Therapists must be careful to couch explanations in terms clients can understand. One exception to this is that therapists sometimes teach elements of the theory to clients as a way to empower them to better understand their own circumstances.

Client-centered practice requires that therapists share their views of the client's situation. Sharing such information gives the client critical information for engaging in the collaborative process. The optimal goal of a client-centered relationship is to allow clients to determine their own vision of the future under the professional guidance of the therapist.

One of the biggest challenges to client-centered practice is a disparity in the therapist's and the client's perspectives (McGavin, 1998; Missiuna & Pollack, 2000; Sumsion & Smyth, 2000). In the event of such a disagreement, it becomes necessary to negotiate with the client. Arriving at a common perspective is important because it helps to ensure that the therapist and the client are committed to a shared vision of therapy.

While the client is viewed as an equal and active collaborator, it is the therapist's responsibility to initiate this step and to facilitate action on the part of the client. Occupational therapists have full responsibility for contributing ideas, suggestions, and cautions as well as defining boundaries beyond which therapists must not go, regardless of a client's wishes (E. Townsend, personal communication, November 4, 1997). The therapist must provide clients with reasonable visions of the likely outcomes of certain decisions and gently challenge the client's perspective if it appears to be unreasonable. The process of communicating this step will be illustrated by returning to the example of Ruth.

*R*uth: Part 2

Communicating the therapist's conceptualization to Ruth was particularly challenging, since Ruth had already lost faith in rehabilitation. The therapist realized it would be necessary to reframe the experience of being in the hospital and reengage Ruth in a therapeutic process that would be meaningful enough for her to want to stay in the hospital and work to improve her abilities.

The therapist began by validating Ruth's experience and her concerns about staying in the hospital. The therapist explained how she appreciated Ruth's experience of therapy as only making her feel more ineffective, her feeling that she had no control over her privacy and choices, and her boredom with the hospital routine. The therapist also advised Ruth of the difficult challenges Ruth would face if she discharged herself home without further therapy.

The therapist negotiated that she would arrange to change Ruth's routine to be more satisfying and would support her to make choices consistent with her abilities. The therapist gave Ruth a vision of how her experience of therapy could be different and the kinds of meaningful occupations in which she could engage as part of therapy. Finally, she shared information about improvements she believed Ruth could realize in therapy and how they would affect her ability to live at home and regain important parts of her life.

Reluctantly, Ruth initially committed to stay 2 more weeks after negotiating with the therapist to determine specific goals that focused on improving her ability to return to live at home. The therapist acted swiftly to put in place what had been negotiated. Ruth ended up staying 4 weeks and making gains that significantly improved her performance of self-care and domestic occupational forms/tasks before being successfully discharged home.

While the therapist was successful in sharing her conceptualization with Ruth, other clients may reject the therapist's opinion at this stage. Sometimes the therapist or the client chooses to terminate the therapeutic relationship when they cannot agree. Other times, negotiation may mean that the therapist supports the client in a decision that the therapist perceives as less than optimal but that is more desirable than terminating therapy.

For example, Ruth was competent to make her own decisions. Therefore, if Ruth had made an informed deci-

sion to discharge herself, the therapist would have supported her to make the transition home with the least risk. The therapist would also have documented the areas of concern, along with the strategies and environmental supports that were put in place to facilitate Ruth's discharge.

Documenting One's Conceptualization of a Client

Documentation of the therapist's conceptualization of the client is important because it provides the rationale for the goals and therapeutic strategies. The note that was written in the medical record concerning Ruth follows.

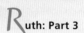

Ruth: Part 3

Current Situation

Ruth stated that she didn't want to be involved in therapy and planned to discharge herself home. If she returned home, she would be extremely limited and at risk for requiring institutional placement.

Assessment

Ruth was assessed through informal interview and two separate observations of her personal care routine.

Strengths

Can identify what is important.

It was also important for Ruth to be able to return home and to complete her personal care routine herself, as she strongly values privacy and independence.

Process Skills

Ruth's process skills were effective. Notably, she could think through how to complete some aspects of the activities by compensating for her motor skills deficits.

Challenges

Role Loss

Ruth is demoralized by the loss of her previous routine and the roles she had as a friend, caretaker, home maintainer, and religious participant.

Motor Skills

She was extremely limited in her ability to complete self-care activities due to motor skill deficits. She was unsafe transferring from one surface to another, and was unable to walk independently due to lack of balance. The risk was greater when she was walking as part of some larger activity. Her walking difficulty also limited her ability to move objects around her environment while doing activities. She could not bend and reach for objects from a standing position. She is unable to use her affected arm within activities. This reduced her ability to complete parts of activities in her usual manner. She became quickly fatigued.

Motivation

Ruth overestimates her abilities (or ignores the risk involved), which leads her to make decisions to do things beyond her current abilities, threatening her safety. Ruth justifies her choices by saying she will never get better if she doesn't try things. Ruth found it extremely painful to face her limitations and felt that therapy underscored her limitations. She also felt that staff members were overprotective and interfered with her choices and privacy.

Conclusion

Prior to the CVA, Ruth lived alone independently and was very active. Now, she feels that she had lost control over her life and access to the things she valued and enjoyed doing. Ruth's experience in rehabilitation was that she could not enact her most important values and she does not feel that rehabilitation has helped her progress. Given Ruth's limited motor skills and choosing to engage in activities that put her at risk, would make it difficult to facilitate a successful discharge at this stage. Home support services would not be sufficient to support Ruth with personal care and homemaking activities.

Ruth is a good candidate to continue in rehabilitation for the following reasons:

- Her stroke was recent and she was beginning to show motor gains.

- She had strong process skills and could readily learn to problem solve how to perform safely.

- She was very motivated to return to and remain in her home and had a successful history of independent living.

Action and Outcome

The above reasoning was shared with Ruth to attempt to convince her to remain in rehabilitation. After much negotiation, Ruth agreed to an occupational therapy program of 2 weeks with specific goals aimed at a successful discharge home.

As the note illustrates, documentation of the therapist's conceptualization of the client's situation serves to communicate critical information to others and to illustrate the therapist's rationale for action.

Developing Your Conceptualization of a Client's Situation

Just as there is no single format for documentation, there are many ways to develop your conceptualization of a client's situation. One way to begin is to use structured reflective questions as shown in *Figure 23.1*.

Using these reflective questions can improve one's conceptualization of a client and along with it one's communication and documentation. Using this kind of structured process can help one with the following:

- Organizing thoughts more clearly along the lines of the underlying theory

- Relating different components of information gathered to create a conceptualization of the client

- Identifying information not yet gathered that could contribute to an understanding of the client's situation.

*A*rchie

The following case formulation was developed by an occupational therapist who had a few years of experience but was new to using MOHO. She was frustrated by the task of documenting her conceptualizations of the clients and brought her documentation to the first author for feedback. They began by examining the OT's inpatient note for the multidisciplinary team. This note reported the results of an interview using the Occupational Circumstances Assessment-Interview and Rating Scale (OCAIRS) (see Chapter 17) with Archie, an adult male admitted to an inpatient mental health unit for the first time with a diagnosis of schizophrenia. It was as follows, as shown in *Figure 23.2.*

The occupational therapist who wrote the note identified that she lacked structure in her thinking. She stated she came away from the interview with the client and wrote down what she could remember. It was clear that the note was primarily descriptive and offered little synthesis that would reflect a theory-based conceptualization of the client, and it was hard to understand what the OT was going to do following the encounter. To structure her thinking, the therapist used reflective questions (*Fig. 23.3*).

Putting what she had learned from Archie into this format allowed her to organize her thoughts and identify additional information from the interview that she did not include in her original note. When going through the reflective questions, she identified important additional information. The therapist knew the information but had not documented it fully. Archie's note was reconstructed for educational purposes by the therapist, as shown in *Figure 23.4.*

This second conceptualization was a synthesis rather than a description of facts, as was displayed in the first conceptualization. The theory was used to understand the client's situation and build arguments as to why the situation was not supporting this client's occupational participation. It is interesting to note that the therapist knew all of the information displayed in the second conceptualization and excluded it because she did not see its relevance in the building an understanding of the client's situation.

FIGURE 23.1 Reflective questions for developing a conceptualization of a client.

✔ Which structured and/or unstructured assessment(s) were used?

✔ What is the state of this person's occupational identity?

✔ What is the over all state of this person's occupational competence?

✔ What critical personal factor(s) [personal causation, values, interests, roles, habits, performance capacity] put this person at risk or prevent this person from engaging in needed/desired occupations?

✔ What critical personal factor(s) [personal causation, values, interests, roles, habits, performance capacity] support this client engagement in needed/desired occupations?

✔ How do environmental factors contribute to this situation?

✔ What is the succinct conclusion statement?

FIGURE 23.2 Initial note written about Archie.

Initial contact: Spoke to Archie about Occupational Therapy role and discussed issues around his current disorganised daily routine and his subjective lack of motivation. Archie plans to attend college next August to pursue a qualification in social care. He has strong values associated with the worker role and currently feels unable to achieve satisfactory role performance due to external influences and a chaotic lifestyle. Archie anticipates that many difficulties will resolve once his new accommodation is in place and plans to find work to support himself to be independent. Archie agreed to consider the balance of work, leisure, and self-care when living independently and to ensure a structured lifestyle to support his short- and long-term goals. He is considering community resources that will support him in structuring his week on discharge.

FIGURE 23.3 Reflective questions for developing a conceptualization of a client: Archie.

Which structured and/or unstructured assessment(s) were used?
Occupational Circumstances Assessment–Interview and Rating Scale (OCAIRS)

What is the state of this person's occupational identity?
Archie has a strong occupational identity as a home maintainer and worker and he has clear goals of moving from brother's home, going to college, and gardening.

What is the overall state of this person's occupational competence?
Archie is currently unable to do what he wants, but appears capable if he has a supportive context.

What critical personal factor(s) [personal causation, values, interests, roles, habits, performance capacity] put this person at risk or prevent this person from engaging in needed/desired occupations?
Archie has a disorganised daily routine (habits) within the ward. He doesn't think personal care activities are important (values) and therefore doesn't have a habit pattern to support a morning routine (habits). Since there are no enjoyable activities (interests) for him to do in the ward, he sees no reason to plan a daily routine (habits). He is not motivated (volition) to focus on the ward routine as he believes he can establish a new routine once he has a new living situation and a job. However, his current choices (volition), and daily ward routine (habits), will not allow him to attain his goal. Archie indicated he will consider changing his routine (habits) and community supports (social environment) on discharge.

What critical personal factor(s) [personal causation, values, interests, roles, habits, performance capacity] support this client engagement in needed/desired occupations?
Archie has identified goals (values) which include in the short term moving from his brother's accommodation to living alone. Archie has strong values associated with being a worker (roles) and has a long term goal (values) of attending college next August to pursue a qualification in social care. Archie finds gardening enjoyable (interests) and wants to do this again in the future (values).

How do environmental factors contribute to this situation?
Opportunities on the ward do not allow him to address his goals; he currently feels bored. He feels unable to fulfil his goal of being a worker on discharge due to living with a brother who has mental illness and a chaotic lifestyle (social environment). Archie anticipates that many difficulties will resolve when he has a new place to live (physical environment) and an appropriate work environment (social environment).

What is the succinct conclusion statement?
"Archie has a strong set of values that have lead to him identifying short term and long term goals; however, his current choices and routines are not supportive of this goal attainment".

FIGURE 23.4 Archie's note reformulated.

Results of the Initial Interview

After being oriented to occupational therapy, Archie was interviewed using a standardized occupational therapy interview; he was conversational and cooperative during the assessment.

Findings

Strengths: Archie identifies goals which include, in the short term, moving from his brother's apartment to living alone. Archie has strong values associated with being a worker and has a long term goal of attending college next August to pursue a training in social care. Archie finds gardening enjoyable and wants to do this again in the future.
Challenges: Archie has a disorganized daily routine within the ward. He states he doesn't think personal care activities are important and therefore doesn't have a habit pattern to support a morning self-care routine. He states there are no enjoyable activities to do in the ward leading to his decision not to plan his day into a routine. Moreover, he is not motivated to focus on current routine as he believes he can readily reorganize his routine once he has a new place to live and a job. He also feels it would be difficult to work after discharge if he lived with his brother who has mental illness and leads a chaotic lifestyle.
Conclusion: Archie's anticipation that many difficulties will resolve once he has a living situation and a new job are supported by his past history of working and living independently. Nonetheless, his current choices and daily ward routine are continuing the lack of organization in his life prior to hospitalization and will contribute to a further deterioration of his habits, making it more difficult for him to attain his goals on discharge.

Summary

Archie has a strong set of values that have led to him identifying short term and long term goals; however his current choices and routine are not supportive of goal attainment.

Communicating Goals and Strategies of Therapy

Having a clear conceptualization of the client's occupational situation provides a foundation for identifying appropriate occupational changes for clients and their environments. Each client's conceptualization leads to an argument for the kinds of changes needed and the occupational engagement and therapeutic strategies that that will support achieving the desired change.

SETTING AND DOCUMENTING GOALS

It is helpful to think of the setting and documentation of goals as a three-step process (*Fig. 23.5*). The first step, as indicated earlier, is to create a conceptualization of the client's situation that emphasizes strengths and problems/challenges. The latter provide a framework for thinking about what needs to change. Therapists will find the Therapeutic Reasoning Table following Section 2 helpful for thinking about client and environmental change that a given client needs. Once one has identified (as much as possible in collab-

oration with the client) the areas of desired or needed change, these change statements can be translated into therapy goals.

LONG- AND SHORT-TERM GOALS

Long-term goals generally specify the overall anticipated outcomes of occupational therapy. Because they

FIGURE 23.5 Steps in setting therapy goals.

A. Conceptualizing the client's situation

B. Identifying with/for client (depending on ability of client to engage in process) personal and environmental changes that will support the client's occupational participation

C. Set Measurable Goals

project further into the future, they may have to be adjusted as the therapy unfolds. Long-term goals are accomplished through a series of short-term goals. Typically, short-term goals imply a sense of sequencing and priority (Trombly, 1995).

Long-term goals are most useful for evaluating the outcome of therapy, and short-term goals enable the therapist to review therapy and determine that appropriate progress is being made. Creating both long-term and short-term goals is helpful because it provides an understanding of what is being worked on immediately and what overall outcome is desired.

Creating Measurable Goals

To be measurable, a goal should contain these elements:

- Action: What the client will do to demonstrate that the occupational goal has been achieved
- Setting: The specific setting where the client will do it (e.g., in the ward or at the client's home)
- Degree: The circumstances under which the client will do it (e.g., independently, with physical support, with verbal cueing, using adaptive equipment, using compensatory techniques)
- Time frame: The period within which the client will be able to do it.

A goal with these elements clearly indicates what therapy aims to accomplish and provides a way of determining whether clients are achieving their goals. *Figure 23.6* provides examples of possible measurable goals. The table is not exhaustive, and the goals are not meant to be exemplars of possible goals but may be used as a starting point for developing your own measurable goals.

Two examples of client scenarios and goals related to MOHO concepts follow. Each goal contains elements associated with a measurable goal.

*B*eatrice and Jack

. . . .

Personal Causation Goal

Following a stroke, a client, Beatrice, stated that she was anxious about her occupational performance.

Having assessed Beatrice's motor and process skills, the occupational therapist noted from other informal observations that Beatrice's personal causation was leading her to avoid choosing to do things that were well within her performance capacity. Consequently, the therapist identified the following goal:

Within 7 days, Beatrice will improve her personal causation as evidenced by independently choosing to engage in personal and domestic occupational forms/tasks in line with her performance capacities in the ward setting.

Role-Related Goal

Jack, a 42-year-old client in a community-based work rehabilitation program for persons with psychiatric impairments, reported that he received negative feedback from the supervisor in a business in which he was placed for work training. Discussion with Jack and with the supervisor indicated that Jack was unaware of many of the subtle role-related expectations in the work setting. The therapist concluded that for Jack to meet worker role performance demands, he had to identify and internalize appropriate expectations for the worker role in this setting. The following goal was established:

Following three on-the-job coaching sessions, Jack will independently demonstrate consistent compliance with the expectations of the worker role at his work placement as judged by his supervisor.

Communicating and Documenting Clients' Occupational Engagement and Therapist's Strategies

Communicating and documenting the plan of therapy means not only specifying goals but how those goals will be reached. Obviously, the occupational therapist must decide how goals will be accomplished as part of therapeutic reasoning prior to implementing therapy. The Therapeutic Reasoning Table following Section 2 will help therapists think about and formulate types of occupational engagement and therapeutic strategies that should make up the therapy plan. Additionally,

F I G U R E   2 3 . 6 . **Examples of Measurable Goals Corresponding to MOHO Concepts**

Volition	• Within [timeframe], [client] will be *able to identify* [number] of occupational form(s)/task(s) that are significant to his/her occupational life [or role as a xxx] and that are commensurate with his/her current skills and abilities [action] within [setting] independently [degree]
	• Within [timeframe], [client] will be *able to perform* in [name occupational form/task] in line with his/her performance capacity without a verbal report/observation of low confidence [action] within [setting] independently [degree]
	• Within [timeframe], [client] will *make the choice* to engage in [name occupatiopal form/task] having *identified* this as significant to his/her [successful performance of/as a step in the progress towards] his/her performance as a [name role] [action] within [setting] with [degree] support
	• Within [timeframe], [client] will be able to demonstrate *an ability to perform* in [occupational form/task] in line with his/her performance capacity [action] within [setting] independently [degree]
	• Within [timeframe], [client] will be able to demonstrate *an ability to choose* to ask for help and use equipment where necessary [action] within [setting] independently [degree]
	• Within [timeframe], [client] will state he/she feels like he/she *is in control* of the occupational outcome while successfully *performing* in [name the occupational forms/tasks] [action], within [setting] with [degree] support
	• Within [timeframe], [client] will be able to *perform in valuable* occupational forms/tasks using adaptive equipment [action], within the [setting], with [degree] support
	• Within [timeframe], [client] will be able to *identify* [number] occupational goals [action], with [degree] support within [setting]
	• Within [timeframe], [OT] will be able to *identify* [number] occupational goals [action], that are based on the OT's understanding [through observation/proxy reports] of the client's occupational needs and wants within [setting]. *(useful with non verbal clients).*
	• Within [timeframe], [client] will be able to *identify* and *choose* to engage in the needed occupational performance to achieve [state goals] [action], with [degree] support within [setting]
	• Within [timeframe], [client] will be able to *sustain performance* in [name occupational form\task] involved in reaching their goal [action], with [degree] support within [setting]
	• Within [timeframe], [client] will be able to *identify* [number] interest(s) to pursue [action], this will be achieved with [degree] support within [setting]
	• Within [timeframe], [client] will be able to *perform in* [number] interests [action], independently [degree] within [setting]
Habituation	• Within [timeframe], [client] will be able to *identify* the responsibilities for roles that are valuable and meaningful to the person [action], this will be achieved with [degree] support within [setting]
	• Within [timeframe], [client] will be able to *plan & meet* the responsibilities for roles that are valuable and meaningful to the person [action], this will be achieved with [degree] support within [setting]
	• Within [timeframe], [client] will be able to *identify* roles that have the potential to be valuable and meaningful to the person [action], this will be achieved with [degree] support within [setting]

(continued)

FIGURE 23.6 *(continued)*

	• Within [timeframe], [client] will be able to *practice* & develop a habit pattern that will support achievement of a single occupational form/task [action], this will be achieved with [degree] support within [setting] • Within [timeframe], [client] will be able to *practice* & develop a habit pattern that will incorporate a new object and/or new way of completing an occupational form/ task [action], this will be achieved independently [degree] within [setting] • Within [timeframe], [client] will be able to *practice* & develop a habit pattern that will support achievement of role performance [action], this will be achieved with [degree] support within [setting]
Skill	• Within [timeframe], [client] will be able to perform within [name the occupational form/task] using [name skills] [action] within [setting], independently [degree] • Within [timeframe], [client] will be able to perform in [name the occupational form/task] using adapted techniques to support lack of skill [action] within [setting], independently [degree]
Performance Capacity	• Within [timeframe], [client] will be able to incorporate damaged/estranged parts of the body into completion of occupational forms/tasks [action], within [setting] independently [degree] • Within [timeframe], [client] will be able to manage symptoms while engaged in [name the occupational forms/tasks] [action] within [setting] with [degree] support
Environment	• Within [timeframe], [client] will be able to *perform* in the occupational forms/tasks they need and/or want to be able to do [action] within [state the physical space] [setting], independently [degree] • Within [timeframe], [client] will be able to *perform* in the occupational form/task using adapted objects or new objects [action] within [setting], independently [degree] • Within [timeframe], [relative] will be able to demonstrate an appropriate level of skill in supporting the client [action] within their [setting], independently [degree] • Within [timeframe], [relative] will be able to understand the client's abilities and limitations [action] within their [setting], with [degree] support • Within [timeframe], [client] will be able to *perform* in [name the occupational form/task] [action] within their physical and social [setting], independently [degree]

the discussions of occupational engagement in Chapter 13 and therapeutic strategies in Chapter 14 will also be of use. The therapy plan should be shared (and to the extent possible negotiated) with the client, relevant family members, and other staff members who might be involved. Moreover, it should be documented in the medical or other intervention record.

We use the examples of Beatrice and Jack who were previously discussed to illustrate how occupational engagement and therapeutic strategies work.

Beatrice and Jack

. . . .

Occupational Engagement and Therapeutic Strategies to Achieve a Personal Causation Goal

Beatrice's personal causation problem was evidenced by her anxiety and her reluctance to choose to do things that were well within her performance capacity. Improving Beatrice's personal causation will require that she experience success in doing more challenging things that she is currently avoiding. Thus Beatrice's occupational engagement will require her to choose more challenging activities and reexamine her thoughts and feelings about her capacity for and effectiveness in performing. To support Beatrice, the occupational therapist will advise Beatrice of occupational forms/tasks she had capacity to perform, encourage her to try to do them, structure the therapy process to ensure success, and provide her feedback on her success.

This plan might be communicated to Beatrice as follows:

> Beatrice, you and I discussed how you sometimes feel anxious about doing things that you probably can do just fine. The best way to overcome this anxiety is to try them out. I will guide you to select things that you can do and make sure they go okay. If you are feeling anxious, just let me know and we will talk about it and do something to make sure you feel okay. After you try out something we will sit down and go over how it went.

The plan could be documented as follows:

Goal: Within 7 days, Beatrice will improve her personal causation as evidenced by independently choosing to engage in personal and domestic occupational forms in line with her performance capacities in the ward setting.

Plan: Advise Beatrice of more challenging tasks she has capacity to perform and encourage her to choose to do them. Structure the therapy

process to ensure success and provide Beatrice feedback on her success.

Occupational Engagement and Therapeutic Strategies to Achieve a Role-Related Goal

Jack's goal was to internalize and comply with his work role expectations. In order to accomplish this goal he will need to identify these expectations and practice the expected behaviors. His therapist will need to coach Jack to understand and comply with the unspoken expectations of the worker role.

This plan might be communicated to Jack as follows:

> Jack, last session we identified that sometimes you are unaware of things you do at work that upset your supervisor. We also noted that you weren't aware that your supervisor expected certain things of you. To help you get on better at work, we are going to review things that your supervisor wants from you and role-play how you can do these things at work. Role playing means that I will pretend to be your boss and we will practice dealing with some of the things that come up at work.

The plan could be documented at follows:

Goal: Following three on-the-job coaching sessions, Jack will independently demonstrate consistent compliance with the expectations of the worker role at his work placement as judged by his supervisor.

Plan: After identifying appropriate work expectations, Jack will role-play relevant situations with coaching from the therapist.

Implementing and Reviewing Therapy

As one implements therapy, it is important to monitor whether the therapy is unfolding as planned and whether progress is being made on goals. Once again, it is important to communicate with the client as therapy unfolds. Feedback to clients concerning their progress helps to solidify commitment to therapy. When clients have attained goals, it is important to recognize their accomplishment and to reinforce the efforts they have put forward to accomplish them. Honest discussion with the client about new problems or lack of progress is equally important to maintain trust in the therapeutic relationship. When clients fail to reach goals, the information should be shared in a supportive context that examines the reasons for failure and facilitates the problem-solving necessary to formulate attainable goals or to ensure future goal attainment.

Documenting Client Progress in Therapy

As the therapist reviews therapy, it is important to maintain an ongoing record of therapeutic interventions and their outcomes. A central element of such documentation is reporting progress on short-term goal attainment. If the guidelines offered for measurable goals are followed, the therapist will already have decided what information to gather, when to gather it, and what criteria to apply to decide whether the client has attained short-term goals.

For instance consider Beatrice and Jack. In the case of Beatrice, the therapist would use informal observation 1 week from the time the goal was established to observe Beatrice's choices of personal care and domestic occupations on the ward. Her criterion for goal attainment is that Beatrice independently makes choices to do things in line with her skills.

In Jack's case, the therapist did not specify a given time but indicated that the evaluation is to follow three job-coaching sessions. According to the goal, the information to be collected is a report from Jack's supervisor, and the criterion of success is that Jack shows consistent compliance with worker role expectations. As these two examples readily illustrate, careful work of creating measurable goals will make the process of collecting information to determine goal attainment relatively straightforward.

A variety of methods of reporting progress are used, but the most common is progress notes in the client's chart or record. SOAP notes are commonly used. SOAP is an acronym for the four components of the note:

- Subjective information
- Objective information
- Assessment results
- Plan (Kettenbach, 1995).

SOAP note for Beatrice

S "I feel more confident to do things now."

O Beatrice was seen for 30 minutes for training in personal occupational forms/tasks at her bedside. Her performance capacities and how they matched to the demands of dressing were discussed with her. When coached to initiate dressing, Beatrice was observed to independently dress her upper body, which was in line with her performance capacity. Beatrice spontaneously asked for support with dressing (donning underwear, shoes, and pants) that could threaten her safety if she attempted to complete them independently.

A Compared to previous sessions, Beatrice appeared more relaxed in both discussing and engaging in personal occupational forms/tasks. Her ability to recognize occupational forms that were within her capabilities has improved over the past week. This improves the likelihood that she can be safely discharged home.

P Continue Beatrice's engagement in personal occupational forms/tasks. Plan a home visit before setting the discharge date to assess Beatrice's ability to manage at home.

SOAP note for Jack

S "I feel I am doing okay."

O Jack's time cards show that he has completed a full work timetable. Jack's supervisor stated that Jack has improved and has shown several behaviors consistent with his worker role. However, Jack has been late four out of five days and has frequently been observed interrupting the work of colleagues with stories unrelated to the job.

A Jack appeared to be happy with his progress following the coaching sessions. He will benefit from a review of time management strategies to foster his ability to get to work on time and a discussion of how his tendency to interrupt coworkers affects the team. A behavioral contract may be useful in changing Jack's behavior if his tendency to disturb coworkers persists after the problem has been addressed.

P Extend the goal timeframe and discuss supervisor's feedback with Jack.

Determining and Documenting the Outcomes of Therapy

The final step in therapy is to assess client outcomes. By collecting information to determine whether clients have attained goals, therapists can determine and document the effectiveness of occupational therapy. Outcomes can be determined by evaluating whether the client has achieved the stated short-term and long-term goals. When goals were not achieved, it is important to document the reason for the lack of success. The following is an example of this kind of documentation.

*B*eatrice

Beatrice attained four of her five short-term goals within the estimated timeframe. The fifth short-term goal, to evaluate Beatrice at home, was being planned and would have provided the information needed to attain the long-term goal of successful discharge home. However, Beatrice fell ill of a chest infection. She will be reassessed when she is well enough for therapy, and goals will be reset.

*J*ack

Jack completed eight coaching sessions and was then able to achieve his stated goal of knowing and meeting work role expectations. It took some time for Jack to hear and understand his supervisor's feedback. A remaining challenge was getting to work on time in the morning. A goal was therefore set for this ongoing challenge. Jack's lack of morning routine contributed to his lateness, and this became the focus of therapy.

Many MOHO evaluations (detailed in Chapters 15 to 18) are designed to be outcome measures and are appropriate for use before and after an intervention. In many cases, they provide clinical occupational profiles that can be compared to understand how a client has changed as a result of therapy. Outcomes of the client's progress can therefore be described in terms of change as measured by one of the assessments.

*S*tructuring Reporting Formats to Include Activities of Daily Living and MOHO

MOHO provides a framework for understanding why a client is not engaging in self-care, productivity, or leisure pursuits. MOHO is a theory-driven activity analysis that can be used in all areas of practice to understand the client's engagement in activities of daily living.

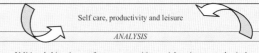

Self care, productivity and leisure

ANALYSIS

Volition, habituation, performance capacities, social environment, physical environment, skills

There are two basic approaches, therefore, to organizing this information for documentation.

In the first approach the therapist would discuss the areas of occupational participation (self-care, productivity, and leisure) and within each describe how the client's volition, habituation, performance capacity, and environment are affecting their ability to engage in activities of daily living. The second approach organizes the discussion around the client's volition, habituation, performance capacity, and environment, discussing the areas of occupational participation (in these areas).

Which approach one uses depends on the client and the site. For example, if the circumstances affecting occupational participation for leisure are quite different from those for work, one might use the first approach to underscore these differences. If occupational therapy services are driven by the concepts of self-care, productivity, and leisure, the first approach promotes this primary concern of occupational therapy.

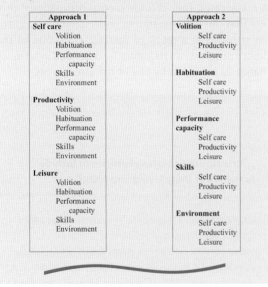

Approach 1	Approach 2
Self care	**Volition**
Volition	Self care
Habituation	Productivity
Performance	Leisure
capacity	
Skills	**Habituation**
Environment	Self care
	Productivity
Productivity	Leisure
Volition	
Habituation	**Performance**
Performance	**capacity**
capacity	Self care
Skills	Productivity
Environment	Leisure
	Skills
Leisure	Self care
Volition	Productivity
Habituation	Leisure
Performance	
capacity	**Environment**
Skills	Self care
Environment	Productivity
	Leisure

Use of MOHO Terminology in Communication and Documentation

The words that are selected to describe therapy are very important. Deciding whether and how to use MOHO terminology in communication and documentation requires consideration of several factors. MOHO

terms, like those of any other professional language, offer benefits and pose challenges.

Occupational therapists acquire the professional languages of several disciplines and theoretical perspectives. The terms resuscitation, repression, and reinforcement reflect medical model, object relations, and behavioral concepts, respectively. Complex conditions or procedures can be conveyed and immediately understood when such professional terminology is used.

A common example of how a professional term can efficiently convey complex information and facilitate communication between professionals is medical diagnosis. The term Alzheimer's dementia conveys the following rather complicated meaning:

> The development of multiple cognitive deficits manifested by both 1) memory impairment (impaired ability to learn new information or recall previously learned information), 2) one (or more) of the following cognitive disturbances: a. aphasia (language disturbance), b. apraxia (impaired ability to carry out motor activities despite intact motor function), c. agnosia (failure to recognize or identify objects despite intact sensory function), d. disturbance in executive functioning (i.e., planning, organizing, sequencing, abstracting). The cognitive deficits in Criteria 1 and 2 each cause a significant impairment in social or occupational functioning and represent a significant decline from a previous level of functioning. The course is characterized by gradual onset and continuing cognitive decline. The cognitive deficits in Criteria 1 and 2 are not due to any of the following: 1) other central nervous system conditions that cause progressive deficits in memory and cognition, 2) systemic conditions that are known to cause dementia, 3) substance-induced conditions. The deficits do not occur exclusively during the course of a delirium. The disturbance is not better accounted for by another Axis I disorder. (American Psychiatric Association, 2000)

As the definition illustrates, use of diagnostic terms allows those who know the meaning of terminology to share common perspectives and to convey information succinctly.

Similarly, MOHO terminology can be used to convey complex concepts to those who are familiar with the model. For example, the term volition denotes a complex idea about how persons are motivated toward their occupations. To those who know its meaning, volition conveys several concepts. When someone refers to a volitional problem, those who know the terminology can anticipate that the problem involves the client's values, personal causation, and interests. They can further expect that the problem is manifested in how clients anticipate, choose, experience, and interpret what they do. In this way, MOHO terminology can succinctly convey information.

The major disadvantage of all professional language is that everyone has to have a common understanding of the terms. It is therefore ineffective to use MOHO terms with colleagues, clients, or relatives who do not understand what the words mean. Some MOHO, terms such as volition, personal causation, and habituation have specialist meanings not readily understood. Other terms, such as interests, values, and habits, contain meaning beyond but still consistent with ordinary usage. Still other terms, such as skill, have a meaning within the MOHO context (i.e., a quality of actual occupational performance given person, task, and environment) that may be quite different from that of everyday usage (i.e., underlying capacity). Therefore, therapists should carefully decide when and how they use MOHO terms in communicating to clients, lay persons, and other professionals.

Communication and MOHO Terminology

In these circumstances it is appropriate to use MOHO terms in communication:

- The primary or exclusive audience is other occupational therapists who are familiar with MOHO language
- Clients are empowered by learning the MOHO concepts as a means of increasing understanding and control over their own circumstances
- Other professionals are receptive to becoming familiar with occupational therapy terminology.

MOHO language is intended to facilitate communication of ideas between occupational therapists. It can be particularly helpful when therapists are discussing clients, plans for therapy, and so on. Whereas clients ordinarily require that we communicate to them

in everyday language, some occupational therapists empower their clients to learn basic MOHO language and concepts. In one community occupational therapy program, Reencuentros, in Santiago, Chile, clients are taught the basic language and views of MOHO as part of their therapy. An important lesson from this experience is that client-centered therapy includes not only respecting clients' perspectives but also enriching their understanding of their own situations.

We have routinely used MOHO language both with clients and other professionals in practice contexts with positive results. Most clients are responsive to a therapist's attempts to explain the ideas they are using. Moreover, other professionals are often quite willing to acquire a basic understanding of one's professional terminology. Therapists have often noted to us that they have been surprised by how quickly teams pick up MOHO terms. Often the therapist's lack of confidence in using the terminology, rather than resistance on the part of other professionals, prevents use of MOHO terminology in an interdisciplinary context. Nonetheless, therapists should be sensitive to the demands they put on other professionals for learning their terminology. It is important to decide which terms one would like interdisciplinary colleagues to understand and to take the time to explain them. Finally, a willingness to attend to the perspectives and language of others goes a long way in encouraging them to attend to our own.

Recently, a colleague shared the following experience about introducing MOHO terminology in a psychiatric setting. Initially, the psychiatrist and other team members were skeptical about such terms as volition and personal causation. The therapist asked that the team give him an opportunity to use these and other terms, since they are part of his professional language. The psychiatrist agreed as the leader of the team that he would entertain the idea of the therapist using the terms in team discussions, provided it was clear how these terms added to understanding of the client and planning interdisciplinary care. Within a few months, the psychiatrist had not only learned the terms but also habitually ventured his own observations of client volition and habituation, asking for the therapist's expert opinion.

Using MOHO language in a multidisciplinary context can convey that the occupational therapist has a specific domain of interest and expertise to contribute to the team. For example, a psychologist recently approached the first author of this chapter, upset because she felt that occupational therapists were claiming motivation as their domain. She felt that motivation was a psychological term and area of expertise. This writer explained that occupational therapy's interest in motivation was based on the concept of volition and offered a brief explanation. Following this, the psychologist realized that her concerns with motivation and occupational therapy concerns were actually complementary rather than competitive or duplicative.

Moving Between MOHO Terms and Everyday Terms

Most therapists find it necessary to develop facility in moving back and forth between using MOHO terminology and expressing MOHO concepts in ordinary language. All professionals who wish to be effective in interacting with those who do not share their expertise

must know how to explain themselves in everyday language. *Figure 23.7* lists some common MOHO terms and ways they can be expressed in everyday language. Therapists may wish to expand and modify this table for their own everyday use, particularly when talking with clients and their families.

Documentation and MOHO Terminology

Since written documentation is primarily intended for professional audiences and aims at accuracy and completeness, a strong case for using MOHO terminology can be made. Consider for example the following note in ordinary language: "Edna lacks confidence and is overly dependent."

Using MOHO language makes the definition of the problem more specific:

Edna's personal causation is characterized by lack of a clear sense of her own capacity. As a result,

FIGURE 23.7 MOHO terms and explanations in everyday language.

Concepts from MOHO	Ways of Explaining the Theory/Concept to Clients
Person	
Volition	Your motivation for the things you do in everyday life and for choices you make about what you do with your life.
	Motivation is based on what we perceive to be interesting and valuable and what we believe ourselves capable of doing.
Personal Causation	How effective you feel in accomplishing the activities in your everyday life.
Values	What is important and meaningful to you and what your goals are.
Interests	What you enjoy or find satisfaction in doing.
Habituation	Your lifestyle and typical routine of daily activities.
Roles	The positions in life you hold and the responsibilities associated with them, such as being a spouse, parent, worker, student.
Habits	The routine way of doing activities, and your daily routine.
Performance Capacity	Physical and mental abilities.
	Subjective experience of symptoms of illness/impairment
Environment	
Spaces	The physical places where you work, play/relax, study, take care of yourself, rest and sleep (e.g., classroom, kitchen, bedroom, office).
Objects	Tools, supplies, furniture, appliances, clothes, vehicles, and other things you use, interact with, wear, or otherwise make part of your everyday life.
Occupational Forms	The everyday activities you do.
Social Groups	The people you interact with in daily life (coworkers, classmates, family members, roommates, neighbors, etc).

she anticipates performance situations with anxiety and frequently chooses to avoid doing things for which she has adequate skills. She also habitually seeks advice and help from others, which leads to her being unnecessarily dependent on others.

As the example illustrates, using the terminology of a theoretical model can result in documentation that is more precise and detailed. Moreover, while the first statement describes Edna's behavior, it does not explain it. The second statement offers an explanation that also provides a rationale for the following interventions:

- Advise Edna on a course of therapy that will be graded to be increasingly challenging to her sense of capacity
- Provide Edna with feedback about her occupational performance to enable a more accurate sense of her own capacities
- Encourage Edna to sustain performance in the face of anxiety
- Structure the environment to provide the opportunity for Edna to practice more autonomy.

Precision in language, including the use of theoretical terms, can clarify what we understand clients' difficulties to be and how we plan to address them. One of the best ways to explain occupational therapy is to demonstrate how its concepts frame problems and solutions.

Using and Modifying MOHO Assessment Forms to Report

Most of the MOHO-based assessments discussed in Chapters 15 to 18 have one or more forms associated with them for recording the results of the assessment. In some instances, therapists use these forms as a means for documentation. In fact, these forms were developed with therapists' input to ensure they would be useful for documentation. Nonetheless, in a variety of circumstances therapists cannot use the forms as they appear in the assessment manuals. For instance, a different format may be required by the setting, or therapists may decide on a format that better communicates to an interdisciplinary team. Whatever the reason, modified reporting of standardized MOHO assessments is not uncommon.

In this section we share some formats for reporting results of the Model of Human Occupational Screening Tool (MOHOST) (Parkinson, Forsyth, & Kielhofner, 2006) that have been developed by therapists in various settings. By focusing on the variety of ways that therapists have modified the standardized report form for this assessment, we hope to demonstrate how any of the MOHO-based assessment forms can be modified to suit a local reporting format.

The MOHOST (see Chapter 18) is a flexible assessment that is used for initial evaluation and to document change in clients. To capture a comprehensive picture of the client's occupational status, the MOHOST collects information on volition, habituation, skills, and the environment. The information gleaned from the MOHOST is used to complete a 24-item rating scale. Each item is rated on a four-point scale. This rating provides a quick visual reference of the client's strengths and challenges, and when research now under way is complete, it will also generate an interval-based measure of the client's resources for occupational participation. A short form for recording the information gathered in the MOHOST is shown in *Figure 18-4*. This form is used by many therapists to document the results of the MOHOST. A number of modifications of the form have also been developed. They are discussed next.

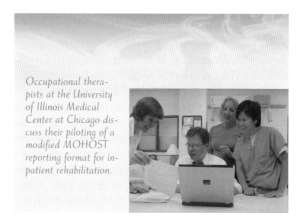

Occupational therapists at the University of Illinois Medical Center at Chicago discuss their piloting of a modified MOHOST reporting format for inpatient rehabilitation.

INPATIENT REHABILITATION SETTING

At the University of Illinois Medical Center at Chicago Hospital and Clinics, occupational therapists working in a physical rehabilitation context decided to adopt the MOHOST as part of their initial assessment. Historically therapists in this setting documented the clients' sensory, motor, and mental capacities and their implications for functional performance. They also completed the Functional Index Measure (Granger & Gresham, 1993), which is required documentation in that institution. When therapists began to work with the MOHOST, they found that it gave them valuable new information but struggled with how to document their use of the MOHOST. Among other things, they had to present the information efficiently, preserving necessary information not included in the MOHOST, and presenting data in a way that would be understood by the interdisciplinary team. After experimenting over several months they arrived at the reporting format shown in *Figure 23.8*. This format allowed them to preserve all of the information in the MOHOST but integrate it with other information therapists were required to collect.

A physical disability acute hospital in Scotland adopted the MOHOST assessment to support its service mission of facilitating successful discharges from acute care into the community. This is a service that completes assessments both within the acute care setting and during a home visit to understand the challenges that may appear for the client after discharge. The acute care ward is fast paced, and practitioners are required to document in a robust but brief way. They complete a MOHOST in acute care and then a MOHOST on the home visit. They then construct a summary sheet with all of the information relevant for discharge planning (*Figure 23.9*).

Mental Health Setting

Occupational therapists at the Northumberland, Tyne and Wear Mental Health NHS Trust who work with older people chose the MOHOST as a standard assessment. They concluded that the MOHOST provided a concise means of demonstrating to others the scope of occupational therapy practice. In practice it became evident that the standard format of MOHOST provided insufficient space in which to articulate the needs of their clients, many of whom have multiple pathologies and complex interrelationships between the various components of occupation.

Thus they adapted the format of MOHOST as follows:

- Space was added for introductory information about the rationale for referral to occupational therapy, the client's general situation and existing support networks, the scope of assessment, and to

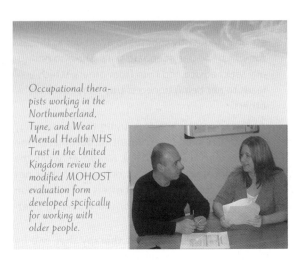

Occupational therapists working in the Northumberland, Tyne, and Wear Mental Health NHS Trust in the United Kingdom review the modified MOHOST evaluation form developed spcifically for working with older people.

record the client's consent to assessment and intervention.
- The inclusion of additional narrative as evidence to support the rating of each section of the MOHOST. When generating narrative, the therapists refer to the expanded criteria given in the MOHOST manual to structure their narrative while including individual comments to reflect each clients' unique circumstances.
- A section for analysis of the MOHOST ratings, a summary of findings, and a plan of intervention arising from that assessment was added. This section links the assessment to planning for intervention.

These adjustments to MOHOST (*Fig. 23.10*) provided the therapists with a format for initial and further assessment, an outcome measure, and a means of reporting to multidisciplinary colleagues the rationale and nature of occupational therapy intervention. Use of this reporting format resulted in better awareness of the role of occupational therapy among the multidisciplinary team; this resulted in increased appropriateness of referrals. Adopting the MOHOST reporting format also resulted in greater emphasis on clients' strengths, resources, and quality of performance rather than performance deficits. Finally, it increased attention to the promotion of health and well-being through occupation.

Industrial Rehabilitation

An occupational therapist working at the University of Illinois Medical Center at Chicago Hospital and Clinics

FIGURE 23.8 Modified MOHOST for an inpatient acute rehabilitation site developed by therapists at University of Illinois Medical Center at Chicago.

Occupational Therapy Inpatient Rehabilitation Evaluation

____Initial   _x__Discharge

Admit Date: 12/27/05   **Discharge Date: 01/28/06**

Diagnosis and HPI: Pt is a 32 y/o female admitted to an OSH on 12/6/04 following motor vehicle accident. Per husband pt was a restrained driver of a car hit by a semi-truck. CT scan revealed right temporal intraparenchymal bleed 2-3 cm/no midline shift. Radiology revealed left clavicular fracture, left humerus fracture, and right femoral fracture. 12/9 pt underwent ORIF of right femur and left humerus. It was noted per team that pt unable to move her left arm or leg and pt complaining of loss of sensation of her left hand. CT scan x 3 (12/6, 12/7, 12/8) revealed no changes. Review of neurological report on 12/12 were positive for left facial droop, fasciculations of left quadriceps, weakness of left side upper>lower and decreased sensation left upper > lower extremities. Pt transferred to UIMC on 12/14. 12/15 CT scan revealed (R) internal capsule and basal ganglia hematoma.

Precautions: WBAT on LE's; No more than 5# on (L)UE.

Occupational Performance History

Prior ADL/IADL Status: Check one box	Independent	Required Assistance
Bathing	x	
Dressing	x	
Transfers	x	
Ambulation	x	
Homemaking	x	
Transportation	x	

Occupational Profile

4= **FACILITATES** participation in occupation leading to positive outcomes
3= **ALLOWS** participation in occupation leading to satisfactory outcomes
2= **INHIBITS** participation in occupation leading to poor outcomes
1= **RESTRICTS** participation in occupation leading to negative outcomes

Admission				Scoring Definitions	Discharge			
4	3	2	1	**Environment**	4	3	2	1
			x	**Physical Space** — self care, productivity and leisure facilities/ privacy & accessibility/stimulation & comfort **4** Space affords a range of opportunities, supports & stimulates valued occupations **3** Space is mostly adequate, allows daily occupations to be pursued **2** Space affords a limited range of opportunities & curtails performance of valued activities **1** Space restricts opportunities & prevents performance of valued activities		x		
		x		**Physical Resources** — finance/equipment & tools/possessions & transport/safety & independence **4** Enables occupational goals to be achieved with ease, equipment & tools are appropriate **3** Generally allows occupational goals to be achieved, may present some obstacles **2** Impedes ability to achieve occupational goals safely, equipment & tools are inadequate **1** Has major impact on ability to achieve occupational goals, lack of equipment leads to high risk		x		
		x		**Social Groups** — family dynamics/friends & social support/work climate/involvement & expectations **4** Social groups offer practical support, values & attitudes support optimal functioning **3** Generally able to offer support but may be some under or over involvement **2** Offer reduced support or detracts from participation, some groups support but not others **1** Do not support functioning due to lack of interest or inappropriate involvement		x		
			x	**Occupational Demands** — activity demands/cultural conventions/construction of activities **4** Demands of activities match well with abilities, interests, energy & time available **3** Generally consistent with abilities, interest, energy, or time available, may present challenges **2** Some clear inconsistencies with abilities and interests, or energy & time available **1** Mostly inconsistent with abilities, construction of activity is under or over-demanding			x	

Current Physical Environment :

[x] Apartment [ ] House [ ] Condo [ ] Nursing Facility [ ] Elevator   [x] Stairs 2nd floor apt with 20 stairs and 1 railing
[x] Tub With Shower   [ ] Shower Stall
Support Next To Toilet: [x]R [ ]L [ ]None
[ ] DMEs/Adaptive Equipment: none

Admission comments: Pt demonstrating slight learned dependency as her level of participation in tasks is inconsistent with her abilities.

Discharge Comments: Pt's home environment will allow participation in most occupations with assistance. Pt's husband, mother, and other family members will provide assistance upon d/c. Bathroom equipment recommendations discussed and

FIGURE 23.8 *(continued)*

husband to purchase tub bench. Pt is not able to participate in all the tasks that she would like.

4	3	2	1	Motivation for Occupation	4	3	2	1
		X		**Appraisal of Ability** —accurate belief in skill & competence/awareness of capacity **4** Accurately assesses own capacities, recognizes strengths, aware of limitations **3** Reasonable tendency to over/under estimate own abilities, recognizes some limitations **2** Difficulty understanding strengths & limitations without support **1** Does not reflect on skills, fails to realistically estimate own abilities		X		
		X		**Expectation of Success** — optimism & hope/self efficacy, sense of control & self identity **4** Anticipates success and seeks challenges, optimistic about overcoming obstacles **3** Has some hope for success, adequate self-belief but has some doubts, may need encouraging **2** Requires support to sustain optimism about overcoming obstacles, poor self-efficacy **1** Pessimistic, feels hopeless, gives up in the face of obstacles, lacks self-control	X			
	X			**Interest** — expressed enjoyment/satisfaction/curiosity/participation **4** Keen, curious, lively, tries new activities, expresses pleasure, perseveres, appears content **3** Has adequate interests that guide choices, has some opportunities to pursue interests **2** Difficulty identifying interests, interest is short-lived, ambivalent about choice of occupations **1** Easily bored, unable to identify interests, apathetic, lacks curiosity even with support	X			
	X			**Choices** — appropriate commitment/readiness for change/sense of value & meaning/goals & preferences **4** Clear preferences & sense of what is important, motivated to work towards occupational goals **3** Mostly able to make choices, may need encouragement to set and work towards goals **2** Difficulties identifying what is important or setting & working towards goals, inconsistent **1** Cannot set goals, impulsive, disorganized; goals are unattainable/unrealistic	X			

Admission Comments: Pt is easily discouraged when faced with challenges and her fear of pain and failure inhibit her engagement in occupational tasks. She overestimates her limitations and underestimates her abilities.
Discharge Comments: Pt is ready and willing to take on new challenges at home. She appears to recognize limitations most of the time; however during her hospital stay she had several incidents of falls.

4	3	2	1	Pattern of Occupation	4	3	2	1
		X		**Routine** — balance/organization of habits/structure/productivity **4** Able to arrange a balanced, organized and productive routine of daily activities **3** Generally able to maintain or follow an organized and productive routine of daily activities **2** Difficulty organizing balanced, productive routines of daily activities without support **1** Empty routine, unable to support responsibilities and goals, erratic/disorganized routine		X		
		X		**Adaptability** — anticipation of change/habitual response to change/tolerance of change **4** Anticipates change, alters actions or routine to meet demand (flexible/accommodating) **3** Generally able to modify behavior, may need time to adjust, hesitant **2** Difficulty adapting to change, reluctant, passive or habitually overreacts to change **1** Rigid, unable to adapt routines or tolerate change	X			
	X			**Responsibility** — role competence/meeting expectations/fulfilling obligations **4** Reliably completes activities and meets the expectations related to role obligations **3** Copes with most responsibilities, meets most expectations, able to fulfill most role obligations **2** Difficulty being able to fulfill expectations & meet role obligations without support **1** Limited ability to meet demands of activities or obligations, unable to complete role activities	X			
		X		**Roles** — role identity/ role variety/belonging/involvement **4** Identifies with a variety of roles, has a sense of identity/belonging that comes from roles **3** Generally identifies with one or more roles and has some sense of belonging from these roles **2** Limited identification of roles, role overload or conflict, poor sense of belonging **1** Does not identify with any role, negligible role demands, no sense of belonging	X			

Primary occupation, roles, & routine prior to admission; Leisure interests & social participation: Pt is a wife, mother, and works in a school as a child welfare attendant. She enjoys gardening and spending time out with her friends.
Admission comments: Pt is limited by pain and the fear of pain.
Discharge comments: Pt has a strong sense of who she is and how her roles play a part in her life. She is able to maintain an organized environment on the rehab unit but will have to re-establish a routine at home and she is able to adapt to new routines without losing effort or motivation.

4	3	2	1	Motor Skills	4	3	2	1
			X	**Posture & Mobility** — stability/alignment/positioning/balance/walking/reaching/transfers **4** Stable, upright, independent, flexible, good range of motion **3** Generally able to maintain posture and mobility in occupation independently or with aids **2** Unsteady at times despite assistive devices/equipment; slow or manages with difficulty **1** Extremely unstable, unable to reach or bend or unable to walk			X	
		X		**Coordination** — manipulation/ease of movement/fluidity/fine motor skills **4** Coordinates body parts with each other, uses smooth fluid movements **3** Some awkwardness or stiffness causing minor interruptions to occupations **2** Difficulty coordinating movements (clumsy/ tremulous/awkward/stiff) **1** Unable to coordinate, manipulate, & use fluid movements			X	
			X	**Strength and Effort** — grip/handling/moving/lifting/transporting/calibrating **4** Grasps, moves & transports objects securely with adequate force and speed **3** Strength and effort are generally sufficient for most tasks **2** Has difficulty with grasping, moving, or transporting objects with adequate force & speed **1** Unable to grasp, move, transport objects with appropriate force & speed			X	
		X		**Energy** — endurance/pace/attention/stamina **4** Maintains appropriate energy levels, able to maintain tempo throughout occupation	X			

FIGURE 23.8 (continued)

			3 Energy may be slightly low or high at times, able to pace self for most tasks		
			2 Difficulty maintaining energy levels (tires easily/evidence of fatigue/distractible/restless)		
			1 Unable to maintain energy level, lacks focus, lethargic, inactive, or highly overactive		

Neuromusculoskeletal functions (ROM, strength, tone, coordination):

Admission: Pt is significantly limited by (L) hemiplegia and pain. Pt has no active movement at (L)UE and only trace at (L)LE. 1 finger subluxation present. PROM WFLs with exception of shoulder ~45 degrees prior to pain. (R)UE WFLs for AROM, strength, and coordination. (R)LE limited due to pain/weakness.

Discharge: PROM: WFLs with exception of shoulder ~70 degrees prior to pain. AROM: ~ 60 degrees of shoulder abd; ~90 elbow flexion; ~25 degrees of elbow extension; ~10 degrees of wrist and finger flexion. Able to use (L)UE as stabilizer but unable to release objects. Pt reports that resting hand splint has eased left wrist pain. Pt has 1 finger subluxation and wears hemi sling to relieve shoulder pain during ambulation.

Sensory Functions (Vision, hearing, pain, sensation):

Admission: Impaired sensation (light touch and proprioception) at (L)UE. Significant pain of (R)LE, (L)UE/LE.

Discharge: Sensation in (L)UE improved with impairment noted at fingertips only. Pt's c/o pain have decreased and are associated mainly with movement of (R)LE and (L) shoulder above 70 degrees flex/abd.

4	3	2	1	Process Skills	4	3	2	1
	X			**Knowledge** – seeking & retaining information/knowing what to do in an activity/ using objects **4** Seeks and retains information, knows how to use tools appropriately **3** Generally able to seek and retain information & knows how to use tools **2** Difficulty knowing how to use tools, difficulty in asking for or retaining information **1** Unable to use knowledge/tools, does not retain information, asks repeatedly for same information	X			
		X		**Planning/Timing** – initiation/completion/sequencing/concentration **4** Sustains concentration, starts, sequences and completes occupation at appropriate times **3** Generally able to concentrate, start, sequence and complete occupations **2** Fluctuating concentration or distractible, difficulty initiating & completing **1** Unable to concentrate, unable to initiate, sequence or complete occupations	X			
	X			**Organization** – arranging space & objects/neatness/preparation/gathering objects **4** Efficiently searches for, gathers & restores tools/objects needed in occupation **3** Generally able to search, gather, & restore needed tools/objects **2** Difficulty searching for, gathering & restoring tools/objects, ineffective locating of items **1** Unable to search for, gather & restore tools and objects, disorganized, marked delay in locating items	X			
		X		**Problem Solving** – judgment/adaptation/decision-making/responsiveness **4** Shows good judgment, anticipates difficulties & generates workable solutions (rational) **3** Generally able to make decisions based on difficulties that arise **2** Difficulty anticipating an adapting to difficulties that arise, seeks reassurance **1** Unable to anticipate and adapt to difficulties that arise and makes inappropriate decisions		X		

Mental functions (attention, memory, problem solving, motor planning, perceptual functions):

Admission: Pt is limited due to feeling overwhelmed and preoccupied by pain. Pt is alert, oriented, and able to follow directions for ADL tasks. No perceptual deficits noted at this time.

Discharge: At times during rehab stay pt demonstrated questionable problem solving abilities, however she is continuing to make improvement in this area.

4	3	2	1	Communication & Interaction Skills	4	3	2	1
X				**Nonverbal Skills** – eye contact/gestures/orientation/proximity **4** Appropriate body language given culture and circumstances **3** Generally able to display appropriate body language **2** Difficulty controlling/displaying appropriate body language (delayed/limited/disinhibited) **1** Unable to display appropriate body language (absent/incongruent/unsafe/aggressive)	X			
X				**Conversation** – disclosing/initiating & sustaining/speech content/language **4** Appropriately initiates, discloses, and sustains conversation (clear/direct/open) **3** Generally able to use language or signing to effectively exchange information **2** Difficulty initiating, disclosing, or sustaining conversation (hesitant/abrupt/limited/irrelevant) **1** Uncommunicative, disjointed, bizarre or inappropriate disclosure of information	X			
X				**Vocal Expression** – intonation/articulation/volume/pace **4** Assertive, articulate, uses appropriate tone, volume and pace **3** Vocal expression is generally appropriate in tone, volume and pace **2** Difficulty expressing self (mumbling/pressured speech/monotone) **1** Unable to express self (incomprehensible/too quiet or loud/too fast)	X			
X				**Relationships** – cooperation/collaboration/rapport/respect **4** Sociable, supportive, aware of others, sustains engagement, friendly, relates well to others **3** Generally able to relate to others & mostly demonstrates awareness of others' needs **2** Difficulty with cooperation or makes few positive relationships **1** Unable to cooperate with others or make positive relationships	X			

Occupational Performance Assessment (FIM)

Activities of Daily Living: (FIM= Functional Independence Measure)

FIM Key **7**=Independent **6**=Modified independent **5**=SBA/Set-up **4**=Min. assist (performs 75% or >)

3=Moderate assist (patient performs 50-75%) **2**=Max assist (dependent but directs care; performs 25-50%)

1=Dependent (25% or less)

ADL	INITIAL STATUS	D/C GOAL	D/C STATUS
Feeding	5	5	6

FIGURE 23.8 (continued)

Grooming	2	4	6
Bathing	2	4	6
UB Dressing	2	5	6
LB Dressing	1	4	5
Toileting	1	4	6
Toilet Transfers	1	4	5
Tub Transfers	1	4	5
Social Interaction	7	7	7
Problem Solving	5	6	6
Memory	6	7	7

IADL	**INDICATE IF THIS AN AREA OF FOCUS**
Homemaking [x] yes [ ] no	
Community Integration [ ]yes [x] not at this time	
Leisure [ ]yes [x] no specific goals for leisure pursuits were identified by the patient at this time	

Functional Mobility (bed mobility, transfers, locomotion):
Admission: Pt requires max assist to stand and transfer. Pt not ambulatory at this time.
Discharge: Pt is able to ambulate with SBA and SBQC; requires assist for occasional loss of balance.

Patient/Family Goals: to regain optimal independence in basic ADL tasks

Summary of Factors Enhancing and Limiting Occupational Performance:
Initial: Pt is motivated but very limited by pain and (L) hemiplegia.
Discharge: Pt remains motivated and optimistic about her progression towards independence. Pt achieved all and surpassed many of her ADL long term goals. Pt has a strong support system with many friends and relatives. She is realistic about her return home stating that it will be difficult but she that she is "up for the challenge". She is limited in occupational performance secondary to limited ROM/strength in LUE/LLE, as well as pain in her RLE with movement.

Treatment plan: Pt will be seen 90 minutes 5 days a week to promote (L) side motor recovery, including optimal positioning and incorporation of (L)UE into functional activities. Pt will explore and practice modified approaches to routine ADL tasks. Treatment sessions will address acquiring new habits to successfully adapt to changed circumstances, enhancing pt understanding of her occupational capacities (strengths and limitations), as well as widening her success in occupational performance by reducing anxiety and fear of failure, and building up her confidence to face occupational demands.

Patient/Family Education (provided/needed): Pt's husband was educated on donning and doffing hemi splint and safe techniques when helping pt with self care routine, transfers and ambulation. Pt was educated in safe techniques in order to navigate space at home and carry out daily activities such as ADL and homemaking tasks. Pt is efficient at explaining and teaching techniques to spouse.

D/C Recommendations: It is recommended that pt obtain a tub bench in order to bathe safely. Pt was issued a raised toilet seat in order to complete toileting and toilet transfers safely. Outpatient OT is recommended to further increase independence and safety in ADL and increase neuromuscular return in LUE for ADL/IADL and community activities.

in an industrial rehabilitation program receives referrals from physicians to evaluate clients for return to work and for need for work-related rehabilitation. For many years the therapist focused primarily on a biomechanical-based work capacity evaluation. However, she noted that many clients had either strengths or problems related to returning to work that were not captured by this approach to assessment and documentation. She decided to modify her industrial evaluation to include the MOHOST. She further developed a brief interview that could be used to gather information relevant to the MOHOST. She uses this interview along with information available from her work capacity evaluation to complete the MOHOST. Since her documentation is primarily read by the referring physician, she wanted to organize it in a fashion that would be easily comprehended. Her document includes these points:

- Information on the injury
- Work-related information such as type of job, time off work, return to work options
- Information not included in the MOHOST, such as sensory and neuromuscular functions.

FIGURE 23.9 An evaluation summary sheet to guide discharge planning, developed by an acute care occupational therapy department in Scotland.

OCCUPATIONAL THERAPY REPORT

Name: Mrs M
Address: 21 Stirling Street, Bridge of Allan
Diagnosis: Cellulitis to both lower legs, Pulmonary fibrosis & Diabetes

---

A: Reason for Referral and Assessment

Mrs M was admitted to Ward 18, Wallace hospital on 9 August 2005 due to a physical collapse at home. Mrs M has completed a period of rehabilitation and no further improvement is anticipated. Mrs M is currently having difficulty performing daily routines within the ward setting due to shortness of breath and lack of confidence in her abilities. Mrs M would like to return home despite limitations and this is supported by her son. This report details the occupational therapy assessment completed in preparation for Mrs M transitioning back to her home environment

---

B: Assessment Structure

Date of assessment:
MOHOST assessment (within ward 18) spanned the period 15th August to 25th August 2005
MOHOST assessment (within her home environment) was completed on 26th August 2005

Data sources for report & evidence based assessment used:
Model of Human Occupation Screening Tool (MOHOST) (within ward 18)
  a) Verbal interview with Mrs M,
  b) Verbal reports from nursing staff on ward 18,
  c) Observations of Mrs M attempting familiar tasks, (washing, dressing)
Model of Human Occupation Screening Tool (MOHOST) (within her home environment)
  a) Verbal interview with Mrs M,
  b) Verbal reports from son, home care support, neighbor (all present on visit)
  c) Observations of Mrs M attempting familiar tasks within her home

Date of report: 27th August 2005

C: Summary of Occupational Therapy Findings

Mrs M is a 75 year old woman who lives alone in a 3 bedroom, two story house. She is a mother and a friend who enjoys reading and television.

Strengths:
- Mrs M values living independently and is, therefore, very motivated to return home
- Mrs M feels much supported by her friends and neighbor (emergency contact) who provide daily valued social contact.
- Mrs M describes a strong relationship with her son and he attends every week and took her out in his car.

Challenges:
- Prior to admission Mrs M was physically limited, requiring home care support four times daily and now states she has less physical ability.
- Mrs M has lost confidence in her limited ability which will make her more anxious about being home and this may affect her mood.
- Mrs M needs to use portable oxygen to mobilise short distances and lacks routines at home that incorporate this into everyday activity.

Recommendations: Before discharge can be arranged the following MUST be in place. They have been agreed with Mrs M & Son
1. **Environmental supports:**
   Provide commode for use downstairs, refer for review of bathing equipment, reinstate previous level of home care support *PLUS* support with preparation of breakfast
2. **Community Rehabilitation:**

FIGURE 23.9 *(continued)*

Refer to support Mrs M re: engage with previous valued roles & related activities
3. **Medical supports:**
    Ward 18 nursing staff to refer to District Nurse for diabetes management and oxygen
    cylinder provision and education

This information is integrated with information that the MOHOST provides in a simple narrative format that is easily read by the physician and that organizes information into logical categories. *Figure 23.11* shows the reporting format.

This section demonstrates that there are many ways of adapting the MOHOST assessment depending on circumstances. This is equally true of all MOHO assessments. The therapist must review the information gained from the MOHO assessment, generate a description of the client's situation, identify measurable goals, and make decisions on how this information should be communicated and documented.

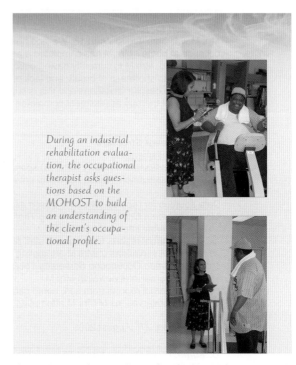

During an industrial rehabilitation evaluation, the occupational therapist asks questions based on the MOHOST to build an understanding of the client's occupational profile.

Conclusion

The strength of using MOHO in clinical thinking is its ability to support robust formulations of the client's complex occupational circumstances. These conceptualizations should then be articulated and documented to ensure strong advocacy for clients. This chapter demonstrated how MOHO and MOHO-based assessments can be used in a flexible manner to communicate to others about clients and to document clients' circumstances and therapeutic outcomes. In addition, a therapist's understanding of a client can be communicated in a manner that fits with local circumstances and contexts.

FIGURE 23.10 An adaptation of the MOHOST by occupational therapists in Northumberland, Tyne, and Wear Mental Health NHS Trust working in older adult mental health services.

NEWCASTLE OLDER PEOPLE'S MENTAL HEALTH SERVICE
OCCUPATIONAL THERAPY ASSESSMENT

Client Information:
Name: *Julie Jones*
Assessor Designation: *Senior Occupational Therapist*
Signature: **Date:** *25/01/2006*
Date of first contact: *17/01/2006*
Date(s) of assessment: *17/01/2006; 23/01/2006*
Assessment settings: *Client's home*
Diagnosis: *Alzheimer's Disease*

Overview:	
Reason for referral Scope of assessment undertaken General situation Relevant clinical & occupational history Consent	*Mrs Jones was referred for Occupational Therapy assessment by her CPN in order to identify Mrs Jones's functional abilities within her home.* *The Model of Human Occupation Screening Tool (MoHOST) was used as a framework to guide assessment. Mrs Jones's friend Harry was present throughout each visit and was able to provide anecdotal information in support.* *Mrs Jones lives alone in warden controlled sheltered accommodation, although spends a significant amount of time with Harry, either at his home within the same complex, or together in her own home. She currently has a care package in place which involves two daily calls to consider: self care, medication prompt, prepare breakfast, housework, laundry, shopping. Harry reports that he carries out the majority of domestic tasks, as well as hot drink and meal preparation, and provides assistance with personal care and toileting as required.*

MOTIVATION FOR OCCUPATION		
Appraisal of ability Understanding of strengths &limitations Self-awareness & realism Belief in skill	**F** **A** **(I)** **R**	*Mrs Jones has little insight into her limitations but was aware of her need for Harry's ongoing support. During discussion, she fluctuated between asserting her independence in all aspects of daily living, to admitting that she does very little for herself. She is generally satisfied and maintains a belief in her own skills, although this is not always realistic.*
Expectation of success Optimism Self-efficacy Sense of control Hope	**F** **A** **(I)** **R**	*She expects success in most areas, although this is generally inappropriate. Her lack of awareness of limitations combined with cognitive impairment mean that she remains optimistic about the future and retains the perception of being in control.*
Interest Expressed enjoyment Satisfaction Curiosity Participation	**F** **A** **(I)** **R**	*Mrs Jones requires significant support and encouragement in order to sustain engagement in activities. She previously had many interests and regularly participated in community activities; however, her involvement has decreased significantly over the last few months. Harry continues to encourage Mrs Jones to attend their local Community Centre for lunch through the week. Day Centre attendance has recently been arranged for both Harry and Mrs Jones to attend twice weekly, and I understand this commenced last week.*

F= Facilitates occupational participation A= Allows occupational participation I= Inhibits occupational participation R= Restricts occupational participation

FIGURE 23.10 *(continued)*

NEWCASTLE OLDER PEOPLE'S MENTAL HEALTH SERVICE
OCCUPATIONAL THERAPY ASSESSMENT

Commitment Values & standards Goals & projects Choices & preferences Sense of purpose	F A Ⓘ R	*Mrs Jones has difficulty identifying how to structure her own time. She is dependent upon others, needing prompts to manage her personal activities of daily living. She looks to Harry to provide her daily structure.*

PATTERN OF OCCUPATION		
Routine Balance Structure Productivity Activity	F A Ⓘ R	*Mrs Jones is reliant on others to provide daily organisation and currently follows a routine enforced by Harry. She tends to get up at the same time (7.00am) each morning and commence her toileting routine; Harry usually arrives to assist with dressing and ensure that any spills/incontinence are cleaned up within the bathroom. He prepares breakfast and a hot drink at this time. Home Care arrives at 8.45 am and their remit is to assist with self care, prompt medication, make breakfast and get any shopping necessary. This formal input has not always been successful to date due to Harry's ongoing involvement in the same tasks, and Mrs Jones's frequent visits to Harry's home, which often coincide with planned Home Carer visits. At lunchtime, Harry heats some tinned soup for the couple in his flat and then they either go out for the afternoon, or watch TV in his flat. In the evening, Harry heats Mrs Jones's meal up in his flat and they eat their meal together. Mrs Jones appears to respond well to eating meals in company and her dietary intake has improved as a result.*
Adaptability Anticipation Flexibility Response to change Frustration tolerance	F A Ⓘ R	*Mrs Jones enjoys her time spent with Harry, but appears to be a passive recipient of daily routines or planned events. She very much relies on Harry's continued input – when this has been withdrawn in the past, she has responded poorly and been unable to adapt to the change in routines, becoming anxious and disorientated.*
Responsibility Awareness Handling expectation Fulfilling obligations Acceptance	F A Ⓘ R	*She has little sense of responsibility, and is content for Harry to continue to care for her.*
Roles Involvement Belonging Response to demand Role variety	F A Ⓘ R	*She derives a sense of belonging and involvement from her friendship with Harry. She looks forward to the regular visits she receives from her family but has little other role variety.*

F= Facilitates occupational participation A= Allows occupational participation   I= Inhibits occupational participation R= Restricts occupational participation

FIGURE 23.10 *(continued)*
NEWCASTLE OLDER PEOPLE'S MENTAL HEALTH SERVICE
OCCUPATIONAL THERAPY ASSESSMENT

COMMUNICATION AND INTERACTION SKILLS		
Non-verbal skills Physicality Eye contact Gestures Orientation	F **(A)** I R	*Although able to convey mood and make needs known with her non-verbal behaviour, at times throughout the assessment she demonstrated questionable awareness of personal space.*
Conversation Disclosing Initiating & sustaining Speech content Language	F A **(I)** R	*Mrs Jones's conversation was repetitive both in content and questions asked. She was able to initiate socially appropriate conversation subjects appropriate to the occasion.*
Vocal expression Intonation Articulation Volume Pace	F **(A)** I R	*Mrs Jones was mostly able to indicate needs.*
Relationships Co-operation Collaboration Rapport Respect	F A **(I)** R	*She is vulnerable to manipulation by others.*

PROCESS SKILLS		
Knowledge Seeking & retaining info Use of knowledge including use of objects Understanding, orientation	F A **(I)** R	*Mrs Jones is disorientated to time and date, although she is orientated with her home. She is dependent upon others to jog her memory regarding appointments or events, despite a calendar prominently positioned in her living room. She does not fully retain information and regularly requires information to be repeated. She is very much lacking in insight, and continues to perceive herself to be fully independent in many ADL activities. During assessment in the kitchen, Mrs Jones was able to select appropriate items and use these as expected.*
Planning Thinking through from beginning to end Timing Concentration	F A **(I)** R	*Assessment highlighted Mrs Jones's difficulty continuing tasks to completion; she began to make a hot drink but became distracted by external cues and did not return to the task. She loses track of time and becomes anxious because of this. Mrs Jones required prompts to commence the task and it is felt that if these prompts were not provided, she would not initiate any tasks.*
Organisation Arranging space & objects Neatness Preparation	F A **(I)** R	*Mrs Jones demonstrated safe and correct use of her electric kettle, filling and plugging this in safely. She loses track of what needs doing and would require constant supervision and prompts in order to complete tasks.*
Problem-solving Judgement Adaptation Decision-making Responsiveness	F A I **(R)**	*Mrs Jones is highly dependent on others for all aspects of daily living activities and she is extremely vulnerable as a result. As she is reliant on others, little is required of her in the way of problem solving, and it is not anticipated that she would manage this alone.*

F= Facilitates occupational participation A= Allows occupational participation I= Inhibits occupational participation R= Restricts occupational participation

FIGURE 23.10 (continued)
NEWCASTLE OLDER PEOPLE'S MENTAL HEALTH SERVICE
OCCUPATIONAL THERAPY ASSESSMENT

MOTOR SKILLS		
Posture & Mobility Stability Walking Alignment Reaching Positioning Bending Balance Transfers	F A (I) R	*Mrs Jones has an awkward gait, although walks unaided. She manages to use the stairs within the complex but relies heavily on the banister rail. She usually uses the lift when with Harry but is not always able to use this correctly when alone. There were no problems identified with transfers, but these were not formally assessed due to Mrs Jones's reluctance to participate. During kitchen activities, she was observed to have some stiffness and increased effort when bending/reaching.*
Co-ordination Manipulation Ease of movement Fluidity Fine motor skills	F A (I) R	*Difficulty was observed when manipulating objects, in particular zips, and Mrs Jones requires assistance with personal care tasks because of this.*
Strength & Effort Grip Lifting Handling Transporting Moving Calibrating	F A (I) R	*Mrs Jones has poor strength for lifting items such as shopping, or even her kettle. She received significant support from Harry because of this.*
Energy Endurance Pace Attention Stamina	F A (I) R	*Mrs Jones tires quickly during activity and becomes short of breath on exertion. Harry reports that she tends to rest or sleep for much of the afternoon.*

ENVIRONMENT		
Physical space Home & Neighbourhood Work &/or leisure facilities Privacy & accessibility Stimulation & comfort	F (A) I R	*Mrs Jones lives in a comfortable warden controlled, sheltered accommodation flat situated on the 2nd floor. Her close friend, Harry, lives nearby within the same complex. The complex is easily accessed and lifts are available to the upper floors. There are laundry facilities on site. The flats are situated in close proximity to local shops and amenities and are well placed to access public transport. Mrs Jones also spends a significant amount of her time in her friend's flat.*
Physical resources Finance Equipment & tools Possessions & transport Safety & independence	F (A) I R	*Physical resources meet all basic needs, but without any luxuries. Access to the flat is via door intercom and Mrs Jones was unable to use this safely which has an impact upon her safety and independence within her home.*
Social groups Family dynamics Friends & social support Expectations & involvement	F A (I) R	*Harry provides significant social input as well as care, but this has proved to be unreliable in the past. Dynamics between Mrs Jones's family, Harry and Mrs Jones are complex. Both Mrs Jones and Harry have recently begun Day Centre attendance twice a week.*
Occupational Demands Social & leisure activities Daily living tasks Domestic &/or work responsibilities	F A (I) R	*Mrs Jones has significantly reduced her involvement in daily activities, and this reduction matches her level of ability. She requires continued supervision and support to maintain her current level of function and ensure safety and wellbeing.*

F= Facilitates occupational participation A= Allows occupational participation I= Inhibits occupational participation R= Restricts occupational participation

FIGURE 23.10 *(continued)*
NEWCASTLE OLDER PEOPLE'S MENTAL HEALTH SERVICE
OCCUPATIONAL THERAPY ASSESSMENT

Summary of Ratings																							
Motivation for Occupation				Pattern of Occupation				Communication & Interaction Skills				Process Skills				Motor Skills				Environment			
Appraisal of abilities	Expectation of success	Interest	Commitment	Routine	Adaptability	Responsibility	Roles	Non-verbal skills	Conversation	Vocal expression	Relationships	Knowledge	Planning	Organisation	Problem-solving	Posture & mobility	Co-ordination	Strength & effort	Energy	Physical Space	Physical resources	Social groups	Occupational demands
F	F	F	F	F	F	F	F	F	F	F	F	F	F	F	F	F	F	F	F	F	F	F	F
A	A	A	A	A	A	A	A	(A)	A	(A)	A	A	A	A	A	A	A	A	A	(A)	(A)	A	A
(I)	(I)	(I)	(I)	(I)	(I)	(I)	(I)	I	(I)	I	(I)	(I)	(I)	(I)	I	(I)	(I)	(I)	(I)	I	I	(I)	I
R	R	R	R	R	R	R	R	R	R	R	R	R	R	R	(R)	R	R	R	R	R	R	R	(R)

SUMMARY & RECOMMENDATIONS

Analysis of the MoHOST highlights Mrs Jones's significant deficits in the majority of Occupational Performance components.

She is currently receiving a significant amount of support and prompts from her friend, Harry, although historically, this has not always been reliable or consistent. She also has a care package in place, which is not always effective due to Mrs Jones's current routines. This level of support is essential to maintain Mrs Jones at home.

Mrs Jones's lack of insight into her limitations combined with her significant global Occupational Performance deficits, demonstrate her vulnerability as well as her need for constant supervision and support in order to maintain her residual function and safety. Without this input, she would be at risk. Her attendance at a Day Centre will provide further routine and social stimulation as well as the opportunity to further monitor her needs in a more structured setting.

F= Facilitates occupational participation A= Allows occupational participation   I= Inhibits occupational participation   R= Restricts occupational participation

FIGURE 23.11 A MOHOST-based reporting format for industrial rehabilitation developed by an occupational therapist at University of Illinois Medical Center at Chicago.

Occupational Therapy Evaluation for Industrial Rehabilitation

Name:	**Sam**
Diagnosis:	**Bilateral calcaneus fractures, closed; Spine fracture at L1;**
Medical History:	**Fracture open reduction, internal fixation of bilateral calcaneal fracture**
Date of injury:	**January 12th 2005**
Cause of injury:	**Patient, who is a carpenter, was at a construction site to lay down wood floors when stairway collapsed and fell approximately 14 feet landing on both his heels.**

Occupational Profile
Environment: *Current Social Environment:* Patient lives in a house which he shares with roommates; He states that he has good social supports and engages in leisure activities and some sports. *Current Physical Environment:* Patient states that there are no physical barriers in his home environment that prevent him from performing his ADL/IADLs; he is able to able to negotiate the environment outside his home such as public transport, communal thoroughfares etc.
Pattern of Occupation: *Job Title:* Carpenter *Employer:* Flooring Company *Length of time off work:* Since January 2005 *Restrictions:* Off work at present
Motivation for Occupation: Patient states he is motivated to return to some form of employment, especially as Carpenter (laying down wood floors); he is aware of his current deficits and that they might prevent him from returning to his original job. An alternative vocation he would consider is that in the field of 'telecommunications'. *Return to work options:* No options currently available since client is still in rehabilitation. *Return to work barriers:* Patient identified pain in his heels and lower back as the only barriers to returning to certain jobs.
Skills: *Motor:* Patient ambulates normally and has a kyphotic posture; He reports no problems with coordination, but decreased fitness levels. He states that prior to injury he was very active, but since then his activity has diminished secondary to pain. *Process Skills:* No apparent limitations. *Communication & Interaction Skills:* Intact. Patient was able to communicate clearly about his previous job, his social situation, and about his work goals.
Performance Capacity *Neuromusculoskeletal Functions:* Range of motion for trunk flexion limited to 110 degrees, Limited ankle eversion and inversion; ankle dorsiflexion slightly limited in right ankle; otherwise WNL; Strength within normal limits for ankle; Grip strength (R) 115 (L) 105 (25th percentile for men in his age group). Tone normal; Pain reported in lower back at 4/10 and pain under both heels and around both malleolus; He wears an orthotic in his shoes for heel support. *Mental Functions:* Patient does report long term memory loss but states that it does not interfere with his ability to function normally. *Sensory Functions:* Intact
ADL/IADL Status: Independent
Treatment Aims: Long term aim: Returning patient to a job whose physical demands match his functional capacity (including work conditioning program). Short term aims: Identify some vocational possibilities; increase motor skills; be able to perform activities without increase in pain or discomfort.

References

American Psychiatric Association. (2000). *Diagnostic and statistical manual of mental disorders* (4th ed., text revision). Washington: Author.

Granger, C.V., & Gresham, G. E. (1993). Functional assessment in rehabilitation medicine. *Physical Medicine and Rehabilitation Clinics of North America, (3),* 417–423.

Kettenbach, G. (1995). *Writing SOAP notes* (2nd ed.). Philadelphia: FA Davis.

McGavin, H. (1998). Planning rehabilitation: A comparison of issues for parents and adolescents. *Physical and Occupational Therapy in Paediatrics, 18 (1),* 69–82.

Missiuna, C., & Pollack, N. (2000). Perceived efficacy and goal setting in young children. *Canadian Journal of Occupational Therapy, 67 (2),* 101–109.

Parkinson, S., Forsyth, K., & Kielhofner, G. (2006). *Model of Human Occupation Screening Tool* (version 2.0). Authors.

Sumsion T., & Smyth G. (2000). Barriers to client centeredness and their resolution. *Canadian Journal of Occupational Therapy, 67,* 15–21.

Trombly, C. A. (Ed.). (1995). *Occupational therapy for physical dysfunction* (4th ed.). Baltimore: Williams & Wilkins.

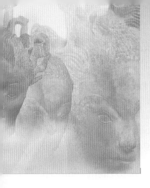

24

Program Development

- Brent Braveman
- Gary Kielhofner
- René Bélanger

The contexts in which occupational therapists work have become progressively complex and demanding. There is increased pressure and scrutiny by consumers, employers, third-party payers, and accrediting bodies to provide high-quality services that are effective and provided at the lowest possible cost. As a result, therapists must be able to propose, create, implement, and evaluate service programs that are efficient and effective.

Program development refers to creating and evaluating an approach to service delivery for a defined client group. Developing a program involves such things as these:

- Specifying clients' needs for occupational therapy
- Indicating the aims or intended outcomes of the program
- Providing a rationale for and detailing the kinds of services that will be included
- Establishing the steps, stages, or processes involved in clients' progression through the program
- Determining how the program will be evaluated.

Completing these and other aspects of developing a program of services can be greatly enhanced when one makes explicit use of a conceptual practice model. A model can enable the program development process by providing the following:

- A theoretical context for framing client problems and for conceptualizing the services and their intended impact
- Empirical evidence to back claims about the relevance and likely impact of services
- Assessments for use in evaluation of the client and in determining the outcomes of the program

- Protocols of service that can be emulated or adapted in the proposed program.

This chapter focuses on how therapists can use MOHO to develop occupational therapy programs. It briefly overviews the steps of program development to provide a context for discussion. Readers looking for in-depth guidance about the steps involved in developing a program are encouraged to use existing resources with that focus (Braveman, 2001; Braveman, Sen, & Kielhofner, 2001; Brownson, 2001; Youngstrom, 1999).

Program Development Process

Discussions of program development in the occupational therapy literature (Braveman & Kielhofner, 2006; Brownson, 2001; Grossman & Bortone, 1986; Youngstrom, 1999) propose similar steps and associated tasks. Building on these works and for the purposes of discussion here, the basic steps of program development include these features:

- Needs assessment
- Program planning
- Program implementation
- Program evaluation.

As shown in *Figure 24.1*, these steps are part of an ongoing process that involves constantly evaluating and improving how the program meets clients' needs by offering the most relevant and effective services. The components of each step identified in *Figure 24.1* are those that most pertain to selecting, creating a rationale for, and implementing a conceptual practice model. This chapter does not focus on financial, logisti-

FIGURE 24.1 The process of program development.

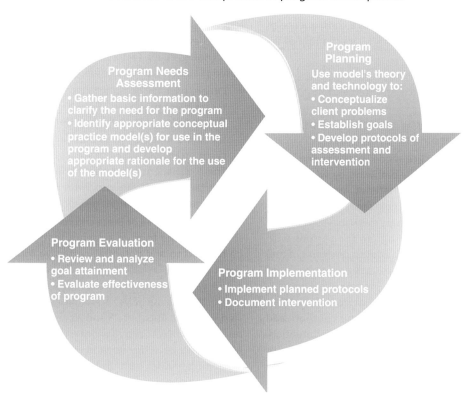

cal, or organizational aspects of program development, which are also essential to a successful program.

As *Figure 24.1* shows, the first step of program development includes selecting and creating the rationale for the model(s) that will inform and shape each subsequent step. Therefore, it is important to determine that one has selected the appropriate model(s) to address clients' needs. Selecting and justifying the conceptual practice model(s) can be facilitated when one reflectively addresses key questions along the way.

Questions to Guide Selecting and Justifying a Conceptual Practice Model

Program development requires active reasoning. In fact, there are parallels between the therapeutic reasoning process discussed in Chapter 11 and program development. The main difference is that the former is concerned with a single client, whereas the latter addresses an entire client group.

This section poses and discusses a series of questions to guide thinking about the model(s) one selects and uses in program development. Answering these questions can:

- Shape the initial choice of the appropriate conceptual practice model(s) for a program
- Validate the choice as the program development process unfolds
- Generate a thorough rationale for the model or models selected.

Question 1: Does the Model Specify the Underlying Mechanisms of Action Necessary to Deal with the Occupational Problems and Challenges Faced by the Client Group?

When developing a program, it is important to specify how the services will achieve changes to address the client's problem and challenges. Therefore, one must consider the underlying mechanism(s) of action of an intervention (Gitlin et al., 2000). The **mechanism of action** refers to the theoretical and empirical account of how a particular change occurs as a consequence of participating in an intervention. The mechanism of action should delineate:

- How change proceeds
- Conditions under which an intervention achieves beneficial results
- Why a change may occur for certain groups of participants and not others.

A conceptual practice model provides the structure for identifying specific pathways by which interventions may function. Sometimes more than one model is chosen because a single model does not adequately address all the necessary mechanisms of action. Consider, for example, a program for persons with head injury that is designed to address problems of motivation, occupational lifestyle, and impairments of performance capacity due to neurological impairments. MOHO would provide accounts for how motivation and lifestyle change through the concepts and propositions associated with volition and habituation. However, it would not provide sufficient guidance for structuring aspects of intervention meant to remediate neurological impairments of performance capacity. In such an instance, MOHO must be used in conjunction with another conceptual practice model that more specifically addresses the mechanisms of action related to facilitate change in nervous system functioning.

Question 2: Is The Evidence Sufficient to Support Application of the Model to the Client Group and the Occupational Problems That They Experience?

Those who receive and pay for occupational therapy services increasingly expect that occupational therapy practice will be evidence based. **Evidence-based practice** refers to conscientious, explicit, and systematic use of available evidence in deciding the kinds of services that will be provided to individuals (Law, 2002; Taylor, 2000; Sackett, Rosenberg, Gray, Haynes, & Richardson, 1996). Before basing programming on a conceptual practice model, one must be sure that there is evidence to support its use with the target client group. Such evidence may exist in the literature. It may reflect others' experience in using the model with a

similar client group. Sometimes it is generated through pilot work that precedes development of the program.

Excellent resources to guide practitioners in finding and evaluating published evidence are now available (Holm, 2000; Taylor, 2000). Basically, evidence-based practice involves considering whether:

- Others have successfully used the model with the target client group
- Others have successfully used the model to address the same kinds of problems faced by the target client group
- There is evidence that the model is effective with the target client group or with the kinds of problems faced by the target group.

Whereas not all of these criteria may be met, there should be some form of evidence that the model will be relevant to and potentially effective for the target client group.

A variety of resources exist for therapists who are considering the use of MOHO for program development. As discussed in Chapters 25 and 26, there is a substantial research base. Moreover, a wide range of programs using MOHO have been described in the literature. These include programs for such diverse clients groups as those with chronic pain (Gusich, 1984; Padilla & Bianchi, 1990), traumatic brain injury (DePoy, 1990), Alzheimer dementia (Oakley, 1987; Olin, 1985), Acquired immune deficiency syndrome (AIDS) (Pizzi, 1984, 1989, 1990a, b; Schindler, 1988), and borderline personality disorder (Salz, 1983). MOHO has guided programs for persons who are homeless and mentally ill (Kavanaugh & Fares, 1995), for battle-fatigued soldiers (Gerardi, 1996), for emotionally disturbed children and adolescents (Reekmans & Kielhofner, 1998; Sholle-Martin, 1987; Weissenberg & Giladi, 1989), and for children with attention deficit hyperactivity disorder (Woodrum, 1993). Moreover, MOHO-based programs have been described for a range of specific contexts, such as a day hospital (Gusich & Silverman, 1991), a work rehabilitation program (Mentrup, Niehaus, & Kielhofner, 1999), prison and correctional settings (Michael, 1991; Schindler, 1990), and early intervention (Schaaf & Mulrooney, 1989).

The MOHO bibliography in Appendix A is a useful resource for identifying publications relevant to a specific target group or context. These publications are often valuable not only because they provide some evidence about others' experiences in using MOHO, but they also provide a wealth of ideas and strategies for building a program for a given client group or context. Additionally, the MOHO Clearinghouse distributes manuals with detailed program protocols. Finally, the MOHO listserv is an excellent resource for communicating with others who have relevant program development experiences. The on-line bibliography is updated regularly, and information about the manuals and listserv may be found on the MOHO Web site. Information on the MOHO Clearinghouse Web site is also provided in Appendix B.

Question 3: Does the Model Fit with the Social, Cultural, Political, Professional, and Financial Contexts in Which the Program Must Be Implemented?

In selecting a conceptual practice model, one must consider whether contextual factors will support or hinder developing the kind of programming necessary to implement the model. For example, reimbursement or funding for the program might limit the type, frequency, or intensity of intervention, influencing how a model can be implemented in a given context. Cultural groups with particular values or expectations may influence how the program can be delivered and whether the concepts of a model are relevant to their concerns. The theories and approaches used by other professionals in the program or in the larger context may or may not be compatible with a particular model. Consideration of such factors can both assure selection of a model that fits with the context and takes necessary action to introduce the model appropriately to the context.

Question 4: Does Implementation of Programming Based on the Model Have any Special Requirements for Space, Equipment, or Personnel?

Before proceeding with program development, practitioners should be aware of the resources required to adequately implement an effective program based on the chosen model. A conceptual practice model may have implications for such things as space, equipment, personnel, or training. For example, MOHO stresses the importance of doing therapy using culturally relevant occupational forms and when possible natural contexts for intervention. This may mean creating the organizational structure and resources for making a range of meaningful occupational forms and social groups available.

Another consideration is whether therapists have adequate training and knowledge to implement a model. Moreover, one should ask whether assessments or written materials that fit the setting are available (e.g., will they have to be adapted or translated to suit the language and culture of the clients?). Thinking about such issues helps to anticipate the necessary resources and activities for implementing a model successfully.

Two Examples of Program Development

The following sections provide two examples of the authors' experiences using MOHO to develop occupational therapy programming. The first example is Employment Options, a vocational rehabilitation program for clients living with HIV or AIDS. This program was developed with federal funding, and its aim was to create, study, and disseminate a model service. The second example is *Programme spécifique d'intervention, premier épisode* (PSI), (Specific Intervention Program, First Episode). PSI was developed at the Hôtel-Dieu de Lévis Hospital in Quebec City, Quebec, Canada. This program offers specialized and integrated services for young clients with schizophrenia. Occupational therapy services are an essential component of this interdisciplinary program.

In each of these instances, using MOHO provided a systematic basis for such things as these:

- Providing a rationale for why the program is needed or why it should be organized in a particular way
- Informing constituencies about the components of a program and how they are intended to work
- Convincing others of the value of investing in the program or including one's concepts and approaches in the program.

Each of the two programs initially had to address lack of knowledge or skepticism about occupational therapy services. To develop these programs successfully, organizers had to gain the trust and confidence of multiple constituencies. Although MOHO was not a guarantee of success, it provided a variety of resources that ultimately helped to shape both programs' success.

The following sections describe each program, following the four basic steps of program development shown in *Figure 24.1*. The discussion focuses on the aspects of each program that demonstrate how MOHO was used and its contributions to the nature and success of the program.

Example 1: Employment Options

In 1997, the Department of Occupational Therapy at the University of Illinois at Chicago (UIC) approached Howard Brown Health Center (HBHC), a community-based health center serving Chicago's gay and lesbian population, to explore whether occupational therapy services might benefit HBHC clients. There were no occupational therapy services and very little knowledge about occupational therapy at the center.

The staff at HBHC asked whether occupational therapy could provide services for an increasing number of their clients with HIV/AIDS who were expressing interest in returning to work. Some of these clients had previously developed serious symptoms and received the recommendation to leave their jobs and receive private or public disability to ensure adequate medical coverage until their death. Other clients, who were unemployed when diagnosed with HIV/AIDS, were not encouraged to pursue employment, given their prognosis. However, new pharmacologic treatments had substantially decreased HIV-related mortality rates while improving health and function, making consideration of work possible for these clients (Feinberg, 1996; Hogg et al., 1997).

Program Needs Assessment

To gain a clearer understanding of their needs, a survey was conducted on 55 HBHC clients. The average respondent was 38 years old and last employed 3.5 years earlier. Some 82% of respondents had already discussed returning to work with their case managers, although none had yet returned to any form of employment.

Respondents identified a number of important barriers to reentering the workplace, including uncertainty over whether:

- Their functional capacity was adequate
- Working might impair their health status
- They could maintain the routine of full-time employment

- Returning to work might negatively affect their health insurance benefits or preclude future eligibility for disability income.

In addition, most respondents described experiencing significant inertia secondary to prolonged illness and interruption of work. They also voiced concerns about how to address the gap in their employment history, facing prejudice because of their diagnosis, and how workplaces would react to their need to manage ongoing symptoms and complex medication regimens.

Since the issues raised by these clients are addressed by MOHO concepts, a pilot program of vocational services based on MOHO was developed and implemented at HBHC with funding from the National AIDS Fund. The pilot program enrolled 20 clients, who received group education sessions and individual occupational therapy. More than 40% of members of the pilot program returned to work within 5 months, and a waiting list for the program soon developed. It became clear that an ongoing service was needed for this client group. Moreover, the pilot program provided evidence that the kind of program envisioned had potential to meet the needs of the clients for vocational services. At the same time, it was clear from communication with other agencies throughout the country that the situation at HBHC reflected a national trend of persons with HIV/AIDS wanting services to assist them to return to work. The Department of Occupational Therapy at UIC and HBHC agreed to enter into a partnership to seek federal funding for a large demonstration program.

Rationale for Selecting MOHO

To obtain federal funding in a research and demonstration grant competition, it was necessary to articulate and justify to an interdisciplinary audience why and how MOHO was to be used as the conceptual practice model for the program. Because of previous applications of MOHO at UIC and elsewhere, it was possible to document that MOHO had been:

- Applied to the study of injured/disabled workers (Azhar, 1996; Corner, Kielhofner, & Lin, 1997; Corner, Kielhofner, & Olson, 1998; Kielhofner & Brinson, 1989; Mallinson, 1998; Munoz & Kielhofner, 1995; Olson, 1998; Salz, 1983; Velozo, Kielhofner, & Fisher, 1998)

- Used for more than a decade to design work-related rehabilitation programs (Mallinson, 1998; Olson, 1998)
- Used to incorporate variables that had been shown to predict success in return to work (Braveman, 1999)
- Applied to rehabilitation services for persons with HIV/AIDS (Pizzi, 1989, 1990a, b; Schindler, 1988, 1990)

These previous applications of MOHO for clients with HIV/AIDS and for addressing return-to-work issues, together with data from the pilot study, were used to justify MOHO as the model for the proposed program. This argument was also complemented by a demonstration that MOHO could effectively be used to conceptualize the problems and needs of the clients and how they would be addressed in the program.

Conceptualizing the Client Group from a MOHO Perspective

The following is a brief overview of how MOHO was used to conceptualize the factors that would influence work success of persons with HIV or AIDS. Data from several sources—including the HBHC survey, the pilot study, literature review, and information from HBHC case managers—were used to inform this conceptualization. *Table 24.1* summarizes these factors and shows them in relation to program goals that will be discussed later.

VOLITION

The target client group was extremely diverse in culture, socioeconomic status, educational background, and work history. Consequently, the role of work in these persons' lives and the identity that they had formed as workers were also extremely diverse. Many persons living with HIV/AIDS whose functional capacity had increased through new medications expressed a desire to return to being self-sufficient and productive. They missed the stimulation, challenges, and feelings of positive self-esteem they experienced at work. Despite their desires for work, most were unsure of their capacity for and had a limited sense of efficacy for returning to work. Many felt they could no longer handle the stress of their former jobs and wondered what new form of work might interest and be meaningful to them. Others, with sporadic work records and a history

of relying on public assistance, had never developed strong vocational interests, established a stable work career, or found meaning in work.

Regardless of background, most shared fears about whether working would negatively influence their health status. They worried about the impact that returning to work would have on their social and health benefits, especially given the costly nature of their life-sustaining medications. They were apprehensive about how peers or supervisors would relate to them and their illness. All of these factors strongly influenced whether they would make the occupational choice to work.

HABITUATION

Clients' work histories varied tremendously, as did their development of worker roles. Many clients had limited experience and were in the second or third generation of a family that relied on public assistance. Even clients who had successful work histories had spent significant time in the sick role, which made return to work a difficult transition. All clients had to face and overcome the barrier of inconsistent work history or gaps in employment that affected their public identity as a worker. Clients in established relationships with partners or families had to renegotiate roles with significant others who had already made substantial sacrifices to accommodate their illnesses.

Clients faced the challenge of overcoming the inertia of habitual inactivity and instituting a routine to support working. Clients who had been habituated to nonproductive lifestyles complicated by drug habits must achieve a productive routine for the first time. The challenge of instituting productive habits was complicated by ongoing symptoms, drug side effects, impairments, and needs to maintain a medication routine.

PERFORMANCE CAPACITY

As noted previously, it was the resurgence of capacity for many persons with HIV/AIDS that opened the possibility of returning to work. Nonetheless, many persons had some ongoing impairment. Many had periodic illness and medication side effects, such as nausea and diarrhea. A common problem, fatigue, was complicated by deconditioning due to prolonged illness and inactivity. Some had neuropathies and mild cognitive impairments.

Together, these underlying impairments and symptoms adversely affected clients' motor and

TABLE 24-1   MOHO-Based Conceptualization of Factors Influencing Vocational Success of Persons Living with AIDS and Corresponding Program Services

	Factors Influencing Vocational Success of Persons Living with AIDS	Employment Options Program Services
Personal Factors	**Volition** • Lack of or need to change work-related interests • Concerns about personal capacity for work and impact of work on health status • Concerns about coping with challenges (e.g., disclosure) • Concerns for optimizing values (i.e., being productive, economic sustenance, maintaining health)	• Self assessment of work interests • Assessment/review of functional capacity • Training and group sessions on coping in the workplace • Economic counseling, benefits management • Peer mentoring and support
	Habituation • Long-term work role disruption • Identification with work versus sick role • Challenges of role transitions • Absence of a functional routine • Routine requirements for managing illness	• Opportunity to reacquire a productive role though volunteer positions, internships, and temporary work experiences • Job coaching to facilitate adjustment to worker role • Structured program schedule to support development of a functional routine
	Performance Capacity • Impairments related to disease, symptoms, and drug side effects • Limited motor, process, and communication/interaction skills	• Support client in identification and request for reasonable accommodations • Skill-building group sessions, volunteer positions, internships and temporary work placement, job coaching, and referral for job training
Environmental Factors	**Workplace** • Negative attitudes/prejudice toward persons with AIDS • Reluctance to accommodate to the challenges of a worker with chronic disability	• Education/consultation for potential/actual employers of clients • Offering employers the National AIDS Fund's "A Positive Workplace" training program (Breuer, 1997)
	Community • Lack of peer network and social support for work • Negative influence of drugs, crime, and poverty • Complicated system of health and social policy	• On the Job Club (drop-in availability for clients to socialize with other clients and program staff) • Determination of economic benefit/impact of returning to work along with counseling and advocacy to ensure continuous medical benefits

process skills. Many clients lacked the communication/interaction skills required in nearly any form of employment. These limitations were complicated by the fact that entering the workplace as a person with HIV/AIDS posed its own special interpersonal challenges. Clients faced the issues of disclosure, dealing with stigma and prejudice, and the need to negotiate accommodations. Those with a poor work history

lacked knowledge and abilities for any specific type of work.

ENVIRONMENT

The context of the workplace could present attitudinal and other barriers to return to work (Weitz, 1990). Although many of the clients were not visibly disabled, they had to disclose their HIV status to request the reasonable accommodations they required to maintain a worker role. By disclosing their HIV status, they increased the visibility of their disease and hence risked the discrimination associated with the stigma of AIDS.

Other contextual factors were community and organizational challenges. Many persons had lost touch with working peers and lacked support networks for work. For many, the neighborhood presence of drugs, crime, and poverty were potential barriers to achieving self-sufficient lifestyles (Billingsley, 1988; Stack, 1974). While facing these hurdles, clients had to navigate a jungle of poorly coordinated systems and service agencies that sometimes functioned at cross-purposes, creating disincentives to self-sufficiency and work.

Program Planning

Once MOHO was used to conceptualize the occupational problems faced by the target client group, it was possible to specify mechanisms of action, that is, to spell out how services would address clients' problems and how they would contribute to clients' successful return to work. *Table 24.1* shows the factors just discussed that influence vocational success and the corresponding program services designed to address each factor. After identifying these program services, it was necessary to consider how they would be organized and sequenced in the program.

The program was organized in four phases to support clients moving through a continuum of development of volition, habituation, and performance capacity. Each of these stages also had different implications for the kind of environments in which service would take place and the kinds of supports clients needed. *Figure 24.2* shows the four phases of the program, briefly described in the following sections.

Phase 1

Clients were initially screened to establish appropriateness of the program for them and to determine necessary problem solving and resources to support program attendance (e.g., child care, transportation). On entry into the program, the client participated in a comprehensive assessment process including:

- The Occupational Performance History Interview—Version 2.0 (OPHI-II)
- The Worker Role Interview (WRI)
- The Occupational Self Assessment (OSA)

- The Assessment of Communication and Interaction Skills (ACIS)
- A fatigue scale.

These evaluations were used in such a way that the therapist and client together formed an appreciation of the client's potential for work and individual needs for services to support return to work.

During this phase, clients also attended individual and group sessions designed to help them explore and develop both work skills and the daily habits needed to support a vocational role. Group sessions included these features:

- Self-assessment exercises
- Vocational planning exercises
- Information sharing related to economics, benefits, the Americans with Disabilities Act (ADA), and other logistics of return to work
- Job search and job skill development exercises
- Peer support groups
- Work task experiences
- Individual therapy sessions addressed each client's unique needs

The aim of phase 1, which lasted 8 weeks, was to provide:

- An opportunity for self-assessment and strengthening and refinement of vocational choice
- A structured routine to develop habits of promptness, consistency, and a commitment to the program
- A forum for sharing critical information about returning to work
- A community of emotional support for return to work
- A context wherein factors that impact on work readiness were identified and addressed
- Opportunities to develop job-relevant skills.

Phase 2

During this phase, clients began participation in volunteer work, an internship, or placement in temporary employment. These opportunities were developed by partnering with businesses in Chicago and were planned to be part-time and combined with continued participation in some components of the group program outlined in phase 1. The duration and intensity of this phase were variable and adjusted to the clients' needs, but typically it ranged from 1 to 3 months.

FIGURE 24.2 Continuum of employment options services.

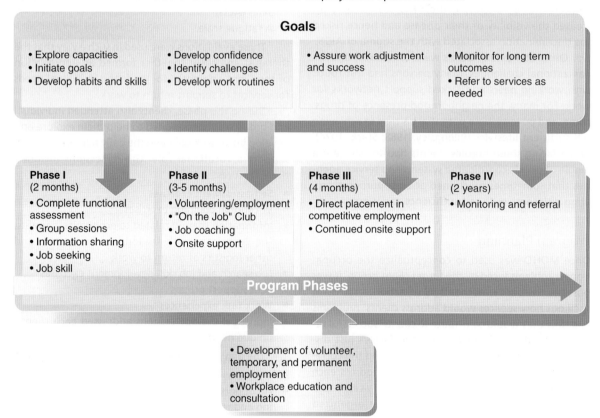

This phase of the program was designed to assist clients to develop confidence in their ability to manage the routine of working. During this phase, the OSA was repeated with clients to allow for self-assessment in this new phase of change and to identify further individual goals.

This phase was also designed to allow clients to face and cope with the challenges associated with working with a chronic disability. Each work, training, or volunteer placement was designed so that clients received assessment and feedback concerning job performance. Project staff worked closely with the volunteer or work supervisor in these placements to assure that the client was receiving appropriate supervision and to support the supervisor in responding to any challenges.

PHASE 3

In this phase, clients were placed in paid jobs developed by the project or were assisted by project staff to

apply for and secure employment. Job analysis and adaptation, as well as on-site job coaching of the client, were provided as needed. Each client participated in the Work Environment Impact Scale at this stage to assess how the work context was influencing the client's performance and well-being. Information gained from this interview was used to assist the client in making personal adjustments to the workplace and in requesting reasonable accommodations.

In addition, employer education, consultation, and trouble-shooting support for the supervisor and coworkers of the client were provided. Clients in this phase could still take advantage of individual meetings with project staff for ongoing support and training. The intensity and duration of this phase varied, but it was planned to average 4 months.

PHASE 4

This phase consisted of long-term follow-up and support. Because AIDS is a chronic condition and periods of illness or functional limitation may occur, it was considered important that project staff be able to intervene and provide support as needed. Consequently, ongoing contact and periodic support through group meetings with others and/or with staff was to be maintained.

Researchers and clinicians at the Department of Occupational Therapy at the University of Illinois at Chicago meet to review Employment Options program outcomes and discuss implications for the newest research program based on MOHO, Enabling Self-Determination.

Program Implementation

The plan of the program was developed as part of the proposal that was funded as a national research and demonstration project for 3 years by the U.S. Department of Education's Rehabilitation Services Administration.[1] Following funding, implementation of Employment Options required developing the specifics of the program, identifying and training appropriate staff, and coordinating and documenting activities to facilitate program evaluation.

As the program was implemented, two occupational therapists already familiar with MOHO were hired. They were provided with training and education to assure their competence in using MOHO concepts and assessments. For example, one staff member was already certified in the ACIS, but the second one had to receive training and certification. Early in the project the therapists presented cases and received supervision from the first two authors of this chapter. A third key member, the vocational placement specialist, was not an occupational therapist. Therefore, specific efforts were made throughout the program planning and implementation to orient her to MOHO and its constructs. As she became more familiar with how clients were conceptualized from the perspective of MOHO and occupational therapy, she was able to provide helpful observations about

the clients that related to key concepts of MOHO. For example, she was able to postulate how a particular client's inaccurate knowledge of capacity, poor sense of self-efficacy, and lack of structured habits and routines acted in combination to prevent the client from following through on recommendations she made. With time, the entire team functioned as a whole to ensure optimal implementation of MOHO-based strategies.

Program Evaluation and Further Program Development

Since this program was funded to investigate its process and outcomes, an extensive program evaluation was also designed and funded with the same grant. It included both a qualitative study of the program implementation and a quantitative study of outcomes. The qualitative component took place within the framework of participatory action research (PAR), a strategy for conducting research that requires subjects to be involved in all phases of research that affects them (National Institute on Disability and Rehabilitation Research, 1995). Data collection for this evaluation ranged from simple strategies, such as conducting evaluations after every group session to obtain feedback, to more complicated strategies, such as conducting periodic interviews with clients and their case managers. This component of the program evaluation allows staff to constantly improve services to better meet the client's needs.

The outcomes of this program were published (Kielhofner, Braveman, Finlayson, Paul-Ward, Goldbaum, & Goldstein, 2004). A total of 129 people originally enrolled in the program, and of these 90 were able to complete at least the first phase of the program. Of these 90, 56% attained employment, and an additional 11% either returned to school or took on volunteer work. Since there was no control group with which to compare the outcomes of the program, findings were compared with typical outcomes of other vocational programs serving persons with multiple impairments and challenges. Based on this comparison, Employment Options appeared to achieve a rate of success as good as that reported in the literature for well-developed programs. Publications based on Employment Options also documented which types of persons benefited from the program, which aspects of the program were most useful, and what kinds of characteristics of clients were associated with successful and unsuccessful outcomes (Braveman, Helfrich,

---

[1]Employment Options for Persons Living with AIDS, Grant #H235A980170, Rehabilitation Services Administration, U.S. Department of Education.

Kielhofner, & Albrecht, 2004; Braveman, Kielhofner, Albrecht, and Helfrich, 2006; Goldstein, Kielhofner, & Paul-Ward, 2004; Kielhofner et al., 2004).

The program evaluation also indicated that one-third of those who enrolled in the program dropped out or were lost to the study. Many factors (including illness, the participant's narrative, and environmental circumstances) contributed to the drop-out rate. Anecdotal data also indicated that for some participants, attending a program that took place some distance from their place of residence and that began immediately with vocational goals was too challenging.

The developers of Employment Options decided to develop a new program, Enabling Self-Determination (Braveman, Kielhofner, Levin, & Josefson, 2007; Paul-Ward, Braveman, Kielhofner, & Levin, 2005), which would be offered in the transitional living facilities where many of the more challenged clients lived. Another federal grant[2] supported a 3-year controlled study of the outcomes of this new combined independent living and vocational program. This program, which is also based on the model of human occupation, uses many of the elements of the previous program in combination with more basic supportive and life skills–oriented services. The results of this study indicated that clients who received the services had much better vocational and independent living outcomes than a control group (Kielhofner, Braveman, Levin, & Fogg, in press).

Example 2: Premiers Épisodes (First Episodes)

The *Programme jeunes adultes: premiers épisodes* (Young Adults Program: First Episodes) was initiated in 1997 as the *Programme spécifique d'intervention, premier épisode* (PSI) in Quebec City, in the Province of Quebec, Canada. It is an interdisciplinary program for young clients having their first psychotic episodes. This example illustrates how MOHO was used to develop the occupational therapy component of this program.

Program Needs Assessment

The program was first developed at Hôtel-Dieu de Lévis Hospital, a general hospital with psychiatric units, on the south shore of Quebec City. Before *Premiers épisodes*

program came into existence, there was no well-coordinated structure between the different multidisciplinary interventions at the hospital. There was also difficulty coordinating the various services offered for schizophrenic clients by other institutions in the region. Some received very specific attention with long-term rehabilitation, whereas others received only little help or no services at all. Moreover, there were no valid, quantitative, and objective data to measure the effects of interventions. The hospital has a mandate for research and teaching and therefore supported the psychiatric department in the idea of developing a program that would represent best practice and assess its own outcomes.

Several other factors also influenced the development of *Premiers épisodes* program. In the implementation of specialized services for clients with psychosis, analytical approaches have given way to the development of cognitive-behavioral therapy approaches (Hansen, Kingdon, & Turkington, 2006) and brief intervention therapies (Cather, 2005). Moreover, a new generation of antipsychotic medications enables better control of the disabling symptoms of schizophrenia, allowing greater expectations for client functioning. Since family members of schizophrenic clients often want to play a more active role in the recovery process, education and support groups have had to be developed. Finally, various community groups supporting the rights of persons with mental illness were lobbying for services to allow the clients to be better informed about their diseases and to participate actively in the intervention process.

As a consequence of these factors, a decision was made to create a specialized program. Three interdisciplinary teams refer clients to *Premiers épisodes* program. Each of these teams works with clients who have a variety of psychiatric problems. When a client meets *Premiers épisodes* criteria (first psychotic episodes), he or she is referred to *Premiers épisodes* program at discharge. Each of the referring teams continues to work with clients after discharge. There is careful coordination between *Premiers épisodes* services and other services given by the referring team.

ASSESSING THE NEEDS OF THE CLIENT GROUP
Although the program officially began in 1997, the groundwork was laid in 1995. A literature search was conducted on early intervention for young psychotic and schizophrenic clients, and a study on client demographics in the area covered by the hospital was under-

[2]Enabling Self Determination, Grant #H235A980170, National Institutes of Disability and Rehabilitation Research.

taken. The literature clearly indicated that schizophrenia is a disease of the brain, genetically influenced and characterized by cognitive deficits, low self-esteem, difficulties in daily functioning, and poor social integration (Brenner, Roder, Hodel, Kienze, Reed, &, 1994; Green, 1996; Harding, 1988; Kaplan, Sadock & Grebb, 1994; Mawrer & Häfner, 1995; Nicole et al., 1999). The social, economic, and human costs of schizophrenia are high, and it is extremely difficult to treat.

The literature review also identified several important points that had to be addressed to make the program efficient and effective:

- Early intervention helps to limit or avoid neurologic deficits, social repercussions, and the progressive degeneration associated with the disease (Harding, 1988; Mawrer & Häfner, 1995; Wyatt, 1991)
- It is important to reduce the period between the appearance of the symptoms of disease and effective therapy (Beiser, Erickson, Fleming & Iacono, 1993; Falloon, 1992; Johnstone, Crow, & Johnson, 1986)
- The complexity of the disease and its multiple facets necessitate an interdisciplinary structure of intervention and specialized care (Nicole et al., 1999).

Premiers épisodes was developed according to guidelines suggested by evidence found in the literature. The goal of the program was to develop a state-of-the-art, specialized, and integrated approach for schizophrenic clients to benefit them during both the initial phase of the disease and subsequent recovery. To accomplish this, it was decided the program should include an optimal combination of interdisciplinary treatment interventions that would:

- Intervene early after the first psychotic episode
- Maintain continuity of care
- Provide innovative and relevant services
- Integrate elements from traditional approaches with newer treatments
- Promote new kinds of therapies as much as possible
- Use of standard clinical tools
- Make optimal use of resources.

Every member of the multidisciplinary team was asked to propose standardized evaluations that would objectify and contribute to understanding the biological, psychological, and social components of each client's condition and to propose corresponding interventions to address identified problems. Within the interdisciplinary team, psychiatrists and nurses covered

the biological areas, psychologists covered the neurocognitive and personality areas, social workers covered family history, and occupational therapists covered occupational areas. It was within this general context of program development that the occupational therapy approach, based on MOHO, was developed. Incorporation of MOHO into the overall program meant that other members of the team had to understand and accept MOHO concepts and that MOHO contributions to the overall program had to be integrated with other theories and approaches used in the interdisciplinary program. This meant that the occupational therapists had to provide an overview of MOHO and its potential contributions to the program for the interdisciplinary team. This introduced the team to the ideas and secured their support for including MOHO as an essential component of this interdisciplinary program. Since 2003, economical constraints in the health system, changes of the structure of the psychiatric department, and a shortage of professional resources have necessitated major changes for the interdisciplinary program, in particular delivery of intervention. Notably, in the midst of constrained resources and organizational changes, the psychiatric department administration left the MOHO-based components intact, since they were considered among the most important parts of *Premiers épisodes*. In the revised program, renamed *Programme jeunes adultes: premiers épisodes* (Young Adults Program: First Episodes), the assessment module was substantially reorganized to accommodate changes in the overall program. MOHO provided a framework for ensuring the continuity of this modified program.

RATIONALE FOR SELECTION OF MOHO

MOHO was chosen and retained as the framework for the occupational therapy component of *Premiers épisodes* because it:

- Furnishes a detailed framework of the occupational functioning of the individual (Hagerdon, 1992)
- Enables precise measurement and useful description of the client's occupational characteristics (Bélanger, Briand, & Rivard, 2006)
- Provides clear links between the occupational problems it helps identify and the intervention strategies to address them (Bonder, 2003)
- Gives specific and detailed guidelines and tools for evaluating a client, a specific language for describ-

ing the difficulties/challenges, and a framework for setting treatment goals and selecting the most appropriate strategy to achieve the desired level of change (Bélanger et al., 2006)

- Allows for a flexible approach to individualize therapy for a client and provides a comprehensive picture of the occupational functioning of the person (Forsyth & Kielhofner, 2003)
- Provides a conceptualization of the process and stages of change that was useful for guiding the sequence of therapy (including deciding when a client is ready to move from one level of change to another) (Bruce & Borg, 2002)
- Offers a solid theoretic view of occupation that clearly helps to explain the occupational functioning of a client faced with his or her first psychotic episode through clearly identified concepts that have been shown to predict later functioning (Henry, 1994; Henry & Coster, 1996).

MOHO is also compatible with cognitive-behavioral and psychoeducational approaches used by other disciplines in the program (Bélanger et al., 2006). Furthermore, MOHO allows the occupational therapist to make valuable, distinct, and specific contributions to the team (Bélanger et al., 2006). For example, MOHO allowed the team to distinguish between the disappearance of the disease's psychotic symptoms and the return to a functional level of occupation. MOHO-based research indicates that remittance of psychotic symptoms does not ensure a return to premorbid levels of functioning (Henry, 1994).

Program Planning

The interdisciplinary team decided to develop *Premiers épisodes* to include two sequential modules. The first module is evaluating and developing a specific intervention plan. The second module is intervention. The first step in developing the occupational therapy component of both modules was to use MOHO to conceptualize a client's occupational situation and to develop related goals.

CONCEPTUALIZING THE CLIENT GROUP FROM A MOHO PERSPECTIVE

MOHO provided a framework for structuring the information gathered from the interdisciplinary team's liter-

ature review and survey, as well as practice experiences with this client group, to create a conceptualization of the occupational problems, challenges, and needs of this population. The following is a brief discussion of how MOHO was used to conceptualize the occupational situation of clients following a first psychotic episode. *Table 24.2* summarizes this information and also shows the major goals of the occupational therapy component of the program. More information on the program's logic, along with the application of MOHO tools in the program, is illustrated in Bélanger et al. (2006) through a detailed case analysis. In addition, this reference outlines how MOHO conceptualizes the occupational performance and participation of clients with schizophrenia.

VOLITION

Problems with motivation are extensively documented in the description of symptoms of schizophrenia (Kaplan et al., 1994; Lalonde & Grunberg, 1988; Nicole et al., 1999). There is a decline in motivation, difficulty in self-determination, loss of interest, and feelings of inadequacy stemming principally from past negative occupational experiences. All of these come to influence volition.

As a result of the disease, clients often have difficulty in evaluating their actual capacity. Clients may be vaguely conscious of their problems, especially those related to communication and social interaction (Pomini, Neis, Brenner, Hodel, & Roder, 1998). Clients tend to feel very ill at ease managing everyday social interaction with emotional content. As a consequence, they often make choices to avoid interaction and isolate themselves from others. Many have difficulties initiating action because they have a long history of experiencing failure in social interaction. Clinical observations have consistently shown that they need to improve their personal causation. They typically shun everyday responsibilities and cannot set life goals for themselves. They often have extreme difficulty achieving a sense of meaning and purpose in their occupational lives. They have also lost most of their past and present interests.

HABITUATION

Roles and habits are ordinarily very disturbed in these clients, although the extent will vary from one client to another. Clients often feel a painful sense of loss and

TABLE 24-2 Conceptualization of Client Problems and Related Strategies to Address Them Within the Premiers Épisodes Program

MOHO Component	Problems and Challenges of Clients	Occupational Therapy Goals
Volition • Personal causation • Values • Interests	• General decline in motivation and loss of interest • Feelings of inadequacy stemming from failures • Difficulty evaluating actual capacity (abilities and limitations), underconfident or overconfident • Vague awareness of problems may lead to choices that isolate self • Difficulty achieving a sense of meaning and purpose in their occupational lives • Difficulty in initiating action and self-determination • Avoidance of responsibilities • Difficulty setting and prioritizing goals • Inability to prioritize among what is important • Avoid decisions to engage in occupations • Difficulty seeking assistance appropriately • Poor concentration leading to difficulty in occupational forms	• Greater expectation of success for engagement in occupational forms • Increase confidence to approach tasks within one's capacity • Develop realistic understanding of abilities and limitations along with acceptance of them • Identify areas in which person can feel sense of accomplishment and meaning • Support choices to engage in occupations with meaning, interest, and social involvement • Develop sense of basic responsibility for self and for productivity according to capacity • Set and pursue realistic life goals • Stimulate interest and desire to do things • More willingness to ask for help when needed • Increase tendency to sustain efforts to realize goals • Increase the ability to identify what is important in a situation • Increase satisfaction and self-esteem from realizing goals • Increase participation in things of interest
Habituation • Roles • Habits	• Roles and habits disturbed • Poor role script • Difficulty meeting role expectations • Sense of loss and emptiness due to lost/absent roles and limited routine • Absence of productive occupation • Minimal participation in home occupational forms • Leisure activities solitary, passive, and simple • Activities of daily living degenerate • Routine bland and discouraging • Difficulty structuring the day due to lack of roles • Reversed day/night cycle isolates self from others • Difficulty imagining self in a variety of roles and kind of life desired • Structured program schedule to support development of a functional routine	• Increase perception of self as involved with roles that are necessary and desirable • Improve organization of daily routine • Improve awareness of responsibilities associated with success in various roles • Increase effectiveness in meeting multiple role expectations of realistic role responsibilities • Increase effectiveness in completing a specific occupation due to acquisition/change in habitual way of doing it

(continued)

TABLE 24-2 *(continued)*

MOHO Component	Problems and Challenges of Clients	Occupational Therapy Goals
Performance Capacity and Skills	• Range of impairments, especially in the area of cognitive processing, attention, memory, concentration, logic inference, and anticipation • Communication/interaction skills affected • Process skills constrained within daily tasks • Performing daily activities is laborious and difficult	• Improve visual perception in social conditions • Develop social adaptive mechanisms to make up for cognitive deficits • Improve skills of the physical domain • Improve capacity to receive, give, and exchange daily information • Improve skills of the relational domain • Improve repertoire of social competence skills • Develop preventive strategies of management of emotions during more intense daily situations • Develop alternative solutions for daily problems encountered
Environment	• Incomprehension, misunderstanding, and impotence to deal with disorganized behaviors on the part of their families and loved ones • Inappropriate family expectations of the client • Overstimulating or abandoning home environment • Negative influences of drugs, alcohol, and physical and psychological abuse • Stigma and prejudice associated with mental illness	• Improve the capacity of the client to express his or her need for assistance and to locate daily difficulties • Improve client's knowledge about the negative effects of drugs and alcohol on psychosis • Improve competence of the client to set limits and to say no • Teach the client how to distinguish and explain to his or her entourage the difference between psychosis and madness

emptiness when they have relinquished roles and been deprived of the many elements of their daily routine. Productive work is almost always absent from their lives. Their participation in occupations in the home is often minimal (Reed, 2003). Their leisure tends to be solitary and passive and to require minimal organization and planning. Performance of activities of daily living can also degenerate in these clients, although it is variable. Finally, the general routine of these clients tends to be bland and discouraging. Many of these clients have reversed day and night cycles that further isolate them from others. Finally, they have difficulty imagining themselves in a variety of roles and do not have an image of the kind of life they would like to lead.

Performance Capacity and Skills

Clients have a range of impairments, especially in the area of cognitive processing, including difficulties with attention, memory, concentration, and problem solving (George & Neufeld, 1985). In more than three-quarters of clients, basic communication and social skills are severely affected (Brenner et al., 1994). They particularly have difficulty exchanging information and adjusting their behavior to others (Pomini et al., 1998). However, clients' communication/interaction skills vary widely, which makes it critical to do a precise evaluation of these skills with each client. The Assessment of Communication and Interaction Skills (ACIS) (see Chapter 15) is very useful for obtaining a specific picture of these patient's communication and interaction skills.

In many young psychotic clients, process skills for daily tasks often are constrained and inefficient within daily tasks. Clinical data from the Assessment of Motor and Process Skills (AMPS) (see Chapter 15) have shown that the skills most likely to be impacted are related to adaptation, temporal organization, spatial organization, and energy level maintenance. All of these skills problems can make daily activities laborious and difficult.

Environmental Contexts

These clients are often faced with incomprehension on the part of their family and loved ones. Since the disease may not be physically visible, people with schizophrenia are often misunderstood and accused of being unmotivated or uncooperative. The family and friends are often unable to deal with the disorganized behaviors and may not know how to respond to these situations. Their expectations of the client are not always appropriate given the nature of the disease. Sometimes the family is overinvolved, whereas in other families clients are more or less abandoned. The emotional intensity of some families can also adversely affect clients.

The clients are often affected by negative influences in their environment, such as drugs, alcohol, or physical and psychological abuse (Bennet, Bellack, & Gearon, 2001). Consumption of drugs and alcohol has an adverse affect on psychotic processes. The stigma and prejudice associated with mental illness in all sectors of society also are barriers for these clients.

Translating the MOHO Conceptualization into Contributions to Program

Since the program was interdisciplinary, the conceptualization of client problems from a MOHO perspective served to identify problems that occupational therapists could address in the program. Corresponding intervention strategies to be used by therapists to address these problems were also identified. They are shown in *Table 24.2*. With this information, the therapists were able to negotiate their contributions to the assessment and intervention modules of *Premiers épisodes*.

Module 1: Assessment

As noted previously, occupational therapy assessment was designed to be part of the first module of *Premiers épisodes*, as shown in *Figure 24-3*. It is a collaborative interdisciplinary assessment process that includes the following:

- A systematic family interview
- A longitudinal clinical history

FIGURE 24.3 The Interdisciplinary Premiers episodes program.

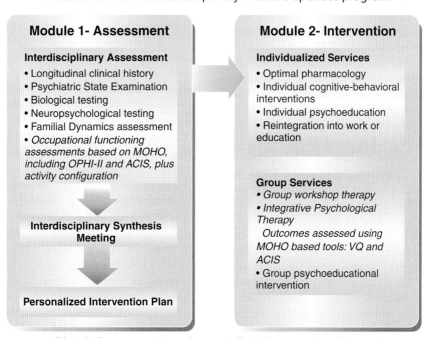

(Note: Italic components are those contributed by occupational therapy.)

- A psychiatric state examination
- Biological testing, including such laboratory tests as an electroencephalogram
- Neuropsychological testing, including cognitive tests, personality tests, diagnostic classification, and intelligence quotient when indicated to provide a complete picture of the client
- Occupational functioning assessments based on MOHO.

These are the assessments that make up the final component during the assessment module:

- Occupational Performance History Interview— Version 2 (OPHI-II)
- The Assessment of Communication and Interaction Skills (ACIS)
- Activity Configuration (Mosey, 1986)

The OPHI-II gives a complete, valid, and detailed functional picture of the patient. Furthermore, this assessment tool provides specific information regarding all areas of occupational functioning. The key forms developed for the three OPHI-II scales also provide measures of global functional changes that occur over the course of therapy. Also, the occupational narrative component of OPHI-II provides important qualitative information on the client's own perception of the past and current situation. The ACIS provides detailed information on communication and interaction skills; this is important, since a major focus of the intervention program is to improve communication and social skills (Bélanger et al., 2006). The assessments included in the occupational functioning component of the assessment module have changed over time. For example, the activity configuration was chosen after initially piloting the Occupational Questionnaire and found that it was too complex for the clients following the first psychotic episode. The activity configuration provides a picture of the client's daily life pattern. Initially, the AMPS was also used in the occupational functioning component. However, Nicole et al. (2006) found that in a cohort of 100 patients who participated in *Premiers épisodes*, the AMPS was not sensitive enough for this population.

Once the assessment process is complete, members of the interdisciplinary team gather for a synthesis meeting. During this meeting, each professional summarizes the assessment results, and the team together develops a specific interdisciplinary intervention plan to decide the combination of interventions that will be most beneficial to the client.

MODULE 2: INTERVENTION

As with assessment, the occupational therapy component of the intervention is fully integrated with the entire interdisciplinary program. The entire structure of the *Premiers épisodes* intervention module is presented in this chapter and shown in *Figure 24-3*. While the components of the program are standard, they are tailored to each client as a result of the personalized plan of intervention developed during the synthesis meeting.

MOHO is an important component of the intervention module of *Premiers épisodes*. MOHO provides specific guidelines for goals of intervention and helps identify the strategies to be undertaken to help the client change (Kielhofner, 2002). Additionally, MOHO integrated well with the other theories and approaches that are used in the program, such as Integrated Psychological Therapy, a cognitive approach developed by Brenner et al. (1994), and individual cognitive-behavioral intervention developed by Kingdon, Turkington, and John (1994), Jackson et al. (1998), Haddock, Morrisson, Hopkins, Lewis, and Tarrier (1998), and Kuipers et al., (1998).

The treatment module may include individual interventions and group interventions. Individual interventions include the following:

- Optimal pharmacology is directed by the psychiatrist and designed to ensure that the best medication approach is used with the client.
- Individual cognitive-behavioral interventions are given by psychiatrists and psychiatric nurses. This intervention is aimed at reducing the impact of positive symptoms of schizophrenia (e.g., delusions or hallucinations) by giving clients cognitive strategies for managing them. Occupational therapy assessment is often used to let the psychiatrists and nurses know how any symptoms are interfering with performance (Hansen et al., 2006).
- Nurses provide to clients and their families individual psychoeducation (Liberman, Wallace, Blackwell, Eckman, Vaccaro, & Kuehmel, 1993) that covers the disease (psychosis) and pharmacology. Since 2003, training on the consequences of abusing substances was also integrated to individual psychoeducation.
- Reintegration into work or education is an individualized component of the program offered by social workers. This component is usually a followup

service for clients who have progressed through the group components of the program and are ready to cope with productive objectives.

In addition to these individualized services, clients can participate in the following group services.

Group Workshop Therapy

Occupational therapy operates group workshop therapy for two to six people at a time. This group meets for 90 minutes. Clients engage in occupational forms that are personally meaningful to them, and intervention is based on MOHO tools and process of occupational change. The aims of this group:

- Engage the client in a significant activity related to his or her current life and stimulate volitional thoughts and feelings (occupational participation, occupational performance, and occupational skills)
- Identify basic challenges he or she may wish to undertake (volition: personal causation, values, and interest)
- Practice motor, process, communication/interaction skills (specific skills with which the client has difficulty).

During this workshop, clients are invited to stop and reflect on the effects of what they do to identify the actions that are most appropriate and that will give satisfactory results. Clients often begin in this group when they are too unstable to handle the demands of the next group, integrative psychological therapy.

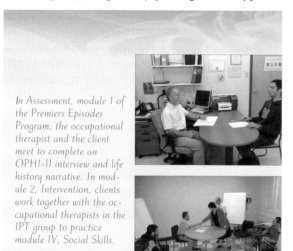

In Assessment, module 1 of the Premiers Episodes Program, the occupational therapist and the client meet to complete an OPHI-II interview and life history narrative. In module 2, Intervention, clients work together with the occupational therapists in the IPT group to practice module IV, Social Skills.

Integrative Psychological Therapy

Integrative psychological therapy (IPT) is a group intervention based on the combined principles of the cognitive-behavioral work of Pomini et al. (1998) and on MOHO. The group focuses simultaneously on difficulties in cognitive functioning, social skills, and emotion management. This group is run by two occupational therapists and consists of 8 to 12 clients who meet twice a week for 1 year. The goal of the IPT group "is to enhance the quality of life of patients by improving their psychosocial functioning and the ability to cope with environmental stressors of daily living" (Briand et al., 2006, p. 463). The group consists of six modules of exercises, organized hierarchically into increasing levels of complexity (Bélanger et al., 2006; Briand et al., 2005). In this manner, the amount of social interaction and emotional content is gradually increased. This program addresses and is designed to enable the clients to improve skills in these areas:

- Cognitive differentiation
- Social perception
- Verbal communication
- Social skills
- Emotional management
- Problem solving.

The group begins with the first two modules, cognitive differentiation and social perception, in which the client aims to improve the quality of data processing and perception. Clinical expediencies have also suggested that these two areas also improve occupational identity (Bélanger et al., 2006). The training then proceeds to more complex verbal competency, social skills, and finally to problem solving.

MOHO was especially helpful for the design of this group because it integrated well with the IPT principles and gave specific assessments and strategies that were not adequately specified in this IPT model. For this group, the ACIS and the VQ are used to identify specific motivation, communication/interaction skill problems, and from them treatment objectives are developed for each client. These assessments also provide a means of measuring client change.

Group Psychoeducational Intervention

This is a group for families of young psychotic clients (Anderson, Hogarty, & Reiss, 1980). Goals of the group are to decrease family isolation and help them to have a positive and active role during intervention and disease evolution. This group is offered only upon request or when clearly indicated as necessary for a client's welfare.

Program Implementation

All key decision makers in the hospital and in the provincial ministry of health strongly supported *Premiers épisodes* program. A detailed plan was needed to lay the groundwork for the program, which required personnel training and new equipment and space. At the beginning of the program, the team was designed to be composed of two psychiatrists, two psychiatric nurses, two neuropsychologists, one social worker, and three occupational therapists, each of whom devoted about half-time effort to the program. Not all members of the team worked exclusively in this program. Since 2003, neuropsychologists, psychiatric nurses, and psychiatrists have not been specifically connected with this program, but they are available upon request. Various members of the team received additional training and certifications to ensure that they had the appropriate competencies for the program. For the occupational therapists, the planning and preparation focused on training in MOHO and the cognitive-behavioral approaches (Hansen et al., 2006; Pomini et al., 1998) that were to be integrated with it.

MOHO experts provided guidance and consultation to the Quebec team on use of the model and its tools. Two training sessions were implemented in Quebec (a total of 4 days) on MOHO. In addition to receiving training in the use of MOHO and relevant assessments, the team received guidance in making translations of the assessments for use in French-speaking Quebec. At the time of this writing, plans are to evaluate the psychometrics of the translations. Practical experience suggests that the translated assessments are effective, and since fall 2005, the rehabilitation department of Laval University has initiated a study of validity for the French translation of OPHI-II. The occupational therapists, along with most other interdisciplinary staff, received training from a team of experts in implementing the cognitive-behavioral approach.

For each of the individual and group interventions, protocols were developed to ensure the quality of the sessions. At this stage, the incorporation of MOHO into the overall program structure called attention to the importance of volition and of the client's interests, values, and personal causation being considered thoroughly in intervention planning (Bélanger et al., 2006). This element served to enhance clients' feelings that they were truly involved in the intervention. Another important element of MOHO, recognized by the interdisciplinary team, was the extent to which assessments like the Volitional Questionnaire and ACIS provided very precise descriptions of volition and skill that could be used to establish specific objectives for the clients in therapy. Moreover, the specific contribution of the OPHI-II allows the team to identify specifically whether the client's occupational identity, occupational competence or occupational behavior setting (environment) are strengths or areas to be addressed in intervention.

Another important step in implementation was to integrate the therapists' use of MOHO with the total team. As noted earlier, the occupational therapists initially presented MOHO concepts to the team during the program planning phase. This served to garner initial support, but at the beginning of this program, some team members remained skeptical and others had very little appreciation of MOHO. However, the therapists' contributions to the team during implementation (i.e., demonstration of what information the assessments yielded and of how MOHO was used in intervention) informed the team more fully about MOHO, made them comfortable with its terminology and concepts, and eventually secured strong support for it as an integral part of this interdisciplinary program. As noted before, circumstances required a major reorganization of the psychiatric department. Despite all the other changes, the use of MOHO and IPT group remain the main core of *Premiers épisodes* program. MOHO is now understood and respected by psychiatrists and other professionals in the psychiatric department, and all occupational therapists in the psychiatric department (adult, psychogeriatric, teenager, inpatients, outpatients and day care hospital) have also decided to integrate MOHO concepts into their work.

Program Evaluation

One component of the evaluation of *Premiers épisodes* program is taking clinical measurements at the beginning and end of the intervention to evaluate the therapeutic effects of the components of the programs, such as the IPT. MOHO assessments are used principally for the measurement of the effects of the IPT. The ACIS and VQ are used to measure the effects of the Brenner IPT group therapy. Measurements are taken at the beginning and at the end of the group.

In 1998, research was initiated to evaluate *Premiers épisodes*. This entailed establishing a longitudinal database that describes in detail the clients who enter the program and that tracks them at 18 and 36 months following entry into the program (Nicole et al., 2006). The data for this research are collected by the psychiatrists, neuropsychologists, and occupational therapists in the program. The fact that occupational therapists collect data for the longitudinal database reflects the respect that MOHO assessments are accorded by the interdisciplinary team.

Part of the goal of the database is to identify initial characteristics of the clients that predict how clients will fare over time. The descriptive evaluation includes data on sociodemographic informational, history of the client, symptoms, neuropsychological functioning, job adaptation and housing, occupational functioning, quality of the client's life and that of his or her family, and the amount and type of services offered to the client. The first results published from this study (Nicole et al., 2006) document the heterogeneity of clients' needs. These findings support the conclusion that a detailed and structured assessment is necessary to identify the specific services each client needs.

Another Quebec-based study,[3] Briand et al. (2006) assessed the outcomes associated with incorporating IPT into nine regular clinical settings. Based on a study of 90 clients, the researchers concluded that clients improved in terms of all overall symptoms, subjective experiences, cognitive and social functioning, and quality of life. This research guided the creation of a Quebec version of the IPT, which better achieves its objectives, particularly those relating to the maintenance and generalization of social learning in the context of a participant's real-life situation (Briand et al., 2005; Briand et al., in press).

Future research will yield more information on how MOHO is best implemented for this client population, and additional studies will examine the outcomes of the services. This research will influence the design of future programs and enable occupational therapists and other professionals to better serve the functional rehabilitation needs of young psychotic patients in their first psychosis.

Conclusion

This chapter outlines a process of program development that emphasizes the importance of using a conceptual practice model. It offers a set of questions to guide the selection and justification of the model(s) to be used in a program. It also indicates four major steps that are ordinarily undertaken in program development. Finally, the authors illustrate how MOHO can be used to guide programs through three detailed examples. These examples illustrate situations in which MOHO was used to plan, implement, and evaluate occupational therapy services.

Key Terms

Evidence-based practice: Conscientious, explicit, and systematic use of available evidence in deciding the kinds of services that will be provided to individuals.

Mechanism of action: Theoretically and empirically accounting for how a particular change occurs as a consequence of participating in an intervention.

Program development: Creating and evaluating an approach to service delivery for a defined client group.

References

Anderson, C. M., Hogarty, G. E., & Reiss, D. J. (1980). Family treatment of adult schizophrenic patients: A psychoeducational approach. *Schizophrenia Bulletin, 6 (3)*, 490–505.

Azhar, F. T. (1996). *The relevance of worker identity to return to work in clients treated for work related injuries.* Unpublished master's thesis, Department of Occupational Therapy, University of Illinois at Chicago.

Beiser, M., Erickson, D., Fleming, J. A. E., & Iacono, W. G. (1993). Establishing the onset of psychotic illness, *American Journal of Psychiatry, 150*, 1349–1354.

Bélanger, R., Briand, C., & Rivard, S. (2006). Le modèle de l'Occupation Humaine (MOH). In : M. J. Manidi, *Ergothérapie comparée en santé mentale et psychiatrie* (pp.

[3]Supported by a grant from the joint program of the fonds de recherche en Santé du Québec, Conseil Québécois de Recherche Sociale, Ministère de la Santé et des Services Sociaux.

111–158). Lausanne: École d'études sociales et pédagogiques ÉÉSP.

Bennet, M. E., Bellack, A. S., & Gearon, J. S. (2001). Treating substance abuse in schizophrenia: An initial report. *Journal of Substance Abuse & Treatment, 20 (2),* 163–175.

Billingsley, A. (1988). *Black families—white America.* New York: Simon & Schuster.

Bonder, B. R. (2003). *Psychopathology and function* (3rd ed.). Thorofare, NJ: Slack.

Braveman, B. (1999). The model of human occupation and prediction of return to work: A review of related empirical research. *Work: A Journal of Prevention, Assessment & Rehabilitation, 12 (1),* 13–23.

Braveman, B. H. (2001). Development of a community-based return to work program for people living with AIDS. *Occupational Therapy in Health Care. 13 (3–4),*113–131.

Braveman, B., Helfrich, C., Kielhofner, G., & Albrecht, G. (2004). The experiences of 12 men with AIDS who attempted to return to work. *Israeli Journal of Occupational Therapy, 13,* 69–83.

Braveman, B., & Kielhofner, G. (2006). Developing evidence-based occupational therapy programming. In B. Braveman (Ed.). *Leading and Managing Occupational Therapy Services: An Evidence-based Approach* (pp. 215–244). Philadelphia: FA Davis.

Braveman, B., Kielhofner, G., Albrecht, G., & Helfrich, C. (2006). Occupational identity, occupational competence and occupational settings (environment): Influence on return to work in men living with HIV/AIDS. *Work: A Journal of Prevention Assessment, and Rehabilitation.* 27(3),267–276.

Braveman, B., Kielhofner, G., Levin, M., & Josefson, J. (2007, April). Enabling self determination in people living with AIDS: Outcomes of a controlled study. Paper presented at the conference of American Occupational Therapy Association, Saint Louis, MO.

Braveman, B. H., Sen, S., & Kielhofner, G. (2001). Community-based vocational rehabilitation programs. In M. Scaffa (Ed.), *Occupational therapy in community-based practice settings* (pp.139–162). Philadelphia: FA Davis.

Brenner, H. D., Roder, V., Hodel, B., Kienze, N., Reed, D., & Liberman, R. P. M. (1994). *Integrated psychological therapy for schizophrenic patients (IPT).* Toronto: Hogrefe.

Briand, C., Vasiliadis, H. M., Lesage, A., Lalonde, P., Stip, E., Nicole, L., Reinhardz, D., Proteau, A., Hamel, V., & Villeneuve, K. (2006). Including integrated psychological treatment as part of standard medical therapy for patients with schizophrenia clinical outcomes. *The Journal of Nervous and Mental Disease.* 194 *(7),* 463–470.

Briand, C., Reinhardz, D., Lesage, A., Nicole, L., Stip, E., & Lalonde, P. (in press). Analyse du contexte de mise en oeuvre d'un programme de réadaptation pour les personnes atteintes de troubles mentaux graves. Healthcare Policy / Politiques de santé.

Briand, C., Bélanger, R., Hamel, V., Nicole, L., Stip, E., Reinharz, D., Lalonde, P., & Lesage, A. D. (2005). Implantation multisite du programme Integrated Psychological Treatment (IPT) pour les personnes souffrant de schizophrénie. Élaboration d'une version renouvelée. *Santé mentale au Québec, 30,* 73–95.

Brownson, C. (2001). Program development for community health: Planning, implementation, and evaluation strategies. In M. Scaffa (Ed.), *Occupational therapy in community-based practice settings* (pp. 95–116). Philadelphia: FA Davis.

Bruce, G. M. A., & Borg, B. (2002). *Psychosocial Frames of Reference Core for Occupation-based Practice.* Thorofare: Slack.

Cather, C. (2005). Functional cognitive-behavioral therapy: A brief, individual treatment for functional impairments resulting from psychotic symptoms in schizophrenia. *Canadian Journal of Psychiatry, 50 (5),* 258–263.

Corner, R., Kielhofner, G., & Lin, F. L. (1997). Construct validity of a work environment impact scale. *Work, 9,* 21–34.

Corner, R., Kielhofner, G., & Olson, L. (1998). *Work Environment Impact Scale (WEIS). (Version 2.0).* Chicago: Model of Human Occupation Clearinghouse, Department of Occupational Therapy, College of Applied Health Sciences, University of Illinois. (Translated and published in Finnish, German, and Swedish).

DePoy, E. (1990). The TBIIM: An intervention for the treatment of individuals with traumatic brain injury. *Occupational Therapy in Health Care, 7 (1),* 55–67.

Falloon, I. R. H. (1992). Early intervention for first episodes of schizophrenia: A preliminary exploration. *Psychiatry, 55,* 4–15.

Feinberg, M. B. (1996). Changing the natural history of HIV disease. *Lancet, 348,* 239–246.

Forsyth, K., & Kielhofner, G. (2003). Model of Human Occupation. In: P. Kramer, J. Hinojosa, & C. Royeen, (Eds.), *Human Occupation: Participation in Life* (pp. 45–86). Philadelphia: Lippincott Williams & Wilkins.

George, L., & Neufeld, R. W. (1985). Cognition and symptomatology in schizophrenia. *Schizophrenia Bulletin, 11 (2),* 264–285.

Gerardi, S. M. (1996). The management of battle-fatigued soldiers: An occupational therapy model. *Military*

Medicine, 161 (8), 483–488.

Gitlin, L. N., Corcoran, M., Martindale-Adams, J., Malone, M. A., Stevens, A., & Winter, L. (2000). Identifying mechanisms of action: Why and how does intervention work? In R. Schulz (Ed.), *Handbook of dementia caregiving: Evidence-based interventions for family caregivers* (pp. 225–248). New York: Springer.

Goldstein, K, Kielhofner, G., & Paul-Ward, A. (2004) Occupational narratives and the therapeutic process. *Australian Occupational Therapy Journal, 51,* 119–124.

Green, M. F. (1996). What are the functional consequences of neurocognitive deficits in schizophrenia? *American Journal of Psychiatry, 153,* 321–330.

Grossman, J., & Bortone, J. (1986). Program development. In S. C. Robertson (Ed.), *SCOPE: Strategies, concepts and opportunities for program development and evaluation* (pp. 91–99). Bethesda, MD: American Occupational Therapy Association.

Gusich, R. (1984). Occupational therapy for chronic pain: A clinical application of the model of human occupation. *Occupational Therapy in Mental Health, 4 (3),* 59–73.

Gusich, R. L., & Silverman, A. (1991). Basava day clinic: The model of human occupation as applied to psychiatric day hospitalization. *Occupational Therapy in Mental Health, 11 (2/3),* 113–134.

Haddock, G., Morrisson, A. P., Hopkins, R., Lewis, S., & Tarrier, N. (1998). Individual cognitive-behavioural interventions in early psychosis. *British Journal of Psychiatry Supplement, 172 (33),* 101–106.

Hagerdon, R. (1992). *Occupational therapy: Foundation for practice, models, frame of reference and care skills.* New York: Churchill.

Hansen, L., Kingdon., D., & Turkington, D. (2006). The ABCs of cognitive-behavioral therapy for schizophrenia. *Psychiatric Times, 23 (7),* 49-54

Harding, C. (1988). Course types in schizophrenia: An analysis of European and American Studies. *Schizophrenia Bulletin, 14 (4),* 633–643.

Henry, A. D. (1994). *Predicting psychosocial functioning and symptomatic recovery of adolescents and young adults with a first psychotic episode: A six-month follow-up study.* Unpublished doctoral dissertation, Boston University.

Henry, A., & Coster, J. (1996). Predictors of functional outcome among adolescents and young adults with psychotic disorders. *American Journal of Occupational Therapy, 50 (3),* 171–181.

Hogg, R. S., O'Shaugnessy, M. V., Gatarac, N., Yip, B., Craib, K., Schecter, M. T., & Mantaner, J. S. (1997). Decline in deaths from new antiretrovirals [letter]. *Lancet, 349,* 1294.

Holm, M. (2000). Our mandate for the new millennium: Evidence-based practice. *American Journal of Occupational Therapy, 54 (6),* 575–585.

Jackson, H., McGorry, P., Edwards, J., Hulbert, C., Francey, S., Maude, D., Cocks, J., Power, P., Harrigan, S., & Dudgeon, P. (1998). Cognitively-oriented psychotherapy for early psychosis (COPE): Preliminary result. *British Journal of Psychiatry Supplement, 172 (23),* 93–100.

Johnstone, E. C., Crow, T. J., & Johnson, A. L. (1986). The Northwick Park study of first episode schizophrenia: Presentation of the illness and problems relating to admission. *British Journal of Psychiatry, 148,* 115–120.

Kaplan, H. I., Sadock, B. J., Grebb, J. A., (1994). *Synopsis of psychiatry: Behavioral sciences clinical psychiatry* (7th ed.). Baltimore: Williams & Wilkins.

Kavanaugh, J., & Fares, J. (1995). Using the model of human occupation with homeless mentally ill patients. *British Journal of Occupational Therapy, 58 (10),* 419–422.

Kielhofner, G. (2002). *A Model of human occupation: Theory and application* (3rd ed.). Baltimore: Lippincott Williams & Wilkins.

Kielhofner, G., Braveman, B., Finlayson, M., Paul-Ward, A., Goldbaum, L., & Goldstein, K. (2004). Outcomes of a vocational program for persons with AIDS. *American Journal of Occupational Therapy, 58,* 64–72.

Kielhofner, G., Braveman, B., Levin, M., & Fogg, L. (In press). A controlled study of services to enhance productive participation among persons with HIV/AIDS. *AJOT.*

Kielhofner, G., & Brinson, M. (1989). Development & evaluation of an aftercare program for young chronic psychiatrically disabled adults. *Occupational Therapy in Mental Health, 9,* 1–25.

Kingdon, D., Turkington, D., & John, C. (1994). Cognitive-behavioral therapy of schizophrenia. *British Journal of Psychiatry, 165 (5),* 695.

Kuipers, E., Fowler, D., Garety, P., Chisholm, D., Freeman, D., Dunn, G., Bebbinton, P., & Hadley, C. (1998). London-East Anglia randomised controlled trial of cognitive-behavioural therapy for psychosis: Follow-up and economic evaluation at 18 months. *British Journal of Psychiatry, 173,* 61–68.

Lalonde, P., & Grunberg, F. (1988). *Psychiatrie clinique approche bio-psycho-sociale.* Québec: Gaëtan Morin Éditeur.

Law, M. (2002). *Evidence-based rehabilitation: A guide to practice.* Thorofare, NJ: Slack.

Liberman, R. P., Wallace, C. J., Blackwell, G., Eckman, T. A., Vaccaro, J. V., & Kuehmel, T. G. (1993). Innovations in skills training for the seriously mentally ill: The UCLA social and independent living skills module. *Innovations and Research, 2 (2),* 43–59.

Mallinson, T. (1998). *Work rehabilitation in mental health programs.* A companion manual to the videotapes "Working it out" and "The write stuff." Chicago: Model of Human Occupation Clearinghouse, Department of Occupational Therapy, College of Applied Health Sciences, University of Illinois.

Mawrer, K., & Häfner, H. (1995). Methodological aspect of onset assessment in schizophrenia. *Schizophrenia Research, 15,* 265–267.

Mentrup, C., Niehaus, A., & Kielhofner, G. (1999). Applying the model of human occupation in work-focused rehabilitation: A case illustration. *Work: A Journal of Prevention, Assessment & Rehabilitation, 12 (1),* 61–70.

Michael, P. S. (1991). Occupational therapy in a prison? You must be kidding! *Mental Health Special Interest Section Newsletter, 14,* 3–4.

Mosey, A. C. (1986). *Psychosocial components of occupational therapy.* New York: Raven.

Munoz, J., & Kielhofner, G. (1995). Program development. In G. Kielhofner (Ed.), *A model of human occupation: Theory and application* (2nd ed.). Baltimore: Williams & Wilkins.

National Institute on Disability and Rehabilitation Research (NIDRR). (1995, April). *Forging collaborative partnerships in the study of disability: A NIDRR conference on participatory action research.* Washington.

Nicole, L., Routhier, G., L'Heureux, S., Bélanger, R., Rivard, P., Bussière G., Duval N., Vignola, A., Cossette, M., & Lesage, A.D. (2006). *A specialized programme for first-episode psychoses: analysis of a 100 patients cohort,* Les Annales médico-psychologiques. Manuscript submitted for publication.

Nicole, L., Pires, A., Routhier, G., Bélanger, R., Bussière, G., L'Heureux, S., Gingras, N., Rivard, P., Chabot, P., Descombes, J., Sylvain, C., Abdal-Baki, A., Duval, N., Vignola, A., & Rhéaume, J. (1999). Schizophrénie, approche spécialisée et continuité de soins: Le programme spécifique d'intervention premier épisode de l'Hôtel-Dieu de Lévis. *Santé Mentale au Québec, 24 (1),* 121–135.

Oakley, F. (1987). Clinical application of the model of human occupation in dementia of the Alzheimer's type. *Occupational Therapy in Mental Health, 7 (4),* 37–50.

Olin, D. (1985). Assessing and assisting the person with dementia: An occupational behavior perspective. *Physical & Occupational Therapy in Geriatrics, 3 (4),* 25–32.

Olson, L. (1998). *Work readiness: Day treatment for the chronically disabled.* Chicago: Model of Human Occupation Clearinghouse, Department of Occupational Therapy, College of Applied Health Sciences, University of Illinois.

Padilla, R., & Bianchi, E. M. (1990). Occupational therapy for chronic pain: Applying the model of human occupation to clinical practice. *Occupational Therapy Practice, 1 (3),* 47–52.

Paul-Ward, A., Braveman, B., Kielhofner, G., & Levin, M. (2005). Developing employment services for individuals with HIV/AIDS: Participatory action strategies at work. *Journal of Vocational Rehabilitation, 22 ,*85–93.

Pizzi, M. A. (1984). Occupational therapy in hospice care. *American Journal of Occupational Therapy, 38,* 252–257.

Pizzi, M. A. (1989). Occupational therapy: Creating possibilities for adults with HIV infection, ARC and AIDS. *AIDS Patient Care, 3,* 18–23.

Pizzi, M.A. (1990a). The model of human occupation and adults with HIV infection and AIDS. *American Journal of Occupational Therapy, 44,* 257–264.

Pizzi, M. A. (1990b). Occupational therapy: Creating possibilities for adults with human immunodeficiency virus infection, AIDS related complex, and acquired immunodeficiency syndrome. *Occupational Therapy in Health Care, 7 (2/3/4),* 125–137.

Pomini, V., Neis, L., Brenner, H. D., Hodel, B., & Roder, V. (1998). Thérapie psychologique des schizophrénies, Sprimont: Mardaga Editeurs.

Reed, K. L. (2003). *Quick Reference to Occupational Therapy* (2nd ed.). Gaithersburg, MD: Aspen.

Reekmans, M., & Kielhofner, G. (1998). Defining occupational therapy services in child psychiatry: An application of the model of human occupation. *Ergotherapie, 5,* 6–13.

Sackett, D. L., Rosenberg, W. M. C., Gray, J. A. M., Haynes, R. B., & Richardson, W. S. (1996). Evidence-based medicine: What it is and what it isn't. *British Medical Journal, 312,* 71–72.

Salz, C. (1983). A theoretical approach to the treatment of work difficulties in borderline personalities. *Occupational Therapy in Mental Health, 3 (3),* 33–46.

Schaaf, R. C., & Mulrooney, L. L. (1989). Occupational therapy in early intervention: A family centered approach. *American Journal of Occupational Therapy, 43,* 745–754.

Schindler, V. J. (1988). Psychosocial occupational therapy intervention with AIDS patients. *American Journal of Occupational Therapy, 42,* 507–512.

Schindler, V. P. (1990). AIDS in a correctional setting. *Occupational Therapy in Health Care, 7 (2/3/4),* 171–183.

Sholle-Martin, S. (1987). Application of the model of human occupation: Assessment in child and adolescent psychiatry. *Occupational Therapy in Mental Health, 7 (2),* 3–22.

Stack, C. B. (1974). *All our kin.* New York: Harper & Row.

Taylor, M. C. (2000). *Evidence-based practice for occupational therapists.* London: Blackwell Science.

Velozo, C., Kielhofner, G., & Fisher, G. (1998). *A user's guide to the Worker Role Interview (WRI).* (Version 9.0). Chicago: Model of Human Occupation Clearinghouse, Department of Occupational Therapy, College of Applied Health Sciences, University of Illinois.

Weissenberg, R., & Giladi, W. (1989). Home economics day: A program for disturbed adolescents to promote acquisition of habits and skills. *Occupational Therapy in Mental Health, 9 (2),* 89–103.

Weitz, R. (1990). Living with the stigma of AIDS. *Qualitative Sociology, 13 (1),* 23–28.

Woodrum, S. C. (1993). A treatment approach for attention deficit hyperactivity disorder using the model of human occupation. *Developmental Disabilities Special Interest Section Newsletter, 16 (1),* 1–2.

Wyatt, R. J. (1991). Neuroleptics and the natural course of schizophrenia. *Schizophrenia Bulletin, 17,* 325–351.

Youngstrom, M. J. (1999). Developing a new occupational therapy program. In K. Jacobs & M. K. Logigian (Eds.), *Function of a manager* (3rd ed.). Thorofare, NJ: Slack.

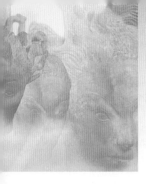

Evidence for Practice from the Model of Human Occupation

- Jessica Kramer
- Patricia Bowyer
- Gary Kielhofner

Occupational therapists are increasingly under pressure from both within and outside the profession to deliver evidence-based practice (Law & Baum, 1998; Lloyd, Basset, & King, 2004; McCluskey & Cusick, 2002). This means that therapists are expected to identify, critique, synthesize, and use evidence as a guide and justification for what they do in practice (Roberts & Barber, 2001; Taylor, 1997).

To a large extent, practicing therapists agree with the importance of evidence-based practice (Bennett et al., 2003; Humphries, Littlejohns, Victor, O'Halloran, & Peacock, 2000; Metcalfe, Lewin, Wisher, Perry, Bannigan, & Moffett, 2001). However, practitioners express concerns about the practicality of using research to guide practice (Dysart and Tomlin, 2002 ; McCluskey and Cusick, 2002; McCluskey, 2003). Practitioners report that research often lacks real-life significance, addresses topics not relevant to practice, and fails to present findings in ways that facilitate their application (Dubouloz, Egan, Vallerand, & Von Zweck, 1999; Sudsawad, 2003).

The Kinds of Evidence Needed to Support Practice

Evidence-based practice is the judicious use of the best available evidence to guide decision making in practice (Sackett, Rosenberg, Muir Gray, Haynes, & Richardson, 1996). As this definition implies, the kind of evidence that is needed differs with the decision a therapist is making (Tickle-Degnen & Bedell, 2003; Tse, Blackwood, & Penman, 2001). This definition also indicates that

therapists must work with available evidence. In cases where there is no or little evidence available from research studies, therapists will need to rely on other forms of evidence. Thus, relevant evidence for practice may include controlled studies of outcomes of services, clinical knowledge presented in case studies, research that explores and develops theory, the expertise of professional peers, and the perspectives of clients (Polatajko & Craik, 2006; Sudsawad, 2006).

MOHO Evidence

The Model of Human Occupation was first published nearly 3 decades ago. Over time, a substantial body of evidence has accumulated. Because MOHO was developed as a practice model, research has always tended to focus on topics relevant to practice. Moreover, in the past decade MOHO developers have embraced the scholarship of practice approach that focuses research on solving practice problems and that looks to practice for questions to be addressed through research (Kielhofner, 2005a, b; Taylor, Fisher, & Kielhofner, 2005). Consequently, most recent MOHO studies have grown out of partnerships between practitioners and researchers, which ensures that the findings are useful to practice settings.

Finding MOHO Evidence

Therapists looking for evidence on a particular topic in the MOHO literature can easily find themselves searching through hundreds of articles and chapters. While it is relatively easy to identify some types of evidence relevant to a topic or question, other relevant evidence may be less apparent. Thus, searching comprehensively for evidence is often a daunting task. To facilitate the location of evidence, the MOHO Clearinghouse Web site includes an evidence-based search engine that enables practitioners to locate citations relevant to practice topics. This search engine is explained in more detail in Appendix B. While the search engine helps identify relevant literature, therapists must still locate the articles and sift through them for the desired evidence.

The Approach of This Chapter

The aim of this chapter is to streamline the process of identifying commonly sought evidence for practice. We have identified some of the most typical questions that practitioners ask when seeking MOHO evidence and synthesized all of the available evidence. The resources in this chapter should never completely substitute for other evidence-based strategies. Since the MOHO literature grows substantially each year, it is likely that when this book is published, there will be evidence beyond the citations included in this chapter. Moreover, because critique is part of the process of using evidence, therapists are encouraged to go beyond the brief descriptions provided here and directly examine the literature they summarize. Finally, this chapter focuses exclusively on evidence generated from published studies. However, there are also other sources of useful evidence. This includes evidence available in the literature, such as case examples and program descriptions. The MOHO Web site provides access to the expertise of occupational therapists who use MOHO through archived listserv discussions coded by topic.

Evidence in this chapter is organized around the following questions:

- What does MOHO research tell us about the occupational lives and needs of people with disabilities?
- What evidence exists for the dependability and utility of MOHO-based assessments?
- What does practice based on MOHO look like?
- What evidence is there that MOHO-based services produce positive outcomes?
- What do clients have to say about MOHO-based services?

The Occupational Lives and Needs of People with Disabilities

From its inception, MOHO research has focused on understanding how both personal and environment factors impact occupational participation. A large number of researchers who use MOHO as a framework for their research have examined the volition, habituation, performance capacity, and/or environments of persons with disabilities in their research, as well as the process of occupational adaptation via the development of occupational competence and occupational identity. MOHO was the first occupational therapy model to incorporate the environment as a major variable in determining occupational participation, and MOHO-based research has sought to better illustrate the concept of environmental impact.

These studies include research that aims to explore or test MOHO concepts, that seeks to identify challenges and needs of disabled persons, and that asks about client or environmental characteristics and their relation to clients' responses to services and the outcomes that are achieved. This type of evidence can be helpful to practitioners in the following ways:

- It can identify factors that are particularly challenging for clients and that should be addressed in therapy,
- It can identify factors that impact the client's involvement in therapy and therefore should be considered when giving services, and
- It can identify factors associated with positive or negative outcomes of therapy that should be recognized as liabilities or strengths and addressed accordingly.

Tables 25.1 to *25.4* list and summarize this research according to the major concepts of MOHO (volition, habituation, environment, and occupational adaptation).

Evidence Concerning the Dependability and Utility of MOHO Assessments

Most of the MOHO-based assessments have been extensively researched. Although the approach to developing MOHO-based assessments has changed over the

TABLE 25.1 Clients' Characteristics Related to Volition

Citation	Outcomes and Findings
Asmundsdottir (2004)	Psychiatric clients reported a low sense of personal causation and efficacy as barriers to return to work.
Aubin, Hachey, & Mercier (1999)	Pleasure (an aspect of volition) in work and rest is positively correlated with subjective quality of life for outpatient psychiatric clients.
Barrett, Beer, & Kielhofner (1999)	A person's volitional narrative influences how a person will participate in and benefit from therapy.
Barris, Dickie, & Baron (1988)	Young adults with eating disorders were more external on dimensions of self-control, young adults with chronic conditions were more internal on dimensions of self control, and adolescents with psychiatric conditions were more external on dimensions of social control compared to community-dwelling adolescents without disabilities.
Barris, Kielhofner, Burch, Gelinas, Klement, & Schultz (1986)	Volitional aspects such as locus of control, importance and value of roles and activities, interests, and enjoyment impact occupational adaptation of adolescents with psychiatric or psychophysiologic conditions and adolescents without disabilities.
Bridle, Lynch, & Quesenberry (1990)	2–8 years after spinal cord injury, persons report difficulty with volition, including less adaptive interests, fewer values and goals, and less adaptive perceptions of abilities and responsibilities.
Chen, Neufeld, Feely, & Skinner (1999)	Volition, specifically perceived self-efficacy, is a main predictor of compliance with home exercise programs among clients with upper extremity impairments and injuries.
Crowe, VanLeit, Berghmans, & Mann (1997)	There were no significant differences in the values reported for various roles by mothers of children with multiple disabilities, mothers of children with Down syndrome, and mothers of typically developing children.
Dickerson & Oakely (1995)	Clients with physical and psychosocial disabilities differed in the value assigned to present and future roles compared to persons without disabilities.
Ebb, Coster, & Duncombe (1989)	The total number of reported strong interests differed between adolescents with psychosocial disabilities staying in hospitals and community-dwelling adolescents without disabilities.
Ekbladh, Haglund, & Thorell (2004)	Persons who returned to work had significantly higher scores on the volitional construct of personal causation (measured by the WRI) compared to persons who did not return to work.
Hachey, Boyer, & Mercier (2001)	Canadian adults with schizophrenia report most value for present roles of friend, worker, and family member, while they anticipate they will most value roles of friend, family member, home maintainer, and hobbyist in the future.
Hakansson, Eklund, Lidfeldt, Nerbrand, Samsioe, & Nilsson (2005)	Women who maintain employment report a significantly greater value for worker role and higher sense of well being than women who report discontinuity in work related to illness.
Helfrich, Kielhofner, & Mattingly (1994)	People with disabilities perceive their life and behavior according to their own narrative account of their life and how the disability has influenced that life.
Jacobshagen (1990)	Interruptions during engagement in craft occupations can affect a person's sense of personal causation and competence for that activity.
Jonsson, Josephsson, & Kielhofner (2001)	Volitional narratives are plastic, and interactions between narratives and actual life events can alter the meaning of and motivation for engaging in occupations.
Jonsson, Josephsson, & Kielhofner (2000)	Volitional narratives are not set scripts for action but represent an active or passive orientation to act in a particular manner depending on the circumstances of an event.
Jonsson, Kielhofner, & Borell (1997)	A person's anticipated future narrative, whether progressive, stable, or regressive, is influenced by how the person experiences and interprets his or her involvement in occupations.

WRI, Worker Role Interview.

(continued)

TABLE 25.1 *(continued)*

Citation	Outcomes and Findings
Katz, Giladi, & Peretz (1988)	Israeli adult psychiatric clients are more interested in ADLs (all clients with psychiatric disabilities) and manual skills (only clients diagnosed with schizophrenia) compared to adults without disabilities.
Katz, Josman, & Steinmetz (1988)	Adolescents hospitalized with psychiatric disabilities expressed more interest in ADLs and less interest in cultural, educational, social, and recreational activities compared to community-dwelling adolescents.
	Locus of control did not differentiate between hospitalized and non hospitalized adolescents.
Lederer, Kielhofner, & Watts (1985)	Fewer incarcerated adolescents reported value for the student, worker, volunteer, and home maintainer role compared to adolescents in the community.
	Incarcerated adolescents often reported value for roles related to risk-taking behavior and self-expression.
Morgan, & Jongbloed (1990)	Volitional factors, such as meaningfulness of an activity, personal standards for performance in an activity, and range of interests, impacted participation in leisure activities after a stroke.
Neville-Jan (1994)	For clients in psychiatric inpatient hospitals, volitional aspects of pleasure and locus of control were significantly related to occupational adaptation when depression was controlled for or not controlled for.
Oakley, Kielhofner, & Barris (1985)	Clients with mental health problems had more external locus of control than persons in the community, but they still reported strong interests.
Peterson, Howland, Kielhofner, Lachman, Assmann, Cote, & Jette (1999)	Sense of self-efficacy related to falls was related to interference with participation and restriction of participation in social and leisure activities in older persons.
Rust, Barris, & Hooper (1987)	Leisure values and personal causation for exercise are predictive of women's exercise behavior.
Scaffa (1991)	Persons attending a program for alcohol abuse reported less participation in cultural and educational interests and fewer avocational interests compared to persons not in treatment for alcohol abuse.
Scheelar (2002)	Volition, including interests, personal satisfaction, and value for career, affects an injured firefighter's decision to return to work.
Smith, Kielhofner, & Watts (1986)	Interests, values, and personal causation are positively correlated with life satisfaction for older adults living in the community or in a nursing home.
Smyntek, Barris, & Kielhofner (1985)	Adolescents hospitalized with psychosocial problems had different volition patterns, including lower self-esteem, more external locus of control, decreased competence for rest, and less value assigned to roles, from those of community-dwelling adolescents.
Tham & Borell (1996)	Clients have a strong sense of self-efficacy for engaging in leisure and self-care regardless of the extent of unilateral neglect experienced post CVA.
Watson & Ager (1991)	For adults aged 50 and up living in the community, value for the student role and religious participant roles was negatively related to life satisfaction, while value for home maintainer role was positively related to life satisfaction.
Widen-Holmqvist et al. (1993)	Adults living at home post stroke report a sense of personal causation, values, and interests that are similar to what other adults living in the community report.
Zimmerer-Branum & Nelson (1994)	Nursing home residents were more likely to choose an occupationally embedded exercise over a route exercise, and those who chose occupation-based activities had a higher level of engagement in the activity as demonstrated by the number of repetitions completed.

ADL, activities of daily living; CVA, cerebrovascular accident.

T A B L E   2 5 . 2   Clients' Characteristics Related to Habituation

Citation	Outcomes and Findings
Baker, Curbow, & Wingard (1991)	Role change and role loss were reported by bone marrow transplant survivors, although roles of family member, friend, and home maintainer changed the least before and after the transplant. Retaining any roles and retaining important roles were significantly and positively correlated with satisfaction with life. Retaining roles and important roles was significantly and negatively correlated with negative mood. For men, loss of worker role, family role, and community role was associated with negative quality of life, affect, or mood variables. For women, loss of worker role was associated with decreased quality of life.
Barris, Dickie, & Baron (1988)	Young adults with eating disorders, young adults with chronic conditions, and adolescents with psychiatric disorders anticipated fewer future roles than did community-dwelling young persons without disabilities. Adolescents with psychiatric disorders had fewer past roles than did community-dwelling young persons without disabilities.
Barris, Kielhofner, Burch, Gelinas, Klement, & Schultz (1986)	Aspects of habituation, such as number of past roles and time spent in ADLs, work, and play activities influence the occupational adaptation of adolescents with psychiatric disabilities, psychophysiologic conditions, and adolescents without disabilities.
Branholm & Fugl-Meyer (1992)	Across age cohorts and gender, involvement in family, leisure, and vocational roles was related to life satisfaction. Persons experienced changes in role engagement based on gender and age-related life circumstances according to social and cultural customs.
Bridle, Lynch, & Quesenberry (1990)	2–8 years after spinal cord injury, persons report difficulty with habituation, including less adaptive organization of daily routines and less adaptive life roles.
Crowe, VanLeit, Berghmans, & Mann (1997)	Role engagement, complexity, and related expectations may change over time for mothers of children with and without disabilities. Mothers of children with Down syndrome and mothers of children with multiple disabilities reported engagement in fewer present roles than mothers of typically developing children. However, mothers of all children report role loss upon the birth of their children, although mothers of children with Down syndrome report the most role loss.
Davies Hallet, Zasler, Maurer, & Cash (1994)	Persons with traumatic brain injuries experience role changes after injury, including role loss (worker and hobby roles) and role gain. There was a significant relationship between the number of role changes and a score on a disability scale.
Dickerson & Oakley (1995)	Clients with physical and psychosocial disabilities had patterns of role involvement that differed from those of community-dwelling persons without disabilities. Clients with physical and psychosocial disabilities reported engagement in fewer roles, which may be indicative of their inpatient status. Clients with psychosocial disabilities do not differ in anticipated patterns of future role engagement from community-dwelling persons, but clients with physical disabilities report a significantly different anticipated future role engagement, particularly in worker and hobbyist roles.
Duellman, Barris, & Kielhofner (1986)	There is a significant positive relationship between the number of organized activities offered by the nursing home and the number of present and future roles reported by older adults living in nursing homes.
Ebb, Coster, & Duncombe (1989)	The total number of reported current and future roles differs between adolescents with psychosocial disabilities staying in the hospital and community-dwelling adolescents without disabilities.

(continued)

TABLE 25.2 *(continued)*

Citation	Outcomes and Findings
Ekbladh, Haglund, & Thorell (2004)	Persons who returned to work were better able to appraise their work expectations related to the worker role than persons who did not return to work.
Eklund (2001)	Roles such as friend, hobbyist, family member, worker, and caregiver are associated with quality of life for clients with mental health problems at admission, discharge, or followup.
Elliott & Barris (1987)	There is a significant positive relationship between the number of roles and the meaningfulness of those roles and life satisfaction for community-dwelling adults. Involvement in meaningful roles leads to a sense of satisfaction with life and enables persons to fulfill their need for mastery and meet expectations of society.
Frosch et al. (1997)	Caregivers of persons with a TBI reported significant changes in engagement in roles from the past to the present. There was a positive trend between number of role changes and the behavioral effects of the TBI survivor and an inverse trend between the number of role changes and caregiver use of support systems.
Hachey, Boyer, & Mercier (2001)	Adults with schizophrenia report more involvement in roles in the past than in the present but anticipate they will be involved in more roles in the future. Adults with schizophrenia also report more role loss than role gain from past to present. Family member, friend, home maintainer, and hobbyist were the most frequently reported roles engaged in by the adults.
Hammel (1999)	For people with disabilities, roles are entered, developed, and exited over time on an individual basis, and the meaning, importance, and definition of roles can change according to an individual's role development process.
Horne, Corr, & Earle (2005)	First-time mothers report a change in roles and routines resulting in periods of occupational imbalance after the birth.
Katz, Giladi, & Peretz (1988)	There are significant differences in role performance between Israeli adult psychiatric clients and adults without disabilities with regard to their patterns of engagement in a profession and patterns of engagement in ADLs, play, recreation, rest, and sleep.
Katz, Josman, & Steinmetz (1988)	Role engagement was significantly different between adolescents hospitalized with psychiatric conditions and community-dwelling adolescents: hospitalized adolescents were more likely to engage in social activities and recreation at home and were more likely to change schools because of problems associated with their hospitalization.
Lee, Strauss, Wittman, Jackson, & Carstens (2001)	The caregiving role and value for the caregiving role is associated with feelings of sorrow when caregivers care for adults with mental health problems at time of the person's diagnosis and in the present. However, high levels of engagement in the hobbyist role are associated with lower levels of sorrow at the time of the person's diagnosis.
Morgan & Jongbloed (1990)	Clients returning home after a stroke report a shift in role balance and routine and report that they altered roles because of changed performance capacity. This included engagement in leisure roles.
Muñoz, Karmosky, Gaugler, Lang, & Stayduhar (1999)	While parents undergo role adaptation when parenting a child with a disability, this role shift occurs differently for mothers and fathers and does not inherently result in a strain on roles. Role adaptations can include a loss of roles (worker, friend), an expansion of roles (caregiver), or the acquisition of new roles (religious participant, advocate). Fathers reported less role disruption than mothers.
Oakley, Kielhofner, & Barris (1985)	Clients with mental health conditions report fewer roles and more role disruption than people without disabilities.
Rosenfeld (1989)	Occupational routines are disrupted and task pressures change after a disaster such as a house fire.

(continued)

TABLE 25.2 *(continued)*

Citation	Outcomes and Findings
Rust, Barris, & Hooper (1987)	Women's exercise behavior can be predicted by the number of roles they are engaged in, the internalization of the exerciser role, and their exercise habits.
Scaffa (1991)	Persons attending a program for alcohol abuse reported less time engaged in work activities, more time engaged in alcohol activities, and less time awake compared to persons living in the community.
Smith, Kielhofner, & Watts (1986)	The amount of time spent engaged in occupations of work and recreation is positively correlated with life satisfaction for older adults living in nursing homes and the community.
Smyntek, Barris, & Kielhofner (1985)	Adolescents hospitalized with psychosocial problems reported fewer present roles and less time spent doing ADLs than community adolescents on a typical Saturday; this may be related to the hospital environment.
Watson & Ager (1991)	Frequency of engagement in the home maintainer role was positively correlated with life satisfaction for adults aged 50 and up living in the community.
Weeder (1986)	People with schizophrenia attending a day program have different patterns of occupational engagement in daily activities such as sleep, leisure, and work during weekdays and weekends from those of people living in the community.
Widen-Holmqvist et al. (1993)	For adults living in the community after a stroke, engagement in activities was limited to home-based leisure activities and self-care activities.

TBI, traumatic brain injury; ADL, activities of daily living.

TABLE 25.3 Environmental Impact and Characteristics Influencing Occupation Participation

Citation	Outcomes and Findings
Ay-Woan, Sarah, LyInn, Tsyr-Jang, & Ping-Chaun (2006)	Environmental assessment should be considered for clients experiencing depression, as the environmental aspects of the OSA predicted quality of life for adult Taiwanese clients with mental health disabilities.
Bridle, Lynch, & Quesenberry (1990)	2–8 years after a spinal cord injury, persons report less adaptive environmental influences that then impact occupational adaptation, mainly within the physical environment.
Duellman, Barris, & Kielhofner (1986)	The environment of a nursing home, particularly the number of organized activities provided by the home, is positively correlated with older adults' perception of engagement in roles.
	People perceive themselves as actively engaged in their environment when opportunities to participate are provided.
Ekbladh, Haglund, & Thorell (2004)	Persons who returned to work perceived the physical work setting to be more supportive of return to work than persons who did not return to work.
Hemmingsson, Borell, & Gustavsson (1999)	Task expectations and demands of schoolteachers associated with their classroom management style can influence a student's ability to participate in school tasks independently.
Kjellberg (2002)	The environment, including national legislation, attitudes, and forms of routines and activities, was a barrier or a support to participation for persons with intellectual disabilities.
Molyneaux-Smith, Townsend, & Guernsey (2003)	The environment (including objects, social environment, and government policies) can be a barrier or a support to reengagement in vocational roles after injury.
Scheelar (2002)	The work social environment can affect an injured firefighter's willingness and ability to return to work.
Tham & Kielhofner (2003)	Social support and cues from the environment enable women with left neglect to engage in occupations and support participation.

OSA, Occupational Self-Assessment.

TABLE 25.4 Client Occupational Adaptation, Identity, and Competence Characteristics

Citation	Outcomes and Findings
Aubin, Hachey, & Mercier (1999)	Perceived competence in ADLs and rest is positively correlated with subjective quality of life for outpatient psychiatric clients.
Ay-Woan, Sarah, LyInn, Tsyr-Jang, & Ping-Chaun (2006)	Perceived competence and ability to engage in occupations (as measured by the OSA) can impact quality of life for adult Taiwanese clients with mental health disabilities.
Barris, Dickie, & Baron (1988)	MOHO concepts have varying degrees of usefulness in explaining clients' performance, depending on the client's diagnosis (i.e., eating disorder, psychiatric condition, or chronic condition).
Barris, Kielhofner, Burch, Gelinas, Klement, & Schultz (1986)	There is no simple linear relationship between inner traits, such as volition and habituation, and occupational behavior. These factors interact to influence occupational adaptation of adolescents with psychophysiologic conditions, psychiatric conditions, or those without a disability.
Braveman & Helfrich (2001)	A disability can impact occupational identity and competence in various ways, which in turn impacts an individual's life narrative.
Bridle, Lynch, & Quesenberry (1990)	Occupational adaptation, including occupational competence, occupational identity, and environment, can be affected by a spinal cord injury even 2–8 years post injury.
Gregory (1983)	Engagement in occupations, particularly the amount the activity was engaged in, the enjoyment felt for the activity, the competency for the activity, and the meaningfulness of the activity, was positively correlated with life satisfaction for adults who were retired.
Haglund, Thorell, & Walinder (1998b)	Occupational adaptation and participation (as measured by the OCAIRS) is different for clients with depression, schizophrenia, and bipolar disorder; clients with depression exhibit the highest levels of occupational adaptation.
Levin & Helfrich (2004)	Homeless teenage mothers' sense of occupational identity as a mother was influenced by their own mother and by their willingness to fulfill the identity. This identity influences other aspects of their lives.
	Homeless teenage mothers did not feel a strong sense of occupational competence in the mother role, although they had personal standards for performance and goals related to that role.
Mallinson, Mahaffey, & Kielhofner (1998)	Occupational adaptation occurs when an individual has a strong sense of occupational competence and an occupational identity over time.
Peterson et al. (1999)	Occupational performance may reflect not just physical ability but also volitional status, as in the case of older adults who report low self-efficacy related to falling and a corresponding restriction of activity.
Restall & Magill-Evans (1994)	Participation in play for children with autism is significantly different from that of children without autism. However, the two groups of children were not significantly different on the number of play material categories used, imitation, space management, or material management during play.

ADL, activities of daily living; OSA, Occupational Self-Assessment; OCAIRS, Occupational Circumstances Assessment—Interview and Rating Scale.

years, the contemporary approach is to use item response theory (Velozo, Forsyth, & Kielhofner, 2006) as a basis for establishing the internal validity and measurement soundness. This process, which ordinarily takes upward of 3 years, results in the creation of key forms that allow the ordinal data obtained from rating scales to be converted to interval data (Kielhofner, Dobria, Forsyth, & Basu, 2005; Velozo et al., 2006). Traditional psychometric approaches (Kielhofner, 2006) are also used to test the reliability and validity of MOHO-based assessments. Finally, because MOHO research emphasizes the scholarship of practice, research often aims to examine the utility of the assessment from practitioner and consumer perspectives. *Tables 25.5* to *25.20* present and summarize the research underlying each assessment. Research is presented in chronological order to illustrate the development of each assessment over time.

Evidence Concerning the Nature of MOHO Practice

A few studies have focused on the process of therapy based on MOHO. These studies provide evidence about the dynamics of therapy and about factors that may contribute to positive outcomes of therapy. The publications are summarized in *Table 25.21*. Another source of information about what MOHO practice looks like are many articles and chapters that describe programs based on MOHO or that present case examples illustrating the use of MOHO. The citations for this type of evidence for practice can be found in the MOHO bibliography in Appendix A.

Evidence Concerning the Outcomes of MOHO-Based Practice

One of the most important kinds of evidence concerns outcomes that result from services based on MOHO. *Table 25.22* includes the results of studies published to date. This type of research is one of the fastest-growing areas of MOHO research, so therapists looking for evidence should also check the literature or the MOHO

Clearinghouse Web site for the most recent studies. Also, outcomes research is the most challenging and costly to conduct, so such studies may not be available for a particular population. In this instance, other forms of evidence, such as the expertise of occupational therapists as documented in descriptions of programs and case examples, are the next best sources of evidence for practice.

Client Perspectives on MOHO Services

Client satisfaction with service is an important indicator of the quality of services. Disabled scholars have critiqued occupational therapists' approaches to practice and interpretation of practice outcomes (Abberley, 1995; Giangreco, 1999). Disabled persons have also asserted that health care professionals' imagined experience of disability is quite different from the reality of living with a disability. As a result, the evidence base for practice may be flawed if research lacks the assessments of outcomes that are meaningful to people with disabilities (Basnett, 2001). Similarity, clients who were recipients of occupational therapy services have stressed that listening to their concerns would lead to better provision of services (Corring & Cook, 1999). The evidence generated by occupational therapy clients regarding their experience of MOHO-based therapy services is summarized in *Table 25.23*.

Summary

This chapter provided summaries of much of the MOHO-related evidence available to support practice. As noted earlier, this chapter focused on research evidence, but there are may other sources of relevant and useful evidence. Additionally, the resources in this chapter are designed to give the reader a quick and accessible overview of what evidence exists. We have not critiqued the rigor of the studies, which is an important step in evidence-based practice. Therapists who wish to use evidence summarized in this chapter should go to the original research and form their own opinions about the extent of confidence that should be placed in each study.

TABLE 25.5 ACIS Evidence Summary

Citation	Findings
Forsyth, Lai, & Kielhofner (1999)	ACIS items are a valid representation of the construct of communication and interaction skills, clients with mental health problems (although not clients with autism) are measured in a valid way using ACIS, and therapists use ACIS in a consistent and interchangeable manner.
	ACIS can be administered in a valid manner in a range of social situations.
Kjellberg (2002)	ACIS scores did not have a systematic relationship with a person's level of intellectual impairment or level of dependence, interdependence, or independence in work or leisure.
Haglund & Henriksson (2003)	Expert panel judged 60% of ACIS items to be aligned with items in ICIDH-2; 30% of ACIS items had a correlation of at least .60 with aligned ICIDH-2 items.
Kjellberg, Haglund, Forsyth, & Kielhofner (2003)	The items and rating scale in a Swedish version of ACIS validly represent the construct of communication/interaction skills and met fit criteria. The continuum of communication/interaction skills as represented by the items replicates previous findings in the English version. Therapists assessed clients with learning disabilities, mental health disabilities, and neurologic disorders in a consistent and interchangeable manner.
Haglund & Thorell (2004)	The study confirms that communication and interaction skills are context dependent for clients with schizophrenia and mood disorders, as clients had at least one item rating that changed across settings.
	There did not appear to be a relationship between the importance or inherent fun of each activity setting and the ACIS ratings as reported by clients.

ACIS, Assessment of Communication and Interaction Skills; ICIDH-2, International Classification of Impairment, Disability, and Handicap.

TABLE 25.6 AOF Evidence Summary

Citation	Findings
Watts, Kielhofner, Bauer, Gregory, & Valentine (1986)	AOF can be used reliably with older adult clients with mental health conditions and community-dwelling older adults. AOF has shown evidence of concurrent validity and can discriminate between clients in institutions and community-dwelling older adults.
Brollier, Watts, Bauer, & Schmidt (1988a)	The AOF has concurrent validity with the Global Assessment Scale when used with clients diagnosed with schizophrenia. The AOF may be sensitive to a client's socioeconomic status.
Brollier, Watts, Bauer, & Schmidt (1988b)	A panel of occupational therapy experts determined that the AOF had content validity and covered the domain of content for 6 MOHO components.
Watts, Brollier, Bauer, & Schmidt (1989)	The AOF has concurrent validity with the OCAIRS when used with clients diagnosed with schizophrenia.
Viik, Watts, Madigan, & Bauer (1990)	AOF can discriminate between adult clients just entering rehabilitation for alcohol abuse and persons with 1 year of sobriety.
Lycett (1992)	A revised version of AOF identified important information when used as an evaluation method in 9 of 16 elderly clients. A revised version of AOF influenced 5 of the elderly client's treatment plans. A revised version of AOF was rated as most useful by clients who had experienced a stroke and who required longer treatment stays.
Widen-Holmqvist et al.	The AOF can be used by adults living in the community to report their sense (1993) of volition after a stroke.
Grogan (1994)	The AOF can be used with adult clients with mental health conditions to show change related to engagement in OT intervention as well as changes related to symptoms.
Eklund (1996a)	AOF components of volition, habituation, and performance all clustered on the health side of a continuum of wellness of the x-axis of a PCA analysis. On the y-axis, AOF component of habituation appeared in the middle of the cluster of health variables. Volition appeared at the top of the cluster of health variables. The AOF concept of performance appeared most removed from the other health variables.
Eklund (1996b)	The AOF can be used to assess intervention outcomes for Swedish clients with mental health disabilities.
Eklund & Hansson (1997)	The AOF can be used to assess the long-term impact of occupational therapy service on everyday occupational functioning of clients with mental health disabilities 1 year after discharge from therapy.
Eklund (1999)	AOF can be used with adult clients with mental health conditions to demonstrate outcomes after an occupational therapy intervention in volition, habituation, communication, and interaction skills.

AOF, Assessment of Occupational Functioning; PCA, Principal Component Analysis

TABLE 25.7 The COSA and Its Predecessor, the Child SAOF Evidence Summary

Citation	Findings
Keller, Kafkes, & Kielhofner (2005)	COSA items coalesce to form a valid construct of occupational competence. Clients aged 8–17 who received OT or did not receive OT used the competence scale in a reliable and valid way but did not frequently use the lowest rating category.
	COSA items also coalesce to form a valid construct of value (importance) of occupations. Again, clients used the value scale in a reliable and valid way but did not frequently use the lowest rating scale category.
	Recommend revision of rating scale.
Keller & Kielhofner (2005)	With a revised four-point scale, COSA items represent a valid and more sensitive construct of occupational competence. Clients aged 8–17 with neurologic, mental health, orthopedic, medical, and developmental diagnoses were able to use the competence scale in a valid and reliable manner.
	With a revised four-point scale, 20 of the 24 COSA items are part of a valid and more sensitive construct of value (importance) of occupations. Clients used the value scale in a valid and reliable manner.
	Item hierarchies, or the continuum of occupational competence and value items, replicated content of hierarchies in the previous study.
	Recommend future research on revised items.
Knis-Matthews, Richard, Marquez, & Mevawala, (2005)	Adolescent females with mental health–related diagnoses and challenges can use the Child SAOF to identify priorities for therapy, including family concerns, health, and wellness.

COSA, Child Occupational Self-Assessment; Child SAOF, Child Self-Assessment of Occupational Functioning; OT, occupational therapy.

TABLE 25.8 Interest Checklist Evidence Summary

Citation	Findings
Rogers, Weinstein, & Figone (1978)	When high school students from the United States use the NPI Interest Checklist, four constructs emerge: ADLs, manual skills, cultural/educational, and physical sports. Social/recreational items are distributed throughout, signifying a more complex theoretic construct.
Oakley, Kielhofner, & Barris (1985)	Adults with mental health problems and adults living in the community can use the Interest Checklist to report interests as one part of a battery of assessments to measure MOHO concepts of volition and habituation.
Katz (1988)	When adult psychiatric clients from Israel completed the Interest Checklist, four constructs emerged, and they explained most of the variance in their responses: sports and physical tasks, intellectual and musical activities, social activities, and motor manual tasks and housekeeping.
Katz, Giladi, & Peretz (1988)	Israeli adults both in psychiatric hospitals and in the community can use the Interest Checklist to report their patterns of interests, and the Interest Checklist reveals different patterns of interests between the two groups.
Katz, Josman, & Steinmetz (1988)	Israeli adolescents hospitalized for psychiatric conditions and community-dwelling adolescents used the Interest Checklist to report their patterns of interests.
Ebb, Coster, & Duncombe (1989)	The Interest Checklist was used with male adolescents with psychosocial disabilities and without disabilities. The Interest Checklist differentiated between the two groups on number of strong interests.
Scaffa (1991)	The Interest Checklist was used with adults with alcoholism attending a substance abuse program and community-dwelling adults without identified substance abuse problems. The Interest Checklist found significant differences between the groups in frequency of engagement in interest and range of interests.
Widen-Holmqvist et al. (1993)	Adults living in the community after a stroke used the Interest Checklist to compare engagement in interests and leisure activities before and after stroke.
Heasman, & Atwal (2004)	The Interest Checklist was used as part of an individualized intervention program for adults with psychiatric disabilities to create an action plan to begin engagement in one new leisure activity.
Horne, Corr, & Earle (2005)	New mothers used the Interest Checklist to report changes in patterns of engagement in interests after the birth of their first child.

NPI, Neuropsychiatric Institute; ADL, activities of daily living.

TABLE 25.9 MOHOST and SCOPE Evidence Summary

Citation	Findings
Forsyth et al. (in press)	The MOHOST items belong to a valid construct of occupational participation, although two environmental items may represent a separate construct. The MOHOST can be used by therapists in the U. K. and U. S. to rate clients with physical and psychiatric disabilities in a valid and reliable manner.
Kielhofner, Fogg, Braveman, Forsyth, & Kramer (2007).	The MOHOST can be described as representing a six-dimensional model of occupational adaptation: volition, habituation, process skills, motor skills, communication/interaction skills, and the environment.
Bowyer, Kramer, Kielhofner, Maziero-Barbosa, & Girolami (2007)	The items on the SCOPE represent a valid construct of occupational participation. The SCOPE can be used by occupational therapists, physical therapists, and speech language pathologists to rate young clients with disabilities aged 2–21 years with a range of disabilities in a similar and reliable manner.

MOHOST, Model of Human Occupation Screening Tool; SCOPE, Short Child Occupational Profile.

TABLE 25.10 OCAIRS Evidence Summary

Citation	Findings
Kaplan (1984)	The OCAIRS has almost perfect interrater reliability overall, and there was a strong relationship between sum of component ratings and sum of global assessment ratings.
Brollier, Watts, Bauer, & Schmidt (1988a)	Evidence for the concurrent validity of the OCAIRS was provided by its correlation with the Global Assessment Scale when used with clients with schizophrenia.
	OCAIRS may be sensitive to SES, as correlations were lower when SES was controlled for.
Watts, Brollier, Bauer, & Schmidt (1989)	Evidence for criterion validity of the OCAIRS was provided by the assessment's high correlation with a similar MOHO-based assessment, the Assessment of Occupational Functioning, when used with clients with schizophrenia.
Haglund & Henriksson (1994)	Evidence of content validity of the Swedish version of the OCAIRS is provided by at least 60% agreement of therapists when matching items to domains.
	Interrater reliability of 6 occupational therapists for rating inpatient psychiatric clients and community-dwelling clients with chronic muscular pain exceeded 60% for 14 OCAIRS domains.
	Variance among raters and client scores is high, and only some OCAIRS items differentiate between inpatient psychiatric and community-dwelling chronic pain clients.
Henriksson (1995a)	OCAIRS interview can be used internationally (Sweden and USA) with women with Fibromyalgia to better understand their encounters within the health care system, interactions with others, and consequences of living with Fibromyalgia.
Henriksson (1995b)	OCAIRS interview can be used internationally (Sweden and United States) to understand the strategies women with fibromyalgia use to cope with pain and ADLs, including adjusting routines and changing their life situation and attitudes.
Henriksson & Burckhardt (1996)	The OCAIRS has a stable meaning across two countries, as the mean scores for women with fibromyalgia from the U. S. and from Sweden were almost identical, although women in the U. S. working full time reported more stress, more exhaustion, and less satisfaction than the Swedish women.
Haglund (1996)	There was no significant difference between 38 Swedish occupational therapists' decision to include or exclude a videotaped client from therapy services based on results of a standard interview versus the OCAIRS interview.
	For therapists who had worked in psychiatry for more than 1.5 years, there was no significant difference in the recommendation for therapy.
Haglund, Thorell, & Walinder (1998a)	A revised Swedish OCAIRS improved interrater agreement with Swedish psychiatry clients. Low to moderate intercorrelations between components indicate that it assesses different domains of participation.
Haglund, Thorell, & Walinder (1998b)	The Swedish OCAIRS may discriminate between the occupational participation of clients with different mental health conditions, as ratings from the Swedish OCAIRS are significantly different for clients with depression, schizophrenia, and bipolar disorder. Clients with depression have the highest occupational participation scores.
Lai, Haglund, & Kielhofner (1999)	Most items on the OCAIRS represent a valid construct of occupational adaptation and can differentiate between clients with different levels of occupational adaptation. (Clients with unipolar affective disorder tended to be more adaptive, and clients with schizophrenia tended to be less adaptive.) While five of six therapists did not differ significantly from each other when rating clients using the OCAIRS, the meaning of the five-point rating varied across items.
Heasman & Atwal (2004)	The OCAIRS can be used as an initial interview to identify leisure goals for young adult clients (aged 20 +) with mental health disabilities attending a day program.

OCAIRS, Occupational Circumstances Assessment—Interview and Rating Scale; ADL, activities of daily living; SES, socioeconomic status.

TABLE 25.11 OPHI-II Evidence Summary

Citation	Findings
Kielhofner, Harlan, Bauer, & Maurer (1986)	The OPHI had acceptable overall interrater and test-retest reliability when used with clients with disabilities seen in inpatient and outpatient settings. It may also be able to detect change over time.
Kielhofner & Henry (1988)	The OPHI had moderate test-retest and interrater reliability when used by therapists in the U. S. and Canada to rate adolescent, adult, and older adult clients with psychiatric and physical disabilities. Past and present scales appear to represent two different constructs. Therapists indicated they would use the OPHI regularly or for some clients.
Bridle, Lynch, & Quesenberry, (1990)	The OPHI can be used to reveal changes in occupational adaptation (in roles and routines, volition, and environment) 2–8 years after spinal cord injury.
Kielhofner, Henry, Walens, & Rogers (1991)	Therapists using an eclectic approach and therapists using a MOHO approach interpreted the OPHI scales in a similar and dependable manner when rating psychiatric clients after attending a workshop on the assessment. One exception was that therapists using a MOHO approach did not use the OPHI present scale in an acceptable manner.
Lynch & Bridle (1993)	The OPHI had acceptable construct validity (and co-varied with the Multidimensional Pain Inventory Scales and the Center for Epidemiological Studies Depression Scale), and the OPHI-II can reveal changes in occupational performance over time as a result of a spinal cord injury.
Neistadt (1995)	13% of 269 directors of adult physical disability settings that served adolescents, adults, and older adults reported that therapists used the OPHI to identify client priorities (in a total of 35 facilities).
Kielhofner & Mallinson (1995)	The types of questions asked by therapists conducting an OPHI interview influenced the type of response; questions about change, motives, and specific circumstances elicited narrative responses. Therapists who let the OPHI interview go where the client's responses led, who asked clients to elaborate their responses, who waited until clients finished their responses, and who showed a genuine interest in a client's response were better able to elicit narrative during the OPHI interview.
Mallinson, Kielhofner, & Mattingly (1996)	The OPHI interview can be used with men and women with mental health disabilities to elicit metaphors that explain their life history.
Fossey (1996)	The OPHI can be used with British clients attending a psychiatric day program to identify turning points in their life narrative, and the narrative summary can be used to convey information about the client's life history to other professionals.
Mallinson, Mahaffey, & Kielhofner, (1998)	Analysis of the OPHI items reveals three constructs of occupational adaptation: occupational competence, occupational identity, and environments/settings. Items rearranged into these three constructs demonstrate good psychometric properties. Revisions to the OPHI are recommended, and new items should be added to strengthen each construct.
Kielhofner, Mallinson, Forsyth, & Lai (2001)	The items of each OPHI-II scale validly measure the underlying constructs of occupational competence, occupational identity, and occupational behavior settings (environment) for an international sample of people with physical, psychiatric, or no known disabilities. The OPHI-II validly measures the occupational adaptation of persons and is sensitive enough to detect differences in occupational adaptation among persons. An international group of therapists can use the OPHI-II in a valid way by using the administration manual.

(continued)

TABLE 25.11 *(continued)*

Citation	Findings
Buning, Angelo, & Schmeler (2001)	The OPHI-II can be used to capture the positive changes in past to present occupational performance of adults who use powered mobility devices.
Braveman & Helfrich (2001)	The OPHI-II can be used to better understand the experiences and sense of occupational competence and occupational identity of men with AIDS returning to work.
Graff, Vernooij-Dassen, Hoefnagels, Dekker, & de Witte (2003)	The OPHI-II was used to gather information from older adults with cognitive impairments regarding their past and present needs, interests, habits, and roles as part of an intervention to support older adults with cognitive impairments living at home and their caregivers.
Gray & Fossey (2003)	The OPHI-II can be used to understand the experiences of Australian men and women living with chronic fatigue syndrome.
Levin & Helfrich (2004)	The OPHI-II can be used to understand the experiences of homeless teenage mothers in the United States. It explicated the identity of homeless adolescent mothers and found their identity was influenced by their development, role choices, and future desire to engage in the mother role.
Goldstein, Kielhofner, & Paul-Ward (2004)	The OPHI-II can be used to explore the narratives of men with AIDS participating in a return-to-work program.
Chan (2004)	The OPHI-II can be used to understand how Chinese men with chronic obstructive pulmonary disease experience the disease process and engagement in occupations.
Farnworth, Nihitin, & Fossey (2004)	The OPHI-II interview was used to elicit the perspectives of clients in a forensic setting regarding their life on the ward.
Braveman, Helfrich, Kielhofner, & Albrecht (2004)	The OPHI-II was used to better understand how men with AIDS experienced returning to work over a 12-month period when they were engaged in a return-to-work study program.
Chaffey & Fossey (2004)	Mothers who were caregivers of adult sons with schizophrenia described their experiences and the meaning of their caregiving using the OPHI-II.
Kielhofner, Braveman, Finlayson, Paul-Ward, Goldbaum, & Goldstein (2004)	The OPHI-II narrative slope predicted outcomes of clients with AIDS (and other difficulties, such as mental health conditions and substance abuse) who participated in a return-to-work program. Clients with progressive narrative slopes were twice as likely to have a successful outcome in the program of employment, school, or volunteer work.
Ingvarsson & Theodorsdottir (2004)	The OPHI-II can be used as part of individualized vocational rehabilitation program to better understand clients' strengths and problems and to set individualized goals.
Apte, Kielhofner, Paul-Ward, & Braveman, (2005)	Therapists and most clients view the OPHI-II interview and narrative slope as a meaningful and rapport-building part of therapy.
Kielhofner, Dobria, Forsyth, & Basu (2005)	The OPHI-II key forms, developed using an international sample of more than 700 people with physical, psychiatric, or no known disabilities, allow therapists to derive a corresponding calibration, or measure, for each OPHI-II total raw score, derived for each of the three OPHI-II scales.
Levin, Kielhofner, Braveman, & Fogg (in press)	A more positive narrative slope generated by the OPHI-II was associated with a higher likelihood of being employed or engaged in other productive engagement. This relationship peaked between 3 and 6 months post intervention.

OPHI-II, Occupational Performance History Interview—II.

TABLE 25.12 The OQ and the NIH Activity Record (ACTRE) Evidence Summary

Citation	Findings
Smyntek, Barris, & Kielhofner (1985)	The OQ was used to assess the self-efficacy and habits of nonpsychotic adolescents with psychiatric disabilities and adolescents living in the community.
Furst, Gerber, Smith, Fisher, & Schulman (1987)	This study modified the OQ to create the NIH Activity Record, which was used with adults with rheumatoid arthritis to assess changes in patterns of physical activity and rest.
Ebb, Coster, & Duncombe (1989)	The OQ was used with male adolescents with or without disabilities to talk about their typical routines. The OQ did not differentiate differences in typical days between groups.
Keilhofner & Brinson (1989)	The OQ can be used to identify client goals as part of a MOHO-based intervention program that helps young people discharged from psychiatric hospitalizations make the transition back to the community.
Aubin, Hachey, & Mercier (1999)	French version of OQ was successfully used with clients with schizophrenia and similar diagnoses to report feelings of competence in everyday activities.
Gerber & Furst (1992)	The NIH Activity Record is a valid measure of adults' perceptions of arthritis symptoms during participation in daily activities.
Aubin, Hachey, & Mercier (2002)	The French version of the OQ can be used by adult clients with severe mental health problems to assess the importance and enjoyment of their daily activities and routine.
Pentland, Harvey, & Walker (1998)	Canadian men with spinal cord injuries used the OQ to report their use of time for sleep, personal care, productive activities, and leisure.
Henry, Costa, Ladd, Robertson, Rollins, & Roy (1996)	The OQ can be used to have U. S. college students report their patterns of and feelings about time use.
Smith, Kielhofner, & Watts (1986)	The OQ can be successfully used to analyze relationship between volition and engagement in everyday occupations and quality of life for older adults living in nursing homes and community settings.
Widen-Holmqvist et al. (1993)	Adults living in the community after a stroke can use the OQ to report their engagement in interests, leisure activities, and social activities.
Packer, Foster, & Brouwer (1997)	The NIH Activity Record can be used to examine differences in the daily routines of Canadians with and without chronic fatigue syndrome.
Leidy & Knebel (1999)	A modified version of the NIH Activity Record can be used by adults with chronic obstructive pulmonary disease, chronic bronchitis, or emphysema to assess their daily routines and performance in activities.

OQ, Occupational Questionnaire; NIH Activity Record (ACTRE), National Institutes of Health Activity Record.

TABLE 25.13 The OSA and Its Predecessor, the SAOF, Evidence Summary

Citation	Findings
Henry, Baron, Mouradian, & Curtin (1999)	A self-assessment of occupational functioning has acceptable test-retest reliability, internal consistency, and ability to discriminate between young psychiatric clients and college students without disabilities.
Venable, Hanson, Shechtman, & Dasler (2000)	There is a correlation between the OSA competence scores and a measure of functional status for adults over age 60 living in the community. This reveals that as less assistance is needed in daily activities, people report a higher sense of occupational competence.
Kielhofner & Forsyth (2001)	The OSA competence items represent a valid construct of occupational competence, can be used in a reliable way by clients internationally, and validly measure the occupational competence of international clients.
	The OSA value items represent a valid construct of value for occupations, can be used in a reliable way by clients internationally, and validly measure the occupational values of international clients.
	The OSA environmental items do not demonstrate acceptable psychometric properties and should be used with caution to gather clinical information.
Fisher & Savin-Baden (2001)	The OSA can be used as part of the evaluation for an individualized therapy program for young people in psychosis.
Bjorklund & Henriksson (2003)	Older adults living in the community and receiving home services can use OSA to report on their ability to do occupations and the occupations' importance.
	The OSA can also be used by Swedish older adults living in the community to identify environmental supports and barriers.
Sviden, Tham, & Borell (2004)	Older adults in Sweden attending social or rehabilitation day programs used the OSA to report levels of perceived competence.
Gorde, Helfrich, & Finlayson (2004)	The OSA can be used to better understand the priorities of women who have been victims of domestic abuse. OSA competence scores may be weakly related to feelings of depression and impaired self-reference.
Kielhofner, Braveman, Finlayson, Paul-Ward, Goldbaum, & Goldstein (2004)	The OSA can be used as part of an initial evaluation during a MOHO-based return-to-work program for adults with HIV.
Crist, Fairman, Muñoz, Hansen, Sciulli, & Eggers (2005)	The OSA can be used to measure the occupational competence and values of incarcerated men and women.
	Incarcerated men and women report different patterns of dissatisfaction with their occupational lives using the OSA (as reflected in the greatest discrepancies between occupational competence and value ratings for each item).
Ay-Woan, Sarah, LyInn, Tsyr-Jang, & Ping-Chaun (2006)	The OSA can be used with adult Taiwanese clients with depression to reflect on occupational competence and the environment.
	OSA scores predicted quality-of-life scores of adult Taiwanese clients with depression.
Kielhofner, Forsyth, & Iyenger (2007)	The OSA competence items and value items can be used in a reliable manner by an international sample of clients and are sensitive enough to measure clients accurately.
	The OSA competence items coalesce to represent a valid construct of occupational competence, and the meaning of the continuum of occupational competence remained stable over a series of three studies.

(continued)

TABLE 25.13 *(continued)*

Citation	Findings
	The OSA value items coalesce to represent a valid construct of value for occupations, and the meaning of the continuum of value for occupations remained stable over a series of three studies and may reflect an international hierarchy of values.
Sousa (2006)	The Portuguese version of the OSA had good reliability and internal consistency when used by psychiatric adult clients. It measured the constructs of occupational competence and value.
	The OSA may be used across hospitals to measure differences in the occupational competence, values, performance capacity, habituation, and volition between clients from different settings.

OSA, Occupational Self-Assessment; SAOF, Self-Assessment of Occupational Functioning.

TABLE 25.14 The Pediatric Interest Profiles Evidence Summary

Citation	Findings
Hann, Regele, Walsh, Fontana, & Bentley (1994)	The 80-item checklist pilot study version of the Adolescent Leisure Interest Profile had items that are meaningful to students in junior high and high school in the U. S.
Andrews, Bleecher, Genoa, Molloy, Monahan, & Sargent (1995)	A series of studies were used to develop the items for the Kid Play Profile and the Preteen Play Profile by having children aged 6–12 complete the profiles and through an expert occupational therapy review.
Brophy, Caizzi, Crete, Jachym, Kobus, & Sainz (1995)	The Adolescent Leisure Interest Profile can be used reliably over time by adolescents aged 14–19.
Beck et al. (1996)	Young children in the U. S. successfully completed a 19-item pilot study version of the Kid Play Profile with pictures and used the assessment in a consistent manner.
Budd et al. (1997)	The Kid Play Profile items can be used reliably over time by children aged 6–9.
Henry (1998)	Adolescents aged 12–21 who have disabilities can use the Adolescent Leisure Interest Profile over time in a reliable way.
	There were significant differences between the different groups of adolescents with disabilities and adolescents without disabilities in the amount of interest, frequency of engagement, and amount of enjoyment for leisure activities.
Henry (2000)	In the pilot study, children aged 9–11 completed a 53-item version of the Preteen Play Profile with pictures, with questions about frequency and feelings of competence in a consistent manner.
	The Preteen Play Profile can be used reliably over time by children aged 9 and 10.

TABLE 25.15 The PVQ Evidence Summary

Citation	Findings
Andersen, Kielhofner, & Lai (2005)	The PVQ items represent a valid construct of volition and reflect a volitional continuum of exploration, competency, and achievement.
	The PVQ can be used to validly measure young clients' volition.
	Environments of classroom, playground, and playroom are appropriate contexts to assess volition.
	Therapists may not be interchangeable when rating young clients with the PVQ.
Harris & Reid (2005)	The PVQ can be used to assess volition of children with CP engaged in therapeutic activities, such as a virtual reality game.
Reid (2005)	The PVQ can be used to measure volition of children with CP engaged in therapeutic activities, such as a virtual reality game.
	Average PVQ scores are significantly correlated with the Test of Playfulness average motivation scores. Scores for the PVQ items "Stays engaged," "Tries to produce effects," "Is task directed," "Initiates actions," "Shows preferences," "Expresses mastery pleasure," and "Organizes and modifies environment" were significantly correlated with Test of Playfulness average motivation score.

PVQ, Pediatric Volitional Questionnaire; CP, cerebral palsy.

TABLE 25.16 The Role Checklist Evidence Summary

Citation	Findings
Lederer, Kielhofner, & Watts (1985)	Incarcerated adolescents and adolescents living in the community used Role Checklist to report the value for roles. The Role Checklist was able to capture different patterns of value for roles between the two groups.
Oakley, Kielhofner, & Barris (1985)	Adult clients with mental health problems can use the Role Checklist to report on role continuity and role disruption.
Smyntek, Barris, & Kielhofner (1985)	The Role Checklist can be used with adolescents with or without psychosocial problems to assess differences in role engagement and value for roles in the two groups.
Barris, Kielhofner, Burch, Gelinas, Klement, & Schultz (1986)	The Role Checklist can be used to examine differing patterns of occupational engagement (including role engagement) between adolescents with psychophysiologic diagnoses, psychiatric diagnoses, and adolescents without disabilities.
Duellman, Barris, & Kielhofner (1986)	The Role Checklist can be used by older adults in nursing homes to report the number of anticipated future roles to better understand their sense of occupational engagement while in the nursing home.
Oakley, Kielhofner, Barris, & Reichler (1986)	The Role Checklist has content validity. The Role Checklist has good reliability, although older persons' responses to sections I and II may be more consistent.
Elliott & Barris (1987)	Role Checklist was used by older adults without disabilities living in the community to report past and present role engagement. It was able to capture changes in role engagement over time.
Rust, Barris, & Hooper (1987)	The Role Checklist and a modified version can be used by college women to report engagement in exercise and related roles.
Barris, Dickie, & Baron (1988)	The Role Checklist can be used to assess different patterns of past and future role engagement between matched peer groups and these groups: female young adults with eating disorders, adolescents with psychiatric disabilities, and young adults with chronic conditions.
Ebb, Coster, & Duncombe (1989)	Adolescent males with psychosocial disabilities and adolescents living in the community without disabilities can use the Role Checklist to report role engagement. The Role Checklist can be used to discriminate between the two groups of adolescents.
Baker, Curbow, & Wingard (1991)	Role checklist was used to have survivors of BMT report whether they engaged in roles before and after BMT and to rate importance of each role.
Watson & Ager (1991)	The Role Checklist was modified to include ratings of role importance, frequency of engagement, and change in values for roles over time. It was effectively used by older adults in the community in several age cohorts.
Branholm & Fugl-Meyer (1992)	The Role Checklist can be used effectively across age cohorts and by males and females living in Sweden to examine differences in role engagement with respect to age and gender.
Egan, Warren, Hessel, & Gilewich (1992)	The Role Checklist was completed by Canadian older adults post hip fracture before and 3 weeks after discharge to assess participation and performance.
Hallett, Zasler, Maurer, & Cash (1994)	People living in the community after experiencing a brain injury can use the Role Checklist to report role loss and value of roles.
Dickerson & Oakley (1995)	The Role Checklist was used by adults with physical or psychosocial disabilities and by adults without disabilities living in the community to report on role engagement. Role checklist was able to detect difference between all groups on the number of roles engaged in the present and future and difference in value of roles.

(continued)

T A B L E 2 5 . 1 6 *(continued)*

Citation	Findings
Hachey, Jummoorty, & Mercier (1995)	The French version of the Role Checklist was translated using parallel back translation, and the instrument had moderate interlanguage and intralanguage test-restest reliability when used with bilingual psychiatric clients in Canada.
Kusznir, Scott, Cooke, & Young (1996)	A modified version of the Role Checklist was used effectively by adults in a bipolar clinic to report involvement in life roles and the importance of those roles.
Larsson & Branholm (1996)	The Role Checklist was used by Swedish adults in a neurologic rehabilitation center to identify goals for therapy.
Crowe, VanLeit, Berghmans, & Mann (1997)	The Role Checklist was used by mothers of children with multiple disabilities, mothers of children with Down syndrome, and mothers of typically developing children to report changes in role engagement after the birth of their child.
Frosch et al. (1997)	The Role Checklist was used only to detect changes in role engagement in past and present roles for caregivers of persons with traumatic brain injury.
Muñoz, Karmosky, Gaugler, Lang, & Stayduhar (1999)	In part of a qualitative study, the Role Checklist was used to examine perceptions of role involvement and role meaningfulness in parents of children with cerebral palsy.
Eklund (2001)	The Role Checklist was used with occupational therapy clients with psychotic and nonpsychotic conditions to report on role engagement and value of roles over time, including at admission, discharge, and at 1 year followup.
Lee, Strauss, Wittman, Jackson, & Carstens (2001)	The Role Checklist was used by caregivers of adults with mental illness to illuminate relationship between role engagement in past and present and caregiver sorrow.
Hachey, Boyer, & Mercier (2001)	The French version of the Role Checklist can be used to explore engagement in and value of roles for persons with schizophrenia.
Colon & Haertlein (2002)	The Spanish version of the Role Checklist had acceptable intralanguage test-retest reliability.
Corr & Wilmer (2003)	The Role Checklist was used by participants aged 34–55 who experienced a stroke. The Role Checklist revealed that work was important to these individuals.
Corr, Phillips, & Walker (2004)	Adults who experienced a stroke and who attended a day program used the Role Checklist to assess role engagement.
Schindler (2004)	The Role Checklist was used within a larger study to identify incarcerated or recently released men's engagement in roles and to identify roles to develop during an intervention.
Horne, Corr, & Earle (2005)	The Role Checklist was used with mothers to report changes in role engagement after the birth of their first child.
Schindler & Baldwin (2005)	The Role Checklist was used by adult psychiatric clients to identify roles to address while engaged in an intervention to acquire roles.
Hakansson, Eklund, Lidfeldt, Nerbrand, Samsioe, & Nilsson (2005)	The Role Checklist can be used to discern difference in value of the worker role between Swedish women who are continuously healthy and working and women who report discontinuity in work related to illness.
Cordeiro, Camelier, Oakley & Jardim (2007)	The Brazilian Portuguese version of the Role Checklist can be used in a reliable manner to gather information about occupational role engagement and the value of those roles.

BMT, bone marrow transplant.

TABLE 25.17 SSI Evidence Summary

Citation	Findings
Hemmingsson & Borell (1996)	The SSI content areas are sensitive and specific and can be used to appropriately identify accommodation needs of students with physical disabilities in regular and special class-rooms. Interrater reliability of SSI is acceptable, and expert review clarified relevant content areas.
Hemmingsson & Borell (2000)	The SSI can be used to determine the accommodation needs and unmet needs of students with physical disabilities in Sweden, where 98% of students reported a need for accommodations and 83.3% of students reported an unmet need.
	Accommodations most frequently needed were in writing, classroom work, and personal assistance, and most frequently reported unmet needs were in reading, remembering, and speaking.
Prellwitz & Tham (2000)	Students with restricted mobility completed the SSI interview and reported few major difficulties with the physical environment of their Swedish primary schools but had difficulties with the social environment, such as teaching situations, social contact with peers, dealing with their personal assistant, and bullying.
Hemmingsson & Borell (2002)	Swedish students aged 10–19 with physical disabilities identified unmet needs using the SSI, and these unmet needs were categorized according to MOHO environmental concepts of spaces, objects, occupational forms, and social groups.
	SSI revealed differences in needs and unmet needs among students with and without personal assistants and younger and older students.
Hemmingsson, Kottorp, & Bernspang (2004)	The SSI represents a valid construct of student-environment fit and need for accommodations for students with physical disabilities aged 8–19 in regular and special education classrooms. Items do not fully cover the range of student environment fit and the needs of students who are most able; however, most students were validly measured by the SSI.

SSI, School Setting Interview.

TABLE 25.18 The VQ Evidence Summary

Citation	Findings
Chern, Kielhofner, de las Heras, & Magalhaes (1996)	Series of two studies: Study 1: Items are a valid representation of construct of volition but require further development to reflect the volitional continuum. Can be used to measure volition of clients with psychiatric disabilities or developmental delays.
	Study 2: Revised VQ items are a valid representation of the construct of volition and are distributed along the volitional continuum. VQ can be used to assess volition of clients with psychiatric disabilities and developmental delays but may not accurately measure clients with high levels of volition.
Reid (2003)	The VQ can be used to assess the volition of older adult stroke survivors engaged in intervention and leisure activities, such as a virtual reality experience.
Li & Kielhofner (2004)	The VQ items coalesce to represent a valid, sensitive construct of volition and represent a volitional continuum of exploration, competency, and achievement.
	The VQ can be used to measure the volition of clients with psychiatric disabilities and HIV or AIDS in a valid manner.
	Therapists use the VQ rating scale in a consistent and valid manner but are not interchangeable when assessing client's volition using the VQ.

VQ, Volitional Questionnaire.

TABLE 25.19 The WEIS Evidence Summary

Citation	Findings
Corner, Kielhofner, & Lin (1997)	The WEIS items coalesce to represent a valid construct of the impact of the work environment on worker performance.
	The WEIS can be used to assess the impact of the environment on the performance of workers with psychiatric disabilities in a valid and reliable way.
Kielhofner, Lai, Olson, Haglund, Ekbadh, & Hedlund (1999)	WEIS items coalesce to represent a valid construct environmental impact on work performance, can be used to assess clients in a valid manner, and can be used in a valid and reliable way by therapists across cultures (United States and Sweden).

WEIS, Work Environment Impact Scale.

TABLE 25.20 The WRI Evidence Summary

Citation	Findings
Biernacki (1993)	When using the WRI to evaluate clients with upper extremity injuries, occupational therapists with experience in rehabilitation demonstrated high test-retest reliability. However, some items did not meet standards for reliability, and further development of the assessment was recommended.
Haglund, Karlsson, & Kielhofner (1997)	The items and rating scale on a Swedish version of the WRI can be used in a valid manner and represent a continuum of psychosocial ability to return to work. However, environmental items should be revised to ensure they validly represent the construct of psychosocial ability to return to work.
Velozo, Kielhofner, Gern, Lin, Lai, & Fischer (1999)	A series of three studies:
	Study 1: WRI items represent a valid, sensitive construct of psychosocial ability to return to work, represent a continuum of psychosocial ability to return to work, and can measure clients in a valid way. However, environmental items should be revised to ensure they validly represent the construct of psychosocial ability to return to work.
	Study 2: Revised WRI items represent a valid, increasingly sensitive construct of psychosocial ability to return to work and measure an increased number of clients in a valid manner, including clients with diverse physical injuries. Only one environmental item continues not to have acceptable statistics. Items represent continuum of psychosocial ability to return to work and replicate past item hierarchies.
	Study 3: When the WRI was used with clients with back injuries, no variables were significant predictors of return to work.
Ekbladh, Haglund, & Thorell (2004)	For a variety of Swedish clients with musculoskeletal, connective tissue, and mood disorders, WRI personal causation items ("Assess abilities and limitations," "Expectations of job success," and "Takes responsibility"), one role item ("Appraises work expectations"), and one environmental item ("Perception of work setting") have tentative predictive validity for return to work.
Jackson, Harkess, & Ellis (2004)	The use of two standardized work assessments, the WRI and the Valpar Component Work Samples, by skilled occupational therapists with clients with physical and mental health disabilities improved the reporting of clients' work abilities across 12 domains that include physical demands, environment, and personal characteristics.
Asmundsdottir (2004)	The WRI can be used with psychiatric clients who are looking to return to work to enable them to express their attitudes and opinions about work.
	Findings from WRI interviews can be used to inform work rehabilitation program services.
Ingvarsson & Theodorsdottir (2004)	The WRI can be used as an initial evaluation that considers psychosocial and environmental factors affecting return to work as part of a successful vocational rehabilitation program for clients with a variety of disabilities.

(continued)

TABLE 25.20 *(continued)*

Citation	Findings
Kielhofner, Braveman, Finlayson, Paul-Ward, Goldbaum, & Goldstein (2004)	The WRI can be used as a part of an initial evaluation in a successful return-to-work program based on MOHO for individuals with AIDS.
Fenger & Kramer (in press)	The items and rating scale in an Icelandic version of the WRI coalesce to represent a valid and sensitive construct of psychosocial ability to return to work, measure clients in a valid manner, and can be used by therapists in a valid manner. Items represent continuum of psychosocial ability to return to work and replicate past item hierarchies. However, two environmental items may not represent the construct of psychosocial ability to return to work, and therapists are not interchangeable when using the Icelandic version of the WRI.
Forsyth et al. (2006)	Across countries (U. S., Iceland, and Sweden), the WRI items validly define the construct of psychosocial ability to return to work. Items represent continuum of psychosocial ability to return to work and replicate past item hierarchies. Most clients are validly measured by the WRI across countries, and the WRI is a sensitive instrument across countries. Therapists across countries can use the WRI consistently to assess clients.

All four environmental items on the WRI exceed acceptable statistics and may represent a separate construct of psychosocial ability to return to work. |

WRI, Worker Role Interview.

TABLE 25.21 Evidence Concerning the Nature of MOHO Practice

Citation	Outcome/Findings/Implications
Apte, Kielhofner, Paul-Ward, & Braveman (2005)	Therapists reported that completing the OPHI-II interview and narrative slope was a rapport-building process that can be adjusted according to characteristics of clients and their life situation to engage clients in collaborative goal setting.
Barrett, Beer, & Kielhofner (1999)	Therapy is more effective when therapists are aware of clients' narrative and the related meaning of change to their client and when therapists respect that narrative in the therapy process.
Braveman, Helfrich, Kielhofner, & Albrecht (2004)	For adults with HIV/AIDS, returning to work is a personal decision about what is best for that person's future and requires individualized service and ongoing support. Even clients with many concerns can be supported to return to work.
Durand, Vachon, Loisel, & Berthelette (2003)	Work rehabilitation programs based on MOHO concepts can be successfully implemented and can enable clients to meet program goals.
Eklund (1996b)	Client's psychological engagement in a day program intervention, as rated by staff, was positively related to clients' volition and habituation.
Fossey (1996)	Therapists' explanations of the purpose of the OPHI-II reflected their own professional values and intended purpose of the interview. Therapists became more flexible and developed their own interview style and process as they gained experience with the assessment and interview skills.
Goldstein, Kielhofner, & Paul-Ward (2004)	Therapists should adjust their approach based on each client's occupational narrative. Clients with a progressive narrative may require support and structure to reach their goals, while clients with a regressive narrative need support to identify attainable goals that they can successfully achieve.
Helfrich & Kielhofner (1994)	Clients perceive occupational therapy intervention as relevant or meaningful based on their own volitional narratives and life events prior to beginning therapy. Clients' views of occupational therapy and its meaning may be incompatible with therapists' view of occupational therapy.
Kielhofner & Barrett (1998)	The occupational forms/tasks used in therapy must relate to the larger context of the client's life. Misunderstanding can occur in goal setting when an implied progressive therapy narrative does not match client's volitional narrative.
Mallinson, Kielhofner, & Mattingly (1996).	Clients use deep metaphors to explain and interpret their life circumstances and guide their actions during life history interviews; e.g., metaphors of momentum evoke images of speed, inertia, and deceleration to describe progression and direction of life, while metaphors of entrapment describe feelings of restriction and confinement and reveal a conflict between desires and reality.
Muñoz, Lawlor, & Kielhofner (1993)	Therapists feel that MOHO is an occupation-focused and well-developed model, and they use main MOHO concepts to guide therapy and convey the purpose of occupational therapy to others.
Tham & Borell (1996)	Motivation to engage in training and intervention may be related to how closely aligned the intervention is with the client's personal view of the situation. An individual's view of the future and the presence of goals may motivate them to participate in intervention.
Tham & Kielhofner (2003)	Women in rehabilitation with left neglect relied on the social environment to negotiate their new experiences and to move forward with their rehabilitation.

OPHI-II, Occupational Performance History Interview—II.

TABLE 25.22 Evidence Concerning Outcomes of MOHO-Based Services

Citation	Type of study	Sample Information	Description of Intervention	Findings & Clinical Implications
Brown & Carmichael (1992)	Group study; quasi-experimental	33 Canadian clients from a large psychiatric hospital Diagnosis: 18 schizophrenia, 7 personality disorders, 8 affective disorders. 16 females, 17 males	Assertiveness training sought to improve communication/interaction skills. Influence of volition and environment also considered. Session topics: asking questions, self-esteem, assertiveness techniques, nonverbal communication, making requests. Group met 2× a week for 90-min × 7 weeks. Average group size: 8 clients, 2 leaders. Assessments completed during initial and final sessions.	Participation in an assertiveness training intervention based on MOHO increases client assertiveness and self-esteem.
Corcoran & Gitlin (2001)	Quasi-experimental. Random assignment to intervention group.	100 caregivers of persons with dementia in U.S. Caregivers were aged 23–87, mean age 59.3 years. 77% of caregivers were Caucasian. 73% of caregivers were female. Those being cared for: mean age 78.5, moderate impairments in self-care, average of 20 behavioral difficulties as reported by caregivers.	Intervention based on the conception of the environment as objects, social, tasks, culture (per MOHO); focused on ADLs, toileting, leisure, IADLs, safety, mobility, wandering, communication, catastrophic reactions, caregiver concerns (fatigue). 5 90-min home visits in 2 months. Therapist and caregiver worked together to identify environmental strategies to resolve behavior concerns. First 3 sessions focused on education of person-environment interaction, problem solving. Last 2 sessions reinforced techniques, helped generalize new skills to emerging problem areas.	Individualized intervention focused on environment, as described by MOHO, can generate useful strategies to decrease problem behaviors of people with dementia living at home: 220 problem areas identified by caregivers addressed in intervention Caregivers tried a total of 1068 strategies, used 869 successfully. Of strategies used, 343 were modifications at task level; 200 at object level; 326 at social group level.
DeForest, Watts, & Madigan (1991)	Pretest, intervention, posttest. No control group.	6 adolescent males in U.S. residential juvenile corrections facility. 4 African American, 2 Caucasian. Aged 13–15.	Participation in 3 crafts (leather, wood, clay) for total of 12 hours over 6 days. 3 days between each pretest and intervention; 3 days between each intervention and posttest.	Participation in crafts increases personal causation and belief in skill for engaging in occupations.

Gitlin, Winter, Corcoran, Dennis, Schinfeld, & Hauck (2003)	Pretest, intervention, posttest with control group. Stratified, random assignment to group.	89 caregivers in experimental group. Mean age 60.4 (SD = 13.6 years). 42.7% Caucasian, 53.9 % African American, 3.4% other. 24.7% male, 75.3% female. 41.9% educated beyond high school. Mean age of care recipient 80.2 years, 71.9% female. 101 caregivers in control group. No significant difference between groups at baseline.	Environmental Skill Building Program seeks to provide caregivers with strategies and problem-solving skills to modify environment (as conceptualized on MOHO concepts of physical, task, and social layers) to make caregiving easier and reduce care recipient problem behaviors.	Individualized intervention focused on environment, as described by MOHO, can improve the experience of giving care to a person with dementia at home. This includes a decrease in assistance needed from others in caregiving, less upset, improved ability to manage caregiving, less time spent in caregiving. Outcomes differ according to gender of caregiver.
Graff, Vernooij-Dassen, Hoefnagels, Dekker, & de Witte (2003)	Single group pretest-posttest design.	12 older individuals and caregivers from Netherlands returning home or to a residential home from the hospital. Older adults were aged 69–88, average age 79.9 years. 8 females, 4 males. Primary caregivers: 8 females, 3 males.	Intervention guidelines, based in part on MOHO, identified clients' needs, interests, beliefs, habits, roles, skills, and environmental supports and barriers. Intervention occurred twice a week for 2 weeks in hospital and twice a week for 5 weeks at home. Same therapist at hospital and at home. Intervention used environmental strategies, education, problem solving, coping strategies.	Participation in home-based interventions based on occupation-based models of practice, such as MOHO, can improve older adults' motor and process skills, decrease need for assistance, increase sense of competence and satisfaction when performing everyday activities, and increase caregiver competence.
Ingvarsson & Theodorsdottir (2004)	Program evaluation	70 individuals attended program since its beginning in 2000. 45 women, 25 men with range of disabilities. Age range 18–59 years (mean age 39 years). Five clients discharged themselves for various reasons without completing program.	Day program in outpatient clinic based on MOHO, Canadian Model of Occupational Performance, cognitive behavioral approaches. Participants attend average of 8–16 weeks. Initial assessment: COPM, WRI; further assessment as needed with OPHI-II, AMPS, standardized measures of strength, dexterity, depression. Goals set with client; program individualized for client. 1st 2 weeks education and training in seminars on ergonomics.	Results from first 6-month followup after discharge with 39 clients: 25% attending adult education 25% employed 20% looking for work 10% receiving disability benefits

(continued)

TABLE 25.22 *(continued)*

Citation	Type of study	Sample Information	Description of Intervention	Findings & Clinical Implications
			Morning, clients participate in 3-hour continuous work (work hardening) of their choice (office or workshop). Afternoon, clients attend groups or individual therapy. Groups include stress management seminar, goal-setting group, self-awareness group, relaxation.	
Josephsson, Backman, Borell, Bernspang, Nygard, & Ronnberg (1993)	Single-subject case design	4 clients at psychogeriatric day care unit of a Swedish geriatric hospital. 3 diagnosed with Alzheimer and one with multiinfarct dementia. 3 females, 1 male Ages 65–74	Individualized program based on MOHO, developed for each client; relied on procedural motor skills rather than higher-order cognitive functions. One ADL was chosen that was motivating, a habitual part of routine, and that the client was beginning to have difficulty with. Subjects trained for 9 sessions with environmental support (external, verbal, physical).	Individualized ADL training for clients with dementia that relies on procedural motor skills may improve process skills when environmental support is provided: One client showed no changes. Two clients showed improved performance in process skills. One client demonstrated improvement in process skills with and without environmental support and at 2-month followup.
Kielhofner, Braveman, Finlayson, Paul-Ward, Goldbaum, & Goldstein (2004)	Quasi-experimental.	Convenience sample of 129 persons with AIDS. Aged 24–61 years, mean age 41. 82.2% male, 16.3% female, 1.5% transgender. 39.5% Caucasian, 44.2% African American, 10.8% Hispanic, 5.5% other. 44% substance abuse, 84% mental illness, 26% physical disability.	4-phase intervention based on MOHO to address volition, habitation, performance capacity, community and workplace environments: Phase 1: 8 weeks. Initial screening with OPHI- II, WRI, and OSA. Self-assess and refine vocation choice, develop job skills, gather information, receive support. Weekly group sessions, peer support, and work task experiences. Phase 2: Productive roles: volunteering, internship, temporary positions. Job coaching as needed. Continued some group programming.	Participating in a MOHO community-based return-to-work program leads to productive outcomes: 67% of participants who completed program were working, volunteering, or in school. Persons with progressive slopes were twice as likely to have a successful outcome.

Author (year)	Design	Participants	Intervention	Findings
			Phase 3: Job placement or support for job application. Job coaching, individual support, employer education as needed. Individual meetings with staff. Phase 4: Long-term followup, support with peers and staff to sustain employment.	MOHO-based intervention that supports transition to community decreases recidivism, increases time engaged in work activities. Interventions in small group formats supportive to clients. To maximize goal achievement, interventions should be flexible to meet needs of clients.
Kielhofner & Brinson (1989)	Posttest only. Random assignment to experimental or control group. Program evaluation.	34 clients ending inpatient hospitalization in U. S., at least 2 previous psychiatric hospitalizations. Experimental group had 16 participants; control group had 14 participants.	12-week program, 36 sessions of 1.5–2 hours, three times a week. Modules throughout based on MOHO. 1st month: explore roles, skills, interests. Participants set long-term goal in self-care, leisure, productivity. 2nd month: practice skills in community. Goal setting continued, achieving goals in groups and during homework. 3rd month: select a group work activity to raise money for outing.	
Kielhofner, Braveman, Levin, and Fogg (in press)	Posttest control group.	38 persons in transitional living in community in model research program: 31 males, 7 females. 27 African American, 8 Caucasian, 1 Native American/Alaskan, 2 Hispanic/Latino. Aged 24–59 years; mean age 42.7 years. All had primary diagnosis of HIV/AIDS. 26 persons in transitional living in community in standard intervention, or control group: 20 males, 6 females. 19 African American, 6 Caucasian, 1 Hispanic/Latino.	MOHO-based individualized program: 4-phase continuum of services to increase independent living, employment. Each phase focused on supporting development of personal skills, habits, confidence, attention to environmental interventions and supports. Vocational components included early placement in actual work contexts, integrated attention to vocational and mental health needs, consumer-focused menu of choices and paths, continuous comprehensive assessment, ongoing support as necessary for ultimate success. Individual and group interventions to	Compared to clients who received a standard educational intervention, clients who received MOHO-based intervention achieved significantly better independent living and employment outcomes: Participants with MOHO-based services were at least twice as likely to be employed 3, 6, and 9 months after the end of treatment than were control participants.

(continued)

TABLE 25.22 (continued)

Citation	Type of study	Sample Information	Description of Intervention	Findings & Clinical Implications
		Aged 31–56; mean age 42.6 . years All had primary diagnosis of HIV/AIDS.	build capacity for ADLs, in prepara- tion for living independently.	

COPM, ; WRI, Worker Role Interview; OPHI-II, Occupational Performance History Interview—II; AMPS, ; OSA, Occupational Self-Assessment; ADL, activities of daily living; IADL, instrumental activities of daily living.

TABLE 25.23 Evidence Concerning Client Perspectives on MOHO-Based Services

Citation	Findings
Apte, Kielhofner, Paul-Ward, & Braveman (2005)	Most clients with AIDS participating in a return-to-work program report that the OPHI-II enables them to communicate with their therapists and allows the therapist to better understand their circumstances. Clients found the narrative slope helpful and motivating, and some expressed a desire to create the narrative slope and/or keep a copy of the narrative slope as a visual motivator.
Ecklund (1996b)	Clients' positive perceptions of the relationship between them and their main therapist in a psychiatric day program was associated with better mental health and MOHO-based outcomes:
	Clients who reported that their relationship with their therapist improved during the course of intervention had significant differences in global mental health and habituation scores from those of clients who reported that their relationship with their therapist declined.
	Clients' perceptions of their relationship with their main therapist was positively related to global mental health, volition, habituation, and communication/interaction skills.
Farnworth, Nihitin, & Fossey (2004)	Clients in forensic mental health wards created challenges for themselves to keep themselves occupied, found their own personal meanings in occupations, and enjoyed occupational therapy groups that had an outcome (i.e., cooking group).
Fisher & Savin-Baden (2001)	MOHO is a person-centered framework that facilitates integrated service models that are acceptable to young adult mental health consumers and their families. These clients felt supported and felt that they had a voice in their services.
Heasman & Atwal (2004)	About 50% of adult clients with mental illness achieved leisure goals when attending a day program based on MOHO. Clients reported that lacks of followup, motivation, and social support were barriers to successful achievement of leisure goals.
Linddahl, Norrby, & Bellner (2003)	For clients with psychiatric disabilities in a Swedish work rehabilitation program, the hardest volitional item on a MOHO-based assessment was saying no when there is something you do not want to do.
	Clients felt that the hardest habituation item on a MOHO-based assessment was taking a leadership role in a group.
	Clients felt that the hardest communication/interaction skill item on a MOHO-based assessment was keeping up a conversation.
	Client felt the hardest process skill item on a MOHO-based assessment was working against the clock.
	Clients felt the hardest motor skill item on a MOHO-based assessment was maintaining physical persistence while performing activities.

OPHI-II, Occupational Performance History Interview—II.

References

Abberley, P. (1995). Disabling ideology in health and welfare: The case of occupational therapy. *Disability and Society, 10,* 221–232.

Andersen, S., Kielhofner, G., & Lai, J. (2005). An examination of the measurement properties of the Pediatric Volitional Questionnaire. *Physical and Occupational Therapy in Pediatrics, 25 (1/2),* 39–57.

Andrews, P. M., Bleecher, R., Genoa, A. M., Molloy, P., Monahan, K., & Sargent, J. (1995). *Leisure interests of children.* Unpublished manuscript, Worcester State College, Worcester, MA.

Apte, A., Kielhofner, G., Paul-Ward, A., & Braveman, B. (2005). Therapists' and clients' perceptions of the occupational performance history interview. *Occupational Therapy in Health Care, 19,* 173–192.

Asmundsdottir, E. E. (2004). The Worker Role Interview: A powerful tool in Icelandic work rehabilitation. *WORK: A Journal of Prevention, Assessment & Rehabilitation, 22 (1),* 21–26.

Aubin, G., Hachey, R., & Mercier, C. (2002). The significance of daily activities in persons with severe mental disorders [French]. *Canadian Journal of Occupational Therapy, 69,* 218–228.

Aubin, G., Hachey, R., & Mercier, C. (1999). Meaning of daily activities and subjective quality of life in people with severe mental illness. *Scandinavian Journal of Occupational Therapy, 6,* 53–62.

Ay-Woan, P., Sarah, C. P., Lylnn, C., Tsyr-Jang, C., & Ping-Chaun, H. (2006). Quality of life in depression: Predictive models. *Quality of Life Research, 15,* 39–48.

Baker, F., Curbow, B., & Wingard, J. R. (1991). Role retention and quality of life of bone marrow transplant survivors. *Social Science & Medicine, 32,* 697–704.

Barrett, L., Beer, D., & Kielhofner, G. (1999). The importance of volitional narrative in treatment: An ethnographic case study in a work program. *Work: A Journal of Prevention, Assessment & Rehabilitation, 12 (1),* 79–92.

Barris, R., Dickie, V., & Baron, K. B. (1988). A comparison of psychiatric patients and normal subjects based on the model of human occupation. *The Occupational Therapy Journal of Research, 8,* 3–23.

Barris, R., Kielhofner, G., Burch, R. M., Gelinas, I., Klement, M., & Schultz, B. (1986). Occupational function and dysfunction in three groups of adolescents. *Occupational Therapy Journal of Research, 6,* 301–317.

Basnett, I. (2001). Health care professionals and their attitudes towards and decisions affecting disabled people. In G. L. Albrecht, K. D. Seelman, & M. Bury (Eds.), *Handbook of disability studies* (pp. 450–467). Thousand Oaks, CA: Sage.

Beck, D., Benson, S., Curet, J., Froehlich, D., McCrary, L., Rasmussen, L., & Skowyra, K. (1996). *Pilot study of a child's play interest profile.* Unpublished manuscript, Worcester State College, Worcester, MA.

Bennett, S., Tooth, L., McKenna, K., Rodger, S., Ziviani, J., Mickan, S., & Gibson, L. (2003). Perceptions of evidence-based practice: A survey of occupational therapists. *Australian Journal of Occupational Therapy, 50,* 13–22.

Biernacki, S. D. (1993). Reliability of the Worker Role Interview. *American Journal of Occupational Therapy, 47,* 797–803.

Bjorklund, A., & Henriksson, M. (2003). On the context of elderly persons' occupational performance. *Physical and Occupational Therapy in Geriatrics, 21 (3),* 49–58.

Bowyer, P., Kramer, J., Kielhofner, G., Maziero-Barbosa, V., & Girolami, G. (2007). The measurement properties of the Short Child Occupational Profile (SCOPE). *Physical and Occupational Therapy in Pediatrics, 27(4).*

Branholm, I., & Fugl-Meyer, A. R. (1992). Occupational role preferences and life satisfaction. *Occupational Therapy Journal of Research, 12,* 159–171.

Braveman, B., & Helfrich, C.A. (2001). Occupational identity: Exploring the narratives of three men living with AIDS. *Journal of Occupational Science, 8,* 25–31.

Braveman, B., Helfrich, C., Kielhofner, G., & Albrecht, G. (2004). The experiences of 12 men with AIDS who attempted to return to work. *The Israel Journal of Occupational Therapy, 13 (3),* E69–E83.

Bridle, M. J., Lynch, K. B., & Quesenberry, C. M. (1990). Long term function following the central cord syndrome. *Paraplegia, 28,* 178–185.

Brollier, C., Watts, J. H., Bauer, D., & Schmidt, W. (1988a). A concurrent validity study of two occupational therapy evaluation instruments: The AOF and OCAIRS. *Occupational Therapy In Mental Health, 8 (4),* 49–60.

Brollier C., Watts, J. H., Bauer, D., & Schmidt, W. (1988b). A content validity study of the Assessment of Occupational Functioning. *Occupational Therapy in Mental Health, 8 (4),* 29–47.

Brophy, P., Caizzi, D., Crete, B., Jachym, T., Kobus, M., & Sainz, C. (1995). *Preliminary reliability study of the Adolescent Leisure Interest Profile.* Unpublished manuscript, Worcester State College, Worcester, MA.

Brown, G. T., & Carmichael, K. (1992). Assertiveness training for clients with a psychiatric illness: A pilot study. *British Journal of Occupational Therapy, 55,* 137–140.

Budd, P., Ferraro, D., Lovely, A., McNeil, T., Owanisian, L., Parker, J., et al. (1997). *Pilot study of the revised child's play interest profile.* Unpublished manuscript, Worcester State College, Worcester, MA.

Buning, M. E., Angelo, J. A., & Schmeler, M. R. (2001). Occupational performance and the transition to powered mobility: A pilot study. *American Journal of Occupational Therapy, 55,* 339–344.

Chaffey, L., & Fossey, E. (2004). Caring and daily life: Occupational experiences of women living with sons diagnosed with schizophrenia. *Australian Occupational Therapy Journal, 51,* 199–207.

Chan, S. (2004). Chronic obstructive pulmonary disease & engagement in OT. *The American Journal of Occupational Therapy, 58,* 408–415.

Chen, C., Neufeld, P. S., Feely, C. A., & Skinner, C. S. (1999). Factors influencing compliance with home exercise programs among patients with upper-extremity impairment. *American Journal of Occupational Therapy, 53,* 171–180.

Chern, J., Kielhofner, G., de las Heras, G., & Magalhaes, L. C. (1996). The Volitional Questionnaire: Psychometric development and practical use. *American Journal of Occupational Therapy, 50,* 516–525.

Colon, H., & Haertlein, C. (2002). Spanish translation of the Role Checklist. *American Journal of Occupational Therapy, 56,* 586–589.

Corcoran, M. A., & Gitlin, L. A. (2001). Family caregiver acceptance and use of environmental strategies provided in an occupational therapy intervention. *Physical and Occupational Therapy in Geriatrics, 19 (1),* 1–20.

Cordeiro, J. R., Camelier, A., Oakley, F., & Jardim, J. R. (2007). Cross-cultural reproducibility of the Brazilian Portuguese version of the Role Checklist for persons with chronic obstructive pulmonary disease. *American Journal of Occupational Therapy, 61,* 33–40.

Corner, R., Kielhofner, G., & Lin, F. L. (1997). Construct validity of a work environment impact scale. *Work, 9 (1),* 21–34.

Corr, S., Phillips, C. J., & Walker, M. (2004). Evaluation of a pilot service designed to provide support following stroke: a randomized cross-over design study. *Clinical Rehabilitation, 18 (1),* 69–75.

Corr, S., & Wilmer, S. (2003). Returning to work after a stroke: An important but neglected area. *British Journal of Occupational Therapy, 66,* 186–192.

Corring, D., & Cook, J. (1999). Client centred care means that I am a valued human being. *Canadian Journal of Occupational Therapy, 66,* 71–82.

Crist, P., Fairman, A., Muñoz, J. P., Hansen, A. M. W., Sciulli, J., & Eggers, M. (2005). Education and practice collaborations: a pilot case study between a university faculty and county jail practitioners. *Occupational Therapy in Health Care, 19 (1/2),*193–210.

Crowe, T. K., VanLeit, B., Berghmans, K. K., & Mann, P. (1997). Role perceptions of mothers with young children: The impact of a child's disability. *American Journal of Occupational Therapy, 51,* 651–661.

Davies Hallet, J., Zasler, N., Maurer, P., & Cash, S. (1994). Role change after traumatic brain injury in adults. *American Journal of Occupational Therapy, 48,* 241–246.

Dickerson, A. E., & Oakely, F. (1995). Comparing the roles of community-living persons and patient populations. *American Journal of Occupational Therapy, 49,* 221–228.

DeForest, D., Watts, J. H., & Madigan, M. J. (1991). Resonation in the model of human occupation: A pilot study. *Occupational Therapy in Mental Health, 11 (2/3),* 57–71.

Dubouloz, C., Egan, M., Vallerand, J., & VonZweck, C. (1999). Occupational therapists' perceptions of evidence based practice. *American Journal of Occupational Therapy, 53,* 445–453.

Duellman, M. K., Barris, R., & Kielhofner, G. (1986). Organized activity and the adaptive status of nursing home residents. *American Journal of Occupational Therapy, 40,* 618–622.

Durand, M., Vachon, B., Loisel, P., & Berthelette, D. (2003). Constructing the program impact theory for an evidence-based work rehabilitation program for workers with low back pain. *Work: A Journal of Prevention, Assessment & Rehabilitation, 21,* 233–242.

Dysart, A. M., & Tomlin, G. S. (2002). Factors related to evidence-based practice among US occupational therapy clinicians. *American Journal of Occupational Therapy, 56,* 275–284.

Ebb, E. W., Coster, W. J., & Duncombe, L. (1989). Comparison of normal and psychosocially dysfunctional male adolescents. *Occupational Therapy in Mental Health, 9 (2),* 53–74.

Egan, M., Warren, S. A., Hessel, P. A., & Gilewich, G. (1992). Activities of daily living after hip fracture: Pre- and post discharge. *Occupational Therapy Journal of Research, 12,* 342–356.

Ekbladh, E., Haglund, L., & Thorell, L. (2004). The Worker Role Interview: Preliminary data on the predictive validity of return to work clients after an insurance medicine investigation. *Journal of Occupational Rehabilitation, 14 (2),* 131–141.

Eklund, M. (2001). Psychiatric patients' occupational roles: changes over time and associations with self-rated quality of life. *Scandinavian Journal of Occupational Therapy, 8,* 125–130.

Eklund, M. (1999). Outcome of occupational therapy in a psychiatric day care unit for long-term mentally ill patients. *Occupational Therapy in Mental Health, 14 (4),* 21–45.

Eklund, M. (1996a). Patient experiences and outcome of treatment in psychiatric occupational therapy: Three cases. *Occupational Therapy International, 3,* 212–239.

Eklund, M. (1996b). Working relationship, participation, and outcome in a psychiatric day care unit based on occupational therapy. *Scandinavian Journal of Occupational Therapy, 3,* 106–113.

Eklund, M., & Hansson, L. (1997). Stability of improvement in patients receiving psychiatric occupational therapy: A one-year follow-up. *Scandinavian Journal of Occupational Therapy, 4,* 15–122.

Elliott, M., & Barris, R. (1987). Occupational role performance and life satisfaction in elderly persons. *Occupational Therapy Journal of Research, 7,* 215–224.

Farnworth, L., Nihitin, L., & Fossey, E. (2004). Being in a secure forensic psychiatry unit: Every day is the same, killing time or making the most of it. *British Journal of Occupational Therapy, 67,* 1–9.

Fenger, K., & Kramer, J. M. (In press). Worker Role Interview: Testing the psychometric properties of the Icelandic version. *Scandanavian Journal of Occupational Therapy.*

Fisher, A., & Savin-Baden, M. (2001). The benefits to young people experiencing psychosis, and their families, of an early intervention programme: Evaluating a service from the consumers' and the providers' perspectives. *British Journal of Occupational Therapy, 64,* 58–65.

Forsyth, K., Braveman, B., Kielhofner, K., Ekbladh, E., Haglund, L., Fenger, K. & Keller, J (2006). Psychometric properties of the Worker Role Interview. *Work: A Journal of Prevention, Assessment & Rehabilitation,* 27, 313–318.

Forsyth, K., Lai, J., & Kielhofner, G. (1999). The Assessment of Communication and Interaction Skills (ACIS): Measurement properties. *British Journal of Occupational Therapy, 62,* 69–74.

Forsyth, K., Parkinson, S., Kielhofner, G., Keller, J., Summerfield Mann, L., & Duncan, E. (in press). The measurement properties of the Model of Human Occupation Screening Tool (MOHOST). *British Journal of Occupational Therapy.*

Frosch, S., Gruber, A., Jones, C., Myers, S., Noel, E., Westerlund, A., & Zavisin, T. (1997). The long term effects of traumatic brain injury on the roles of caregivers. *Brain Injury, 11,* 891–906.

Fossey, E. (1996). Using the occupational performance history interview (OPHI): Therapists' reflections. *British Journal of Occupational Therapy, 59,* 223–228.

Furst, G., Gerber, L., Smith, C., Fisher, S., & Schulman, B. (1987). A program for improving energy conservation behaviors in adults with rheumatoid arthritis. *American Journal of Occupational Therapy, 41,* 102–111.

Gerber, L., & Furst, G. (1992). Validation of the NIH Activity Record: A quantitative measure of life activities. *Arthritis Care and Research, 5,* 81–86.

Giangreco, M. F. (1999). *The stairs don't go anywhere! A self advocate's reflection on specialized services and their impact on people with disabilities: An interview with Norman Kunc.* Retrieved 9/7/99 at http://www.normemma.com/arstairs.htm.

Gitlin, L. N., Winter, L., Corcoran, M., Dennis, M. P., Schinfeld, S., & Hauck, W. W. (2003). Effects of the Home Environmental Skill-Building Program on the caregiver–care recipient dyad: 6–month outcomes from the Philadelphia REACH initiative. *The Gerontologist, 43,* 532–546.

Goldstein, K., Kielhofner, G., Paul-Ward, A. (2004). Occupational narratives and the therapeutic process. *Australian Occupational Therapy Journal, 51,* 119–124.

Gorde, M. W., Helfrich, C. A., & Finlayson, M. L. (2004). Trauma symptoms and life skill needs of domestic violence victims. *Journal of Interpersonal Violence, 19,* 691–708.

Graff, M. J. L., Vernooij-Dassen, M. J. F. J., Hoefnagels, W. H. L., Dekker, J., & de Witte, L. P. (2003). Occupational therapy at home for older individuals with mild to moderate cognitive impairments and their primary caregivers: A pilot study. *OTJR: Occupation, Participation, and Health, 23,* 155–164.

Gray, M. L., & Fossey, E. M. (2003). Illness experience and occupations of people with chronic fatigue syndrome. *Australian Occupational Therapy Journal, 50,* 127–136.

Gregory, M. (1983). Occupational behavior and life satisfaction among retirees. *American Journal of Occupational Therapy, 37,* 548–553.

Grogan, G. (1994). The personal computer: A treatment tool for increasing sense of competence. *Occupational Therapy in Mental Health, 12,* 47–70.

Hachey, R., Boyer, G., & Mercier, C. (2001). Perceived and valued roles of adults with severe mental health problems. *Canadian Journal of Occupational Therapy, 68,* 112–120.

Hachey, R., Jummoorty, J., & Mercier, C. (1995). Methodology for validating the translation of test measurements applied to occupational therapy. *Occupational Therapy International, 2,* 190–203.

Haglund, L. (1996). Occupational therapists' agreement in screening patients in general psychiatric care for occupational therapy. *Scandinavian Journal of Occupational Therapy, 3,* 62–68.

Haglund, L., & Henriksson, C. (2003). Concepts in occupational therapy in relation to the ICF. *Occupational Therapy International, 10,* 253–268.

Haglund, L., & Henriksson, C. (1994). Testing a Swedish Version of OCAIRS on two different patient groups. *Scandinavian Journal of Caring Sciences, 8,* 223–230.

Haglund, L., Karlsson, G., & Kielhofner, G. (1997). Validity of the Swedish version of the Worker Role Interview. *Physical and Occupational Therapy in Geriatrics, 4 (1),* 23–29.

Haglund, L., & Thorell, L. (2004). Clinical perspective on the Swedish version of the Assessment of Communication and Interaction Skills: Stability of assessments. *Scandinavian Journal of Caring Sciences, 18,* 417–423.

Haglund, L., Thorell, L., & Walinder, J. (1998a). Assessment of occupational functioning for screening of patients to occupational therapy in general psychiatric care. *Occupational Therapy Journal of Research, 4,* 193–206.

Haglund, L., Thorell, L., & Walinder, J. (1998b). Occupational functioning in relation to psychiatric diagnoses: Schizophrenia and mood disorders. *Journal of Psychiatry, 52,* 223–229.

Hakansson, C., Eklund, M., Lidfeldt, J., Nerbrand, C., Samsioe, G., & Nilsson, P. M. (2005). Well-being and occupational roles among middle-aged women. *Work: A Journal of Prevention, Assessment & Rehabilitation, 24,* 341–351.

Hallett, J. D., & Zasler, N. D., Maurer, P., & Cash, S. (1994). Role change after traumatic brain injury in adults. *American Journal of Occupational Therapy, 48,* 241–246.

Hammel, J. (1999). The Life Rope: A transactional approach to exploring worker and life role development. *Work: A Journal of Prevention, Assessment, & Rehabilitation, 12,* 47–60.

Hann, J., Regele, K., Walsh, C., Fontana, L., & Bentley, R. (1994). *Item development for a new measure of adolescent leisure interests.* Unpublished manuscript, Worcester State College, Worcester, MA.

Harris, K., & Reid, D. (2005). The influence of virtual reality play on children's motivation. *Canadian Journal of Occupational Therapy, 72,* 21–29.

Heasman, D., & Atwal, A. (2004). The Active Advice pilot project: Leisure enhancement and social inclusion for people with severe mental health problems. *British Journal of Occupational Therapy, 67,* 511–514.

Helfrich, C. & Kielhofner, G. (1994). Volitional narratives and the meaning of occupational therapy. *American Journal of Occupational Therapy, 48,* 319–326.

Helfrich, C., Kielhofner, G., & Mattingly, C. (1994). Volition as narrative: Understanding motivation in chronic illness. *American Journal of Occupational Therapy, 48,* 311–317.

Hemmingsson, H., & Borell, L. (2002). Environmental barriers in mainstream schools. *Child: Care, Health, and Development, 28 (1),* 57–63.

Hemmingsson, H., & Borell, L. (2000). Accommodation needs and student–environment fit in upper secondary school for students with severe physical disabilities. *Canadian Journal of Occupational Therapy, 67,* 162–173.

Hemmingsson, H., & Borell, L. (1996). The development of an assessment of adjustment needs in the school setting for use with physically disabled students. *Scandinavian Journal of Occupational Therapy, 3,* 156–162.

Hemmingsson, H., Borell, L., & Gustavsson, A. (1999). Temporal aspects of teaching and learning: Implications for pupils with physical disabilities. *Scandinavian Journal of Disability Research, 1,* 26–43.

Hemmingsson, H., Kottorp, A., & Bernspang, B. (2004). Validity of the School Setting Interview: An Assessment of the student–environment fit. *Scandinavian Journal of Occupational Therapy, 11,* 171–178.

Henriksson, C. M. (1995a). Living with continuous muscular pain: Patient perspectives. Part I: Encounters and consequences. *Scandinavian Journal of Caring Sciences, 9,* 67–76.

Henriksson, C.M. (1995b). Living with continuous muscular pain: Patient perspectives Part II: Strategies for daily life. *Scandinavian Journal of Caring Sciences, 9,* 77–86.

Henriksson, C., & Burckhardt, C. (1996). Impact of fibromyalgia on everyday life: A study of women in the USA and Sweden. *Disability and Rehabilitation, 18,* 241–248.

Henry, A. (2000). *The Pediatric Interest Profiles.* Retrieved May 30, 2006: *http://www.moho.uic.edu/images/assessments/PIPs%20Manual.pdf.*

Henry, A. (1998). Development of a measure of adolescent leisure interests. *American Journal of Occupational Therapy, 52,* 531–539.

Henry, A. D., Baron, K. B., Mouradian, L., & Curtin, C. (1999). Reliability and validity of the self-assessment of occupational functioning. *American Journal of Occupational Therapy, 53,* 482–488.

Henry, A. D., Costa, C., Ladd, D., Robertson, C., Rollins, J., & Roy, L. (1996). Time use, time management and academic achievement among occupational therapy students. *Work: A Journal of Prevention, Assessment & Rehabilitation, 6,* 115–126.

Horne, J., Corr, S., & Earle, S. (2005). Becoming a mother: Occupational change in first time motherhood. *Journal of Occupational Science, 12,* 176–183.

Humphries, D., Littlejohns, P., Victor, C., O'Halloran, P., & Peacock, J. (2000). Implementing evidence-based practice: Factors that influence the use of research evidence by occupational therapists. *British Journal of Occupational Therapy, 63,* 516 –522.

Ingvarsson, L., & Theodorsdottir, M. H. (2004). Vocational rehabilitation at Reykjalundur Rehabilitation Center in Iceland. *Work: A Journal of Prevention, Assessment & Rehabilitation, 22,* 17–19.

Jackson, M., Harkess, J., & Ellis, J. (2004). Reporting patients' work abilities: how the use of standardised work assessments improved clinical practice in Fife. *British Journal of Occupational Therapy, 67,* 129–132.

Jacobshagen, I. (1990). The effect of interruption of activity on affect. *Occupational Therapy in Mental Health, 10 (20),* 35–45.

Jonsson, H., Josephsson, S., & Kielhofner, G. (2001). Narratives and experiences in an occupational transition: A longitudinal study of the retirement process. *American Journal of Occupational Therapy, 55,* 424–432.

Jonsson, H., Josephsson, S., & Kielhofner, G. (2000). Evolving narratives in the course of retirement: A longitudinal study. *American Journal of Occupational Therapy, 54,* 463–470.

Jonsson, H., Kielhofner, G., & Borell, L. (1997). Anticipating retirement: Narratives concerning an occupational transition. *American Journal of Occupational Therapy, 51,* 49–56.

Josephsson, S., Backman, L., Borell, L., Bernspang, B., Nygard, L., & Ronnberg, L. (1993). Supporting everyday activities in dementia: An intervention study. *International Journal of Geriatric Psychiatry, 8,* 395–400.

Kaplan, K. (1984). Short-term assessment: The need and a response. *Occupational Therapy in Mental Health, 4,* 29–45.

Katz, N. (1988). Interest Checklist: A factor analytical study. *Occupational Therapy in Mental Health, 8,* 45–55.

Katz, N., Giladi, N., & Peretz, C. (1988). Cross-cultural application of occupational therapy assessments: Human occupation with psychiatric inpatients and controls in Israel. *Occupational Therapy in Mental Health, 8,* 7–30.

Katz, N., Josman, N., & Steinmetz, N. (1988). Relationship between cognitive disability theory and the model of human occupation in the assessment of psychiatric and nonpsychiatric adolescents. *Occupational Therapy in Mental Health, 8,* 31–43.

Keller, J., Kafkes, A, & Kielhofner, G. (2005). Psychometric characteristics of the child occupational self assessment (COSA), part one: An initial examination of psychometric properties. *Scandinavian Journal of Occupational Therapy, 12,* 118–127.

Keller, J., & Kielhofner, G. (2005). Psychometric characteristics of the child occupational self assessment (COSA), part two: Refining the psychometric properties. *Scandinavian Journal of Occupational Therapy, 12,* 147–158.

Kielhofner, G. (2006). Developing and evaluating quantitative data collection instruments. In G. Kielhofner, (Ed.), *Research in Occupational Therapy: Methods of Inquiry for Enhancing Practice* (pp. 155–176). Philadelphia: FA Davis.

Kielhofner, G. (2005a). A scholarship of practice: Creating discourse between theory, research and practice. *Occupational Therapy in Health Care, 19,* 7–17

Kielhofner, G. (2005b). Scholarship and practice: Bridging the divide. *American Journal of Occupational Therapy, 59,* 231–239.

Kielhofner, G. & Barrett, L. (1998). Meaning and misunderstanding in occupational forms: A study of therapeutic goal setting. *American Journal of Occupational Therapy, 52,* 345–353.

Kielhofner, G., Braveman, B., Finlayson, M., Paul-Ward, A., Goldbaum, L., & Goldstein, K. (2004). Outcomes of a vocational program for persons with AIDS. *American Journal of Occupational Therapy, 58,* 64–72.

Kielhofner, G., Braveman, B., Levin, M., & Fogg, L. (in press) A controlled study of services to enhance productive participation among persons with HIV/AIDS. *American Journal of Occupational Therapy.*

Kielhofner, G., & Brinson, M. (1989). Development and evaluation of an aftercare program for young chronic psychiatrically disabled adults. *Occupational Therapy in Mental Health, 9,* 1–25.

Kielhofner, G., Dobria, L., Forsyth, K., & Basu, S. (2005). The construction of keyforms for obtaining instantaneous measures from the occupational performance history interview rating scales. *Occupational Therapy Journal of Research, 25,* 23–32.

Kielhofner, G., Fogg, L., Braveman, B., Forsyth, K., & Kramer, J. (2007). A factor analytic study of the Model of Human Occupation Screening Tool of hypothesized variables. [Manuscript in preparation].

Kielhofner, G., & Forsyth, K. (2001). Measurement properties of a client self-report for treatment planning and documenting therapy outcomes. *Scandinavian Journal of Occupational Therapy, 8,* 131–139.

Kielhofner, G., Forsyth, K., & Iyenger, A. (2007). *Creating a client self-report measure: Part 1, Assuring validity and sensitivity.* [Unpublished manuscript. University of Illinois at Chicago, Chicago, Illinois.]

Kielhofner, G., Harlan, B., Bauer, D., & Maurer, P. (1986). The reliability of a historical interview with physically disabled respondents. *American Journal of Occupational Therapy, 40,* 551–556.

Kielhofner, G., & Henry, A. D. (1988). Development and investigation of the Occupational Performance History Interview. *American Journal of Occupational Therapy, 42,* 489–498.

Kielhofner, G., Henry, A. D., Walens, D., & Rogers, E. S. (1991). A generalizability study of the Occupational Performance History Interview. *Occupational Therapy Journal of Research, 11,* 292–306.

Kielhofner, G., Lai, J.S., Olson, L., Haglund, L., Ekbadh, E., & Hedlund, M. (1999). Psychometric properties of the Work Environment Impact Scale: A cross-cultural study. *Work: A Journal of Prevention, Assessment, and Rehabilitation, 12,* 71–77.

Kielhofner, G., & Mallinson, T. (1995). Gathering narrative data through interviews: Empirical observations and suggested guidelines. *Scandinavian Journal of Occupational Therapy, 2,* 63–68.

Kielhofner, G., Mallinson, T., Forsyth, K., & Lai, J. S. (2001). Psychometric properties of the second version of the

Occupational Performance History Interview (OPHI-II). *American Journal of Occupational Therapy, 55,* 260–267.

Kjellberg, A. (2002). More or less independent. *Disability and Rehabilitation, 10, 24 (16),* 828–840.

Kjellberg, A., Haglund, L., Forsyth. K., & Kielhofner, G. (2003). The measurement properties of the Swedish version of the Assessment of Communication and Interaction Skills. *Scandinavian Journal of Caring Sciences, 17,* 271–277.

Knis-Matthews, L., Richard, L., Marquez, L., & Mevawala, N. (2005). Implementation of occupational therapy services for an adolescent residence program. *Occupational Therapy in Mental Health, 21,* 57–72.

Kusznir, A., Scott, E., Cooke, R. G., & Young, L. T. (1996). Functional consequences of bipolar affective disorder: An occupational therapy perspective. *Canadian Journal of Occupational Therapy, 63,* 313–322.

Lai, J., Haglund, L., & Kielhofner, G. (1999). Occupational case analysis interview and rating scale. *Scandinavian Journal of Caring Sciences, 13,* 276–273.

Larsson, M., & Branholm, I. (1996). An approach to goal-planning in occupational therapy and rehabilitation. *Scandinavian Journal of Occupational Therapy, 3,* 14–19.

Law, M., & Baum, C. (1998). Evidence-based practice occupational therapy. *Canadian Journal of Occupational Therapy, 65,* 131–135.

Lederer, J., Kielhofner, G., & Watts, J. H. (1985). Values, personal causation and skills of delinquents and non delinquents. Occupational Therapy in Mental Health *5,* 59–77.

Lee, A. L., Strauss, L., Wittman, P., Jackson, B., & Carstens, A. (2001). The effects of chronic illness on roles and emotions of caregivers. *Occupational Therapy in Health Care, 14,* 47–60.

Leidy, N. K., & Knebel, A. R. (1999). Clinical validation of the functional performance inventory in patients with chronic obstructive pulmonary disease. *Respiratory Care, 44,* 932–939.

Levin, M., Kielhofner, G., Braveman, B., & Fogg, L. (In press). Narrative Slope as a Predictor of Work and other Occupational Participation. *Scandanavian Journal of Occupational Therapy.*

Levin, M., & Helfrich, C. (2004). Mothering role identity and competence among parenting and pregnant homeless adolescents, *Journal of Occupational Science, 11,* 95–104.

Li, Y., & Kielhofner, G. (2004). Psychometric properties of the Volitional Questionnaire. *The Israel Journal of Occupational Therapy, 13,* E85–E98.

Linddahl, I., Norrby, E., & Bellner, A. (2003). Construct validity of the instrument DOA: A dialogue about ability related to work. *Work: A Journal of Prevention, Assessment & Rehabilitation, 20,* 215–224.

Lloyd, C., Basset, H., & King, R. (2004). Occupational therapy and evidence-based practice in mental health. *British Journal of Occupational Therapy, 67,* 83–88.

Lycett, R. (1992). Evaluating the use of an occupational assessment with elderly rehabilitation patients. *British Journal of Occupational Therapy, 55,* 343–346.

Lynch, K. & Bridle, M. (1993). Construct validity of the Occupational Performance Interview. *Occupational Therapy Journal of Research, 13,* 231–240.

Mallinson, T., Kielhofner, G., & Mattingly, C. (1996). Metaphor and meaning in a clinical interview. *American Journal of Occupational Therapy, 50,* 338–346.

Mallinson, T., Mahaffey, L., & Kielhofner, G. (1998). The occupational performance history interview: Evidence for three underlying constructs of occupational adaptation. *Canadian Journal of Occupational Therapy, 65,* 219–228.

McCluskey, A. (2003). Occupational therapists report a low level of knowledge, skill and involvement in evidence-based practice. *Australian Occupational Therapy Journal, 50,* 3–12.

McCluskey, A., & Cusick, A. (2002). Strategies for introducing evidence-based practice and changing clinical behaviour: A manager's toolbox. *Australian Occupational Therapy Journal, 49,* 63–70.

Metcalfe, C., Lewin, R., Wisher, S., Perry, S., Bannigan, K., & Moffett, J. K. (2001). Barriers to implementing the evidence base in four NHS therapies: Dietitians, occupational therapists, physiotherapists, speech and language therapists. *Physiotherapy, 87, Part 8,* 433–441.

Molyneaux-Smith, L., Townsend, E., & Guernsey, J. R. (2003). Occupation disrupted: Impacts, challenges, and coping strategies for farmers with disabilities. *Journal of Occupational Science, 10,* 14–20.

Morgan, D., & Jongbloed, L. (1990). Factors influencing leisure activities following a stroke: An exploratory study. *Canadian Journal of Occupational Therapy, 57,* 223–229.

Muñoz, J. P., Karmosky, A., Gaugler, J., Lang, K., & Stayduhar, M. (1999). Perceived role changes in parents of children with cerebral palsy. *Mental Health Special Interest Section Quarterly, 22 (4),* 1–3.

Muñoz, J. P., Lawlor, M., & Kielhofner, G. (1993). Use of the Model of Human Occupation: A survey of therapists in psychiatric practice. *Occupational Therapy Journal of Research, 13,* 117–139.

Neistadt, M. E. (1995). Methods of assessing clients' priorities: A survey of adult physical dysfunction settings. *American Journal of Occupational Therapy, 49,* 428–436.

Neville-Jan, A. (1994). The relationship of volition to adaptive occupational behavior among individuals with varying degrees of depression. *Occupational Therapy in Mental Health, 12 (4)*, 1–18.

Oakley, F., Kielhofner, G., & Barris, R. (1985). An occupational therapy approach to assessing psychiatric patients' adaptive functioning. *American Journal of Occupational Therapy, 30*, 147–154.

Oakley, F., Kielhofner, G., Barris, R., & Reichler, R. K. (1986). The Role Checklist: Development and empirical assessment of reliability. *Occupational Therapy Journal of Research, 6*, 157–170.

Packer, T. L., Foster, D. M., & Brouwer, B. (1997). Fatigue and activity patterns of people with chronic fatigue syndrome. *Occupational Therapy Journal of Research, 17*, 186–199.

Pentland, W., Harvey, A. S., & Walker, J. (1998). The relationships between time use and health and well-being in men with spinal cord injury. *Journal of Occupational Science, 5 (1)*, 14–25.

Peterson, E., Howland, J., Kielhofner, G., Lachman, M. E., Assmann, S., Cote, J., & Jette, A. (1999). Falls self-efficacy and occupational adaptation among elders. *Physical and Occupational Therapy in Geriatrics, 16 (1/2)*, 1–16

Polatajko, H. J., & Craik, J. (2006). Editorial: In search of evidence: strategies for an evidence-based practice process. *OTJR: Occupation, Participation, and Health, 26 (1)*, 2–3.

Prellwitz, M., & Tham, M. (2000). How children with restricted mobility perceive their school environment. *Scandinavian Journal of Occupational Therapy, 7*, 165–173.

Reid, D. T. (2005). Correlation of the Pediatric Volitional Questionnaire with the Test of Playfulness in a virtual environment: The power of engagement. *Early Child Development and Care,175 (2)*, 153–164.

Reid, D. (2003). The influence of a virtual reality leisure intervention program on the motivation of older adult stroke survivors: a pilot study. *Physical & Occupational Therapy in Geriatrics, 21 (4)*, 1–19.

Restall, G., & Magill-Evans, J. (1994). Play and preschool children with autism. *American Journal of Occupational Therapy, 48*, 113–120.

Roberts, A. E. K., & Barber, G. (2001). Applying research evidence to practice. *British Journal of Occupational Therapy, 64*, 223–227.

Rogers, J., Weinstein, J., & Figone, J. (1978). The Interest Checklist: An empirical assessment. *American Journal of Occupational Therapy, 32*, 628–630.

Rosenfeld, M. S. (1989). Occupational disruption and adaptation: A study of house fire victims. *American Journal of Occupational Therapy, 43*, 89–96.

Rust, K., Barris, R., & Hooper, F. (1987). Use of the model of human occupation to predict women's exercise behavior. *Occupational Therapy Journal of Research, 7*, 23–35.

Sackett, D.L., Rosenberg, W. M. C., Muir Gray, J. A., Haynes, R. B., & Richardson, W. S. (1996). Evidence based medicine: what it is and what it isn't. *British Medical Journal, 312*, 71–72.

Scaffa, M. E. (1991). Alcoholism: An occupational behavior perspective. *Occupational Therapy in Mental Health, 11*, 99–111.

Scheelar, J. F. (2002). A return to the worker role after injury: Firefighters seriously injured on the job and the decision to return to high-risk work. *Work: A Journal of Prevention, 19*, 181–184.

Schindler, V. P. (2004). Evaluating the effectiveness of role development: Quantitative data. *Occupational Therapy in Mental Health, 20 (3/4)*, 79–104.

Schindler, V. P., & Baldwin, S. A. M. (2005). Role development: Application to community-based clients. *Israeli Journal of Occupational Therapy, 14*, E3–18.

Smith, N., Kielhofner, G., & Watts, J. (1986). The relationship between volition, activity pattern and life satisfaction in the elderly. *American Journal of Occupational Therapy, 40*, 278–283.

Smyntek, L., Barris, R., & Kielhofner G. (1985). The model of human occupation applied to psychosocially functional and dysfunctional adolescents. *Occupational Therapy in Mental Health, 5 (1)*, 21–39.

Sousa, S. (2006). *Reliability and validity of the Occupational Self Assessment with psychiatric inpatients in Portugal.* [Manuscript submitted for publication].

Sudsawad, P. (2006). Definition, evolution, and implementation of evidence-based practice in occupational therapy. In G. Kielhofner, (Ed.), *Research in Occupational Therapy: Methods of Inquiry for Enhancing Practice* (pp. 656–662). Philadelphia: FA Davis.

Sudsawad, P. (2003). *Rehabilitation practitioners' perspectives on research utilization for evidence-based practice.* Paper presented at the American Congress of Rehabilitation Medicine conference, October 24, 2003, Tucson, Arizona.

Sviden, G. A., Tham, K., & Borell, L. (2004). Elderly participants of social and rehabilitative day centres. *Scandinavian Journal of Caring Sciences,18*, 402–409.

Taylor, M. C. (1997). What is evidence-based practice? *British Journal of Occupational Therapy, 60*, 470–474.

Taylor, R. R., Fisher, G., & Kielhofner, G. (2005). Synthesizing research, education, and practice according to the scholarship of practice model: Two faculty examples. *Occupational Therapy in Health Care, 19 (1/2)*, 107–122.

Tham, K., & Borell, L. (1996). Motivation for training: A case study of four persons with unilateral neglect. *Occupational Therapy in Health Care, 10 (3)*, 65–79.

Tham, K., & Kielhofner, G. (2003). Impact of the social environment on occupational experience and performance among persons with unilateral neglect. *American Journal of Occupational Therapy, 57,* 403–412.

Tham, K., & Borell, L. (1996). Motivation for training: A case study of four persons with unilateral neglect. *Occupational Therapy in Health Care, 10 (3),* 65–79.

Tickle-Degnen, L., & Bedell, G. (2003). Heterarchy and hierarchy: A critical appraisal of the "levels of evidence" as a tool for clinical decision-making. *The American Journal of Occupational Therapy, 57,* 234–237.

Tse, S., Blackwood, K., & Penman, M. (2001). From rhetoric to reality: Use of randomised controlled trials in evidence-based occupational therapy. *Australian Occupational Therapy Journal, 47,* 181–185.

Velozo, G., Forsyth, K., & Kielhofner, G. (2006). Objective measurement: The influence of item response theory on research and practice. In G. Kielhofner, (Ed.), *Research in Occupational Therapy: Methods of Inquiry for Enhancing Practice* (pp. 177–200). Philadelphia: FA Davis.

Velozo, C. A., Kielhofner, G., Gern, A., Lin, F. L., Lai, J., & Fischer, G. (1999). Worker role interview: Toward validation of a psychosocial work-related measure. *Journal of Occupational Rehabilitation, 9,* 153–168.

Venable, E., Hanson, C., Shechtman, O., & Dasler, P. (2000). The effects of exercise on occupational functioning in the well elderly. *Physical and Occupational Therapy in Geriatrics, 17 (4),* 29–42.

Viik, M. K., Watts, J. H., Madigan, M. J., & Bauer, D. (1990). Preliminary validation of the Assessment of Occupational Functioning with an alcoholic population. *Occupational Therapy in Mental Health, 10,* 19–33.

Watts, J. H., Brollier, C., Bauer, D., & Schmidt, W. (1989). A comparison of two evaluation instruments used with psychiatric patients in occupational therapy. *Occupational Therapy in Mental Health, 8,* 7–27.

Watts, J. H., Kielhofner, G., Bauer, D., Gregory, M., & Valentine, D. (1986). The Assessment of Occupational Functioning: A screening tool for use in long-term care. *American Journal of Occupational Therapy, 40,* 231–240.

Watson, M. A., & Ager, C. L. (1991). The impact of role valuation and performance on life satisfaction in old age. *Physical and Occupational Therapy in Geriatrics, 10 (1),* 27–62.

Weeder, T. (1986). Comparison of temporal patterns and meaningfulness of the daily activities of schizophrenic and normal adults. *Occupational Therapy in Mental Health, 6,* 27–45.

Widen-Holmqvist, L., de Pedro-Cuesta, J., Holm, M., Sandsrom, B., Hellblom, A., Stawiarz, L., & Bach-y-Rita, P. (1993). Stroke rehabilitation in Stockholm: Basis for late intervention in patients living at home. *Scandinavian Journal of Rehabilitation Medicine, 25,* 173–181.

Zimmerer-Branum, S., & Nelson, D. (1994). Occupationally embedded exercise versus rote exercise: A choice between occupational forms by elderly nursing home residents. *American Journal of Occupational Therapy, 49,* 397–402.

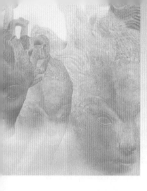

26

Research: Investigating MOHO

● Gary Kielhofner

Since MOHO was first published nearly 30 years ago, about 200 studies based on or related to it have been published. It is not possible to synthesize this diverse body of research in a single discussion. Therefore, this chapter aims to characterize the kinds of research that has investigated MOHO and place it in a framework for thinking about what research is needed to examine any conceptual practice model. This chapter addresses the following questions:

● Why is research important to a conceptual practice model like MOHO?
● What kinds of research have been undertaken to study MOHO?
● What kinds of evidence have MOHO-based studies provided about the model and its application in practice?
● What kind of research is still needed?

Drawing Conclusions from Research: Rigor and Cumulative Evidence

The studies presented in this chapter characterize types of MOHO-based research. The discussions will focus on what the findings have revealed and how they have been used to develop theory and practice rather than the details of research designs, statistics, or other methodologic issues that bear on the rigor of the studies. Nonetheless, methodologic rigor is critical to consider in deciding how much credibility to give any study. The findings from any investigation must always be looked at in light of its methodology. There are excellent resources for critiquing studies and their relevance to occupational therapy practice (e.g., Crombie, 1996; Helewa & Walker, 2000; Holm, 2000; Taylor, 2000). An evaluation of evidence from studies of MOHO should always consider the strengths and limitations of each investigation.

It is also important to keep in mind that no single study provides definitive evidence. Rather, conclusions can be drawn only from cumulative findings across many studies with different research designs, methods, and samples. With the growing research base of MOHO, it is increasingly possible to consider the results from several studies that have addressed a given issue in different ways.

Thus, it is both the rigor of individual studies and the consistency of cumulative evidence across studies that ultimately determines what research has to say about MOHO. Whenever evidence has been used to alter some aspect of MOHO, it has been based on whether the evidence is both sound and consistent across studies.

Integration of Applied and Basic Research Within Conceptual Practice Models

Conceptual practice models like MOHO offer theory to explain certain phenomena. Additionally, each model generates a technology for application (e.g., assessments and intervention strategies) for use in practice. As shown in *Figure 26.1*, research in a model includes both testing of a model's theoretical accuracy and examination of its practical utility. Consequently, the research can be referred to as encompassing both basic and applied aims. Basic research aims to test the explanations offered by a theory, whereas applied research examines the practical results of using theory to solve problems (Mosey, 1992a, b).

As illustrated in *Figure 26.1*, a model naturally integrates basic and applied research concerns. The term **basic research** refers to investigations or aspects of investigations that aim to test the theoretical arguments

FIGURE 26.1 How research raises questions and tests and refines theory and technology in a conceptual practice model.

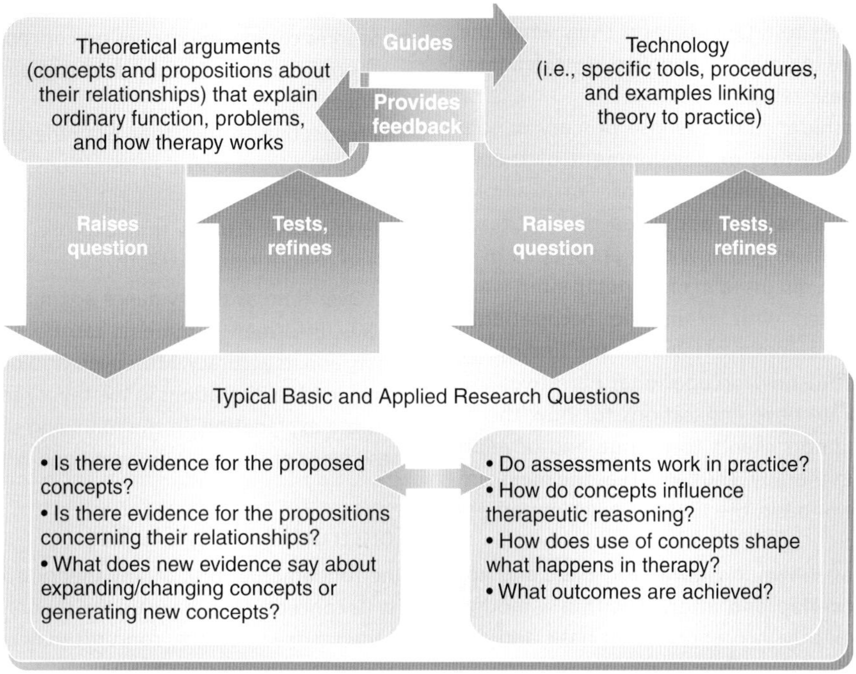

proposed in MOHO. Such research examines whether the theory is supported by evidence. This kind of research yields findings that may lead one to have confidence in the theory and/or to eliminate, change, or expand the theory. Thus, basic research is ordinarily guided by the following broad questions:

- Is there evidence for the model's concepts?
- Is there evidence for the model's propositions?
- What does new evidence say about the theory, and does it point to the need to change it?

These types of questions are concerned with testing and improving the accuracy and adequacy of the explanations offered in the model's theory.

Investigations or aspects of investigations that aim to test the practical utility of the theory and related technology for application are **applied research**. Such studies ordinarily address the following types of broad questions, as shown in *Figure 26.1*:

- Do assessments based on a model provide dependable and useful information when applied in practice?
- How do a model's concepts influence therapeutic reasoning?

- When the model's concepts are operationalized practice, how do they shape what occurs in therapy?
- What outcomes are achieved from therapy based on the model?

As can be seen from these questions, applied studies are primarily concerned with how well a model works in practice.

Although one can distinguish basic from applied research in studies that have examined MOHO, it is important to recognize these points:

- Many MOHO-based studies incorporate both basic and applied research aims.
- When studies are undertaken within the framework of a conceptual practice model, they tend to have both applied and basic relevance, no matter what their primary aim.

For example, some studies that primarily sought to examine the dependability of an assessment tool have identified new concepts that were later incorporated into the theory. One instance is a study by Mallinson, Mahaffey, and Kielhofner (1998) that sought to understand how the Occupational Performance History Interview (OPHI) rating scales worked. This study provided the first evidence for the concept of occupational identity that was subsequently added to MOHO theory. Thus, while the original purpose of the study was applied, it yielded findings relevant to basic research concerns.

In similar fashion, studies whose primary or sole purpose was the testing or development of theory have contributed to applied concerns. For example, some MOHO-based research addressed the nature of occupational narratives and how they are shaped over time. These studies, discussed in more detail later, were primarily concerned with examining occupational identity and its development. However, the findings of these studies about how occupational narratives are shaped and change have implications for how therapists can best support clients to change and develop their narratives in therapy. Thus, whereas the main aim of the research was basic, the findings have immediate applied relevance.

Therefore, as shown in *Figure 26.1*, basic and applied research overlap and interact within a model. Many studies explicitly incorporate both basic and applied purposes. Moreover, when studies are undertaken with primarily applied or basic aims, their findings tend to be relevant for both applied and basic purposes.

Types of Basic Research on MOHO

As noted previously, the purpose of basic research on a model is to test and develop theory. Within a theory, the web of concepts and propositions about the relationships between concepts create a logically interconnected explanation of the phenomena addressed by the theory. Since no study can ever test all of the concepts or propositions of MOHO theory at once, studies necessarily partition chunks of the theory and derive research questions from it. Translating theory into testable research questions can be done by asking whether evidence exists for the concepts included in the theory and for the postulated relationships between the concepts. It also involves asking whether the theory can account for and predict the kinds of phenomena it seeks to explain. Therefore, basic research on MOHO includes the following kinds of studies:

- Construct validity studies that seek to verify MOHO concepts

- Correlative studies that examine the accuracy of relationships between constructs proposed in MOHO theory
- Studies comparing groups on concepts from MOHO theory to test whether they explain group differences
- Prospective studies that examine the potential of MOHO concepts and propositions to predict future behavior or states
- Qualitative studies that explore MOHO concepts and propositions in depth

Over time as the evidence accumulates across such studies, informed judgments can be made about the theory and its accuracy. Moreover, findings from such research lead to alterations in the theory to create a more accurate explanation. In the following sections, each of these types of studies is discussed and illustrated.

Construct Validity Studies

One fundamental task of any theory is to clearly identify its concepts that make up the theory. In early stages of theory development, concepts may be incompletely defined, too narrow, or too broad. Additionally, theories may include unnecessary concepts or fail to include concepts that capture critical phenomena.

In any theoretical tradition, a necessity of empirical study of the concepts is methods to gather information on the construct. Such studies usually have an applied purpose, since they examine tools that are designed to capture information on the intended construct. Nonetheless, these studies are equally important for validating the underlying concept (Benson & Schell, 1997). Consequently, they address the basic scientific purpose of gathering evidence about how well a concept corresponds to the phenomenon it references.

Studies that were part of developing measures of MOHO concepts have been critical to generating evidence about the concepts. In many instances, these studies have led to refinement of the definitions of the concepts. Occasionally, such studies have even pointed toward new concepts. Recall the earlier mention of one example of how the concept of occupational identity emerged from research that was also designed to examine the Occupational Performance History Interview (OPHI) (Mallinson et al., 1996). In that case, the research pointed out that the concept of occupational adaptation actually encompassed two discrete phenomena that were later represented in the concepts of occupational identity and competence.

Some further examples are as follows. Early research on the Assessment of Motor and Process Skills (AMPS) (Doble, 1991; Pan & Fisher, 1994) resulted in a critical change in the concept of skill. Originally, skill was equated with underlying capacity, but the research efforts to develop measures of skill resulted in a redefinition of skill as a quality of the performance itself. The research that was part of developing the Role Checklist (Oakley, Kielhofner, Barris, & Reichler, 1986) helped refine the definition of role and the range of roles identified in the theory.

Many MOHO studies are primarily characterized as psychometric or instrument development studies. However, most of these studies have also substantially contributed to testing and clarifying concepts. Moreover, in the earlier stages of developing a conceptual model of practice, it is important to do such research, since it not only refines concepts but also creates operational measures of concepts that can be used in other types of basic studies.

Correlational Studies

MOHO theory specifies relationships between variables that can be tested in research. The following is an example. Volition includes the concepts of personal causation, values, and interests. A proposition of MOHO theory is that a person's values, interests, and personal causation lead to activity and occupational choices. The theory also proposes that over time these choices result in a pattern of occupational participation. As shown in *Figure 26.2*, one can logically derive from these two propositions that one's personal causation, values, and interests should bear a relationship to one's pattern of occupational participation.

An example of a study that tested this relationship is Neville-Jan's (1994) examination of the correlation between volition and patterns of occupation among 100 individuals with varying degrees of depression. This study found, as expected, a relationship between the adaptiveness of the subjects' routines and measures of their personal causation and interests. Another example is a study by Peterson et al. (1999) of the relationship between personal causation (feelings of efficacy related

to falling) and pattern of occupational engagement in 270 older adults. They found, as expected, that lowered self-efficacy for falls was related to reduced leisure and social occupations, mediated by the elders' choices to restrict what they did. These two studies thus provided evidence in support of the propositions noted earlier.

Correlational studies are also helpful in identifying concepts that do not hold up under scrutiny. For example, the concept of values previously included a subconcept of temporal orientation (Kielhofner, 1985). The study by Neville-Jan (1994) failed to find an expected relationship between extent of future orientation and adaptiveness in the subjects' occupational participation. Kavanaugh (1982) also failed to find a relationship between future orientation and interaction with the environment among adults with mental retardation. The findings of these two studies, combined with those of other basic and applied studies (Duellman, Barris, & Kielhofner, 1986; Muñoz, Lawlor, & Kielhofner, 1993), led to the elimination of temporal orientation from the concept of values.

Correlational research also has important implications for intervention. When the concepts in a theory have been shown to be important for explaining actions that may be targets of intervention, therapists can have greater confidence that it is worth their efforts to evaluate and address them in therapy. For example, the evidence that lack of self-efficacy for falls leads to unnecessary curtailment of doing things suggests that assessing and addressing the fear of falling could have a positive impact on persons' occupational participation.

Comparative Studies

Comparative studies test the explanatory value of MOHO concepts by asking whether distinctly different groups differ on variables derived from these concepts. The logic of such studies derives from the fact that MOHO concepts are aimed at explaining occupational adaptation. For example, MOHO argues that environmental impact, volition, habituation, and performance capacity (and their subconcepts) contribute to occupational adaptation. Therefore, groups whose occupational adaptation is clearly different should demonstrate some differences on environmental impact, values, personal causation, interests, roles, habits, and performance capacity.

FIGURE 26.2 Example questions addressed in correlational research.

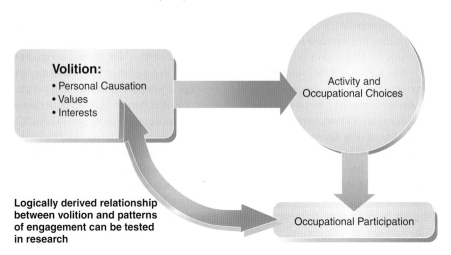

When such hypothesized differences are found, they lend support to the explanatory value of the concepts. When differences are not found, the evidence can suggest that the theory is not useful for explaining why the individuals belonging to the two or more groups differ in their occupational adaptation. Also, when groups are compared on several variables derived from MOHO, the fact that some concepts distinguish the groups while others do not can be helpful in refining how the theory is used to explain the occupational adaptation of particular groups.

The following are some examples of comparative studies. Dickerson and Oakley (1995) compared 1020 community-living adults with 292 adults who had physical or psychologic impairments. They found that persons with disabilities had fewer roles and fewer anticipated future roles. Ebb, Coster, and Duncombe (1989) compared 18 nondisabled male adolescents with 15 who had psychosocial impairments. They also found differences between the groups in the number of current and anticipated future roles. Lederer, Kielhofner, and Watts (1985) compared 15 delinquent and 15 nondelinquent adolescents and found that fewer delinquent adolescents valued student and worker roles highly and that more delinquents assigned no value to the volunteer and home maintainer role. These studies support the MOHO assertion that problems of occupational adaptation involve a disruption or failure of roles.

Barris, Dickie, and Baron (1988) compared 66 adolescents and young adults who had chronic physical impairments, psychiatric impairments, or eating disorders with 86 adolescents and adults who did not have impairments. They found differences in personal causation, values, roles, and family environment across these groups. Barris, Kielhofner, Burch, Gelinas, Klement, and Schultz (1986) studied 30 adolescents. Two groups had either psychophysiologic illness or psychiatric diagnoses. A third group included subjects not being treated for any medical or emotional problems. Personal causation, values, roles, and habit patterns were shown to be factors that effectively discriminated the three groups. These two studies provided evidence for expected differences in volition and habituation and indicated that MOHO concepts can effectively explain differences in the occupational adaptation of groups.

In addition to studies that examine different groups of persons, some studies examine the same group across time to compare when they did and did not have disabilities. Davies Hallet, Zasler, Maurer, and Cash (1994) examined 28 adolescents and adults following traumatic brain injury, comparing their roles before and after the onset of disability. They found that subjects tended to lose the worker, hobbyist, and friend roles, although some subjects also gained the roles of home maintainer, family member, and religious participant. Studies such as this one are useful for revealing information about the kinds of disability-related changes that occur over time.

Although aimed at testing and refining theory, these types of studies have important implications for practice. They constitute a form of needs assessment. That is, they identify areas of likely problems in certain client groups. This information is helpful for knowing what should be addressed in therapy. For example, the study of adolescents indicates that adolescents who are identified as being delinquent tend to experience alienation from roles valued by most members of society. This information suggests that a program for such adolescents should consider addressing the development of role identification.

Predictive Studies

Predictive studies ask whether MOHO concepts can explain and anticipate future behavior or states in subjects. The logic of these studies is similar to that of correlational studies. Predictive studies are generally more rigorous tests of theory than correlational studies, since they add the element of temporal directionality to the questions. Such studies test whether the status of a variable derived from MOHO concepts can accurately predict what a client will do or what kind of status a subject will have at a later time.

Rust, Barris, and Hooper (1987) found that roles and leisure values, along with an exercise-specific variable derived from the concept of personal causation, were predictors of women's exercise behavior. A further example of this type of research is Henry's (1994) follow-up study of adolescents and young adults following a first psychotic episode. She found that occupational adaptation (OPHI) and a self-report checklist predicted psychosocial functioning and symptomatic recovery of subjects 6 months later. In another predictive study, Chen, Neufeld, Feely, and Skinner (1999) asked whether volition, habituation, and performance capacity variables would predict compliance in 62 outpatient clients at an orthopedic upper extremity rehabilitation facility. They found that while roles and physical capacity were not related, personal causation–related variables (perceived self-efficiency and health locus of control) were predictors of compliance. Ekbladh, Haglund, and Thorell (2004) found that personal causation predicted return to work among persons who attended an insurance medicine investigation center.

Studies such as the last three, which examine the ability of MOHO concepts and explain and predict health- or intervention-related outcomes, are also important to inform intervention. For example, if personal causation is consistently shown in ongoing research to predict compliance, it follows that outpatient services relying heavily on client compliance may improve their impact by addressing personal causation. Similarly, if occupational adaptation as captured by the OPHI-II and client self-report predicts psychosocial functioning and symptomatic recovery, practitioners might be encouraged to administer the OPHI-II and self-reports such as the Occupational Self-Assessment (OSA) in practice to identify for remediation specific problems of occupational adaptation that might otherwise later compromise functioning.

Finally, since personal causation was shown to predict return to work, rehabilitation efforts aimed at this objective should address client's personal causation.

Qualitative Research That Examines and Explicates Theory

Whereas most quantitative studies are designed to test whether concepts hold up under empiric scrutiny, qualitative studies often seek to go beyond this aim. That is, they also examine phenomena in depth to see how adequately a theory explains it. Such research then often tends to further explicate theory. That is, it reveals a richer, deeper dimension to the phenomena addressed by the theory, thereby allowing the theory to be altered to better fit the phenomena. Such research leads to expanding or refining concepts and postulates. It can also result in new concepts and postulates.

The following three investigations that are part of a longitudinal qualitative study exemplify this approach. As shown in *Figure 26.3*, the studies were concerned with the role of narrative in occupational adaptation. The central postulate was that persons understand their occupational lives in terms of narrative and seek to influence how their occupational narrative unfolds.

In this multiple-year study, Jonsson, Kielhofner, and Borell (1997) first examined a group of 32 older persons just before retirement. The study underscored

FIGURE 26.3 Example theory explicating research: three sequential studies of occupational narratives.

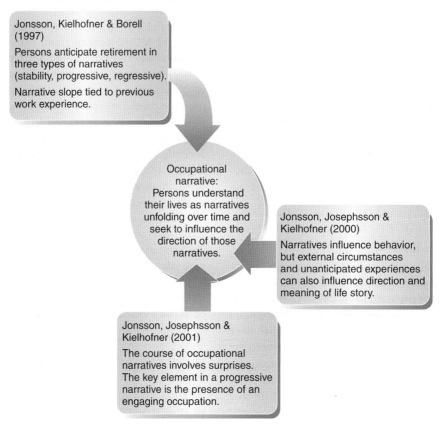

Jonsson, Kielhofner & Borell (1997)

Persons anticipate retirement in three types of narratives (stability, progressive, regressive).

Narrative slope tied to previous work experience.

Occupational narrative: Persons understand their lives as narratives unfolding over time and seek to influence the direction of those narratives.

Jonsson, Josephsson & Kielhofner (2000)

Narratives influence behavior, but external circumstances and unanticipated experiences can also influence direction and meaning of life story.

Jonsson, Josephsson & Kielhofner (2001)

The course of occupational narratives involves surprises. The key element in a progressive narrative is the presence of an engaging occupation.

two things. First, the way that elders anticipated retirement could be seen as progressive (things will get better after retirement), regressive (things will get worse), or stability (things will be the same) narratives. Second, the kind of narrative with which each person anticipated retirement was closely tied to work experience. Someone who did not like work was likely to tell a progressive narrative in which retirement would be a release from a negative experience. This study lent support to the hypothesis that persons made sense of their occupational lives in terms of narratives and provided some insight into how persons formed their occupational narratives.

In the next investigation, Jonsson, Josephsson, and Kielhofner (2000) examined how these narratives shaped and were influenced by what happened as these persons retired. They found that the direction that retirees' lives took reflected interaction between their original narrative and unfolding events and cir-

cumstances. Subjects' narratives readied them to respond in particular ways to what happened. At the same time, what happened could also nudge the narrative in one direction or another. Although occupational narratives tended to be resilient—that is, to maintain their own plot—they could also change in response to changed circumstances. The study also identified that some persons were much more active in attempting to change the shape of their narrative (e.g., avoid an undesired outcome or affect a desired one) than others. Thus, the original postulate that persons seek to continue their narratives was somewhat attenuated by this finding. In fact, the extent to which persons are motivated by their narratives appeared to vary according to their tendency either to actively shape or to respond to the events of their lives.

The third study (Jonsson, Josephsson, & Kielhofner, 2001), which followed the subjects further into retirement, yielded two findings. First, elders' narratives often had to deal with surprising turns of events. Quite unanticipated things happened. This included not only events but also how some persons felt about their situations. Interestingly, elders were often surprised at their own reactions and experiences. One example is that elders had anticipated being highly motivated to do things once they could do only what they wanted. Paradoxically, they found it more difficult to find the energy to get things done.

The second major finding of this study was that constructing a positive life story required these elders to find and participate in an engaging occupation. Engaging occupations evoked a passion or strong feeling and were a central feature in occupational narratives. They were infused with positive meaning connected to interest (i.e., pleasure, challenge, enjoyment), personal causation (i.e., challenge, indication of one's competence), and value (i.e., something worth doing, something important, a contribution to family or society). This study thus provided more information about how narratives unfold and about what is critical to the construction of a positive narrative.

Taken together these three studies validated the postulate that persons made sense of their lives and anticipated their futures through narrative. Even more important, the studies offered additional insights into how occupational narratives figure in persons' lives and into how they are constructed. In this way, the studies provided information that enriched and allowed the theory to be extended further. Finally, the studies' findings provided information useful to therapists who were attempting to help their clients construct positive occupational narratives.

Types of Studies Characterizing MOHO-Based Applied Research

Applied research addresses questions on a continuum of events that occur in providing individual services or in a program, as shown in *Figure 26.4*. This means that the types of applied research fall in the following categories:

- Psychometric studies leading to development of structured assessments
- Studies of how concepts influence therapeutic reasoning and practice
- Studies that examine what happens in therapy
- Outcomes studies.

These types of applied research are examined next.

Psychometric Studies Leading to Development of Structured Assessments

As discussed in Chapter 12, research that supports development of structured assessments seeks to ensure the dependability of those methods (Benson & Schell, 1997). A dependable information-gathering method is reliable and yields consistent information in different circumstances, at different times, with different clients, and when different therapists administer it. For example, Biernacki (1993) examined the inter-rater reliability of the Worker Role Interview (WRI) by comparing the ratings of three different therapists who interviewed 30 adults receiving rehabilitation. She also interviewed 20 of the subjects a second time to test-retest reliability. The study found the assessment to have good inter-rater and test-retest reliability.

A dependable information-gathering method must also provide the information it is intended to provide. MOHO concepts point toward certain phenomena. Assessments must capture information on these specific phenomena to ensure the validity of the decisions based on the assessment findings.

Studies that build validity often begin by examining whether the content of an assessment is coherent and representative of what is intended to be gathered (i.e., content validity). Thus, items on an assessment may be examined for the extent to which they cohere to reflect the underlying concept. Sometimes this is done by gathering the opinions of experts. For example, Brollier, Watts, Bauer, and Schmidt (1989) examined content validity of the Assessment of Occupational Functioning (AOF) by asking 15 occupational therapists to match the 25 items in the assessment to MOHO concepts of volition, personal causation, interests, roles, habits, and skills. Based on the responses of these therapists, the researchers concluded that the AOF adequately covered the domain of content of the six concepts.

Another approach to examining content validity is statistical analysis of the items to determine whether they coalesce to identify an underlying trait. Forsyth, Lai, and Kielhofner (1999) examined 52 therapists' ratings of 117 subjects and found evidence that the items on the Assessment of Communication and Interaction Skills (ACIS) coalesced well to capture this area of skill.

FIGURE 26.4 Applied research questions.

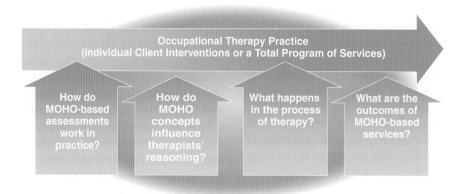

As noted in the discussion of basic research, studies such as these also serve to provide evidence about the underlying concept the assessment is designed to capture. Thus, they have both the applied purpose of developing an assessment for use in therapy and the basic purpose of providing evidence about the concept on which the assessment gathers information.

Other research that examines validity asks whether the assessments correlate with measures of concepts which are expected to concur and whether it diverges from those with which no relationship is expected. Brollier, Watts, Bauer, and Schmidt (1988) demonstrated that the AOF was correlated, as expected, with a well-known measure of adaptation, the Global Assessment Scale (GAS), when both were administered to 41 persons with a primary diagnosis of schizophrenia.

Another way of examining the validity of decisions based on assessments is to determine whether they can differentiate between groups of people. An example of this type of study is an investigation by Viik, Watts, Madigan, and Bauer (1990) in which the AOF was administered to 24 adults undergoing inpatient treatment for alcoholism and 24 adults with at least 1 year of alcohol abstinence and attendance at Alcoholics Anonymous meetings. The rater who scored the AOF was unaware of the subjects' group membership. AOF scores correctly sorted all but 3 of 48 subjects into the correct group.

In addition to studies that examine reliability and validity, some studies examine the clinical utility of assessments. For example, Fossey (1996) examined the

use of the OPHI by British therapists who were assessing persons with psychiatric disabilities. She concluded that the therapists found the interview useful for planning intervention, but she also made recommendations for improving the utility of the assessment.

The development of any MOHO assessment ordinarily involves a series of studies. These studies not only provide evidence about the reliability, validity, and utility of each assessment but also contribute to the ongoing improvement of the assessment. Some of the assessments are quite extensively studied, whereas others are still in development, as noted in Chapters 15 to 18.

Studies of How MOHO Theory Influences Therapeutic Reasoning

Chapter 11 emphasized that therapists should actively use MOHO theory and technology in their therapeutic reasoning. An important area of research is to examine how therapists use the theory and related tools in practice. One such investigation is a survey by Muñoz, Lawlor, and Kielhofner (1993) that examined the use of MOHO among 50 skilled occupational therapists and identified which concepts therapists most actively used in their practices.

A study by Oakley, Kielhofner, and Barris (1985) examined how information from MOHO-based assessments influenced therapists' ability to make judgments about clients. In this study, the results of a battery of MOHO-based assessments on 30 persons hospitalized for psychiatric illness were given to a therapist who was blind to the identities of the clients. The therapist reviewed the assessment results and rated each subject on a scale of adaptiveness. The therapist's judgment was found to be an excellent predictor of the patients' adaptive behaviors as rated by nursing staff. This study provides evidence that therapists who use MOHO concepts and assessments can effectively discriminate between levels of adaptive potential in clients.

Studies that scrutinize the use of theory by therapists examine how the theory affects practice. These studies also highlight which concepts in the theory are most helpful to therapists (Lee, Taylor, Keilhofner, & Fisher, in press). Thus, such studies provide critical information about how the theory can be altered to be more relevant to practitioners.

Studies That Examine What Happens in Therapy

It is important not only to understand whether interventions based on a model of practice work, but also to know why they do or do not work. Studies that examine the impact of interventions increasingly focus on identifying the underlying mechanism of change (Gitlin, Corcoran, Martindale-Adams, Malone, Stevens, & Winter, 2000). Examining what goes in therapy to improve services before they are more formally tested is often an important prelude to designing intervention outcome studies.

The following studies examined what happened in therapy. Helfrich and Kielhofner (1994) examined how clients' occupational narratives influenced the meaning they assigned to occupational therapy. This study showed how the meanings of therapy intended by therapists were often not received by or in concert with clients' meaning. The findings underscored the importance of therapists knowing the client's narrative and organizing therapy as a series of events that enter into that narrative.

Kielhofner and Barrett (1997) examined occupational therapists' use of goal setting in therapy. Their findings illustrate that therapists actively worked both to give substance to the occupational form of goal setting and to surround it with an implied progressive narrative in which the client makes short-term efforts to affect the long-term outcomes of the narrative. At the same time, clients' assigned meaning to therapy is based on their own narratives. When the two narratives did not coincide, therapists ended up encouraging clients toward attitudes and performances that did not resonate with their experience of reality.

Studies such as these illuminate, from the perspective of MOHO concepts, aspects of the dynamics of therapy. They provide specific information about how therapy can be improved to meet client needs and support clients to achieve desired change. More studies that carefully examine what goes on in therapy are needed to illuminate the dynamics of therapy and more clearly illuminate the nature of client change.

Outcomes Studies

Outcomes research is concerned with the results of applying MOHO in practice. Such studies examine whether therapy based on the model's theory and technology for application produces desirable outcomes. The development of outcomes studies follows a process (Case-Smith, 1999) in which a variety of the research strategies are integrated over time into an ongoing program of research, culminating in large-scale studies. The following is an example of this process.

At the University of Illinois at Chicago, investigators several years ago began to develop measures of psychosocial and environmental factors relevant to work success (Haglund, Karlsson, Kielhofner, & Lai, 1997; Kielhofner, Lai, Olson, Haglund, Ekbladh, & Hedlund 1999; Velozo et al., 1999). They developed, implemented, and documented work programs based on MOHO (Kielhofner, Braveman, Baron, Fisher, Hammel, & Littleton, 1999; Mallinson, LaPlante, & Hollman-Smith, 1998; Mentrup, Neihaus, & Kielhofner, 1999; Olson & Kielhofner, 1998). With funding from the American Occupational Therapy Foundation, a preliminary outcomes study of one of these work programs was conducted (Barrett, Beer, & Kielhofner, 1999; Kielhofner & Barrett, 1997). Subsequently, another foundation grant supported a pilot project that applied and investigated the approach with persons living with AIDS. Building on the experience and expertise developed over several years, investigators have undertaken two federally funded multiyear research and demonstration projects to investigate the outcomes of a MOHO-based work programs: Employment Options[1]

---

[1]Employment Options: A Program Leading to Employment of Persons Living with AIDS (Rehabilitation Services Administration, U.S. Department of Education, Grant no. DED H235A980170-00).

and an independent living and employment program, Enabling Self-Determination[2] (see Chapter 24). Studies of these programs have provided evidence of positive outcomes and are noted in Chapter 25.

Discussion

This chapter seeks to identify why research on a conceptual practice model is important and to characterize the kinds of studies that have examined and contributed to the development of MOHO. In the course of the discussion, types of both basic and applied research that examine MOHO were identified. Only a few of the approximately 200 published studies are used as examples.

Anyone who wishes to have a fuller appreciation of the research in a particular area should review the relevant studies directly. A bibliography of published work can be found on the MOHO Web site at *www.moho.uic.edu* under the Scholarship menu bar.

One of the most important things about MOHO research, as with research on any model, has been the establishment of a tradition of research. Within a research tradition, two important things occur:

- Findings are cumulative
- The approach to conducting research on the model is refined and becomes more sophisticated.

Cumulative Findings

As already noted, no single study can ever provide the definitive evidence to answer a research question. Therefore, it is important to generate cumulative findings (Christiansen, 1981, 1990). Over time, a growing body of evidence can be used to scrutinize and refine the theoretical arguments and the various technologies for application. This results in the following:

- More and more accurate explanations of the phenomena the model addresses
- Greater effectiveness in the model's application.

In the end, this is the fundamental purpose of research on a model. It improves the ability of the model to explain some phenomena and to generate practical actions to address those phenomena.

Refinement of Research Methodologies

Nearly 3 decades ago, when MOHO was first introduced, it was not clear how it would be studied. The research generated by a wide range of investigators has demonstrated a variety of ways in which the model can be studied. For example, the previous discussions illustrate that MOHO is being studied with a range of quantitative and qualitative research methods, and the body of research includes a number of different kinds of studies that address both basic and applied questions. The fact that many research strategies are being used to investigate this model is an important strength. Different research approaches provide different kinds of evidence that when taken together provide greater scrutiny of and insight into MOHO.

Over time, MOHO-based research has grown more sophisticated and rigorous. As one develops a tradition of research within a model, studies are able to build on the findings of previous studies, refine their approaches and methods, and provide more precise results. For example, early studies often used instruments to gather data that were relevant to but not specifically developed to capture MOHO concepts. Now that many tools have been developed for gathering data on MOHO concepts, more precise studies are possible.

Key Terms

Applied research: Investigations or aspects of investigations that aim to test the practical utility of the theory and related technology for application.

Basic research: Investigations or aspects of investigations that aim to test the theoretic arguments proposed in the model.

References

Barrett, L., Beer, D., & Kielhofner, G. (1999). The importance of volitional narrative in treatment: An ethnographic case study in a work program. *Work: A Journal of Prevention, Assessment & Rehabilitation, 12 (1),* 79–92.

Barris, R., Dickie, V., & Baron, K. (1988). A comparison of psychiatric patients and normal subjects based on the model of human occupation. *Occupational Therapy Journal of Research, 8,* 3–37.

Barris, R., Kielhofner, G., Burch, R. M., Gelinas, I., Klement, M., & Schultz, B. (1986). Occupational function and dysfunction in three groups of adolescents. *Occupational Therapy Journal of Research, 6,* 301–317.

---

[2]Enabling Self Determination, Grant #H235A980170, National Institutes of Disability and Rehabilitation Research.

Benson, J., & Schell, B. A. (1997). Measurement theory: Application to occupational and physical therapy. In Van Deusen J., & Brunt D. (Eds.), *Assessment in occupational therapy and physical therapy*. Philadelphia: Saunders.

Biernacki, S. D. (1993). Reliability of the Worker Role Interview. *American Journal of Occupational Therapy, 47,* 797–803.

Brollier, C., Watts, J. H., Bauer, D., & Schmidt, W. (1988). A content validity study of the Assessment of Occupational Functioning. *Occupational Therapy in Mental Health, 8 (4),* 29–47.

Case-Smith, J. (1999). Developing a research career: Advice from occupational therapy researchers. *American Journal of Occupational Therapy, 53,* 44–50.

Chen, C., Neufeld, P. S., Feely, C. A., & Skinner, C. S. (1999). Factors influencing compliance with home exercise programs among patients with upper-extremity impairment. *American Journal of Occupational Therapy, 53,* 171–180.

Christiansen, C. (1981). Toward resolution of crisis: Research requisites in occupational therapy. *Occupational Therapy Journal of Research, 1,* 115–124.

Christiansen, C. (1990). The perils of plurality. *Occupational Therapy Journal of Research, 10,* 259–265.

Crombie, I. K. (1996). *The pocket guide to critical appraisal.* London: BMJ.

Davies Hallet, J., Zasler, N., Maurer, P., & Cash, S. (1994). Role change after traumatic brain injury in adults. *American Journal of Occupational Therapy, 48,* 241–246.

Dickerson, A. E., & Oakley, F. (1995). Comparing the roles of community-living persons and patient populations. *American Journal of Occupational Therapy, 49,* 221–228.

Doble, S. E. (1991). Test-retest and inter-rater reliability of a process skills assessment. *Occupational Therapy Journal of Research, 11,* 8–23.

Duellman, M. K., Barris, R., & Kielhofner, G. (1986). Organized activity and the adaptive status of nursing home residents. *American Journal of Occupational Therapy, 40,* 618–622.

Ebb, E. W., Coster, W., & Duncombe, L. (1989). Comparison of normal and psychosocially dysfunctional male adolescents. *Occupational Therapy in Mental Health, 9,* 53–74.

Ekbladh, E., Haglund, L., & Thorell, L.-H. (2004). The Worker Role Interview: Preliminary data on the predictive validity of return to work of clients after an insurance medicine investigation. *Journal of Occupational Rehabilitation, 14 (2),* 131–141.

Forsyth, K., Lai, J., & Kielhofner, G. (1999). The assessment of communication and interaction skills (ACIS): Measurement properties. *British Journal of Occupational Therapy, 62 (2),* 69–74.

Fossey, E. (1996). Using the occupational performance history interview (OPHI): Therapists' reflections. *British Journal of Occupational Therapy, 59 (5),* 223–228.

Gitlin, L. N, Corcoran, M., Martindale-Adams, J., Malone, M. A., Stevens, A., & Winter, L. (2000). Identifying mechanisms of action: Why and how does intervention work? In R. Schulz (Ed.), *Handbook of dementia caregiving: Evidence-based interventions for family caregivers.* New York: Springer.

Haglund, L., Karlsson, G., Kielhofner, G., & Lai, J. S. (1997). Validity of the Swedish version of the Worker Role Interview. *Scandinavian Journal of Occupational Therapy, 4,* 23–29.

Helewa, A., & Walker, J. M. (2000). *Critical evaluation of research in physical rehabilitation: Towards evidence-based practice.* Philadelphia: Saunders.

Helfrich, C., & Kielhofner, G. (1994). Volitional narratives and the meaning of occupational therapy. *American Journal of Occupational Therapy, 48,* 319–326.

Henry, A. D. (1994). *Predicting psychosocial functioning and symptomatic recovery of adolescents and young adults with a first psychotic episode: A six-month follow-up study.* Unpublished doctoral dissertation, Boston University.

Holm, M. (2000). The 2000 Eleanor Clarke Slagle Lecture. Our mandate for the new millennium: Evidence-based practice. *American Journal of Occupational Therapy, 54,* 575–585.

Jonsson, H., Josephsson, S., & Kielhofner, G. (2001). Narratives and experience in an occupational transition: A longitudinal study of the retirement process. *American Journal of Occupational Therapy, 55,* 424–432.

Jonsson, H., Josephsson, S., & Kielhofner, G. (2000). Evolving narratives in the course of retirement: A longitudinal study. *American Journal of Occupational Therapy, 54,* 463–470.

Jonsson, H., Kielhofner, G., & Borell, L. (1997). Anticipating retirement: The formation of narratives concerning an occupational transition. *American Journal of Occupational Therapy, 51,* 49–56.

Kavanaugh, M. (1982). *Person-environment interaction: The model of human occupation applied to mentally retarded adults.* Unpublished masters thesis, Virginia Commonwealth University.

Kielhofner, G. (1985). *A model of human occupation: Theory and application* (2nd ed.). Baltimore: Williams & Wilkins.

Kielhofner, G., & Barrett, L. (1997). Meaning and misunderstanding in occupational forms: A study of therapeutic goal-setting. *American Journal of Occupational Therapy, 52 (5),* 345–353.

Kielhofner, G., Braveman, B., Baron, K., Fischer, G., Hammel, J., & Littleton, M. (1999). The model of human occupation: understanding the worker who is injured or disabled. *Work: A Journal of Prevention, Assessment & Rehabilitation, 12,* 3–11.

Kielhofner, G., Lai, J. S., Olson, L., Haglund, L., Ekbladh, E., & Hedlund, M. (1999). Psychometric properties of the work environment impact scale: A cross-cultural study. *Work: A Journal of Prevention, Assessment & Rehabilitation, 12,* 71–77.

Lederer, J., Kielhofner, G., & Watts, J. (1985). Values, personal causation and skills of delinquents and non delinquents. *Occupational Therapy in Mental Health, 5,* 59–77.

Lee, S., Taylor, R., Kielhofner, G., & Fisher, G. (in press). Theory use in practice: A national survey of therapists who use the Model of Human Occupation. *American Journal of Occupational Therapy.*

Mallinson, T., Kielhofner, G., & Mattingly, C. (1996). Metaphor and meaning in a clinical interview. *American Journal of Occupational Therapy,* 50, 338–346.

Mallinson, T., LaPlante, D., & Hollman-Smith, J. (1998). *Work rehabilitation in mental health programs.* Chicago: Model of Human Occupation Clearinghouse, Department of Occupational Therapy, College of Applied Health Sciences, University of Illinois.

Mallinson, T., Mahaffey, L., & Kielhofner, G. (1998). The occupational performance history interview: Evidence for three underlying constructs of occupational adaptation. *Canadian Journal of Occupational Therapy, 65,* 219–228.

Mentrup, C., Niehaus, A., & Kielhofner, G. (1999). Applying the model of human occupation in work-focused rehabilitation: A case illustration. *Work: A Journal of Prevention, Assessment & Rehabilitation, 12,* 61–70.

Mosey, A. C. (1992a). *Applied scientific inquiry in the health professions: An epistemological orientation.* Rockville, MD: American Occupational Therapy Association.

Mosey, A. C. (1992b). Partition of occupational science and occupational therapy. *American Journal of Occupational Therapy, 4,* 851.

Muñoz, J., Lawlor, M., & Kielhofner, G. (1993). Use of the model of human occupation in psychiatric practice: A survey of skilled therapists. *Occupational Therapy Journal of Research, 13,* 117–139.

Neville-Jan, A. (1994). The relationship of volition to adaptive occupational behavior among individuals with varying degrees of depression. *Occupational Therapy in Mental Health, 12,* 1–18.

Oakley, F., Kielhofner, G., & Barris, R. (1985). An occupational therapy approach to assessing psychiatric patients' adaptive functioning. *American Journal of Occupational Therapy, 39,* 147–154.

Oakley, F., Kielhofner, G., Barris, R., & Reichler, R. K. (1986). The Role Checklist: Development and empirical assessment of reliability. *Occupational Therapy Journal of Research, 6,* 157–170.

Olson, L. M., & Kielhofner, G. (1998). *Work readiness: Day treatment for persons with chronic disabilities.* Chicago: Model of Human Occupation Clearinghouse, Department of Occupational Therapy, College of Applied Health Sciences, University of Illinois.

Pan, A. W., & Fisher, A. G. (1994). The assessment of motor and process skills of persons with psychiatric disorders. *American Journal of Occupational Therapy, 48,* 775–780.

Peterson, E., Howland, J., Kielhofner, G., Lachman, M. E., Assmann, S., Cote, J., & Jette, A. (1999). Falls self-efficacy and occupational adaptation among elders. *Physical & Occupational Therapy in Geriatrics, 16,* 1–16.

Rust, K., Barris, R., & Hooper, F. (1987). Use of the model of human occupation to predict women's exercise behavior. *Occupational Therapy Journal of Research, 7,* 23–35.

Taylor, M. C. (2000). *Evidence-based practice for occupational therapists.* Osney Mead, Oxford: Blackwell Science.

Velozo, C., Kielhofner, G., Gern, A., Lin, F-L., Azhar, F., Lai, J-S., & Fisher, G. (1999). Worker Role Interview: Validation of a psychosocial work-related measure. *Journal of Occupational Rehabilitation, 9,* 153–168.

Viik, M. K., Watts, J. H., Madigan, M. J., & Bauer, D. (1990). Preliminary validation of the Assessment of Occupational Functioning with an alcoholic population. *Occupational Therapy in Mental Health, 10* (2), 19–33.

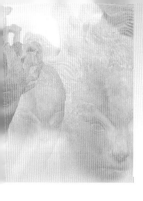

27

The Model of Human Occupation, the ICF, and the Occupational Therapy Practice Framework: Connections to Support Best Practice Around the World

- Jessica Kramer

- Patricia Bowyer

- Gary Kielhofner

In Taiwan, an occupational therapy researcher presents findings from her recent study based on MOHO. She is speaking to an audience of health professionals and doctors who often use the International Classification of Functioning, Disability and Health (ICF) to describe participation outcomes. Therefore, so that other professionals will understand the significance of her outcomes, she must translate MOHO based concepts to the ICF components and domains.

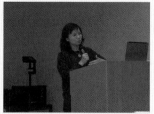

Dr. Ay-Woan Pan presents her MOHO-based research findings to other international health professionals.

A therapist working in a pubic school in the United States has been encouraged by his supervisor to assess students' occupational performance, performance skills, and performance patterns as detailed in the American

Occupational Therapy Association's Occupational Therapy Practice Framework. He must translate findings from MOHO assessments to report his evaluation with the OT Practice Framework Domains and Processes.

An occupational therapist collaborates with other rehabilitation professionals to assess a student's occupational performance. (Photo courtesy of Leon Kirschner, OTR/L.)

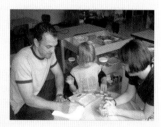

Almost since its inception, MOHO has been used by international therapists working in a variety of contexts. These therapists often work in settings that use classification frameworks to organize rehabilitation and/or occupational therapy service provision. These are two of the most widely influential frameworks affecting occupational therapy:

- The International Classification of Functioning, Disability, and Health (ICF)

- The American Occupational Therapy Association's (AOTA) Occupational Therapy Practice Framework (OT Practice Framework).

This chapter discusses how MOHO is aligned with the ICF and OT Practice Framework to support practitioners who use MOHO along with these frameworks. It also demonstrates how MOHO concepts and assessments correspond with these frameworks.

The World Health Organization's International Classification of Function, Disability, & Health (ICF)

The World Health Organization (WHO) ICF was established to describe how people live with health conditions and to reflect the interaction between personal health factors and contextual factors (WHO, 2001). The ICF was also an attempt to encourage collaboration and understanding among international researchers and health care workers. The ICF was developed by the WHO after the disability community critiqued its predecessor, the International Classification of Impairment, Disability, & Health, for ignoring environmental factors as inhibiting participation (Dahl, 2002; Hemmingsson & Jonsson, 2005). The ICF is intended to provide an international and interdisciplinary framework for talking about health and disability in research, health policy, and service provision (Stuki, Cieza, Ewert, Kostanjsek, Chatterji, & Bedirhan Ustun, 2002).

Internationally, occupational therapy practitioners and researchers may use the ICF to talk with other professionals about their clients. These therapists may want to better understand how MOHO concepts are related to the ICF. This chapter illustrates how MOHO concepts are aligned with ICF components and domains and demonstrates how MOHO-based assessments can be used to gather information about a client's body functions, participation, activity, and environmental factors.

There are several similarities between MOHO and the ICF:

- Both MOHO and the ICF recognize the centrality of participation and activity as an outcome
- Both MOHO and the ICF recognize that health conditions can alter a person's participation
- Both MOHO and the ICF recognize that individual characteristics and the environment determine participation and activity
- Both MOHO and the ICF recognize that these various factors influence each other in a dynamic and nonlinear way.

MOHO and the ICF both explicate broad aspects of engaging in one's everyday life. For example, MOHO describes several levels of doing: participation, performance, and skill (see Chapter 8). These levels of doing are aligned with ICF components of participation and activity, as illustrated in *Table 27.1*.

Beyond these broad concepts of engagement, MOHO concepts are aligned with ICF domains and categories that detail the ways in which that engagement is impacted by personal and environmental factors. In *Table 27.2*, ICF concepts and definitions are listed next to complementary MOHO concepts. The codes provided in parentheses in the "ICF Domain and Category" columns are taken from the ICF and represent some of the specific categories that the MOHO concept is aligned with.

MOHO concepts align with ICF concepts in different ways and at different levels of specificity. As featured in *Table 27.2*, the MOHO concept *volition* is aligned with the ICF category *motivation* under the ICF domain of mental functioning. Motivation, which the ICF defines as the "incentive to act" and "the conscious or unconscious driving force for action," is similar to the MOHO concept of a volitional drive to act. In this instance, the MOHO and ICF concepts are highly similar in a specific way. However, MOHO's concept of occupational performance is broadly similar to the ICF domain *major life area*, as they both refer to carrying out tasks associated with major life roles such as work and education. Here, occupational performance reflects aspects of every category in the domain of *major life area*.

Finally, several MOHO concepts can be aligned with one ICF domain and its categories. For example, MOHO's concept of social groups is aligned with the ICF domain *attitudes* in that social groups considers the attitudes held at the individual level and small group level. However, MOHO's definition of culture is better aligned with the specific *attitude* categories *societal attitudes* and *social norms, practices, and ideologies*. Clinicians or researchers who would like to go deeper to explore the connections between ICF and MOHO concepts are encouraged to refer to the brief ICF glossary in the back of this chapter or to refer directly to the ICF text.

MOHO assessments can also provide information to researchers and clinicians who are using the ICF to communicate with other disciplines. Haglund and Henriksson (2003) conducted research with a panel of

TABLE 27.1 Intersections Between MOHO and the ICF Describing Engagement

MOHO Levels of Doing	ICF Components	Explanation of Intersection
Occupational participation	Participation	While ICF concept of participation encompasses a variety of domains, MOHO defines participation as engagement in work, play, or ADL specific to contexts addressed in occupational therapy.
Occupational performance	Activity	Both involve engagement in a specific task.
Skill		No comparable ICF concept for MOHO concept of skill, a fine-grained examination of performance (i.e., all performance requires exercise of a number of skills) (see Chapter 8)

ADL, activities of daily living.

occupational therapy experts in Sweden to determine how the items on the Assessment of Communication and Interaction Skills (ACIS) were aligned with ICF concepts. This panel found that 60% of the skill items were equivalent to items in the ICIDH-2, which was very similar to the ICF in the categories included in their study. Several of the concepts represented by the ACIS items correlated with more than one ICIDH-2 item, which Haglund and Henriksson (2003) suggest is because the ACIS is a profession-specific assessment and occupational therapy language complements, not replicates, the concepts in the ICF. *Table 27.3* lists MOHO-based assessments that can be used to gather information about the components, domains, and categories previously identified as being aligned with MOHO concepts.

As noted in *Table 27.2*, MOHO is not perfectly aligned with ICF (see also Stamm, Cieza, Machold, Smolen, & Stucki, 2006). This is because the frameworks stem from different theoretic backgrounds. MOHO is an occupational therapy–based practice model, therefore predominantly concerned with people's meaningful participation in culturally and personally relevant occupations. Conversely, the ICF, which attempts to classify function in relation to health, stems from a biopsychosocial perspective (Dahl, 2002; Hemmingsson & Jonsson, 2005) that seeks to understand the effect of disease on function (see the WHO's related *International Classification of Diseases*). The most notable difference between these two theoretic backgrounds is MOHO's concern with the experience and meaning of participation and the recognition of the client as the author of his or her own occupational narratives; the

ICF does not consider the experience of doing and autonomy in doing in the classification (Hemmingsson & Jonsson, 2005).

The purpose of the ICF and MOHO also differ, affecting the extent to which their concepts are aligned. The ICF is an interdisciplinary tool, while MOHO is specific to occupational therapy. In addition, while MOHO seeks both to describe and to explain how occupational adaptation occurs, the ICF is a classification system for describing health and effects of health on participation.

Although the ICF is a powerful tool (Dahl, 2002), it is important to consider its limitations. One unclear aspect of the ICF classification system is that the domains related to the main components of *activity and participation* are listed together and not distinguished as belonging to activity, participation, or both. For example, *learning and applying knowledge* and engaging in *community, social, and civic life* are depicted as equivalent domains, without a clear delineation of either's association with the ICF component of activity or participation. This makes it difficult to determine the exact challenges an individual is facing. For example, if an individual is having difficulty engaging in community life, is it a participation problem or an activity problem? If a client is having difficulty learning and applying knowledge, will it impact activity or participation? This ambiguity in the ICF fails to provide the mechanism to acknowledge that "different kinds of participation can appear in a single life situation" (Hemmingsson & Jonsson, 2005, p. 574). In contrast, MOHO helps therapists to differentiate between observed performance (skill), the execution of a task or

TABLE 27.2 ICF Components, Domains, and Categories and Related MOHO Concepts

ICF Components	ICF Domains & Categories*	MOHO Concept
Body Functions	*Mental functions*	
	Orientation to time (b1140)	Habituation
	Intellectual functions (b117)	Performance capacity
	Confidence (b1266)	Personal causation
	Motivation (b1301)	Volition
	Attention (b140), higher-level cognitive functions (b164), mental functions of language (b167)	Communication/interaction skills
	Higher-level cognitive functions (b164)	Process skills
	Sequencing complex movements (b176)	Motor skills
	Sensory functions and pain	Objective and subjective performance capacity
	Voice and speech functions	Communication/interaction skills
	Articulation (b320)	
	Fluency and rhythm of speech (b330)	
	Alternative vocalization functions (b340)	
	Neuromusculoskeletal and movement-related functions	Objective performance capacity
	Control of voluntary movement functions (b760)	Motor skills
Body Structures		Objective performance capacity
Activity Participation	*Learning and Applying Knowledge*	
	Applying knowledge (d160–179)	Process skills
	General Tasks and Demands	
	Carrying out daily routine (d230)	Habituation
	Handling responsibilities (d2400)	Process skills
	Carrying out single and multiple tasks (d210, d220)	
	Carrying out single and multiple tasks (d210, d220)	
	Carrying out daily routine (d230)	Occupational Competence
	Handling responsibilities (d2400)	Occupational Identity
	Carrying out single and multiple tasks in groups (d2103, d2203)	Communication/interaction skills
	Communication	Communication/interaction skills
	Conversation (d350)	
	Use of communication devices and techniques (d360)	
	Mobility	
	Changing and maintaining body position (d410–d429)	Motor skills
	Carrying, moving, and handling objects (d430–d449)	
	Walking and moving (d450–d469)	
	Moving around using transportation (d470–d489)	Occupational competence
	Self-Care	Occupational performance

*The codes provided in parentheses are taken from the ICF and represent the specific categories that each MOHO concept is aligned with.

(continued)

TABLE 27.2 *(continued)*

ICF Components	ICF Domains & Categories	MOHO Concept
	Domestic Life Acquisition of goods and services (d620) Household tasks (d630–d649) Caring for household objects and assisting others (d650–d669)	Occupational performance Occupational competence Occupational identity Process, motor, and communication/ interaction skills
	Interpersonal Interactions and Relationships General (d710–d729) and particular (d730–d779) interpersonal relationships Particular interpersonal relationships (d730–d779)	Communication/interaction skills Occupational identity
	Major Life Areas	Occupational performance
	Community, Social, and Civic Life Community life (d910) Recreation and leisure (d920) Religion and spirituality (d930) Political life and citizenship (d950)	Occupational participation Occupational competence Occupational identity
Environmental Factors	*Products and Technology*	Physical environment (objects & spaces)
	Natural Environment and Human-Made Changes to the Environment Physical geography (e210) Flora and fauna (e220) Climate (e225) Light (e240) Sound (e250)	Physical environment (objects & spaces)
	Support and Relationships	Social Environment (social groups)
	Attitudes Societal attitudes (e460) Social norms, practices, and ideologies (e465)	Social Environment (social groups) Culture
	Services, Systems, and Policies	Political conditions Economic conditions

TABLE 27.3 ICF Concepts and Related MOHO-based Assessments

ICF Component	ICF domain	ICF Category Examples[a]	ACIS	AMPS	Interest Checklist	MOHOST/SCOPE	OCAIRS	OPHI-II	OQ/ACTRE	OSA/COSA	OT PAL	Role Checklist	SSI	VQ/PVQ	WEIS	WRI
Body functions	Mental functions	Orientation to time, motivation, mental functions of language, higher-level cognitive functions	X		X	X	X	X	X	X	X		X	X		X
	Voice and speech functions	Articulation				X	X									
	Neuromusculoskeletal and movement functions	Control of voluntary movements		X		X	X									
	Learning and applying knowledge	Applying knowledge		X		X	X									
	General tasks and demands	Carrying out daily routine, tasks in groups	X	X		X	X	X	X	X		X	X		X	X
Activity and Participation	Communication	Conversation	X			X	X	X		X		X	X		X	
	Mobility	Carrying, moving, handling objects		X		X	X			X			X			
	Self-care			X		X			X	X		X	X			
	Domestic life	Household tasks	X					X	X	X	X	X				
	Interpersonal interactions, relationships	Interpersonal relationships				X	X	X	X	X		X	X		X	X
	Major life areas					X	X	X	X	X	X	X	X		X	X
	Community, social, civic life	Leisure and recreation			X	X	X	X	X	X		X			X	X
Environmental Factors	Products, technology	Physical geography				X	X						X	X	X	X
	Natural environment, human-made changes to environment					X	X	X					X	X	X	X
	Support, relationships					X	X	X					X	X	X	X
	Attitudes	Societal attitudes				X	X	X					X	X	X	
	Services, systems, policies					X							X		X	

[a]See Table 27-2 for more detailed information on ICF categories.

524

action (performance), and involvement in a life situation (participation) and allows therapists to understand how a personal characteristic or an environmental factor will affect each of these aspects.

Furthermore, the ICF does not take into consideration the complexity of the interaction between the environment and an individual. While the ICF recognizes that the environment contains barriers or facilitators to participation (Hemmingsson & Jonsson, 2005), MOHO provides a framework that enables a therapist to explicate how an environment can simultaneously provide constraints, demands, and resources that facilitate participation. Also, MOHO's concept of environmental impact gives an individualized view of the environment and recognizes that an environmental resource for one individual may be a constraint for another (e.g., raised toilet seat).

Finally, the ICF does not consider how change occurs and how it influences participation. MOHO explains change in many ways: an individual's sense of volition can change through the volitional process and across the volitional continuum; experiences of doing occupations can shift according to life circumstances and an individual's personal narrative; and changes to the physical and social environment may impact participation.

Therapists using the ICF as a guiding framework should also understand the disability community's critiques of the framework. Disabled activists assert that the ICF's biopsychosocial background perpetuates a medical view of disability (Pfeiffer, 2000) and continues to associate disability with health or lack thereof (Barnes, 2003). They also charge that the practice of classifying the function of disabled persons perpetuates labeling, stigmatizing, and oppressing persons with disabilities (Barnes, Mercer, & Shakespeare, 2000).

The AOTA Occupational Therapy Practice Framework

In the United States, using MOHO supports best practice for occupational therapists, as the concepts of MOHO were used to help shape and are directly aligned with the OT Practice Framework as developed by AOTA (2002). This section details the ways in which MOHO and the OT Practice Framework are aligned:

- The way the OT Practice Framework defines occupational therapy
- The specific practice domains for occupational therapists as defined by the OT Practice Framework.

The OT Practice Framework states that occupational therapy consists of evaluation, intervention, and outcomes (AOTA, 2002). This three-phase process directly corresponds with the MOHO process of therapeutic reasoning, outlined in Chapter 11. MOHO's theory-driven process of therapeutic reasoning further supports occupational therapists in evaluation, intervention, and outcomes by describing the specific actions that integrate theory with practice. It also provides a detailed examination of the occupational therapy process. *Table 27.4* shows how each step in therapeutic reasoning is part of the larger occupational therapy process.

The OT Practice Framework calls for a process that is guided by client-centered collaboration and defines a client-centered approach as "an orientation that honors the desires and priorities of clients" (Dunn, 200, p. 4, as cited in AOTA, 2002, p. 630). As noted in Chapter 11, MOHO supports client-centered collaboration because it views each client as a unique individual whose characteristics and context determine the rationale for and nature of therapy. As MOHO-based as-

TABLE 27.4 Alignment of AOTA's OT Practice Framework and MOHO's Therapeutic Reasoning

AOTA Practice Framework Steps	MOHO Therapeutic Reasoning Steps
Evaluation	Generate and use questions to guide information gathering
	Gather information on/with the client using structured and unstructured means
	Create a conceptualization of the client that includes strengths and challenges
Intervention	Identify goals and plan for therapy
	Implement and review therapy
Outcomes	Collect information to assess outcomes

Client-Centered Collaboration in the Assessment Process

When administration of an assessment tool requires the involvement of the client or the client's family or caregivers, an assessment can be said to support a formal collaboration. However, other MOHO assessments offer informal opportunities for therapists to collaborate with clients, their family, and other professionals even if it is not a requirement for the assessment administration. This includes the following:

- Gathering additional information in interviews instead of relying only on observation during the administration of the MOHOST/ SCOPE
- Talking with clients and/or someone who cares about them to identify any meaningful activity that can be observed when administering the ACIS
- Sharing client self-report responses, such as OSA/COSA results, with other professionals during interdisciplinary meetings to ensure that an absent client's voice is heard.

Taking advantage of assessments that offer both formal and informal opportunities for collaboration supports best practice and ensures that the assessment and intervention planning process remains as client driven as possible. Some example opportunities each assessment provides for collaboration are listed in the nearby table.

MOHO Assessment	Formal Collaboration Opportunities	Informal Collaboration Opportunities
ACIS ⟶		Selecting meaningful activity for observation with client
COSA ⟶	Client self-evaluation	Setting goals and intervention plan based on evaluation Sharing information with interdisciplinary team
MOHOST ⟶		Interview with client and caregiver Interview with interdisciplinary team
OCAIRS ⟶	Interview with client	
OPHI-II ⟶	Interview with client	Creating narrative slope with client
OSA ⟶	Client self-evaluation Setting goals and intervention plan based on evaluation	Sharing information with interdisciplinary team
OT PAL ⟶	Teacher interview Parent take-home interview	Interview with student
PVQ ⟶		Working with interdisciplinary team to identify activities for observation
SCOPE ⟶		Interview with client and parent Interview with interdisciplinary team
SSI ⟶	Evaluation conducted in collaboration with student Interview with student Identifying solutions and accommodations with students	Working with interdisciplinary team to identify solutions and accommodations (ie., teachers, other school support staff)

MOHO Assessment	Formal Collaboration Opportunities	Informal Collaboration Opportunities
VQ ⟶		Working with interdisciplinary team to identify activities for observation
WEIS ⟶	Interview with client	Collaborate with client to request accommodations from employer
WRI ⟶	Interview with client	

TABLE 27.5 Alignment of MOHO Concepts and OT Practice Framework (OTPF) Domains

Practice Framework Domain	Related MOHO Concept	Explanation of Alignment
Performance in occupations, Occupational performance	Occupational participation, Occupational performance	MOHO and OTFP definitions of participation both describe engagement in work, play, leisure. MOHO also considers tasks that support engagement in larger life roles in the concept of occupational performance
Performance skills: Communication/interaction Motor Process	Skills: Communication/interaction Motor Process	OTFP definitions of communication/interaction skills and process skills are supported by literature of MOHO-based theory and research Both define skill as something one does while engaging in a specific action MOHO's definition more explicitly considers the impact of the environment on skill
Performance patterns: Habits Roles	Habituation: Habits Internalized role	Both definitions recognize routine as integral to performance patterns Both MOHO and OTPF define habits as automatic responses that support performance Both MOHO and OTPF recognize that roles are delineated by socially defined actions
Context	Environment Environmental Impact Culture	Both definitions recognize that the social groups, physical space, and culture influence the client's context
Activity demands	Environment: Physical Social Occupational forms/Tasks Environmental impact	MOHO considers social and physical demands as an aspect of the environment; OTPF separates activity demands from the environment MOHO concept of environmental impact considers the dynamic relationship between the environment and the individual
Client factors	Performance capacity	MOHO's concept of objective performance capacity is aligned with OTPF's client factors MOHO also considers living with specific capacities in the subjective performance capacity concept of the lived body

sessments focus on participation rather than specific abilities, therapists are able to evaluate a client's whole occupational performance and to better understand each client's unique occupational profile. This supports the development of a top-down and client-centered intervention plan. An additional consideration for therapists working with children and youth is that collaboration occurs *not only* with the child but with their parents or caregivers and often teachers. MOHO assessments have been designed to solicit input and information to support collaboration not only with the client but with all people involved in the client's life. The box "Client-Centered Collaboration in the Assessment Process" outlines the opportunities each MOHO-based assessment offers that support a client-centered occupational therapy process.

The OT Practice Framework outlines six domains that occupational therapists may address to support participation in context. These domains and their alignment with MOHO concepts are presented in *Table 27.5*. Definitions of terms from the OT Practice Framework can be found at the glossary at the end of this chapter. Although MOHO concepts and the OT Practice

Framework domains are highly similar because they share focus on occupation and participation, the purpose of the OT Practice Framework is to describe the domain of practice, not to explain how and why occupational therapy clients have difficulty engaging in everyday life activities. As a result, MOHO definitions and OT Practice Framework domain definitions differ in their specificity, terminology, and scope. Therapists using MOHO can also use information from MOHO-based assessments to gather information relevant to the OT Practice Framework domains, as outlined in *Table 27.6*.

Conclusion

This chapter provided resources to describe how MOHO is aligned with other organizing frameworks, including the ICF and the AOTA OT Practice Framework. MOHO concepts are not in exact alignment with these frameworks because their purposes and theoretic influences differ. However, occupational therapists can use MOHO concepts and assessments to gather information relevant to both of these rehabilitation frameworks.

TABLE 27.6 The OT Practice Framework and Related MOHO-Based Assessments

OTFP Domain	ACIS	AMPS	Interest Checklist	MOHOST/SCOPE	OCAIRS	OPHI-II	OQ/ACTRE	OSA/COSA	OT PAL	Role Checklist	SSI	VQ/PVQ	WEIS	WRI
Occupational performance	X	X	X	X	X	X	X	X	X	X	X	X	X	X
Performance skills	X	X		X	X									
Performance patterns			X	X	X	X	X	X	X	X				X
Context				X	X	X		X			X	X	X	X
Activity demands	X	X		X	X	X			X		X	X	X	X

529

ICF Glossary[1]

Activity: The execution of a task or action by an individual.

Attitudes: The attitudes that are the observable consequences of customs, practices, ideologies, values, norms, factual beliefs and religious beliefs. These attitudes influence individual behavior and social life at all levels, from interpersonal relationships and community associations to political, economic and legal structures.

Body functions: Physiological functions of the body systems

Body structures: Anatomical parts of the body

Communication: This refers to general and specific features of communicating by language, signs and symbols, including receiving and producing messages, carrying on conversations, and using communication devices and techniques.

Community, social, and civic life: Refers to the actions and tasks required to engage in organized social life outside the family, in community, social and civic areas of life.

Domestic life: This refers to carrying out domestic and everyday actions and tasks. Areas of domestic life include acquiring a place to live, food, clothing and other necessities, household cleaning and repairing, caring for personal and other household objects, and assisting others.

Environmental factors: The physical, social, and attitudinal environment in which people live and conduct their lives.

General tasks and demands: Refers to general aspects of carrying out single or multiple tasks, organizing routines and handling stress. Can be used in conjunction with more specific tasks or actions to identify the underlying features of the execution of tasks under different circumstances.

Interpersonal interactions and relationships: This refers to carrying out the actions and tasks required for basic and complex interactions with people (strangers, friends, relatives, family members and partners) in a contextually and socially appropriate manner.

Learning and applying knowledge: Refers to learning, applying the knowledge that is learned, thinking, solving problems, and making decisions.

Major life areas: Refers to carrying out the tasks and actions required to engage in education, work and employment and to conduct economic transactions.

Mental functions: Functions of the brain, both global mental functions, such as consciousness, energy and drive, orientation, and temperament and personality; and specific mental functions, such as attention, memory, organization and planning, language and calculation mental functions.

Occupational Therapy Practice Framework Glossary[2]

Activity demands: The aspects of an activity, which include the objects, space, social demands, sequencing or timing, required actions, and required underlying body functioning and body structures needed to carry out the activity.

Client factors: Those factors that reside within the client and that may affect performance in areas of occupation. Client factors include body functions and body structures.

Communication/interaction skills: Conveying intentions and needs as well as coordinating social behavior to act together with people.

Context: Refers to a variety of interrelated conditions within and surrounding the client that influence performance.

Habits: Autonomic behavior that is integrated into more complex patterns that enable people to function on a day-to-day basis.

Motor skills: Skills in moving and interacting with task, objects, and environment.

Occupational performance: The ability to carry out activities of daily life . . . the accomplishment of the selected activity or occupational resulting from the dynamic transaction among the client, the context, and the activity.

Performance patterns: Patterns of behavior related to daily life activities that are habitual or routine.

Performance skills: Features of what one does, not of what one has, related to observable elements of action that have implicit functional purposes.

Process skills: Skills . . . used in managing and modifying actions en route to the completion of daily life tasks.

Roles: A set of behaviors that have some socially agreed upon function and for which there is an accepted code of norms.

References

American Occupational Therapy Association (2002). Occupational therapy practice framework: Domain and process. *American Journal of Occupational Therapy, 56,* 609–639.

---

[1]These definitions can be found at http://www3.who.int/icf/onlinebrowser/icf.cfm

[2]These definitions can be found in AOTA (2002).

Barnes, C. (2003). Rehabilitation for disabled people: A sick joke? *Scandinavian Journal of Disability Research, 5 (1),* 7–24.

Barnes, C., Mercer, G., & Shakespeare, T. (2000). *Exploring disability: A sociological introduction.* Cambridge, UK: Polity.

Dahl, T. H. (2002). International Classification of Functioning, Disability and Health: An introduction and discussion of its potential to impact on rehabilitation services and research. *Journal of Rehabilitation Medicine, 34,* 201–204.

Haglund, L., & Henriksson, C. (2003). Concepts in occupational therapy in relation to the ICF. *Occupational Therapy International, 10 (4),* 253–268.

Hemmingsson, H., & Jonsson, H. (2005). An occupational perspective on the concept of participation in the International Classification of Functioning, Disability and Health: Some critical remarks. *American Journal of Occupational Therapy, 59,* 569–576.

Pfeiffer, D. (2000). The devils are in the details: ICIDH-2 and the disability movement. *Disability and Society, 15,* 1079–1082.

Stamm, T. A., Cieza, A., Machold, K., Smolen, J. S., & Stucki, G. (2006). Exploration of the link between conceptual occupational therapy models and the International Classification of Functioning, Disability, and Health. *Australian Occupational Therapy Journal, 53,* 9–17.

Stuki, G., Cieza, A., Ewert, T., Kostanjsek, N., Chatterji, S., & Bedirhan Ustun, T. (2002). Clinical commentary: Application of the International Classification of Functioning, Disability and Health (ICF) in clinical practice. *Disability and Rehabilitation, 24 (5),* 281–282.

World Health Organization (2001). *International Classification of Functioning, Disability and Health* (ICF). Geneva: Author.

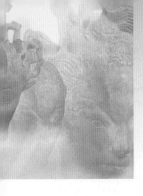

Appendix A

Bibliography

A

Abelenda, J., & Helfrich, C. (2003). Family resilience and mental illness: The role of occupational therapy. *Occupational Therapy in Mental Health, 19 (1)*, 25–39.

Abelenda, J., Kielhofner, G., Suarez-Balcazar, Y., & Kielhofner, K. (2005). The Model of Human Occupation as a conceptual tool for understanding and addressing occupational apartheid. In F. Kronenberg, S. Simo-Algado, & N. Pollard (Eds.), *Occupational Therapy without borders: Learning from the spirit of survivors* (pp. 183–196). London: Elsevier Churchill Livingstone.

Adelstein, L. A., Barnes, M. A., Murray-Jensen, F., & Skaggs, C. B. (1989). A broadening frontier: Occupational therapy in mental health programs for children and adolescents. *Mental Health Special Interest Section Newsletter, 12*, 2–4.

Affleck, A., Bianchi, E., Cleckley, M., Donaldson, K., McCormack, G., & Polon, J. (1984). Stress management as a component of occupational therapy in acute care settings. *Occupational Therapy in Health Care, 1 (3)*, 17–41.

Anderson, S., Kielhofner, G., & Lai, J. S. (2005). An examination of the measurement properties of the pediatric volitional questionnaire. *Physical and Occupational Therapy in Pediatrics, 25 (1/2)*, 39–57.

Apte, A., Kielhofner, G., Paul-Ward, A., & Braveman, B. (2005). Therapists' and clients' perceptions of the occupational performance history interview. *Occupational Therapy in Health Care, 19 (1/2)*, 173–192.

Arnsten, S. M. (1990). Intrinsic Motivation. *American Journal of Occupational Therapy, 44*, 462–463.

Asmundsdottir, E. E. (2004). The worker role interview: A powerful tool in Icelandic work rehabilitation. *Work: A Journal of Prevention, Assessment & Rehabilitation, 22 (1)*, 21–26.

Aubin, G., Hachey, R., & Mercier, C. (1999). Meaning of daily activities and subjective quality of life in people with severe mental illness. *Scandinavian Journal of Occupational Therapy, 6*, 53–62.

Aubin, G., Hachey, R., & Mercier, C. (2002). The significance of daily activities in persons with severe mental disorders [French]. *Canadian Journal of Occupational Therapy, 69*, 218–228.

Ay-Woan, P., Sarah, C. P., LyInn, C., Tsyr-Jang, C., & Ping-Chuan, H. (2006). Quality of life in depression: Predictive models. *Quality of Life Research, 15*, 39–48.

B

Baker, F., Curbow, B., & Wingard, J. R. (1991). Role retention and quality of life of bone marrow transplant survivors. *Social Science and Medicine, 32*, 697–704.

Banks, S., Bell, E., & Smits, E. (2000). Integration tutorials and seminars: Examining the integration of academic and fieldwork learning by student occupational therapists. *Canadian Journal of Occupational Therapy, 67*, 93–100.

Baron, K. (1987). The Model of Human Occupation: A newspaper treatment group for adolescents with a diagnosis of conduct disorder. *Occupational Therapy in Mental Health, 7 (2)*, 89–104.

Baron, K. (1989). Occupational therapy: A program for child psychiatry. *Mental Health Special Interest Section Newsletter, 12*, 6–7.

Baron, K. (1991). The use of play in child psychiatry: Reframing the therapeutic environment. *Occupational Therapy in Mental Health, 11 (2/3)*, 37–56.

Baron, K., Kielhofner, G., Iyenger, A., Goldhammer, V., & Wolenski, J. (2006). *The Occupational Self Assessment (OSA) (Version 2.2)*. Chicago: Model of Human Occupation Clearinghouse, Department of

Occupational Therapy, College of Applied Health Sciences, University of Illinois.

Baron, K., & Littleton, M. J. (1999). The Model of Human Occupation: A return to work case study. *Work: A Journal of Prevention, Assessment, and Rehabilitation, 12,* 37–46.

Barrett, L., Beer, D., & Kielhofner, G. (1999). The importance of volitional narrative in treatment: An ethnographic case study in a work program. *Work: A Journal of Prevention, Assessment, and Rehabilitation, 12,* 79–92.

Barris, R. (1982). Environmental interactions: An extension of the Model of Human Occupation. *American Journal of Occupational Therapy, 36,* 637–644.

Barris, R. (1986). Occupational dysfunction and eating disorders: Theory and approach to treatment. *Occupational Therapy in Mental Health, 6 (1),* 27–45.

Barris, R. (1986). Activity: The interface between person and environment. *Physical and Occupational Therapy in Geriatrics, 5 (2),* 39–49.

Barris, R., Dickie, V., & Baron, K. (1988). A comparison of psychiatric patients and normal subjects based on the Model of Human Occupation. *Occupational Therapy Journal of Research, 8* (1), 3–37.

Barris, R., Kielhofner, G., Burch, R. M., Gelinas, I., Klement, M., & Schultz, B. (1986). Occupational function and dysfunction in three groups of adolescents. *Occupational Therapy Journal of Research, 6,* 301–317.

Barris, R., Oakley, F., & Kielhofner, G. (1988). The Role Checklist. In B.J. Hemphill (Ed.), *Mental Health Assessment in Occupational Therapy: An integrative approach to the evaluative process* (pp. 73–91). Thorofare, NJ: Slack.

Barrows, C. (1996). Clinical interpretation of "Predictors of functional outcome among adolescents and young adults with psychotic disorders." *American Journal of Occupational Therapy, 50,* 182–183.

Basu, S., Jacobson, L., & Keller, J. (2004). Child-centered tools: Using the model of human occupation framework. *School System Special Interest Section Quarterly, 11 (2),* 1–3.

Basu, S., Kafkes, A., Geist, R., & Kielhofner, G. (2002). *The Pediatric Volitional Questionnaire (PVQ) (Version 2.0).* Chicago: Model of Human Occupation Clearinghouse, Department of Occupational Therapy, College of Applied Health Sciences, University of Illinois.

Bavaro, S. M. (1991). Occupational therapy and obsessive-compulsive disorder. *American Journal of Occupational Therapy, 45,* 456–458.

Bernspang, B., & Fisher, A. (1995). Differences between persons with right or left cerebral vascular accident on the Assessment of Motor and Process Skills. *Archives of Physical Medicine and Rehabilitation, 76,* 1144–1151.

Biernacki, S. D. (1993). Reliability of the Worker Role Interview. *American Journal of Occupational Therapy, 47,* 797–803.

Bjorklund, A., & Henriksson, M. (2003). On the context of elderly persons' occupational performance. *Physical and Occupational Therapy in Geriatrics, 21,* 49–58.

Blakeney, A. (1985). Adolescent development: An application to the Model of Human Occupation. *Occupational Therapy in Health Care, 2 (3),* 19–40.

Boisvert, R. A. (2004, May 31). Enhancing substance dependence intervention. *Occupational Therapy Practice,* 11–16.

Borell, L., Gustavsson, A., Sandman, P., & Kielhofner, G. (1994). Occupational programming in a day hospital for patients with dementia. *Occupational Therapy Journal of Research, 14 (4),* 219–238.

Borell, L., Sandman, P., & Kielhofner, G. (1991). Clinical decision making in Alzheimer's disease. *Occupational Therapy in Mental Health, 11 (4),* 111–124.

Bowyer, P., Kramer, J., Kielhofner, G., Maziero Barbosa, V., & Girolami, G. (2007). The measurement properties of the Short Child Occupational Profile (SCOPE). *Physical and Occupational Therapy in Pediatrics,* 27(4), (pages not assigned).

Bowyer, P., Ross, M., Schwartz, O., Kielhofner, G., & Kramer, J. (2005). *The Short Child Occupational Profile (SCOPE) (Version 2.1).* Chicago: Model of Human Occupation Clearinghouse, Department of Occupational Therapy, College of Applied Health Sciences, University of Illinois.

Branholm, I., & Fulg-Meyer, A. R. (1992). Occupational role preferences and life satisfaction. *Occupational Therapy Journal of Research, 12 (3),* 159–171.

Braveman, B. (1999). The Model of Human Occupation and prediction of return to work: A review of related empirical research. *Work: A Journal of Prevention, Assessment, and Rehabilitation, 12,* 13–23.

Braveman, B. (2001). Development of a community-based return to work program for people with AIDS. *Occupational Therapy in Health Care, 13 (3/4),* 113–131.

Braveman, B., & Helfrich, C. (2001). Occupational identity: Exploring the narratives of three men living with AIDS. *Journal of Occupational Science, 8 (2),* 25–31.

Braveman, B., Helfrich, C., & Kielhofner, G. (2003). The narratives of 12 men with AIDS: Exploring return to work. *The Journal of Occupational Rehabilitation, 13 (3),* 143–157.

Braveman, B., Helfrich, C., Kielhofner, G., & Albrecht, G. (2004). The experiences of 12 men with AIDS who attempted to return to work. *The Israel Journal of Occupational Therapy, 13,* E69–E83.

Braveman, B., & Kielhofner, G. (2006). Developing evidence-based occupational therapy programming. In B. Braveman (Ed.), *Leading and managing occupational therapy services: An evidence-based approach* (pp 215–244). Philadelphia: FA Davis.

Braveman, B., Kielhofner, G., Albrecht, G., & Helfrich, C. (2006). Occupational identity, occupational competence, and occupational settings (environment): Influence on return to work in men living with HIV/AIDS. *Work: A Journal of Prevention, Assessment, and Rehabilitation,* 27(3), 267–276.

Braveman, B., Robson, M., Velozo, C., Kielhofner, G., Fisher, G., Forsyth, K., & Kerschbaum, J. (2005). *Worker Role Interview (WRI) (Version 10.0).* Chicago: Model of Human Occupation Clearinghouse, Department of Occupational Therapy, College of Applied Health Sciences, University of Illinois.

Braveman, B., Sen, S., & Kielhofner, G. (2001). Community-based vocational rehabilitation programs. In M. Scaffa (Ed.), *Occupational therapy in community-based practice settings* (pp. 139–162). Philadelphia: FA Davis.

Briand, C., Bélanger, R., Hamel, V., Nicole, L., Stip, E., Reinharz, D., Lalonde, P., & Lesage, A.D. (2005). Implantation multisite du programme Integrated Psychological Treatment (IPT) pour les personnes souffrant de schizophrénie. Élaboration d'une version renouvelée. *Santé mentale au Québec, 30,* 73–95.

Bridgett, B. (1993). Occupational therapy evaluation for patients with eating disorders. *Occupational Therapy in Mental Health, 12 (2),* 79–89.

Bridle, M. J., Lynch, K. B., & Quesenberry, C. M. (1990). Long term function following the central cord syndrome. *Paraplegia, 28,* 178–185.

Broadley, H. (1991). Assessment guidelines based on the Model of Human Occupation. *World Federation of Occupational Therapists: Bulletin, 23,* 34–35.

Brollier, C., Watts, J. H., Bauer, D., & Schmidt, W. (1988). A content validity study of the Assessment of Occupational Functioning. *Occupational Therapy in Mental Health, 8 (4),* 29–47.

Brollier, C., Watts, J. H., Bauer, D., & Schmidt, W. (1988). A concurrent validity study of two occupational therapy evaluation instruments: The AOF and OCAIRS. *Occupational Therapy in Mental Health, 8 (4),* 49–59.

Brown, G. T., Brown, A., & Roever, C. (2005). Paediatric occupational therapy university programme curricula in the United Kingdom. *British Journal of Occupational Therapy, 68,* 457–466.

Brown, T., & Carmichael, K. (1992). Assertiveness training for clients with psychiatric illness: A pilot study. *British Journal of Occupational Therapy, 55,* 137–140.

Bruce, M., & Borg, B. (1993). The Model of Human Occupation. In *Psychosocial Occupational Therapy: Frames of Reference for Intervention* (Second ed., pp. 145–175). Thorofare, NJ: Slack.

Buning, M. E., Angelo, J. A., & Schmeler, M. R. (2001). Occupational performance and the transition to powered mobility: A pilot study. *American Journal of Occupational Therapy, 55,* 339–344.

Burke, J. P. (1998). Commentary: Combining the Model of Human Occupation with cognitive disability theory. *Occupational Therapy in Mental Health, 8,* xi–xiii.

Burke, J. P., Clark, F., Dodd, C., & Kawamoto, T. (1987). Maternal role preparation: A program using sensory integration, infant-motor attachment, and occupational behavior perspectives. *Occupational Therapy in Health Care, 4,* 9–21.

Burrows, E. (1989). Clinical practice: An approach to the assessment of clinical competencies. *British Journal of Occupational Therapy, 52,* 222–226.

Burton, J. E. (1989). The Model of Human Occupation and occupational therapy practice with elderly patients, part 1: Characteristics of Aging. *British Journal of Occupational Therapy, 52,* 215–218.

Burton, J. E. (1989). The Model of Human Occupation and occupational therapy practice with elderly patients, part 2: Application. *British Journal of Occupational Therapy, 52,* 219–221.

C

Cermak, S. A., & Murray, E. (1992). Nonverbal learning disabilities in the adult framed in the Model of Human Occupation. In N. Katz (Ed.), *Cognitive rehabilitation: Models for intervention in occupational therapy* (pp. 258–291). Boston: Andover Medical Publishers.

Chaffey, L., & Fossey, E. (2004). Caring and daily life: Occupational experiences of women living with sons diagnosed with schizophrenia. *Australian Occupational Therapy Journal, 51,* 199–207.

Chan, S. C. C. (2004). Chronic obstructive pulmonary disease and engagement in occupation. *American Journal of Occupational Therapy, 58(4),* 408–415.

Chen, C., Neufeld, P. S., Feely, C. A., & Skinner, C. S. (1999). Factors influencing compliance with home exercise programs among patients with upper-extremity impairment. *American Journal of Occupational Therapy, 53,* 171–180.

Chern, J., Kielhofner, G., de las Heras, C., & Magalhaes, L. (1996). The Volitional Questionnaire: Psychometric development and practical use. *American Journal of Occupational Therapy, 50,* 516–525.

Cole, M. (1998). A model of human occupation approach. In *Group dynamics in occupational therapy: The theoretical basis and practice application of group treatment* (2nd ed., pp. 268–290). Thorofare, NJ: Slack.

Colon, H., & Haertlein, C. (2002). Spanish translation of the role checklist. *American Journal of Occupational Therapy, 56,* 586–589.

Corner, R., Kielhofner, G., & Lin, F. L. (1997). Construct validity of a work environment impact scale. *Work, 9* (1), 21–34.

Corr, S., Phillips, C. J., & Walker, M. (2004). Evaluation of a pilot service designed to provide support following stroke: A randomized cross-over design study. *Clinical Rehabilitation, 18* (1), 69–75.

Corr, S., & Wilmer, S. (2003). Returning to work after a stroke: An important but neglected area. *British Journal of Occupational Therapy, 66,* 186–192.

Coster, W. J., & Jaffe, L. E. (1991). Current concepts of children's perceptions of control. *American Journal of Occupational Therapy, 45,* 19–25.

Crist, P., Fairman, A., Muñoz, J. P., Hansen, A. M. W., Sciulli, J., & Eggers, M. (2005). Education and practice collaborations: A pilot case study between a university faculty and county jail practitioners. *Occupational Therapy in Health Care, 19 (1/2),* 193–210.

Crowe, T. K., VanLeit, B., Berghmans, K. K., & Mann, P. (1997). Role perceptions of mothers with young children: The impact of a child's disability. *American Journal of Occupational Therapy, 51,* 651–661.

Cubie, S., & Kaplan, K. (1982). A case analysis method for the model of human occupation. *American Journal of Occupational Therapy, 36,* 645–656.

Cull, G. (1989). Anorexia nervosa: A review of theory approaches to treatment. *Journal of New Zealand Association of Occupational Therapists, 40 (2),* 3–6.

Curtin, C. (1990). Research on the Model of Human Occupation. *Mental Health-Special Interest Section Newsletter, 13 (2),* 3–5.

Curtin, C. (1991). Psychosocial intervention with an adolescent with diabetes using the Model of Human Occupation. *Occupational Therapy in Mental Health, 11 (2/3),* 23–36.

D

Davies Hallet, J., Zasler, N., Maurer, P., & Cash, S. (1994). Role change after traumatic brain injury in adults. *American Journal of Occupational Therapy, 48 (3),* 241–246.

de las Heras, C. G., Dion, G. L., & Walsh, D. (1993). Application of rehabilitation models in a state psychiatric hospital. *Occupational Therapy in Mental Health, 12 (3),* 1–32.

de las Heras, C. G., Geist, R., Kielhofner, G., & Li, Y. (2003). *The Volitional Questionnaire (VQ) (Version 4.0).* Chicago: Model of Human Occupation Clearinghouse, Department of Occupational Therapy, College of Applied Health Sciences, University of Illinois.

de las Heras, C. G., Llerena, V., & Kielhofner, G. (2003). *Remotivation process: Progressive intervention for individuals with severe volitional challenges. (Version 1.0)* Chicago: Department of Occupational Therapy, University of Illinois.

DeForest, D., Watts, J. H., & Madigan, M. J. (1991). Resonation in the model of human occupation: A pilot study. *Occupational Therapy in Mental Health, 11(2/3),* 57–75.

DePoy, E. (1990). The TBIIM: An intervention for the treatment of individuals with traumatic brain injury. *Occupational Therapy in Health Care, 7 (1),* 55–67.

DePoy, E., & Burke, J. P. (1992). Viewing cognition through the lens of the model of human occupation. In N. Katz (Ed.), *Cognitive Rehabilitation: Models for intervention in occupational therapy* (pp. 240–257). Stoneham, MA: Butterworth-Heinemann.

Dickerson, A. E., & Oakley, F. (1995). Comparing the roles of community-living persons and patient population. *American Journal of Occupational Therapy, 49,* 221–228.

Dion, G. L., Lovely, S., & Skerry, M. (1996). A comprehensive psychiatric rehabilitation approach to severe and persistent mental illness in the public sector. In S. M. Soreff (Ed.), *Handbook for the treatment of the seriously mentally ill* . Seattle: Hogrete & Huber.

Doble, S. (1988). Intrinsic motivation and clinical practice: The key to understanding the unmotivated client. *Canadian Journal of Occupational Therapy, 55,* 75–81.

Doble, S. (1991). Test-retest and inter-rater reliability of a process skills assessment. *Occupational Therapy Journal of Research, 11(1),* 8–23.

Doughton, K. J. (1996). Hidden talents. *O. T. Week, 10 (26),* 19–20.

Duellman, M. K., Barris, R., & Kielhofner, G. (1986). Organized activity and the adaptive status of nursing home residents. *American Journal of Occupational Therapy, 40,* 618–622.

Duran, L. J., & Fisher, A. G. (1996). Male and female performance on the assessment of motor and process skills. *Archives of Physical Medicine and Rehabilitation, 77,* 1019–1024.

Dyck, I. (1992). The daily routines of mothers with young children: Using a sociopolitical model in research. *Occupational Therapy Journal of Research, 12 (1),* 17–34.

E

Early, M., & Pedretti, L. (1998). A frame of reference and practice models for physical dysfunction. In M. Early (Ed.), *Physical dysfunction practice skills for the occupational therapy assistant.* (pp. 17–30). St. Louis: Mosby.

Ebb, E. W., Coster, W. J., & Duncombe, L. (1989). Comparison of normal and psychosocially dysfunctional male adolescents. *Occupational Therapy in Mental Health, 9 (2),* 53–74.

Ecklund, M. (1996). Working relationship, participation, and outcome in a psychiatric day care unit based on occupational therapy. *Scandinavian Journal of Occupational Therapy, 3,* 106–113.

Egan, M., Warren, S. A., Hessel, P. A., & Gilewich, G. (1992). Activities of daily living after hip fracture: Pre- and post discharge. *Occupational Therapy Journal of Research, 12,* 342–356.

Ekbladh, E., Haglund, L., & Thorell, L. (2004). The Worker Role Interview: Preliminary data on the predictive validity of return to work clients after an insurance medicine investigation. *Journal of Occupational Rehabilitation, 14,* 131–141.

Eklund, M. (1996). Patient experiences and outcome of treatment in psychiatric occupational therapy-three cases. *Occupational Therapy International, 3 (3),* 212–239.

Eklund, M. (1996). Working relationship, participation, and outcome in a psychiatric day care unit based on occupational therapy. *Scandinavian Journal of Occupational Therapy, 3,* 106–113.

Eklund, M. (1999). Outcome of occupational therapy in a psychiatric day care unit for long-term mentally ill patients. *Occupational Therapy in Mental Health, 14 (4),* 21–45.

Eklund, M. (2001). Psychiatric patients' occupational roles: Changes over time and associations with self-rated quality of life. *Scandinavian Journal of Occupational Therapy, 8,* 125–130.

Eklund, M., & Hansson, L. (1997). Stability of improvement in patients receiving psychiatric occupational therapy: A one-year follow-up. *Scandinavian Journal of Occupational Therapy, 4,* 15–22.

Elliott, M., & Barris, R. (1987). Occupational role performance and life satisfaction in elderly persons. *Occupational Therapy Journal of Research, 7,* 215–224.

Ennals, P., & Fossey, E. (2007). The occupational performance history interview in community mental health case management: Consumer and occupational therapists perspectives. *Australian Occupational Therapy Journal, 54,* 11–21.

Esdaile, S. A. (1996). A play-focused intervention involving mothers of preschoolers. *American Journal of Occupational Therapy, 50,* 113–123.

Esdaile, S. A., & Madill, H. M. (1993). Causal attributions: Theoretical considerations and their relevance to occupational therapy practice and education. *British Journal of Occupational Therapy, 56,* 330–334.

Evans, J., & Salim, A. A. (1992). A cross-cultural test of the validity of occupational therapy assessments with patients with schizophrenia. *American Journal of Occupational Therapy, 46,* 695.

F

Farnworth, L., Nikitin, L., & Fossey, E. (2004). Being in a secure forensic psychiatry unit: Every day is the same, killing time to making the most of it. *British Journal of Occupational Therapy, 67,* 1–9.

Fisher, A. G. (1993). The assessment of IADL motor skills: An application of many-faceted Rasch analysis. *American Journal of Occupational Therapy, 47,* 319–329.

Fisher, A. G., Liu, Y., Velozo, C. A., & Pan, A. W. (1992). Cross-cultural assessment of process skills. *American Journal of Occupational Therapy, 46,* 876–885.

Fisher, A., & Savin-Baden, M. (2001). The benefits to young people experiencing psychosis, and their families, of an early intervention programme: Evaluating a service from the consumers' and the providers' perspectives. *British Journal of Occupational Therapy, 64,* 58–65.

Fisher, G. (2004). The residential environment impact survey. *Developmental Disabilities Special Interest Section Quarterly, 27 (3),* 1–4.

Fisher, G. S. (1999). Administration and application of the Worker Role Interview: Looking beyond functional capacity. *Work: A Journal of Prevention, Assessment, and Rehabilitation,* 12, 25–36.

Forsyth, K., Braveman, B., Kielhofner, G., Ekbladh, H., Haglund, H., Fenger, K., & Keller, J. (2006). Psychometric properties of the Worker Role Interview. *Work: A Journal of Prevention, Assessment & Rehabilitation,* 27, 313–318.

Forsyth, K., Deshpande, S., Kielhofner, G., Henriksson, C., Haglund, L., Olson, L., Skinner, S., & Kulkarni, S. (2005). The *Occupational Circumstances Assessment Interview and Rating Scale (OCAIRS) (Version 4.0).* Chicago: Model of Human Occupation Clearinghouse, Department of Occupational Therapy, College of Applied Health Sciences, University of Illinois.

Forsyth, K., Duncan, E. A. S., & Mann, L. S. (2005). Scholarship of practice in the United Kingdom: An oc-

cupational therapy service case study. *Occupational Therapy in Health Care, 19,* 17–29.

Forsyth, K., & Kielhofner, G. (2003). Model of Human Occupation. In: P. Kramer, J. Hinojosa, & C. Royeen, (Eds.), *Human Occupation: Participation in Life* (pp. 45–86). Philadelphia: Lippincott Williams & Wilkins.

Forsyth, K., Lai, J., & Kielhofner, G. (1999). The assessment of communication and interaction skills (ACIS): Measurement properties. *British Journal of Occupational Therapy, 62,* 69–74.

Forsyth, K., Melton, J., & Mann, L. S. (2005). Achieving evidence-based practice: A process of continuing education through practitioner-academic partnership. *Occupational Therapy in Health Care, 19 (1/2),* 211–227.

Forsyth, K., Parkinson, S., Kielhofner, G., Keller, J., Summerfield Mann, L., & Duncan, E. (in press). The measurement properties of the Model of Human Occupation Screening Tool (MOHOST). *British Journal of Occupational Therapy.*

Forsyth, K., Salamy, M., Simon, S., & Kielhofner, G. (1998). *The Assessment of Communication and Interaction Skills (version 4.0).* Chicago: Department of Occupational Therapy, University of Illinois.

Forsyth, K., Summerfield-Mann, L., & Kielhofner, G. (2005). A Scholarship of practice: Making occupation-focused, theory-driven, evidence-based practice a reality. *British Journal of Occupational Therapy, 68,* 261–268.

Fossey, E. (1996). Using the occupational performance history interview (PHI):Therapists' reflections. *British Journal of Occupational Therapy, 59,* 223–228.

Fougeyrollas, P., Noreau, L., & Boschen, K. A. (2002). Interaction of environment with individual characteristics and social participation: Theoretical perspectives and applications in persons with spinal cord injury. *Topics in Spinal Cord Injury Rehabilitation, 7,* 1–16.

Froelich, J. (1992). Occupational therapy interventions with survivors of sexual abuse. *Occupational Therapy in Health Care, 8 (2/3),* 1–25.

Frosch, S., Gruber, A., Jones, C., Myers, S., Noel, E., Westerlund, A., & Zavisin, T. (1997). The long term effects of traumatic brain injury on the roles of caregivers. *Brain Injury, 11,* 891–906.

Furst, G., Gerber, L., Smith, C., Fisher, S., & Shulman, B. (1987). A program for improving energy conservation behaviors in adults with rheumatoid arthritis. *American Journal of Occupational Therapy, 41,* 102–111.

G

Gerardi, S. M. (1996). The management of battle fatigued soldiers: An occupational therapy model. *Military Medicine, 161,* 483–488.

Gerber, L., & Furst, G. (1992). Scoring methods and application of the Activity Record (ACTRE) for patients with musculoskeletal disorders. *Arthritis Care and Research, 5*(3), 151–156.

Gerber, L., & Furst, G. (1992). Validation of the NIH Activity Record: A quantitative measure of life activities. *Arthritis Care and Research, 5*(2), 81–86.

Gillard, M., & Segal, M. E. (2002). Social roles and subjective well-being in a population of nondisabled older people. *Occupational Therapy Journal of Research, 22,* 96.

Gitlin, L. N., Winter, L., Corcoran, M., Dennis, M. P., Schinfeld, S., & Hauck, W.W. (2003). Effects of the Home Environmental Skill-Building Program on the caregiver-care recipient dyad: 6–month outcomes from the Philadelphia REACH initiative. *The Gerontologist, 43,* 532–546.

Goldstein, K., Kielhofner, G., & Paul-Ward, A. (2004). Occupational narratives and the therapeutic process. *Australian Occupational Therapy Journal, 51,* 119–124.

Gorde, M. W., Helfrich, C. A., & Finlayson, M. (2004). Trauma symptoms and life skill needs of domestic violence victims. *Journal of Interpersonal Violence, 19,* 691–708.

Graff, M. J. L., Vernooij-Dassen, M. J. F. J., Hoefnagels, J. D., Dekker, J. & de Witte, L. P. (2003). Occupational therapy at home for older individuals with mild to moderate cognitive impairments and their primary caregivers: A pilot study. *Occupational Therapy Journal of Research, 23 (4),* 155–163.

Gray, M. L., & Fossey, E. M. (2003). Illness experience and occupations of people with chronic fatigue syndrome. *Australian Occupational Therapy Journal, 50,* 127–136.

Gregory, M. (1983). Occupational behavior and life satisfaction among retirees. *American Journal of Occupational Therapy, 37,* 548–553.

Grogan, G. (1991). Anger management: A perspective for occupational therapy (part 1). *Occupational Therapy in Mental Health, 11 (2/3),* 135–148.

Grogan, G. (1991). Anger management: A perspective for occupational therapy (part 2). *Occupational Therapy in Mental Health, 11 (2/3),* 149–171.

Grogan, G. (1994). The personal computer: A treatment tool for increasing sense of competence. *Occupational Therapy in Mental Health, 12,* 47–60.

Guidetti, S., & Tham, K. (2005). Therapeutic strategies used by occupational therapists in self-care training: A qualitative study. *Occupational Therapy International, 9,* 257–276.

Gusich, R. L. (1984). Occupational therapy for chronic pain: A clinical application of the model of human occupation. *Occupational Therapy in Mental Health, 4 (3),* 59–73.

Gusich, R. L., & Silverman, A. L. (1991). Basava day clinic: The model of human occupation as applied to psychiatric day hospitalization. *Occupational Therapy in Mental Health, 11 (2/3),* 113–134.

H

Hachey, R., Boyer, G., & Mercier, C. (2001). Perceived and valued roles of adults with severe mental health problems. *Canadian Journal of Occupational Therapy, 68,* 112–120.

Hachey, R., Jumoorty, J., & Mercier, C. (1995). Methodology for validating the translation of test measurements applied to occupational therapy. *Occupational Therapy International, 2 (3),* 190–203.

Haglund, L. (1996). Occupational therapists agreement in screening patients in general psychiatric care for OT. *Scandinavian Journal of Occupational Therapy, 3,* 62–68.

Haglund, L. (2000). Assessment in general psychiatric care. *Occupational Therapy in Mental Health, 15,* 35–47.

Haglund, L., Ekbladh, E., Lars-Hakan, T., & Hallberg, I. R. (2000). Practice models in Swedish psychiatric occupational therapy. *Scandinavian Journal of Occupational Therapy, 7,* 107–113.

Haglund, L., & Henriksson, C. (1994). Testing a Swedish version of OCAIRS on two different patient groups. *Scandinavian Journal of Caring Sciences, 8,* 223–230.

Haglund, L., & Henriksson, C. (1995). Activity: From action to activity. *Scandinavian Journal of Caring Sciences, 9,* 227–234.

Haglund, L., & Henriksson, C. (2003). Concepts in occupational therapy in relation to the ICF. *Occupational Therapy International, 10,* 253–268.

Haglund, L., Karlsson, G., & Kielhofner, G. (1997). Validity of the Swedish version of the Worker Role Interview. *Physical and Occupational Therapy in Geriatrics, 4 (1–4),* 23–29.

Haglund, L., & Kjellberg, A. (1999). A critical analysis of the model of human occupation. *Canadian Journal of Occupational Therapy, 66,* 102–108.

Haglund, L., & Thorell, L. (2004). Clinical perspective on the Swedish version of the assessment of communication and interaction skills: Stability of assessments. *Scandinavian Journal of Caring Sciences, 18,* 417–423.

Haglund, L., Thorell, L., & Walinder, J. (1998). Assessment of occupational functioning for screening of patients to occupational therapy in general psychiatric care. *Occupational Therapy Journal of Research, 18 (4),* 193–206.

Haglund, L., Thorell, L., & Walinder, J. (1998). Occupational functioning in relation to psychiatric diagnoses: Schizophrenia and mood disorders. *Journal of Psychiatry, 52,* 223–229.

Hahn-Markowitz, J. (2004). Advancing practice through scholarship. *The Israel Journal of Occupational Therapy, 13,* E130–E134.

Hakansson, C., Eklund, M., Lidfeldt, J., Nerbrand, C., Samsioe, G., & Nilsson, P. M. (2005). Well-being and occupational roles among middle-aged woman. *Work: A Journal of Prevention, Assessment & Rehabilitation, 24,* 341–351.

Hallett, J.D., & Zasler, N.D., Maurer, P., & Cash, S. (1994). Role change after traumatic brain injury in adults. *American Journal of Occupational Therapy, 48,* 241–246.

Hammel, J. (1999). The life rope: A transactional approach to exploring worker and life role development. *Work: A Journal of Prevention, Assessment, and Rehabilitation, 12,* 47–60.

Harris, K., & Reid, D. (2005). The influence of virtual reality play on children's motivation. *Canadian Journal of Occupational Therapy, 72,* 21–29.

Harrison, H., & Kielhofner, G. (1986). Examining reliability and validity of the Preschool Play Scale with handicapped children. *American Journal of Occupational Therapy, 40,* 167–173.

Harrison, M., & Forsyth, K. (2005). Developing a vision for therapists working within child and adolescent mental health services: Poised of paused for action? *British Journal of Occupational Therapy, 68,* 1–5.

Heasman, D., & Atwal, A. (2004). The active advice pilot project: Leisure enhancement and social inclusion for people with severe mental health problems. *British Journal of Occupational Therapy, 67,* 511–514.

Helfrich, C., & Aviles, A. (2001). Occupational therapy's role with domestic violence: Assessment and intervention. *Occupational Therapy in Mental Health, 16 (3/4),* 53–70.

Helfrich, C., & Kielhofner, G. (1994). Volitional narratives and the meaning of occupational therapy. *American Journal of Occupational Therapy, 48,* 319–326.

Helfrich, C., Kielhofner, G., & Mattingly, C. (1994). Volition as narrative: an understanding of motivation in chronic illness. *American Journal of Occupational Therapy, 48,* 311–317.

Hemmingsson, H., & Borell, L. (1996). The development of an assessment of adjustment needs in the school setting for use with physically disabled students. *Scandinavian Journal of Occupational Therapy, 3,* 156–162.

Hemmingsson, H., Borell, L., & Gustavsson, A. (1999). Temporal aspects of teaching and learning: Implications for pupils with physical disabilities. *Scandinavian Journal of Disability Research, 1,* 26–43.

Hemmingson, H., Kottorp, A., & Bernspang, B. (2004). Validity of the school setting interview: An assessment of the student-environment fit. *Scandinavian Journal of Occupational Therapy, 11,* 171–178.

Hemmingsson, H., & Borell, L. (2000). Accommodation needs and student-environment fit in upper secondary school for students with severe physical disabilities. *Canadian Journal of Occupational Therapy, 67,* 162–173.

Hemmingsson, H., & Borell, L. (2002). Environmental barriers in mainstream schools. *Child: Care, Health, and Development, 28 (1),* 57–63.

Hemmingsson, H., Egilson, S., Hoffman, O., & Kielhofner, G. (2005). *School Setting Interview (SSI) (Version 3.0).* Swedish Association of Occupational Therapists. Nacka, Sweden.

Henriksson, C. M. (1995). Living with continuous muscular pain: Patient perspectives: part I. *Scandinavian Journal of Caring Sciences, 9,* 67–76.

Henriksson, C. M. (1995). Living with continuous muscular pain: Patient perspectives: part II. *Scandinavian Journal of Caring Sciences, 9,* 77–86.

Henriksson, C., & Burckhardt, C. (1996). Impact of fibromyalgia on everyday life: A study of women in the USA and Sweden. *Disability and Rehabilitation, 18,* 241–248.

Henriksson, C., Gundmark, I., Bengtsson, A., & Ek, A. C. (1992). Living with fibromyalgia. *Clinical Journal of Pain, 8,* 138–144.

Henry, A. D. (1998). Development of a measure of adolescent leisure interests. *American Journal of Occupational Therapy, 52,* 531–539.

Henry, A. D. (2000). *The Pediatric Interest Profiles: Surveys of play for children and adolescents.* Unpublished manuscript, Model of Human Occupation Clearinghouse, Department of Occupational Therapy, University of Illinois at Chicago.

Henry, A. D., Baron, K., Mouradian, L., & Curtin, C. (1999). Reliability and validity of the self-assessment of occupational functioning. *American Journal of Occupational Therapy, 53,* 482–488.

Henry, A. D., Costa, C., Ladd, D., Robertson, C., Rollins, J., & Roy, L. (2006). Time use, time management and academic achievement among occupational therapy students. *Work: A Journal of Prevention, Assessment, and Rehabilitation, 6,* 115–126.

Henry, A. D., & Coster, W. J. (1996). Predictors of functional outcome among adolescents and young adults with psychotic disorders. *American Journal of Occupational Therapy, 50,* 171–181.

Henry, A. D., & Coster, W. J. (1997). Competency beliefs and occupational role behavior among adolescents: Explication of the personal causation construct. *American Journal of Occupational Therapy, 51,* 267–276.

Hocking, C. (1989). Anger management. *Journal of New Zealand Association of Occupational Therapists, 40 (2),* 12–17.

Hocking, C. (1994). Objects in the environment: A critique of the model of human occupation dimensions. *Scandinavian Journal of Occupational Therapy, 1,* 77–84.

Horne, J., Corr, S., & Earle, S. (2005). Becoming a mother: Occupational change in first time motherhood. *Journal of Occupational Science, 12,* 176–183.

Howie, L., Coulter, M., & Feldman, S. (2004). Crafting the self: Older persons' narratives of occupational identity. *American Journal of Occupational Therapy, 58,* 446–454.

Hubbard, S. (1991). Towards a truly holistic approach to occupational therapy. *British Journal of Occupational Therapy, 54,* 415–418.

Hurff, J. M. (1984). Visualization: A decision-making tool for assessment and treatment planning. *Occupational Therapy in Health Care, 1 (2),* 3–23.

I

Ingvarsson, L., & Theodorsdottir, M. H. (2004). Vocational rehabilitation at Reykjalundur rehabilitation center in Iceland. *Work: A Journal of Prevention, Assessment, and Rehabilitation, 22,* 17–19.

J

Jackoway, I., Rogers, J., & Snow, T. (1987). The role change assessment: An interview tool for evaluating older adults. *Occupational Therapy in Mental Health, 7 (1),* 17–37.

Jackson, M., Harkess, J., & Ellis, J. (2004). Reporting patients' work abilities: How the use of standardised work assessments improved clinical practice in Fife. *British Journal of Occupational Therapy, 67,* 129–132.

Jacobshagen, I. (1990). The effect of interruption of activity on affect. *Occupational Therapy in Mental Health, 10 (2),* 35–45.

Jongbloed, L. (1994). Adaptation to a stroke: The experience of one couple. *American Journal of Occupational Therapy, 48,* 1006–1013.

Jonsson, H. (1993). The retirement process in an occupational perspective: A review of literature and theories. *Physical and Occupational Therapy in Geriatrics, 11 (4),* 15–34.

Jonsson, H., Borell, L., & Sadlo, G. (2000). Retirement: An occupational transition with consequences for temporality, balance, and meaning of occupations. *Journal of Occupational Science, 7 (1),* 29–37.

Jonsson, H., Josephsson, S., & Kielhofner, G. (2000). Evolving narratives in the course of retirement: A longitudinal study. *American Journal of Occupational Therapy, 54,* 463–470.

Jonsson, H., Josephsson, S., & Kielhofner, G. (2001). Narratives and experiences in an occupational transition: A longitudinal study of the retirement process. *American Journal of Occupational Therapy, 55,* 424–432.

Jonsson, H., Kielhofner, G., & Borell, L. (1997). Anticipating retirement: The formation of narratives concerning an occupational transition. *American Journal of Occupational Therapy, 51,* 49–56.

Josephsson, S., Backman, L., Borell, L., Bernspang, B., Nygard, L., & Ronnberg, L. (1993). Supporting everyday activities in dementia: An intervention study. *International Journal of Geriatric Psychiatry, 8,* 395–400.

Josephsson, S., Backman, L., Borell, L., Hygard, L., & Bernspang, B. (1995). Effectiveness of an intervention to improve occupational performance in dementia. *Occupational Therapy Journal of Research, 15 (1),* 36–49.

Jungersen, K. (1992). Culture, theory, and the practice of occupational therapy in New Zealand/Aotearoa. *American Journal of Occupational Therapy, 46,* 745–750.

K

Kaplan, K. (1984). Short-term assessment: The need and a response. *Occupational Therapy in Mental Health, 4 (3),* 29–45.

Kaplan, K. (1986). The directive group: Short term treatment for psychiatric patients with a minimal level of functioning. *American Journal of Occupational Therapy, 40,* 474–481.

Kaplan, K. (1988). *Directive group therapy: Innovative mental health treatment.* Thorofare, NJ: Slack.

Kaplan, K., & Eskow, K. G. (1987). Teaching psychosocial theory and practice: The model of human occupation as the medium and the message. *Mental Health-Special Interest Section Newsletter, 10 (1),* 1–5.

Kaplan, K., & Kielhofner, G. (1989). *Occupational Case Analysis Interview and rating scale.* Thorofare, NJ: Slack.

Katz, N. (1985). Occupational therapy's domain of concern: Reconsidered. *American Journal of Occupational Therapy, 39,* 518–524.

Katz, N. (1988). Interest checklist: A factor analytical study. *Occupational Therapy in Mental Health, 8 (1),* 45–56.

Katz, N. (1988). Introduction to the collection (MOHO). *Occupational Therapy in Mental Health, 8 (1),* 1–6.

Katz, N., Giladi, N., & Peretz, C. (1988). Cross-cultural application of occupational therapy assessments: Human occupation with psychiatric inpatients and controls in Israel. *Occupational Therapy in Mental Health, 8 (1),* 7–30.

Katz, N., Josman, N., & Steinmetz, N. (1988). Relationship between cognitive disability theory and the model of human occupation in the assessment of psychiatric and non psychiatric adolescents. *Occupational Therapy in Mental Health, 8 (1),* 31–44.

Kavanagh, J., & Fares, J. (1995). Using the model of human occupation with homeless mentally ill patients. *British Journal of Occupational Therapy, 58,* 419–422.

Kavanagh, M. R. (1990). Way station: A model community support program for persons with serious mental illness. *Mental Health-Special Interest Section Newsletter, 13 (1),* 6–8.

Keller, J., & Forsyth, K. (2004). The model of human occupation in practice. *The Israel Journal of Occupational Therapy, 13,* E99–E106.

Keller, J., Kafkes, A., & Kielhofner, G. (2005). Psychometric characteristics of the Child Occupational Self Assessment (COSA), part 1: An initial examination of psychometric properties. *Scandinavian Journal of Occupational Therapy, 12,* 118–127.

Keller, J., Kafkes, A., Basu, S., Federico, J., & Kielhofner, G. (2005). *The Child Occupational Self Assessment (Version 2.1).* Chicago: Model of Human Occupation Clearinghouse, Department of Occupational Therapy, College of Applied Health Sciences, University of Illinois.

Keller, J., & Kielhofner, G. (2005). Psychometric characteristics of the Child Occupational Self-Assessment (COSA), part 2: Refining the psychometric properties. *Scandinavian Journal of Occupational Therapy, 12,* 147–158.

Kelly, L. (1995). What occupational therapists can learn from traditional healers. *British Journal of Occupational Therapy, 58,* 111–114.

Keponen, R., & Kielhofner, G. (2006) Occupation and meaning in the lives of women with chronic pain. *Scandinavian Journal of Occupational Therapy,* 13(4), 211–220.

Khoo, S. W., & Renwick, R. M. (1989). A model of human occupation perspective on mental health of immigrant women in Canada. *Occupational Therapy in Mental Health, 9 (3),* 31–49.

Kielhofner, G. (1980). A model of human occupation, part 2: Ontogenesis from the perspective of temporal adaptation. *American Journal of Occupational Therapy, 34,* 657–663.

Kielhofner, G. (1980). A model of human occupation, part 3: Benign and vicious cycles. *American Journal of Occupational Therapy, 34,* 731–737.

Kielhofner, G. (1984). An overview of research on the model of human occupation. *Canadian Journal of Occupational Therapy, 51,* 59–67.

Kielhofner, G. (1985). *A model of human occupation: Theory and application* (2nd ed.). Baltimore: Williams & Wilkins.

Kielhofner, G. (1986). A review of research on the model of human occupation: part 1. *Canadian Journal of Occupational Therapy, 53,* 69–74.

Kielhofner, G. (1986). A review of research on the model of human occupation: part 2. *Canadian Journal of Occupational Therapy, 53,* 129–134.

Kielhofner, G. (1992). The future of the profession of occupational therapy: Requirements for developing the field's knowledge base. *Journal of Japanese Association of Occupational Therapists, 11,* 112–129.

Kielhofner, G. (1993). Functional assessment: Toward a dialectical view of person-environment relations. *American Journal of Occupational Therapy, 47,* 248–251.

Kielhofner, G. (1995). A meditation on the use of hands. *Scandinavian Journal of Caring Sciences, 2,* 153–166.

Kielhofner, G. (1995). *A model of human occupation: Theory and application.* (2nd ed.) Philadelphia: Lippincott Williams & Wilkins.

Kielhofner, G. (1999). From doing in to doing with: The role of environment in performance and disability. *Toimintaterapeutti, 1,* 3–9.

Kielhofner, G. (1999). Guest editorial. *Work: A Journal of Prevention, Assessment, and Rehabilitation, 12,* 1.

Kielhofner, G. (2002). *The model of human occupation: Theory and application* (3rd ed.). Philadelphia: Lippincott Williams & Wilkins.

Kielhofner, G. (2004). The model of human occupation. In G. Kielhofner (Ed.), *Conceptual foundations of occupational therapy* (3rd ed., pp. 147–170). Philadelphia: FA Davis.

Kielhofner, G. (2005). A Scholarship of practice: Creating discourse between theory, research and practice. *Occupational Therapy in Health Care, 19 (1/2),* 7–17.

Kielhofner, G. (2005). Scholarship and Practice: Bridging the Divide. *American Journal of Occupational Therapy, 59,* 231–239.

Kielhofner, G., & Barrett, L. (1998). Meaning and misunderstanding in occupational forms: A study of therapeutic goal setting. *American Journal of Occupational Therapy, 52,* 345–353.

Kielhofner, G., & Barrett, L. (1998). Theories derived from occupational behavior perspectives. In M. E. Neistadt & E. B. Crepeau (Eds.), *Willard and Spackman's occupational therapy* (9th ed., pp. 525–535). Philadelphia: Lippincott.

Kielhofner, G., Barris, R., & Watts, J. H. (1982). Habits and habit dysfunction: A clinical perspective for psychosocial occupational therapy. *Occupational Therapy in Mental Health, 2 (2),* 1–21.

Kielhofner, G., & Brinson, M. (1989). Development and evaluation of an aftercare program for young and chronic psychiatrically disabled adults. *Occupational Therapy in Mental Health, 9 (2),* 1–25.

Kielhofner, G., Braveman, B., Baron, K., Fischer, G., Hammel, J., & Littleton, M. J. (1999). The model of human occupation: Understanding the worker who is injured or disabled. *Work: A Journal of Prevention, Assessment, and Rehabilitation, 12,* 3–11.

Kielhofner, G., Braveman, B., Finlayson, M., Paul-Ward, A., Goldbaum, L., & Goldstein, K. (2004). Outcomes of a vocational program for persons with AIDS. *American Journal of Occupational Therapy, 58,* 64–72.

Kielhofner, G., Braveman, B., Levin, M., & Fogg, L. (in press). A controlled study of services to enhance productive participation among persons with HIV/AIDS. *American Journal of Occupational Therapy.*

Kielhofner, G., & Burke, J. P. (1980). A model of human occupation, part 1: Conceptual framework and content. *American Journal of Occupational Therapy, 34,* 572–581.

Kielhofner, G., & Burke, J. P., & Heard, I. C. (1980). A model of human occupation, part 4. Assessment and intervention. *American Journal of Occupational Therapy, 34,* 777–788.

Kielhofner, G., Dobria, L., Forsyth, K., & Basu, S. (2005). The construction of keyforms for obtaining instantaneous measures from the occupational performance history interview rating scales. *Occupational Therapy Journal of Research, 25 (1),* 23–32.

Kielhofner, G., & Fisher, A. (1991). Mind-brain relationships. In A. Fisher, E. Murray, & A. C. Bundy (Eds.), *Sensory Integration: Theory and Practice* (pp. 27–45). Philadelphia: FA Davis.

Kielhofner, G., & Forsyth, K. (1997). The Model of Human Occupation: An overview of current concepts. *British Journal of Occupational Therapy, 60,* 103–110.

Kielhofner, G., & Forsyth, K. (2001). Measurement properties of a client self-report for treatment planning and documenting therapy outcomes. *Scandinavian Journal of Occupational Therapy, 8,* 131–139.

Kielhofner, G., Harlan, B., Bauer, D., & Maurer, P. (1986). The reliability of a historical interview with physically disabled respondents. *American Journal of Occupational Therapy, 40,* 551–556.

Kielhofner, G., & Henry, A. D. (1988). Development and investigation of the Occupational Performance History Interview. *American Journal of Occupational Therapy, 42,* 489–498.

Kielhofner, G., Henry, A. D., Walens, D., & Rogers, E. S. (1991). A generalizability study of the Occupational Performance History Interview. *Occupational Therapy Journal of Research, 11,* 292–306.

Kielhofner, G., Lai, J., Olson, L., Haglund, L., Ekbadh, E., & Hedlund, M. (1999). Psychometric properties of the work environment impact scale: a cross-cultural study. *Work: A Journal of Prevention, Assessment, and Rehabilitation, 12,* 71–77.

Kielhofner, G., & Mallinson, T. (1995). Gathering narrative data through interviews: Empirical observations and suggested guidelines. *Scandinavian Journal of Occupational Therapy, 2,* 63–68.

Kielhofner, G., Mallinson, T., Crawford, C., Nowak, M., Rigby, M., Henry, A., & Walens, D. (2004). *Occupational Performance History Interview-II (OPHI-II) (Version 2.1).* Chicago: Model of Human Occupation Clearinghouse, Department of Occupational Therapy, College of Applied Health Sciences, University of Illinois.

Kielhofner, G., Mallinson, T., Forsyth, K., & Lai, J. S. (2001). Psychometric properties of the second version of the Occupational Performance History Interview (OPHI-II). *American Journal of Occupational Therapy, 55,* 260–267.

Kielhofner, G., & Neville, A. (1983). *The Modified Interest Checklist.* Unpublished manuscript, Model of Human Occupation Clearinghouse, Department of Occupational Therapy, University of Illinois at Chicago.

Kielhofner, G., & Nicol, M. (1989). The model of human occupation: A developing conceptual tool for clinicians. *British Journal of Occupational Therapy, 52,* 210–214.

Kjellberg, A. (2002). More or less independent. *Disability and Rehabilitation, 24,* 828–840.

Kjellberg, A., Haglund, L., Forsyth, K., & Kielhofner, G. (2003). The measurement properties of the Swedish version of the assessment of communication and interaction skills. *Scandinavian Journal of Caring Sciences, 1,* 271–277.

Knis-Matthews, L., Richard, L., Marquez, L., & Mevawala, N. (2005). Implementation of occupational therapy services for an adolescent residence program. *Occupational Therapy in Mental Health, 21 (1),* 57–72.

Krefting, L. (1985). The use of conceptual models in clinical practice. *Canadian Journal of Occupational Therapy, 52,* 173–178.

Kusznir, A., Scott, E., Cooke, R. G., & Young, L. T. (1996). Functional consequences of bipolar affective disorder: An occupational therapy perspective. *Canadian Journal of Occupational Therapy, 63,* 313–322.

Kyle, T., & Wright, S. (1996). Reflecting the model of human occupation in occupational therapy documentation. *Canadian Journal of Occupational Therapy, 63,* 192–196.

L

Lai, J. S., Haglund, L., & Kielhofner, G. (1999). Occupational case analysis interview and rating scale. *Scandinavian Journal of Caring Sciences, 13,* 276–273.

Lancaster, J. M. M. (1991). Occupational therapy treatment goals, objectives, and activities for improving low self-esteem in adolescents with behavioral disorders. *Occupational Therapy in Mental Health, 11 (2/3),* 3–22.

Larsson, M., & Branholm, I. S. (1996). An approach to goal-planning in occupational therapy and rehabilitation. *Scandinavian Journal of Caring Sciences, 3,* 14–19.

Lederer, J., Kielhofner, G., & Watts, J. H. (1985). Values, personal causation and skills of delinquents and non delinquents. *Occupational Therapy in Mental Health, 5 (2),* 59–77.

Lee, A. L., Strauss, L., Wittman, P., Jackson, B., & Carstens, A. (2001). The effects of chronic illness on roles and emotions of caregivers. *Occupational Therapy in Health Care, 14 (1),* 47–60.

Lee, S. Taylor, R. R., Keilhofner, G., & Fisher, G. (in press). Theory use in practice: A national survey of therapists who use the model of human occupation. *American Journal of Occupational Therapy.*

Leidy, N. K., & Knebel, A. R. (1999). Clinical validation of the functional performance inventory in patients with chronic obstructive pulmonary disease. *Respiratory Care, 44,* 932–939.

Levin, M., & Helfrich, C. (2004). Mothering role identity and competence among parenting and pregnant homeless adolescents. *Journal of Occupational Science, 11,* 95–104.

Levin, M., Kielhofner, G., Braveman, B., & Fogg, L. (in press). Narrative slope as a predictor of return to work and other occupational participation. *Scandinavian Journal of Occupational Therapy.*

Levine, R. (1984). The cultural aspects of home care delivery. *American Journal of Occupational Therapy, 38,* 734–738.

Levine, R., & Gitlin, L. N. (1990). Home adaptations for persons with chronic disabilities: An educational model. *American Journal of Occupational Therapy, 44,* 923–929.

Levine, R., & Gitlin, L. N. (1993). A model to promote activity competence in elders. *American Journal of Occupational Therapy, 47,* 147–153.

Li, Y., & Kielhofner, G. (2004). Psychometric properties of the volitional questionnaire. *The Israel Journal of Occupational Therapy, 13,* E85–E98.

Linddahl, I., Norrby, E., & Bellner, A. L. (2003). Construct validity of the instrument DOA: A dialogue about ability related to work. *Work: A Journal of Prevention, Assessment, and Rehabilitation, 20,* 215–224.

Lycett, R. (1992). Evaluating the use of an occupational assessment with elderly rehabilitation patients. *British Journal of Occupational Therapy, 55,* 343–346.

Lynch, K., & Bridle, M. (1993). Construct validity of the Occupational Performance Interview. *Occupational Therapy Journal of Research, 13,* 231–240.

Lyons, M. (1984). Shaping up: The model of human occupation as a guide to practice. *Proceedings of the 13th Federal Conference of the Australian Association of Occupational Therapists, 2,* 95–100.

M

Mackenzie, L. (1997). An application of the model of human occupation to fieldwork supervision and fieldwork issues in New South Wales. *Australian Occupational Therapy Journal, 44,* 71–80.

Mallinson, T., LaPlante, D., & Hollman-Smith, J. (1998). *Work rehabilitation in mental health programs.* Chicago: Model of Human Occupation Clearinghouse, Department of Occupational Therapy, College of Applied Health Sciences, University of Illinois.

Mallinson, T., Mahaffey, L., & Kielhofner, G. (1998). The occupational performance history interview: Evidence for three underlying constructs of occupational adaptation. *Canadian Journal of Occupational Therapy, 65,* 219–228.

Mallison, T., Kielhofner, G., & Mattingly, C. (1996). Metaphor and meaning in a clinical interview. *American Journal of Occupational Therapy, 50,* 338–346.

Maynard, M. (1987). An experiential learning approach: Utilizing historical interview and an occupational inventory. *Physical and Occupational Therapy in Geriatrics, 5 (2),* 51–69.

Mentrup, C., Niehous, A., & Kielhofner, G. (1999). Applying the model of human occupation in work-focused rehabilitation: A case illustration. *Work: A Journal of Prevention, Assessment, and Rehabilitation, 12,* 61–70.

Michael, P. S. (1991). Occupational therapy in a prison? You must be kidding! *Mental Health-Special Interest Section Newsletter, 14,* 3–4.

Mocellin, G. (1992). An overview of occupational therapy in the context of the American influence on the profession: part 1. *British Journal of Occupational Therapy, 55,* 7–12.

Mocellin, G. (1992). An overview of occupational therapy in the context of the American influence on the profession: part 2. *British Journal of Occupational Therapy, 55,* 55–60.

Molyneaux-Smith, L., Townsend, E., & Guernsey, J. R. (2003). Occupation disrupted: Impacts, challenges, and coping strategies for farmers with disabilities. *Journal of Occupational Science, 10,* 14–20.

Moore-Corner, R., Kielhofner, G., & Olson, L. (1998). *Work Environment Impact Scale (WEIS) (Version 2.0).* Chicago: Model of Human Occupation Clearinghouse,

Department of Occupational Therapy, College of Applied Health Sciences, University of Illinois.

Morgan, D., & Jongbloed, L. (1990). Factors influencing leisure activities following a stroke: An exploratory study. *Canadian Journal of Occupational Therapy, 57,* 223–229.

Muñoz, J. P. (1988). A program for acute inpatient psychiatry. *Mental Health-Special Interest Section Newsletter, 11,* 3–4.

Muñoz, J. P., Karmosky, A., Gaugler, J., Lang, K., and Stayduhar, M. (1999). Perceived role changes in parents of children with cerebral palsy. *Mental Health Special Interest Section Quarterly, 22*(4), 1–3.

Muñoz, J. P., Lawlor, M., & Kielhofner, G. (1993). Use of the model of human occupation: A survey of therapists in psychiatric practice. *Occupational Therapy Journal of Research, 13,* 117–139.

N

Nave, J., Helfrich, C., & Aviles, A. (2001). Child witnesses of domestic violence: A case study using the OT PAL. *Occupational Therapy in Mental Health, 16,* 127–140.

Neistadt, M. E. (1995). Methods of assessing clients' priorities: A survey of adult physical dysfunction settings. *American Journal of Occupational Therapy, 49,* 428–436.

Neville, A. (1985). The model of human occupation and depression. *Mental Health-Special Interest Section Newsletter, 8* (1), 1–4.

Neville-Jan, A. (1994). The relationship of volition to adaptive occupational behavior among individuals with varying degrees of depression. *Occupational Therapy in Mental Health, 12,* 1–18.

Neville-Jan, A., Bradley, M., Bunn, C., & Gheri, B. (1991). The model of human occupational and individuals with co-dependency problems. *Occupational Therapy in Mental Health, 11 (2/3),* 73–97.

O

Oakley, F., Kielhofner, G., & Barris, R. (1985). An occupational therapy approach to assessing psychiatric patients' adaptive functioning. *American Journal of Occupational Therapy, 39,* 147–154.

Oakley, F., Kielhofner, G., Barris, R., & Reichter, R. K. (1986). The Role Checklist: Development and empirical assessment of reliability. *Occupational Therapy Journal of Research, 6,* 157–170.

Oakley, F. (1987). Clinical application of the model of human occupation in dementia of the Alzheimer's type. *Occupational Therapy in Mental Health, 7 (4),* 37–50.

Olin, D. (1984). Assessing and assisting the person with dementia: An occupational behavior perspective. *Physical and Occupational Therapy in Geriatrics, 3 (4),* 25–32.

Olson, L. M., & Kielhofner, G. (1998). *Work readiness: Day treatment for persons with chronic disabilities.* Chicago: Model of Human Occupation Clearinghouse, Department of Occupational Therapy, College of Applied Health Sciences, University of Illinois.

P

Packer, T. L., Foster, D. M., & Brouwer, B. (1997). Fatigue and activity patterns of people with chronic fatigue syndrome. *Occupational Therapy Journal of Research, 17,* 187–199.

Padilla, R. (1998). Application of occupational therapy theories with elders. In H. Lohman, R. Padilla, & S. Byers-Connon (Eds.), *Occupational therapy with elders: Strategies for the certified occupational therapist assistant.* (pp. 63–79). St. Louis: Mosby.

Padilla, R., & Bianchi, E. M. (1990). Occupational therapy for chronic pain: Applying the model of human occupation to clinical practice. *Occupational Therapy Practice, 2,* 47–52.

Parkinson, S., Forsyth, K., & Kielhofner, G. (2006). *The Model of Human Occupation Screening Tool (Version 2.0).* Authors: University of Illinois at Chicago, Chicago, Illinois.

Paul-Ward, A., Braveman, B., Kielhofner, G., & Levin, M. (2005). Developing employment services for individuals with HIV/AIDS: Participatory action strategies at work. *Journal of Vocational Rehabilitation, 22,* 85–93.

Pentland, W., Harvey, A. S., & Walker, J. (2006). The relationships between time use and health and well-being in men with spinal cord injury. *Journal of Occupational Science, 5 (1),* 14–25.

Peterson, E., Howland, J., Kielhofner, G., Lachman, M. E., Assmann, S., Cote, J., & Jette, A. (1999). Falls self-efficacy and occupational adaptation among elders. *Physical and Occupational Therapy in Geriatrics, 16 (1/2),* 1–16.

Pizzi, M. A. (1984). Occupational therapy in hospice care. *American Journal of Occupational Therapy, 38,* 257.

Pizzi, M. A. (1989). Occupational therapy: Creating possibilities for adults with HIV infection, ARC and AIDS. *AIDS Patient Care, 3*, 18–23.

Pizzi, M. A. (1990). Occupational therapy: Creating possibilities for adults with human immunodeficiency virus infection, AIDS related complex, and acquired immunodeficiency syndrome. *Occupational Therapy in Health Care, 7 (2/3/4)*, 125–137.

Pizzi, M. A. (1990). The model of human occupation and adults with HIV infection and AIDS. *American Journal of Occupational Therapy, 44*, 257–264.

Platts, L. (1993). Social role valorisation and the model of human occupation: A comparative analysis for work with learning disability in the community. *British Journal of Occupational Therapy, 56*, 278–282.

Prellwitz, M., & Tamm, M. (2000). How children with restricted mobility perceive their school environment. *Scandinavian Journal of Occupational Therapy, 7*, 165–173.

Provident, I. M., & Joyce-Gaguzis, K. (2005). Brief report: Creating an occupational therapy level II fieldwork experience in a county jail setting. *American Journal of Occupational Therapy, 59*, 101–106.

R

Reekmans, M., & Kielhofner, G. (1998). Defining occupational therapy services in child psychiatry: An application of the model of human occupation. *Ergotherapie, 5*, 6–11.

Reid, C. L., & Reid J. K. (2000). Care giving as an occupational role in the dying process. *Occupational Therapy in Health Care, 12 (2/3)*, 87–93.

Reid, D. (2003). The influence of a virtual reality leisure intervention program on the motivation of older adult stroke survivors: A pilot study. *Physical & Occupational Therapy in Geriatrics, 21 (4)*, 1–19.

Reid, D. T. (2005). Correlation of the Pediatric Volitional Questionnaire with the Test of Playfulness in a virtual environment: The power of engagement. *Early Child Development and Care, 175*, 153–164.

Restall, G., & Magill-Evans (1994). Play and preschool children with autism. *American Journal of Occupational Therapy, 48*, 113–120.

Roitman, D. M., & Ziv, N. (2004). Application of the Model of Human Occupation in a geriatric population in Israel: Two case studies. *Israeli Journal of Occupational Therapy, 13*, E24–E28.

Rosenfeld, M. S. (1989). Occupational disruption and adaptation: A study of house fire victims. *American Journal of Occupational Therapy, 43*, 89–96.

Rust, K., Barris, R., & Hooper, F. (1987). Use of the model of human occupation to predict women's exercise behavior. *Occupational Therapy Journal of Research, 7*, 23–35.

S

Salz, C. (1983). A theoretical approach to the treatment of work difficulties in borderline personalities. *Occupational Therapy in Mental Health, 3 (3)*, 33–46.

Scaffa, M. E. (1991). Alcoholism: an occupational behavior perspective. *Occupational Therapy in Mental Health, 11*, 99–111.

Scarth, P. P. (1983). Services for chemically dependent adolescents. *Mental Health Special Interest Section Newsletter, 13*, 7–8.

Schaff, R. C., & Mulrooney, L. L. (1989). Occupational therapy in early intervention: A family centered approach. *American Journal of Occupational Therapy, 43*, 745–754.

Scheelar, J. F. (2002). A return to the worker role after injury: Firefighters seriously injured on the job and the decision to return to high-risk work. *Work: A Journal of Prevention, 19*(2), 181–184.

Schindler, V. J. (1988). Psychosocial occupational therapy intervention with AIDS patients. *American Journal of Occupational Therapy, 42*, 507–512.

Schindler, V. P. (1990). AIDS in a correctional setting. *Occupational Therapy in Health Care, 7*, 171–183.

Schindler, V. P. (2004). Occupational therapy in forensic psychiatry: Role development and schizophrenia. *Occupational Therapy in Mental Health, 20*, 57–104.

Schindler, V. P. (2004). Evaluating the effectiveness of role development: Quantitative data. *Occupational Therapy in Mental Health, 20*, 79–104.

Schindler, V. P., & Baldwin, S. A. M. (2005). Role development: Application to community-based clients. *The Israel Journal of Occupational Therapy, 14*, E3–E18.

Sepiol, J. M., & Froehlich, J. (1990). Use of the role checklist with the patient with multiple personality disorder. *American Journal of Occupational Therapy, 44*, 1008–1012.

Series, C. (1992). The long-term needs of people with head injury: A role for the community occupational therapist? *British Journal of Occupational Therapy, 55*, 94–98.

Shimp, S. L. (1989). A family-style meal group: Short-term treatment for eating disorder patients with a high level of functioning. *Mental Health Special Interest Section Newsletter, 12 (3)*, 1–3.

Shimp, S. L. (1990). Debunking the myths of aging. *Occupational Therapy in Mental Health, 10 (3)*, 101–111.

Sholle-Martin, S. (1987). Application of the model of human occupation: Assessment in child and adolescent psychiatry. *Occupational Therapy in Mental Health, 7 (2)*, 3–22.

Sholle-Martin, S., & Alessi, N. E. (1990). Formulating a role for occupational therapy in child psychiatry: A clinical application. *American Journal of Occupational Therapy, 44*, 871–881.

Simmons, D. (1999). The psychological system in adolescence. In *Pediatric Therapy: A systems approach* (pp. 430–432). Philadelphia: FA Davis.

Simo-Algado, S., & Cardona, C. E. (2005). The return of the corn men. In F.Kronenberg, S. Simo-Algado, & N. Pollard (Eds.), *Occupational therapy without borders: Learning from the spirit of survivors* (pp. 336–350). London: Elsevier Churchill Livingstone.

Simo-Algado, S., Mehta, N., Kronenberg, F., Cockburn, L., & Kirsh, B. (2002). Occupational therapy intervention with children survivors of war. *Canadian Journal of Occupational Therapy, 69*, 205–217.

Skold, A., Josephsson, S., & Eliasson, A. C. (2004). Performing bimanual activities: The experiences of young persons with hemiplegic cerebral palsy. *American Journal of Occupational Therapy, 58*, 416–425.

Smith, H. (1987). Mastery and achievement: Guidelines using clinical problem solving with depressed elderly clients. *Physical and Occupational Therapy in Geriatrics, 5*, 35–46.

Smith, N., Kielhofner, G., & Watts, J. (1986). The relationship between volition, activity pattern and life satisfaction in the elderly. *American Journal of Occupational Therapy, 40*, 278–283.

Smith, R. O. (1992). The science of occupational therapy assessment. *Occupational Therapy Journal of Research, 12 (1)*, 3–15.

Smyntek, L., Barris, R., & Kielhofner, G. (1985). The model of human occupation applied to psychoso-cially functional and dysfunctional adolescents. *Occupational Therapy in Mental Health, 5 (1)*, 21–40.

Sousa, S. (2006). *Reliability and validity of the Occupational Self Assessment with psychiatric inpatients in Portugal.* [Manuscript submitted for publication].

Spadone, R. A. (1992). Internal-external control and temporal orientation among Southeast Asians and White Americans. *American Journal of Occupational Therapy, 46*, 713–719.

Stamm, T. A., Cieza, A., Machold, K., Smolen, J. S., & Stucki, G. (2006). Exploration of the link between conceptual occupational therapy models and the International Classification of Functioning, Disability and Health. *Australian Occupational Therapy Journal, 53*, 9–17.

Stein, F., & Cutler, S. (1998). Theoretical models underlying the clinical practices of psychosocial occupational therapy. In *Psychological occupational therapy: A holistic approach.* (pp. 150–152). San Diego: Singular.

Stofell, V. (1992). The Americans with Disabilities Act of 1990 as applied to an adult with alcohol dependence. *American Journal of Occupational Therapy, 46*, 640–644.

Sviden, G. A., Tham, K., & Borell, L. (2004). Elderly participants of social and rehabilitative day centres. *Scandinavian Journal of Caring Sciences, 18*, 402–409.

T

Tatham, M. (1992). Leisure facilitator: The role of the occupational therapist in senior housing. *Journal of Housing for the Elderly, 10 (1/2)*, 125–138.

Tayar, S. G. (2004). Description of a substance abuse relapse prevention programme conducted by occupational therapy and psychology graduate students in a United States women's prison. *British Journal of Occupational Therapy, 67*, 159–166.

Taylor, R. R., Fisher, G., & Kielhofner, G. (2005). Synthesizing research, education, and practice according to the scholarship of practice model: Two faculty examples. *Occupational Therapy in Health Care, 19 (1/2)*, 107–122.

Taylor, R. R., & Kielhofner, G. W. (2003). An occupational therapy approach to persons with chronic fatigue syndrome, part 2: Assessment and intervention. *Occupational Therapy in Health Care, 17*, 63–88.

Taylor, R. R., Kielhofner, G., Abelenda, J., Colantuono, K., Fong, R., Heredia, R. et al. (2003). An approach to persons with chronic fatigue syndrome based on the Model of Human Occupation, part 1: Impact on occupational performance and participation. *Occupational Therapy in Health Care, 17,* 47–62.

Tham, K., & Borell, L. (1996). Motivation for training: A case study of four persons with unilateral neglect. *Occupational Therapy in Health Care, 10 (3),* 65–79.

Tham, K., Borell, L., & Gustavsson, A. (2000). The discovery of disability: A phenomenological study of unilateral neglect. *American Journal of Occupational Therapy, 54,* 398–406.

Tham, K., & Kielhofner, G. (2003). Impact of the social environment on occupational experience and performance among persons with unilateral neglect. *American Journal of Occupational Therapy, 57,* 403–412.

Townsend, S. C., Carey, P. D., Hollins, N. L., Helfrich, C., Blondis, M., Hoffman, A., Collins, L., Knudson, J., & Blackwell, A. (2001). *The Occupational Therapy Psychosocial Assessment of Learning (OT PAL). (Version 1.0)* Chicago: Model of Human Occupation Clearinghouse. Department of Occupational Therapy, University of Illinois.

V

Velozo, C. A. (1993). Work evaluations: Critique of the state of the art of functional assessment of work. *American Journal of Occupational Therapy, 47,* 203–209.

Velozo, C. A., Kielhofner, G., Gern, A., Lin, F. L., Lai, J., & Fischer, G. (1999). Worker role interview: Toward validation of a psychosocial work-related measure. *Journal of Occupational Rehabilitation, 9,* 153–168.

Venable, E., Hanson, C., Shechtman, O., & Dasler, P. (2000). The effects of exercise on occupational functioning in the well elderly. *Physical and Occupational Therapy in Geriatrics, 17 (4),* 29–42.

Viik, M. K., Watts, J., Madigan, M. J., & Bauer, D. (1990). Preliminary validation of the Assessment of Occupational Functioning with an alcoholic population. *Occupational Therapy in Mental Health, 10*(2), 19–33.

W

Wallenbert, I., & Jonsson, H. (2005). Waiting to get better: A dilemma regarding habits in daily occupations after stroke. *American Journal of Occupational Therapy, 59,* 218–224.

Watson, M. A., & Ager, C. L. (1991). The impact of role valuation and performance on life satisfaction in old age. *Physical and Occupational Therapy in Geriatrics, 10 (1),* 27–48.

Watts, J., Brollier, C., Bauer, D., & Schmidt, W. (1989). The Assessment of Occupational Functioning: The second revision. *Occupational Therapy in Mental Health, 8 (4),* 61–87.

Watts, J., Kielhofner, G., Bauer, D., Gregory, M., & Valentine, D. (1986). The Assessment of Occupational Functioning: A screening tool for use in long-term care. *American Journal of Occupational Therapy, 40,* 240.

Watts, J. H., Brollier, C., Bauer, D., & Schmidt, W. (1989). A comparison of two evaluation instruments used with psychiatric patients in occupational therapy. *Occupational Therapy in Mental Health, 8,* 7–27.

Watts, J. H., Hinson, R., Madigan, M. J., McGuigan, P. M., & Newman, S. M. (1999). The Assessment of Occupational Functioning: Collaborative version. In B. J. Hempill-Pearson (Ed.), *Assessments in occupational therapy in mental health.* Thorofare, NJ: Slack.

Weeder, T. (1986). Comparison of temporal patterns and meaningfulness of the daily activities of schizophrenic and normal adults. *Occupational Therapy in Mental Health, 6 (4),* 27–45.

Weissenberg, R., & Giladi, W. (1989). Home economics day: A program for disturbed adolescents to promote acquisition of habits and skills. *Occupational Therapy in Mental Health, 9 (2),* 89–103.

Widen-Holmqvist, L., de Pedro-Cuesta, J., Holm, M., Sandstrom, B., Hellblom, A., Stawiarz, L. et al. (1993). Stroke rehabilitation in Stockholm: Basis for late intervention in patients living at home. *Scandinavian Journal of Rehabilitation Medicine, 25,* 175–181.

Wienringa, N., & McColl, M. (1987). Implications of the model of human occupation for intervention with native Canadians. *Occupational Therapy in Health Care, 4 (1),* 73–91.

Woodrum, S. C. (1993). A treatment approach for attention deficit hyperactivity disorder using the model of human occupation. *Developmental Disabilities Special Interest Section Newsletter, 16 (1),* 5–12.

Y

Yeager, J. (2000). Functional implications of substance use disorders. *Occupational Therapy Practice, 5,* 36–39.

Yelton, D., & Nielson, C. (1991). Understanding Appalachian values: Implications for occupational therapists. *Occupational Therapy in Mental Health, 11 (2/3)*, 173–195.

Z

Zimmer-Branum, S., & Nelson, D. (1994). Occupationally embedded exercise versus rote exercise: A choice between occupational forms by elderly nursing home residents. *American Journal of Occupational Therapy, 49*, 397–402.

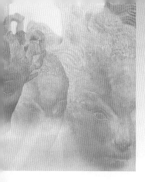

Introduction to the MOHO Clearinghouse and Web Site

- Sun Wook Lee
- Annie Ploszaj

MOHO Clearinghouse

The MOHO Clearinghouse was established more than 10 years ago to serve as a repository of information on MOHO. Today it also distributes a wide variety of information related to MOHO through printed and electronic medium. The mission of the clearinghouse is to support scholarship and practice based on MOHO.

The clearinghouse is a not-for-profit organization directed by Dr. Gary Kielhofner and staffed by research assistants and fellows, who are doctoral and master's students, postdoctoral fellows, and international scholars in residence. It is in the Department of Occupational Therapy at the University of Illinois at Chicago (UIC). The clearinghouse is the center of international communication for clinicians, students, and scholars to share information and experiences about MOHO.

The clearinghouse also sponsors research and development projects that create and test practice resources. All profits from sales (e.g., assessments, intervention manuals, and videotapes) are reinvested in ongoing research projects designed to benefit practice. Over the years these projects have resulted in a wide range of practice resources, especially assessment manuals. The focus for the future of clearinghouse projects will be resources for intervention. For example, intervention manuals and practice resources are being developed by students and researchers for use with pediatric MOHO-based assessments.

The clearinghouse is constantly developing and is open for anyone who wants to participate at any level.

To contact the MOHO Clearinghouse please e-mail *moho_c@yahoo.com.*

Visiting Scholars

The MOHO Clearinghouse is privileged to have international scholars and fellows who visit the University of Illinois at Chicago (UIC) to collaborate with professionals, contribute to ongoing research at the clearinghouse, and enhance their learning experience. The following are two personal accounts of scholars who worked in the clearinghouse to develop their professional work related to MOHO.

Kristjana Fenger

"I came to stay for 4 months at UIC in the spring of 2005. As an assistant professor at the University of Akureyri, Iceland, I was teaching and translating occupational therapy concepts from English to Icelandic. I was also translating assessments. One assessment I translated was the Worker Role Interview. I was working in cooperation with other Icelandic occupational therapists collecting data for the validation of that translation. In order to show that the assessment was valid, I needed to learn Rasch analysis. It was also important for me

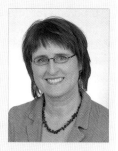

Visiting scholar Kristjana Fenger, who visited the MOHO Clearinghouse from Iceland.

to have the opportunity to discuss MOHO with experts, since that is the conceptual practice model on which the assessment was built. During my visit at UIC I had the opportunity to take a course in Rasch analysis, work with my data in cooperation with the head research assistant of the MOHO Clearinghouse, Jessica Kramer, and publish an article on the research I conducted. I had the opportunity to discuss MOHO during a course offered that spring in advanced MOHO theory. This visit also gave me connections around the world, which allowed me the opportunity to write a book chapter in cooperation with Dr. Braveman and Dr. Kielhofner [professors at UIC] and take part in research across different countries. This was a great learning experience."

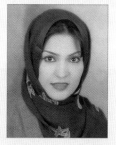

Farzaneh Yazdani, a scholar from the University of Jordan Rehabilitation College, who enjoyed her experience visiting and collaborating with the MOHO Clearinghouse.

Farzaneh Yazdani

"I came to the MOHO Clearinghouse when I was a lecturer and PhD candidate at the University of Jordan Rehabilitation College. I had hopes of being able to discuss my research idea with professionals in MOHO theory. I also hoped to further develop my idea through attending Dr. Kielhofner's lecture, learning about the available tools related to the model, and working with people who have experience with the practical use of

the model on a daily basis. My basic idea was "Studying university students' Subjective Well Being (SWB) through the Model of Human Occupation." I was interested in studying whether and how MOHO can contribute in students' SWB. Through group discussion I was able to decide on the best methodology to use for my study as well as develop a more clear focus which allowed me to complete my proposal. I found that during my experience at the clearinghouse, the greatest help to me was being able to share my ideas, think out loud in the company of other scholars, and receiving advice and opinions of MOHO-based researchers. The results of my study revealed a way to write an intervention plan for university students to improve their mental health. I completed my PhD and I am now an assistant professor at the same university. Currently, I am implementing another research study to examine the same issue among disabled university students."

MOHO Clearinghouse Web Site: *www.moho.uic.edu*

The Web site is one of the key elements of the clearinghouse. It provides a range of up-to-date information and resources that may be beneficial to students, scholars, and clinicians, again serving to connect these individuals in support of scholarship of practice. The scholarship of practice is a dialectic in which theory and research is brought to bear on practice and in which practice guides the development of theory and research (Apte, Kielhofner, Paul-Ward & Braveman, 2005; Crist & Kielhofner, 2005; Forsyth, Summerfield-Mann & Kielhofner, 2005; Kielhofner, 2005; Kielhofner, Braveman, Finlayson, Paul-Ward, Goldbaum, & Goldstein, 2004). The following are key elements of how the scholarship of practice is incorporated into activities within the MOHO Clearinghouse:

- The clearinghouse has a commitment to conducting research that directly contributes to practice

- The clearinghouse supports partnerships between academic and practice settings
- The clearinghouse works to create synergies that advance practice and scholarship simultaneously.

Another important dimension of the scholarship of practice is educating students, fellows, and international scholars to become practice scholars. The clearinghouse functions as a community of learning in which those in academic roles partner with those in practice roles to address real-world practice challenges. Consequently, the scholarship of practice guides the MOHO Clearinghouse to be a dynamic center that integrates research, practice development, and learning.

How the Web Site Can Be Beneficial for a Student, Scholar, or Clinician

The Web site is designed to be an information source. It provides:

- Background information about MOHO
- Practitioner perspectives about their personal experiences using MOHO in practice
- Resources for locating evidence-based practice related to MOHO
- Information about ongoing research

- Access to the e-store to purchase assessments and programs for intervention
- Information about translated assessments
- Listserv discussions about current issues related to MOHO in practice or in research.

How to Find Information on the MOHO Web Site

The following is a guide that will describe link by link how to access information from the MOHO Web site.

HOME PAGE

Welcome to the MOHO Clearinghouse Web site (*Fig. B.1*)!

ABOUT MOHO

Intro to MOHO

This page provides basic background information about the development of the theory of MOHO and a brief explanation of what phenomena it explains and its application to practice.

Practitioner Perspectives

Practitioners and scholars from around the world report their personal experiences with the use of MOHO.

FIGURE B.1 This view of the Web site's home page demonstrates the various links available to its users.

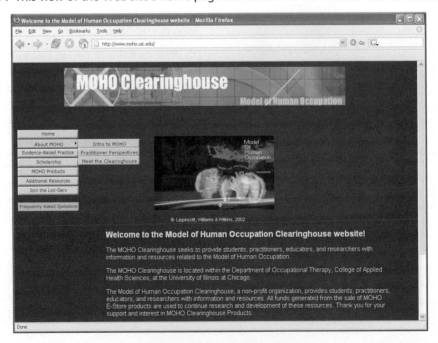

Meet the Clearinghouse

This page, which is under development, will include photos and information about who makes up the clearinghouse and its mission.

EVIDENCE-BASED PRACTICE

This link provides access to the evidence-based practice search engine and comprehensive list of MOHO-based literature and research. Users can narrow their search by criteria such as topic or practice setting (*Fig. B.2*). Also found on this page are archived listserv discussions organized by topic that contain dialog between students, clinicians, and scholars about specific queries related to the use of MOHO.

SCHOLARSHIP

Reference Lists

This resource is a comprehensive bibliography of close to 400 English-language articles, books, and chapters that discuss MOHO. This alphabetic bibliography is a constantly growing list of resources.

Ongoing Research

A list of current research projects is found here, along with contact information for anyone interested in becoming involved in a specific project.

MOHO PRODUCTS

Assessments

This page is one of the most visited links of the Web site, as it provides information about all MOHO-related assessments, as well as .pdf files of sample pages from various assessments (*Fig. B.3*). This page also provides you with the *Buy Now* link, which takes you to the home page of the MOHO e-store, where you can buy products online (*Fig. B.4*).

Programs and Interventions

Various MOHO-based programs and interventions are described here, along with a link to the e-store to purchase these products.

FIGURE B.2 A view of the search criteria found under the link to *Evidence-Based Practice Search*.

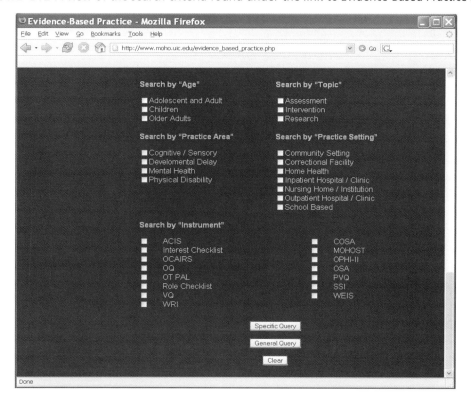

FIGURE B.3 A view of the *Assessments* link. Clicking on *Buy Now* link takes users to the MOHO Clearinghouse e-store, shown in *Figure B.4*.

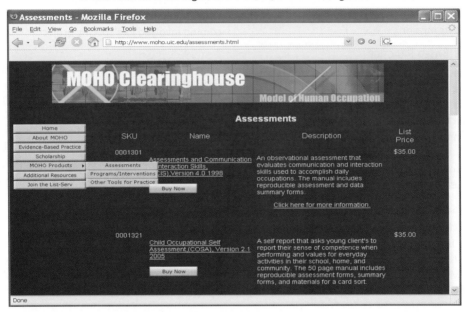

FIGURE B.4 The MOHO e-store where assessments can be purchased online.

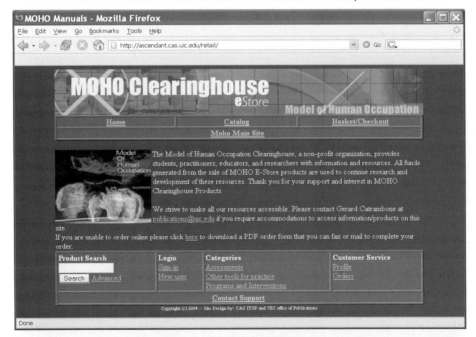

Other Tools for Practice

This link provides the most current information about purchasing e-moho, an electronic documentation and treatment planning tool. E-moho is new and developing software that makes assessment administration, treatment planning, and documentation more efficient and more client centered.

ADDITIONAL RESOURCES

MOHO-Related Resources

This page provides information to request or download free resources, links to MOHO resources that are available for purchase through other companies, and MOHO-related Web links. This page also provides you with a list of MOHO assessments that have been translated into other languages, along with contact information on how to obtain those translated assessments (*Fig. B.5*).

OT Links

Various links to occupational therapy Web sites both nationally and internationally are here.

e-MOHO Support

E-moho information, directions, and frequently asked questions are on this page.

JOIN THE LISTSERV

The last link provides you with the opportunity to join the MOHO listserv. This active listserv allows students, clinicians, and scholars from around the world to post intellectually stimulating messages containing information and experiences related to MOHO, as well as questions about the use of MOHO in practice or in research.

FIGURE B.5 Link to *MOHO-Related Resources* that lists all of the languages of MOHO assessment translations.

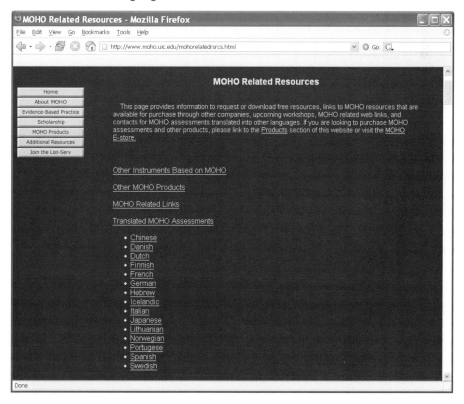

References

Apte, A., Kielhofner, G., Paul-Ward, A. & Braveman, B. (2005). Therapists' and clients' perceptions of the Occupational Performance History Interview. *Occupational Therapy in Health Care, 19,* 173–192.

Crist, P., & Kielhofner, G. (Eds.). (2005). *The Scholarship of Practice: Academic-Practice Collaborations for Promoting Occupational Therapy.* New York: Hawthorne.

Forsyth, K., Summerfield-Mann, L. & Kielhofner, G. (2005). A scholarship of practice: Making occupation-focused, theory-driven, evidence-based practice a reality. *British Journal of Occupational Therapy, 68,* 261–268.

Kielhofner, G. (2005). Scholarship of practice: Bridging the divide. *American Journal of Occupational Therapy, 59,* 231–239.

Kielhofner, G., Braveman, B., Finlayson, M., Paul-Ward, A., Goldbaum, L. & Goldstein, K. (2004). Outcomes of a vocational program for persons with AIDS. *American Journal of Occupational Therapy, 58,* 64–72.

INDEX

Note: Page numbers in *italics* refer to illustrations; page numbers followed by "t" refer to tables.

Achievement, 127–128
ACIS. *See* Assessment of
　Communication and Interaction
　Skills (ACIS)
Activity choices, 14, 46
ACTRE. *See* National Institutes of
　Health Activity Record (ACTRE)
Adaptation, occupational. *See*
　Occupational adaptation
Adolescence, MOHO basic concepts,
　131–133
Adolescent Leisure Profile, 254, 256
Adulthood
　later. *See* Older adults
　MOHO basic concepts, 133–135
Advising, as therapeutic strategy,
　189–190
AIDS patients, employment options
　program example, 446–452, *448,*
　448t, *450*
American Occupational Therapy
　Association (AOTA), Occupational
　Therapy Practice Framework
　(OTPF), 525–528, 525t, 527t, 529t,
　530
AMPS. *See* Assessment of Motor and
　Process Skills (AMPS)
Anticipation, 14, 46
AOF-CV. *See* Assessment of
　Occupational Functioning-
　Collaborative Version (AOF-CV)
Applied research
　described, *507,* 507–508
　research questions, *514*
　types, 513–516
Appraising the self, 39
Assessment, 155–169. *See also* MOHO-
　based assessments; *specific
　instruments*
　client-centered, 164
　combined methods, 288–309
　efficiency of administration, 164
　explaining to clients/peers, 409–410
　holistic and dynamic process, 29, *30*
　information gathering decisions,
　　156–164

interdisciplinary approach, 164
interview, 262–287. *See also* Interview
　assessments
nature of process, 29
noncomprehensive, case illustration,
　155–156
non–MOHO-based, 164
observational, 217–223. *See also*
　Observational assessments
piloting, 167
psychometric studies and, 513–514
purpose, 29, 155
selection
　role of diagnosis, 164–165
　steps in choosing, 166–169, *168*
self-report, 237–261. *See also* Self-
　report assessments
strategy, development, 167, 169,
　169
structured, 159–164, 160t–163t
theory-based questions, 157
unstructured, 157–159
Assessment of Communication and
　Interaction Skills (ACIS), 223–226
administration, 223–224
alignment with ICF, 520–521, 524t
case example, 224–226, *225*
community-based intervention,
　369–370, *370*
components, 160t
evidence summary, 475t
explaining to clients/peers, 410
long-term setting, 387, 388, 389
ordering copies, 224
recrafting narratives, 328–329,
　330–332
research finding, 513
taxonomy, 103, *104*
Assessment of Motor and Process Skills
　(AMPS), 217–223
administration, 218
case example, 218–223, *220, 221*
components, 160t
ordering copies, 218
psychotic patients, 456
recrafting narratives, 328

research finding, *509*
taxonomy, 103, 104
Assessment of Occupational
　Functioning-Collaborative Version
　(AOF-CV), 288–293
administration, 289
case example, 289–294, *291, 293*
components, 160t
evidence summary, 476t
ordering copies, 289
research finding, 513, 514

Basic research
　described, 506–508, *507*
　types, 508–513, *510, 512*
Behavioral patterning. *See* Habituation
Bodily experience, 71–72
Bodily knowing, 73
Body, lived. *See* Lived body

Capacity
　alterations and limitations, 74–75
　performance. *See* Performance
　　capacity
　personal, 35, 37–38
Cartesian dualism, 70–71
Catastrophic change, 127, 128
Causation, personal. *See* Personal
　causation
Change. *See also* Occupational
　development
　case examples
　　child, 178–181, *180*
　　older adult, 181–182, *183*
　catastrophic, 127, 128
　course of development and, 128
　documenting, 166, 166t
　environment as central factor, 128
　habit formation and, 57
　importance to therapy, 171–172, 178
　key element, 28
　occupational engagement and,
　　171–184. *See also* Occupational
　　engagement
　permanent, 126, *127*
　readiness, 128

Change—*continued*
 stages, 127–128
 systems principle, 28
 therapeutic strategies to support,
  186, 195
 transformational, 127, 128
Child Occupational Self-Assessment
  (COSA). *See also* Short Child
  Occupational Profile (SCOPE)
 case example, 251–254, *252*
 community-based intervention, 358,
  359, 360, *361*
 description and administration, 160t,
  248, *249*
 evidence summary, 477t
 ordering copies, 248
Childhood, MOHO basic concepts,
  129–131
Children
 interest profile. See Kid Play Profile;
  Pediatric Interest Profile (PIP)
 occupational engagement case
  example, 178–181, *180*
 therapeutic reasoning questions,
  145–146
 volitional questionnaire, 231–235. See
  also Pediatric Volitional
  Questionnaire (PVQ)
Choosing/deciding, 45–46. *See also*
  Occupational engagement
 factor in change, 172
 role of disability, 42
Client-centered approach
 assessment, 164
 collaborative opportunities, 526–527
 MOHO process, 3–4, 143–144,
  525–528
 OTPF definition, 525
Client perspectives, on MOHO services,
  474, 497t
Client requirements, MOHO assessment
  administration, 162t–163t
Coaching, as therapeutic strategy,
  192–193
Cognitive impairment. *See also*
  Disability
 case illustrations
  getting control, 347–353, *348, 349,*
   350, 351
  learning to reach out, 344–347, *345*
  recapturing freedom, 340–344, *341,*
   342, 343
  rediscovering volition, 337–340, *339*
 narrative slope examples, 342, *343,*
  348, *348*

Occupation Performance History
  Interview-II (OPHI-II), 341–342,
  342, 347, *349*, 349–350
 Occupational Self Assessment (OSA),
  347, 350–352, *351*
 Role Checklist, 347, 350, *350*
 Snoezelen room, 338
 Volitional Questionnaire (VQ), 338,
  339, 340, *341*, 344, *345*
Collaborative opportunities
 client-centered approach, 526–527
 goal-setting, 149–150
Committing, factor in change, 172–173
Communication and documentation,
  407–434
 assessment process
  informing clients, 407–409
  informing peers, 409, 410
 client change, 166, 166t
 client progress, 422–423
 conceptualization of client, 413–415,
  415, 416, 417
 goals and strategies, *417*, 417–418,
  419
 inpatient note (sample), 415, *416, 418*
 MOHO-modified forms
  industrial rehabilitation, 428, 432,
   434, *440*
  inpatient rehabilitation, 427–428,
   429–433
  mental health setting, 428, *435–439*
 MOHO terminology, 424–434, *426*
 occupational engagement, 418, 420
 reflective questions, 414–415, *415*
 SOAP notes, 422–423
 therapeutic outcomes, 151, 423–424
 therapeutic strategies, 418, 420
Communication skills, 103, 223–226,
  225. See also Assessment of
  Communication and Interaction
  Skills (ACIS)
Community-based intervention
 Assessment of Communication and
  Interaction Skills (ACIS), 369–370,
  370
 case examples
  home-based functioning, 360–365
  increasing motivation, 355–360
  supporting volition, 374–378
  work rehabilitation, 365–374
 Child Occupational Self-Assessment
  (COSA), 358, *359*, 360, *361*
 Model of Human Occupation
  Screening Tool (MOHOST),
  375–377, *377*

narrative slope, 366, *369*
 Occupation Performance History
  Interview-II (OPHI-II), 362, 365,
  366, *367*
 occupational identity, 378
 Occupational Self Assessment (OSA),
  369–370, *371, 372*
 Resident Trainee Employment
  Program (RTEP), 365, 370, 375
 volitional evaluations, 356, 360, 376
 Worker Role Interview (WRI), 365,
  366, *368*
Comparative studies, 509–511
Competence, occupational. *See*
  Occupational competence
Competency, factor in change, 127
Concept studies, 514–515
Conceptual practice model. *See also*
  Model of Human Occupation
  (MOHO)
 as basis for program development,
  442
 selecting and justifying, 443–445
Conceptualization of client
 assessment as prerequisite, 155
 documentation, 413–415, *415, 416, 417*
 informing client, 412–413
 informing other professionals,
  411–412
 therapeutic reasoning, 149
Control parameter, defined, 26
Controlled multisensory intervention,
  338
Correlational studies, 509, *510*
COSA. *See* Child Occupational Self-
  Assessment (COSA)
Crafting occupational life, 110–124
 case illustrations, living with an
  impairment, 113–122, *116, 118,*
  120, 122
 factors influencing, 122–124
 impact of narratives, 112–113
 plot, 110–112
Cultural considerations, MOHO-based
  assessments, 165–166
Cultural messages, 39
Culture
 defined, 95
 impact on persons with disabilities, 96
 influences, 95–96
 milieu and values, 39–40, *40*
 occupational forms/tasks, 92–93, *94*
 overview, 5
 thoughts and feelings, 34–35
 volition and, 34, 95

Daily living activities
  defined, 5
  structuring reporting formats to
    include, 423–424
  transformation, 129
Daily occupations, influence of habits,
  55, 55–57
Data gathering process, 147, 149
Deciding/choosing, 45–46. See also
    Occupational engagement
  factor in change, 172
  role of disability, 42
Decision tree, MOHO-based
    assessments, 168
Development. See Occupational
    development
Disability. See also Cognitive
    impairment
  as central experience, 97
  challenge to interests, 44–45
  choice and, 42
  cultural views, 96
  embodiment/experience, 83
  family impact, 94
  habits and, 57–59
  heterarchical contributions, 30
  impact of environment, 93–95, 97
  impact of objects, 88, 91, 91–92
  impact of spaces, 88, 90, 91–92, 93
  interface with values, 41–42
  lived body experiences, 74–77
  occupational lives and needs of
    people with, MOHO evidence on,
    467, 468t–474t
  occupational participation and,
    102–103
  political and economic conditions,
    96
  positive-identity deficit, 64
  as positive value, 41–42
  roles and, 62–64
  self-esteem deficit, 41
  subjective experience, 83
Documentation. See Communication
    and documentation
Doing, 101–109. See also Occupational
    adaptation; Occupational
    competence; Occupational
    identity
  case examples, 101, 105–106, 105t
  consequences, 106–108
  embedded levels, 104–106, 105t
  impact of narratives, 112
  intersection of MOHO/ICF, 520, 521t
  levels, 101–103

range of, occupation and, 5
Dynamics of occupation, 24–31

Economic conditions, influence on
    occupation, 96
Embodied mind, 72–73
Emergence
  defined, 25
  dynamic interaction, 25
  systems principle, 26
Employment options program, AIDS
    patients, 446–452, 448, 448t,
    450
Encouraging, as therapeutic strategy,
    193–194
Engagement, occupational. See
    Occupational engagement
Engaging occupation, described,
    123–124
Enjoyment, 43–46
Environment, 82–98
  as central factor in change, 128
  culture as pervasive force, 95
  defined, 86, 87
  demands and constraints, 87–96
  factor in MOHO, 4
  habits and, 21, 54, 58
  heterarchical contribution, 30
  impact
    changes in, occupational life and,
      126–127, 128
    described, 21, 88, 89
    on disability experience, 93–95, 97
    on occupation, 20, 21, 85–86, 97
  interface with habituation, 18
  measurable goals, 420
  occupational participation and, 467,
    472t
  opportunities and resources, 86–87
  therapeutic reasoning table, 212, 213
Evidence-based practice, 444
  kinds of evidence needed, 466
  on MOHO. See MOHO evidence
Experience
  described, 14, 46
  interdependency with performance
    capacity, 83
  lived body and disability, 74–82
Exploration, factor in change, 127, 173

Feedback, as therapeutic strategy, 189
Feelings and thoughts. See also Volition
  cultural effect, 34–35
  volitional, 13, 13, 34–35
Flow, 44

Goals
  collaborative approach, 149–150
  communicating, 417, 417–418, 419
  long-term, 417–418
  measurable, 418, 419–420
  negotiating, 190–191
  personal causation, 418, 421
  role-related, 418, 421
  short-term, 418
  steps in setting, 416, 417
Group psychoeducational intervention,
    459–460
Group workshop therapy, 459

Habitat, interdependency with
    habituation, 17, 52–53, 53
Habits. See also Internalized roles
  change and, 57
  daily occupation influences, 55,
    55–57
  defined, 16, 53
  disability factor, 57–59
  effectiveness and efficiency, 54
  environment and, 21, 54, 58
  formation, 57
  occupational performance and, 56
  reconstruction, 59
  roles, 86–88
  routine, 56
  social customs/relevance, 54–55
  style, 57
  therapeutic reasoning table, 209
Habituation, 51–64
  adolescence, 132
  adulthood, 134
  case illustrations, 51–52
  childhood, 131
  client characteristics related to,
    470t–472t
  definitions and explanations, 16, 52
  environmental interface, 18
  habits and roles, 19
  heterarchical contribution, 30
  interdependency with habitat, 52–53,
    53
  internalized roles, 59–60
  later adulthood, 137–138
  measurable goals, 419–420
  role change, 62
  role identification, 60
  role influence on occupation, 60–61
  roles and disability, 62–64
  socialization, 62
  summarized, 17, 18
  whole person concept, 21, 22

Heterarchy
  described, 25, *25*
  systems principle, 26
HIV/AIDS patients, employment options
      program development example,
      446–452, *448,* 448t, *450*
Human occupation. *See* Occupation
Human organization, systems principle,
      27

ICF. *See* International Classification of
      Functioning, Disability, and
      Health (ICF)
ICJEV (Interest Checklist Japanese
      Elderly Version), case example,
      239–241, *240*
Identifying. *See also* Occupational
      engagement
  factor in change, 173–174
  as therapeutic strategy, 188
Identity. *See* Occupational identity
Impairment. *See* Cognitive impairment;
      Disability
Industrial rehabilitation, MOHO-
      modified forms, 428, 432, 434,
      440
Information gathering. *See also*
      Assessment
  adequacy, 156
  client-centeredness, 164
  decisions about, 156–164
  questions, 156, 157
  structured, 159–164, 160t–163t
  therapeutic efficiency, 164
  unstructured, 157–159
Inpatient rehabilitation. *See* Long-term
      setting
Integrative psychological therapy, 459
Interaction skills, 103, 223–226, *225*. *See
      also* Assessment of
      Communication and Interaction
      Skills (ACIS)
Interest Checklist
  components, 160t
  evidence summary, 478t
  long-term setting, 382, *383–385*
Interest Checklist Japanese Elderly
      Version (ICJEV), case example,
      239–241, *240*
Interests, 42–43
  anticipation, 46
  confluence factor, 35
  defined, 12–13, *43*
  failure of, 45
  impairment and, 44–45
  as inspiration, 45–46

patterns, 44
  therapeutic reasoning table, 206
Internalized roles
  described, 16–18
  disability, 62–64
  influence on occupation, 60, *61*
  socialization, 60–62
International Classification of
      Functioning, Disability, and
      Health (ICF)
  glossary, 530
  MOHO comparison, 520–521, 521t,
      522t–523t, 524t, 525
Interpretation of actions, 14, 46
Intervention. *See also* Community-
      based intervention; Long-term
      setting
  controlled multisensory, 338
  group psychoeducational, 459–460
  importance of research studies, 509,
      511, 515–516
  Premier Èpisode module, 458–459
  psychotic patients, 452–461,
      455t–456t, *457*
  Snoezelen Room, 338–340
Intervention planning form, School
      Setting Interview (SSI), *277*
Interview assessments, 262–287
  Occupation Performance History
      Interview-II (OPHI-II), 266–272,
      267
  Occupational Circumstances
      Assessment-Interview and Rating
      Scale (OCAIRS), 262–266, *264*
  School Setting Interview (SSI),
      272–278
  Work Environment Impact Scale
      (WEIS), 283–286
  Worker Role Interview (WRI), 278–283

Kid Play Profile
  case example, 256–258
  description and administration, 254,
      255, 256, 257

Later adulthood. *See* Older adults
Lived body
  concept, 70
  disability and, 74–77
  in perspective, 73
  program sample, 357
  transformation studies
    recapturing self, 75–77
    therapeutic passage, 77–80
    "We," 80–82
  unstructured assessment, 157–158

Long-term setting
  Assessment of Communication and
      Interaction Skills (ACIS), 387, *388,*
      389
  assessment strategy, 167, 169
  case illustrations
    building trust, 379–389
    reclaiming occupational life,
        396–404
    rediscovering volition, 389–396
  Interest Checklist, 382, *383–385*
  MOHO-modified forms, 427–428,
      429–433
  Occupation Performance History
      Interview-II (OPHI-II), 380, *381,*
      382, 398, *399*
  Occupational Self-Assessment
      (OSA)
    Environment section, 391, *394*
    Myself section, 391, *392–393*
  Role Checklist, 398, 400, 402
Lower-functioning clients. *See*
      Cognitive impairment

Meaning, 112
Mechanism of action, 444
Metaphor, in occupational narrative,
      112
Mind-body unity, 70–73
Model of Human Occupation (MOHO).
      See also MOHO *entries*
  as activity analysis, 423–424
  alignment with ICF, 520–525, 521t,
      522t–523t, 524t
  alignment with OTPF, 525–528, 525t,
      527t, 529t
  application with other models, 4
  applied to cognitively impaired
      patients, 337–354
  aspects of person, 12
  characteristics, 1–5
  concepts. *See* MOHO concepts
  evidence-based practice. *See* MOHO
      evidence
  integration of systems theory, 24n1
  for program development, 444–461
  research and dissemination, 2–3
  terminology. *See* MOHO terminology
  theoretical basis, 144
  therapeutic strategies, 185–202
  versatility,
      multinational/multicultural, 1–3
Model of Human Occupation Screening
      Tool (MOHOST), 293–300, *295*
  administration, 294
  case example, 297–300, *298*

community-based intervention, 375–377, *377*
components, 160t
evidence summary, 478t
ordering copies, 294
reporting formats (modified), 427–434
summarized, 303
Modified Interest Checklist, *238,* 238–241
administration, 239
case example (Japanese version), 239–241, *240*
ordering copies, 239
recrafting narratives, 322, *324*
MOHO. *See* Model of Human Occupation (MOHO)
MOHO-based assessments
alignment with ICF, 520–521, 524t
alignment with OTPF, 528, 529t
client-centered approach, 3–4, 143–144, 525–528
client/therapist requirements, 162t–163t
concept overview, 160t–161t
cultural considerations, 165–166
decision tree, *168*
documenting client change and program outcomes, 166, 166t
evidence on utility/dependability, 467, 474, 475t–490t
explaining to clients/peers, 409–410
information-gathering questions, 156, 157
modified forms
industrial rehabilitation, 428, 432, 434, *440*
inpatient rehabilitation, 427–428, *429–433*
mental health setting, 428, *435–439*
structured, 159–164, 160t–163t
target populations, 160t–161t
MOHO-based research, 506–516
applied, *507,* 507–508, 513–516
basic, 506–507, *507,* 508–513
bibliographic resources, 516
cumulative findings, 516
integration of applied and basic, 506–508, *507*
refinement of research methodologies, 516
theory-explicating, 511–513, *512*
MOHO clearinghouse and web site, 550–555
MOHO concepts. *See also specific concepts, e.g.,* Habitation

adolescence, 131–133
adulthood, 133–135
childhood, 129–131
IFC concepts and, 520, 522t–523t
later adulthood, 136–138
OTFP domains and, 527t, 528
MOHO evidence
client perspectives on services, 474, 497t
identifying, 466–467
MOHO-based assessments, 467, 474, 475t–490t
nature of MOHO practice, 474, 491t
occupational lives and needs of people with disabilities, 467, 468t–474t
outcomes of MOHO-based practice, 474, 492t–496t
MOHO terminology
in communication and documentation, 424–434, *426*
and everyday language, moving between, 426, *426*
structuring reporting formats to include, 423–424
MOHO theory
communicating to clients and peers, 407–409
as practice model, 144
questions generated by, *147,* 157, 507
MOHOST. *See* Model of Human Occupation Screening Tool (MOHOST)
Motivation, increasing, community-based intervention example, 355–360
Motor skills
assessment, 217–223. See also Assessment of Motor and Process Skills (AMPS)
taxonomy, 103

Narrative. *See* Occupational narrative
Narrative slope
case samples, *271, 317, 322, 329, 343, 348*
community-based intervention, 366, *369*
National Institutes of Health Activity Record (ACTRE), 241–243, *242*
components, 160t
evidence summary, 482t
Negotiating
factor in change, 174–175
as therapeutic strategy, 190–191

NIH Activity Record. *See* National Institutes of Health Activity Record (ACTRE)

Objects
described, 88, *91*
impact on disabilities, 91–92
Observational assessments, 217–223
communication and interaction skills, 223–226
motor and process skills, 217–223
volition, 226–235
OCAIRS. *See* Occupational Circumstances Assessment-Interview and Rating Scale (OCAIRS)
Occupation
case examples, 11–12
concepts/factors
environment, 21
habituation, 16–18, *17, 19*
integration of, *22*
performance capacity, 18, 20, *20*
volition, 12–16, *13, 15*
defined, 5
dynamics, 24–31
emergence, 26–27
heterarchy, 26–27
influences
environmental, 20, 21, 85–86, 97
habits, *55,* 55–57
objects, 88, 91
political and economic, 96
roles, 60–61, *61*
thoughts and feelings, 13, *13*
patterns, 28
principles, 26, 27, 28
range of doing, 5
Occupation Performance History Interview-II (OPHI-II), 266–272, *267. See also* Community-based intervention; Long-term setting
administration, 267
case example, 268–272, *269, 271*
cognitive impairments, 341–342, *342,* 347. 337–338, *349*
community-based intervention, 362, 365, 366, *367*
components, 160t
evidence summary, 480t–481t
explaining to clients/peers, 409–410
long-term setting, 380, *381,* 382, 398, *399*
obtaining copies, 267–268
recrafting narratives, 315–316, *316,* 321, 326, *327*
research finding, 507–508, 514

Occupational adaptation
adolescence, 132–133
adulthood, 135
childhood, 131
client characteristics related to, 473t
described, *107*, 107–108, *108*
later adulthood, 136–137
rebuilding
realizing values, 326–336, *327,
329–335*
rebuilding identity, 313–319, *316,
317*
from victim to heroine, 319–326,
321–324
research finding, 508–509
role of narrative, 511–513, *512*
tasks, 129
Occupational change. *See* Change;
Occupational development
Occupational choices
defined, 14–15
impact, 46
Occupational Circumstances
Assessment-Interview and Rating
Scale (OCAIRS), 262–266, *264*
administration, 262–263
case example, 263–266, *265*
components, 160t
evidence summary, 479t
obtaining copies, 263
Occupational competence. *See also
Occupational life*
adolescence, 132
adulthood, 135
childhood, 131
client characteristics related to, 473t
described, 107
dimensions, 107
factor in occupational life, 110
impact of disability, 107
later adulthood, 138
narrative element, 113
research finding, 508–509
Occupational development, 126–138.
See also Change
adolescence, 131–133
adulthood, 133–135
childhood, 129–131
fundamental tasks, 129
later adulthood, 136–138
processes of change, 126–127
readiness for change, 128
stages of change, 127–128
trajectory, 128
Occupational engagement, 171–184
case examples

change for child, 178–181, *180*
change for older adult, 181–182,
183
family roles/routines, 175–176
new occupations, 174
sustaining participation, 177–178
worker role, 173
client efforts, 172
defined, 171, 171n1
dimensions, 172–178
choose/decide, 172
commit, 172–173
explore, 173
identify, 173–174
negotiate, 174–175
plan, 175–176
practice, 176–177
reexamine, 177
sustain, 177–178
MOHO/ICF intersections, 520, 521t
therapeutic reasoning and, 171–172,
178
therapeutic supportive strategies, *186*
volition and, *510*
Occupational forms
described, 92–93, *94*, 95
relationship to performance, 103
success in completing, 105t, 106
Occupational identity. *See also* Change;
Occupational development
adolescence, 132–133
adulthood, 135
childhood, 131
client characteristics related to, 473t
defined, 106
dimensions, 106
factor in occupational life, 110
later adulthood, 138
process, 107–108
as research finding, 508
team intervention (sample), 378
Occupational life
background elements, 110
changes in environmental impact,
126–127, *128*
crafting, 110–124
case illustrations, living with an
impairment, 113–122, *116, 118,
120, 122*
factors influencing, 122–124
impact of narratives, 112–113
plot, 110–112
factors influencing, 29–30, *30*
narrative organization, 110–113
processes of change, *127*
reconstruction in long-term setting

building trust, 379–389
reclaiming occupational life,
396–404
rediscovering volition, 389–396
scope of narratives, 113
Occupational narrative
case illustrations, living with an
impairment, 113–122, *116, 118,
120, 122*
defined, 113
factors influencing, 122–124
features, 112–113
meaning, 112
metaphors, 112
narrative slope samples, *111, 116,
118, 120, 122*
nature, 508
perspective on, 122
plot, 110–112, *111*
recrafting case illustrations
realizing values, 326–336, *327,
329–335*
rebuilding identity, 313–319,
316–317
from victim to heroine, 319–326,
321–324
sequential studies, 511–513, *512*
types, 111, *111*
Occupational participation, 101–102
defined, 101–102, 102n2
disability and, 102–103
environment and, 467, 472t
factors influencing, 102
intervention in community context
home-based functioning, 360–365
mental health problems, 374–378
performance capacity, 355–360
work rehabilitation, 365–374
MOHO/ICF similarities, 520, 521t
performance limitations, 102
volition and, *510*
Occupational performance, 102–103
definition, 103
habits and, 56
intersection of MOHO/ICF, 520,
521t
Occupational Questionnaire (OQ),
241–246
case example, 243–244, *245–246*
components, 160t
evidence summary, 482t
ordering copies, 243
Occupational Self Assessment (OSA),
246–254, *247. See also*
Community-based intervention;
Long-term setting

administration, 246, 248
case example, 248–251, *251*
cognitive impairments, 347, 350–352, *351*
community-based intervention, 369–370, *371, 372*
described, 161t
evidence summary, 483t–484t
explaining to clients/peers, 409
long-term setting
    Environment section, 391, *394*
    Myself section, 391, *392–393*
ordering copies, 248
Occupational settings, summarized, 97
Occupational tasks
described, 92–93, *94, 95*
factors influencing, 26–27
relationship to performance, 103
success in completing, 105t, 106
Occupational therapy
aim and effectiveness, 30
assessment as prerequisite, 155
change process, 171–172, 178
classification frameworks, 519–528, 521t–525t, 527t
communicating goals and strategies, *417*, 417–418, *419*
contemporary view, 29n3
documenting outcomes, 151, 423–424
group workshop, 459
implementation, process review, 151
integrative psychological, 459
MOHO practice, research findings, 474, 491t
monitoring/reviewing, 421–424
programs. See Program development
research on dynamics, 515
Occupational Therapy Practice Framework (OTPF), 101
glossary, 530
MOHO comparison, 525–528, 525t, 527t, 529t
Occupational Therapy Psychosocial Assessment of Learning (OT PAL), 161t, 305–308
administration, 304
case example, 305–308, *307, 309*
ordering copies, 304
Older adults
MOHO basic concepts, 136–138
occupational engagement case example, 181–182, *183*
therapeutic reasoning questions, 146–147
OPHI-II. *See* Occupation Performance History Interview-II (OPHI-II)

OQ. *See* Occupational Questionnaire (OQ)
OSA. *See* Occupational Self Assessment (OSA)
OTPF. *See* Occupational Therapy Practice Framework (OTPF)
Outcome studies, 515–516

Participation. *See* Occupational participation
Pediatric Interest Profile (PIP), 254–258, *255. See also* Kid Play Profile
administration, 256
case example, 256–258
evidence summary, 484t
ordering copies, 256
overview, 161t
Pediatric Volitional Questionnaire (PVQ), 231–235
administration, 231–232
case example, 232–235, *234*
described, 161t
evidence summary, 485t
ordering copies, 231
Perception of objects, 72
Performance capacity
adolescence, 132
adulthood, 135
childhood, 131
components, 18, *20*, 68–70, *69, 70*
defined, 18, 20, 68, *69*
factors influencing quality, 26–27
heterarchical contribution, *30*
interdependency with experience, 83
intervention in community context, 355–360
later adulthood, 138
measurable goals, *420*
objective components, 68
principles affecting, 26, 27, 28
spatial dimension, 58–59
subjective experience and, 68–69, 73
temporal dimension, 59
therapeutic reasoning table, 210
transformation factor, 83
whole person concept, 21, 22
Permanent change, 126, *127*
Personal capacity, 35, 37–38
Personal causation
anticipation, 46
conceptualized, *36*
confluence factor, 35
defined, 13
dimensions, 35–39
goals, 418, 421
impact of efforts, 38–39

self-appraisal, 39
self-control, 38
self-efficacy, 38–39
sense of personal capacity, 37–38
therapeutic reasoning table, 205
Personal convictions, 40
Phenomenologic approach to human performance, 70
Physical environment, 212. *See also* Environment
Physical support, as therapeutic strategy, 194–195
Piloting assessments, 167
PIP. *See* Pediatric Interest Profile (PIP)
Planning, factor in change, 175–176
Play
defined, 5
transformation, 129
Plot, 110–112, *111*
Political conditions, influence on occupation, 96
Positive identity, impact of disability, 64
Practicing, factor in change, 176–177
Predictive studies, 511
Preteen Play Profile, 254, 256
Process skills, 103. *See also* Assessment of Motor and Process Skills (AMPS)
Productivity, defined, 5
Program development
compared to therapeutic reasoning, 443
conceptual practice model selection, 443–445
examples, 445–461
    employment options for HIV/AIDS patients, 446–452, *448*, 448t, *450*
    Premier Episodes, 452–461, 455t–456t, *457*
MOHO resources, 444–445
process, *442–443, 443*
therapeutic reasoning parallels, 443
Prospective studies, 508, 511
Psychiatric setting
assessment strategy, 167, *169*
MOHO-modified forms, 428, *435–439*
Psychometric studies, importance, 513–514
Psychotic patients, intervention program example, 452–461, 455t–456t, *457*
PVQ. *See* Pediatric Volitional Questionnaire (PVQ)

Qualitative studies, 511–513, *512*
Questions
  information-gathering, 156
  reflective, 414–415, *415*
  theory-based, *147*, 157, *507*
  therapeutic reasoning, 145–147, *147*

Reasoning. *See* Therapeutic reasoning
Recrafting occupational narratives. *See* Occupational narrative
Reexamining, factor in change, 177
Reflective questions, 414–415, *415*
Rehabilitation
  industrial, MOHO-modified forms, 428, 432, 434, *440*
  inpatient. See Long-term setting
  work, community-based intervention example, 365–374
Resident Trainee Employment Program (RTEP), community-based intervention, 365, 370, 375
Role(s)
  disability and, 62–64
  impact of restrictions, 94–95
  influence on occupation, 60, *61*
  insufficiency, 63
  internalized, 16–18
  personal identity, 60
  social barriers, 63
  socialization, 60–62
  therapeutic reasoning table, 208
Role Checklist, 258–260
  administration, 258–259
  case example, 259–260, *260*
  cognitive impairments, 347, 350, *350*
  description and administration, 161t
  evidence summary, 486t–487t
  long-term setting, 398, *400*, 402
  ordering copies, 259
  recrafting narratives, 320–321, *323*
Role identification, 60
Role-related goal, 418, 421. *See also* Goals

School Setting Interview (SSI), 161t, 272–278
  administration, 273
  case example, 273–278, *275, 277*
  evidence summary, 488t
  ordering copies, 273
SCOPE. *See* Short Child Occupational Profile (SCOPE)
Self-appraisal, 39
Self-control, 38

Self-efficacy, 35, 38–39
Self-esteem, and disability, 41
Self-report assessments, 237–261
  Modified Interest Checklist, 238, 238–241
  National Institutes of Health Activity Record (ACTRE), 241–243, *242*
  Occupational Questionnaire (OQ), 241–246
  Occupational Self Assessment (OSA), 246–254, *247*
  Pediatric Interest Profile (PIP), 254–258, *255*
  Role Checklist, 258–260
Senior citizens. *See* Older adults
Sense of obligation, 41
Sense of personal capacity, 35, 37–38
Short Child Occupational Profile (SCOPE)
  administration, 294
  case example, 300–303, *301*
  description, 294, *296*
  evidence summary, 478t
  illustration of components, 161t
  ordering copies, 297
  summarized, 303
Sick role, 63–64
Skills
  assessment, 217–226. See also Assessment of Communication and Interaction Skills (ACIS); Assessment of Motor and Process Skills (AMPS)
  defined, 103, *103*
  intersection of MOHO/ICF, 520, 521t
  measurable goals, *420*
  therapeutic reasoning table, 211
  types, 103–105, *104*, 105t
Slopes. *See* Narrative slope; Occupational narrative
Snoezelen intervention, case example, rediscovering volition, 337–340, *339*
Snoezelen room, 338
SOAP notes, 422–423
Social barriers, to role performance, 63
Social customs/relevance, habits, 54–55
Social environment. *See also* Environment
  attitudes about disabilities, 93–95
  groups, 92, *93*, 94–95
  therapeutic reasoning table, 213
Social space, 92, *93*

Socialization, described, 60–62
Spaces
  described, 88, *90*
  impact on disabilities, 91–92
SSI. *See* School Setting Interview (SSI)
Structuring, as therapeutic strategy, 191–192
Subjective experience, performance capacity and, 68–69, 73
Sustaining, factor in change, 177–178
Systems theory
  concepts of emergence/heterarchy, 25–27
  control parameter, 26
  discussed, 24n1
  implications for occupational therapy, 29–30, *30*
  key postulates, 31t
  understanding occupation, 26–27

Tasks. *See* Occupational tasks
Terminology. *See* MOHO terminology
Theory-based practice. *See* Conceptual practice model; MOHO-based research; Therapeutic reasoning
Theory-based questions, *147*, 157, *507*
Therapeutic reasoning
  case examples, 150, 152–154, *153*
  client centeredness, 143–144
  illustration of process, 152–154, *153*
  MOHO theory influences on, 514–515
  occupational engagement and, 171–172, 178
  OTPF alignment illustration, 525, 525t
  parallels to program development, 443
  steps, 143–154, *144*
    assessing outcomes, 151
    conceptualizing client, 149
    gathering client information, 147, 149
    generating questions, 145–147, *147*
    identifying goals/plans, 149–150
    implementing therapy, 151
    theory-driven, 144
Therapeutic reasoning table, 149, 178, 195, 202, 204–213
  habits, 209
  interests, 206
  performance capacity, 210
  personal causation, 205
  physical environment, 212
  roles, 208

skills, 211
social environment, 213
values, 207
Therapeutic strategies, 185–202
advising, 189–190
case examples, 196–201, *197, 202*
coaching, 192–193
defined, 185
encouraging, 193–194
feedback, 189
identifying, 188
negotiating, 190–191
physical support as, 194–195
structuring, 191–192
therapeutic use of self and, 185
validating, 185–187
Therapist requirements, MOHO
assessment administration,
162t–163t
Therapy. *See* Occupational therapy
Thoughts and feelings. *See also* Volition
cultural effect, 34–35
volitional, 13, *13*, 34–35
Transformational change, 127, 128
Triangulation, in unstructured
information gathering, 159
Trust building, long-term setting
example, 379–389

Validation
as therapeutic strategy, 185–187
unstructured information, 159
Validity studies, 508–509
Values
anticipation, 46
confluence factor, 35
cultural context, 39–40, *40*

defined, 13
interface with impairment, 41–42
therapeutic reasoning table, 207
Volition, 12–16, 32–47
adolescence, 131–132
adulthood, 133–134
case examples, 32–34
childhood, 129–130
client characteristics related to,
468t–469t
community-based evaluation
intervention, 356, 360, 375
culture and, 34, 95
cycle, 34, *34*
defined, 12, 15–16
dynamic perspective, 35
heterarchical contribution, *30*
later adulthood, 136
measurable goals, *419*
pattern, 15–16
personal causation, values, and
interests, 13–14
personal history, 35
principles affecting, 26, 27, 28
processes, 14–15, *15*, 46–47
rediscovering
cognitively impaired patient,
337–340, *339*
long-term setting example, 389–396
relationship to engagement, *510*
supporting, community-based
intervention example, 374–378
theory-based understanding, *153*
thoughts and feelings, 13, *13*, 34–35
whole person concept, 21, *22*
Volitional Questionnaire (VQ), 226–231
administration, 227

case example, 228–231, *230*
cognitive impairments, 338, *339*, 340,
341, 344, *345*
described, 161t
evidence summary, 488
ordering copies, 231
pediatric, 231–235. See also Pediatric
Volitional Questionnaire (PVQ)
recrafting narratives, 329, *333–335*
Volitional whole, 35

Whole person concept, 21, *22*
Work
defined, 5
transformation, 129
Work Environment Impact Scale (WEIS),
283–286
administration, 283
case example, 284–286, *285–286*
evidence summary, 489t
illustration of components, 161t
ordering copies, 284
Worker Role Interview (WRI), 161t,
278–283
administration, 278
case example, 279–283, *280–281*
community-based intervention, 365,
366, *368*
evidence summary, 489t–490t
ordering copies, 279
research finding, 513
World Health Organization (WHO),
definition of participation, 101

Young Adults Program: First Episodes,
program development example,
452–461, 455t–456t, *457*